普通高等教育“十一五”国家级规划教材
全国高等医药院校规划教材

何深一　主编

人体寄生虫学

Human Parasitology

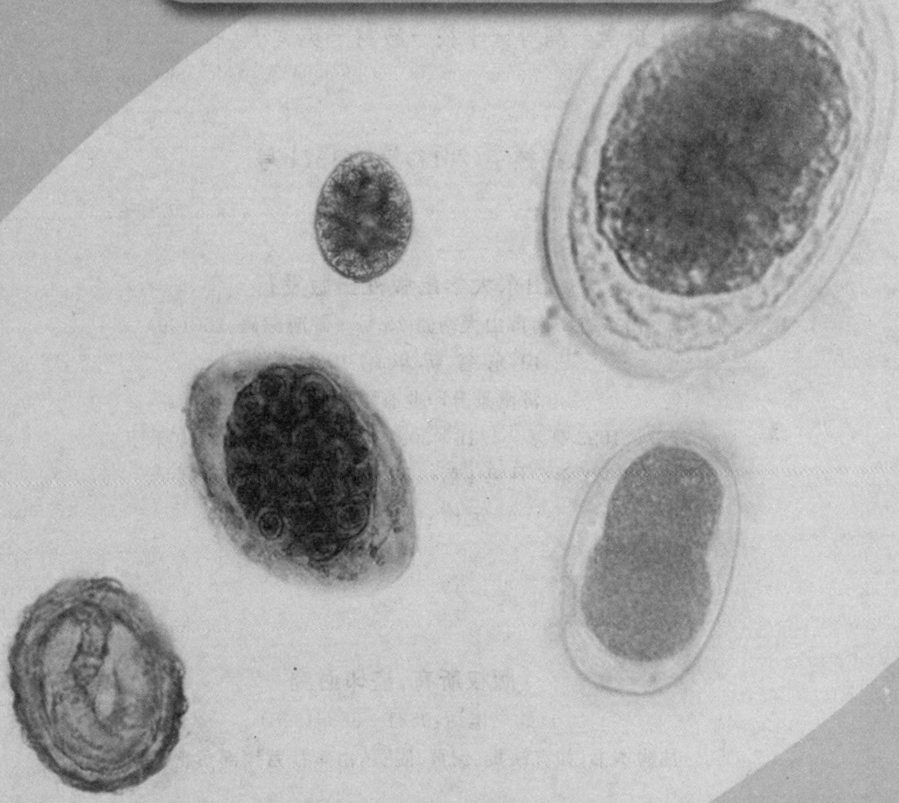

山东大学出版社

内容简介

全书为英文编写，包括总论、医学原虫、医学蠕虫、医学节肢动物、寄生虫病的诊断技术、实验指导和英汉对照词汇等内容。该教材在认真总结五年制、六年制、七年制、八年制和留学生英语教学经验的基础上编写而成，并依据高等医药院校五年制和长学制培养计划，结合国情重点阐述了我国常见的严重危害人体健康的寄生虫和重要病媒节肢动物，同时收录了世界上重要的寄生虫和我国少见的人体寄生虫，共计100余种。本书系统地介绍了寄生虫病实验诊断技术。为配合全英文和双语教学的开展，全部内容用英语表达、描述，插图新颖、实用，并用英文标注。

本教材适合于高等医药院校五年制、长学制临床、基础、预防、口腔、麻醉、影像、护理、药学、检验、法医等专业学生和留学生使用。也可用作医药卫生专业教师、临床医护人员、疾病控制中心人员和科研人员的参考书和专业英语学习的工具书。

图书在版编目(CIP)数据

人体寄生虫学：英文/何深一主编.
—济南：山东大学出版社，2011.5(2012.2重印)
ISBN 978-7-5607-4312-7

Ⅰ.①人…
Ⅱ.①何…
Ⅲ.①医学：寄生虫学－高等－学校－教材－英文
Ⅳ.①R38

中国版本图书馆CIP数据核字(2011)第091571号

山东大学出版社出版发行
(山东省济南市山大南路27号　邮政编码：250100)
山 东 省 新 华 书 店 经 销
济南景升印业有限公司印刷
787×1092毫米　1/16　30.75印张　2插页　710千字
2011年5月第1版　2012年2月第2次印刷
定价：52.00元

《人体寄生虫学》编委会

前 言

《人体寄生虫学》曾于1989年由学苑出版社出版发行，被国内开设英语教学的许多医学院校采用，受到同行和学生的好评。2006年，本书被遴选为普通高等教育“十一五”国家级规划教材。在本书以“十一五”国家级规划教材面世之际，感谢本教材上一版主编王永祥教授及各位编者的努力。

本教材根据教学大纲的要求，将相关专业知识与教学内容融为一体，进行了重新编写，增加了大量内容和图表，编者由上一版的1所院校增加到15所。

全书包括总论、医学原虫、医学蠕虫、医学节肢动物、寄生虫病的诊断技术和实验指导、英汉对照词汇等内容。在突出国内流行广泛、危害严重的主要虫种的基础上，也编入目前国内外逐步受到重视的一些人类致病寄生虫。书中融入本学科比较成熟的新进展，增加重要寄生虫病的临床症状、体征、诊断、治疗和预防措施，以期与临床应用的结合更密切。该教材力求科学性、先进性、系统性和实用性相结合，并将免疫学、病理学、流行病学、传染病学、诊断学、影像学和分子生物学等学科的理论、知识和方法应用于寄生虫学中，既体现出高等医学教材的深度和广度，也注意到寄生虫学的特殊性。内容强调“三基”(基本理论、基本知识、基本技能)，反映国内外本学科的最新进展。在总结各院校教学、科研经验的基础上，体现编者的新见解和教学特色。该教材在认真总结五年制、六年制、七年制、八年制和留学生英语教学经验的基础上编写而成，尽量做到保证专业水准，符合英语习惯，用词准确，通俗易懂。

为了满足全英语教学的需要，书中图表全部采用英文标注，图文并茂，书末附有专业词汇中英文对照，便于学习。新增了寄生虫病常用实验诊断技术，尤其是病原生物学检查技术；绘制了许多新的寄生虫插图；按照大多数院校的教学顺序编排内容，符合实际教学习惯。本书结合我们网站教学和学习内容使用，将收到更好的效果。

山东大学出版社为本教材的出版做了大量工作，并提供经费支持。在此，谨向他们为本教材顺利出版所做的贡献致以诚挚的谢意。

全体编写人员的辛勤劳动，以及山东大学出版社各位领导、策划、责编们的共同努力，是本书顺利出版的重要前提。袁方曙老师为本书绘制了大量图片。由于编者知识水平所限，书中难免存在不足和错误之处，殷切希望同行专家及广大师生批评指正，将发现的问题反馈给我们，以便今后加以修正，我们将不胜感激。

何深一

2010年12月

Preface

This book presents basic descriptions of parasites commonly found to cause human diseases. The book was written to provide information for a full course in human parasitology to address the needs of students and other relevant people in the medical and health science fields.

The book *Human Parasitology* is organized into textbook and laboratory manual.

The textbook consists of seventeen chapters divided into five parts. Parasites are divided into three broad groups, that is, protozoa, helminths and arthropods. Part I begins with an introduction (Chapter One), which provides an overview of human parasitology and commonly used terms. Part II consists of four chapters on helminths worms. Nematodes (roundworms) are discussed in Chapter Four and trematodes (flukes) are discussed in Chapter Five. Cestodes (tapeworms) are included in Chapter Six, and Acanthocephala (thorny-headed worms) are covered in Chapter Seven. Part III consists of five chapters devoted to the protozoa. Intestinal amebae and the free-living amebae, Acathamebae species and Naegleria species, are discussed in Chapter Nine, while the flagellates are discussed in Chapter Ten. Sporozoa are presented in Chapter Eleven; Ciliates are covered in Chapter Twelve. Part IV consists of three chapters devoted to the medically important arthropods. Part V consists of two chapters devoted to the diagnostic techniques. Chapter Sixteen provides more in-depth information on each type of method. Chapter Seventeen presents current information on immunological techniques available to diagnose parasitic infections. A discussion of molecular diagnostic techniques is also included.

We hope that the book will be fruitful and provides the clear, concise, practical, and clinically relevant information necessary to gain an understanding of the pathogenesis of parasitic infections and be able to diagnose these infections in the laboratory for students. Furthermore, we would like to thank Shangdong University Press, for their cooperation and generous support to produce this book.

He Shenyi

December 2010

Contents

TEXTBOOK

LABORATORY MANUAL

TEXTBOOK

Part I Introduction to Human Parasitology

Chapter 1 Basic Conceptions of Human Parasitology

Parasitology, the study of parasites and their relationships to their hosts, is one of the most fascinating areas of biology. Human parasitology is the study of those organisms which parasitize humans, and is a branch of medical science dealing with parasites living in and on the body of humans and with aspects of the host-parasite relationships having medical significance. It is referred to the study of morphology, growth and development of the parasites in the host, the pathogenesis and clinical manifestation caused by the parasites and the diagnosis, and transmission and prevention of the disease. It encompasses elements of medical protozoology, medical helminthology, and medical arthropodology. According to the very broad definition of parasitology, parasites should include the **viruses**, **rickettsiae**, **bacteria**, **fungi**, **protozoa** and **metazoa** (multi-celled organisms) which infect their host species. However, for historical reasons the first four have been incorporated into the discipline of **Microbiology**. Newly developed techniques in biochemistry and cellular and molecular biology have also opened significant new avenues for research on parasites.

There are far more kinds of parasitic than non-parasitic organisms in the world. Even if we exclude the viruses and rickettsiae, which are all parasitic, and the many kinds of parasitic bacteria and fungi, the parasites are still in majority. The study of parasitic disease is timeless and will always be relevant to the practice of modern medicine, especially when considering how easy it is for people to travel from one place in the world to another in just a matter of hours.

Parasitology and Medical Significance

Parasitic infections and diseases are the most common diseases in the world. Therefore, parasitology has an important role on medicine and public health. During our relatively short history on Earth, humans have acquired an amazing number of parasites, about 530 species of helminth worms and over 120 species of protozoa. Many of these are rare and accidental parasites, but we still harbor about 90 relatively common species, of which a small proportion cause some of the most important diseases in the world, inevitably, these are the ones that have received the most attention. According to the WHO 2001 year report, parasitic diseases are still important human diseases. In the world, 210 million people reside in the endemic areas of malaria; 10 million cases of malaria occur every year; 20 million infected individuals were estimated in the world. So TDR/WHO has proclaimed 10 major unconquered human tropical diseases: African trypanosomiasis, Dengue, Leishmaniasis, Malaria, Schistosomiasis, Tuberculosis, Chagas disease, Leprosy, Lymphatic filariasis, and Onchocerciasis. Among them 7 diseases are parasitic.

Parasitism, Parasite and Host

Symbiosis

Two different organisms live together and interact, in this association one partner lives in or on another one's body. It includes 3 types: mutualism, commensalism, and parasitism.

Mutualism is a permanent association between two different organisms, in which life apart is impossible, and the two partners benefit each other, such as termites and flagellates.

The mutual organisms are metabolically dependent on each other; one cannot survive in the absence of the other.

Mutualism describes a relationship in which both partners benefit from the association. Mutualism is usually obligatory, since in most cases physiological dependence has evolved to such a degree that one mutual cannot survive without the other. Termites and their intestinal protistan fauna are an excellent example of mutualism. Termites cannot digest cellulose because they cannot synthesize and secrete the enzyme cellulase. The myriad flagellates in a termite's intestine, however, synthesize cellulase and consequently digest the wood eaten by the host. The termite uses molecules excreted as a by-product of the flagellates' metabolism. If we kill the flagellates by exposing termites to high temperature or high oxygen concentration, then the termites starve to death, even though they continue to eat wood.

Commensalism is the association of two different organisms, in which one partner is benefited while the other neither benefited nor injured.

Commensalism does not involve physiologic interaction or dependency between the two partners, the host and the commensal. The two partners can survive independently. Although at times certain nonpathogenic organisms (e. g. , protozoa) are referred to as commensals, this interpretation is incorrect because they are physiologically dependent on the host and are, therefore, parasites. An example of commensalism is the association between hermit crabs and the sea anemones they carry on their borrowed shells.

Parasitism is the association of two different organisms, in which one partner is benefited while the other is injured, such as *Ascaris lumbricoides* and men.

Parasite

In parasitism, it is the benefited partner. It is an animal organism which lives in or on the host in order to obtain nourishment and shelter from the host as well as does harms to the host.

Parasites may cause mechanical injury, such as boring a hole into the host or digging into its skin or other tissues, stimulating a damaging inflammatory or immune response, or simply robbing the host of nutrition. Most parasites inflict a combination of these conditions on their hosts.

There are many types of parasites.

Most parasites are **obligate parasites**; that is, they cannot complete their life cycle without spending at least part of the time in a parasitic relationship. However, many obligate parasites have free-living stages outside any host, including some periods of time in the external environment within a protective eggshell or cyst.

Facultative parasites are not normally parasitic but can become so when they are accidentally eaten or enter a wound or other body orifice. Two examples are certain free-living amebas, such as *Naegleria fowleri*, and free-living nematodes belonging to the genus *Micronema*. Infection of humans with either of these is extremely serious and usually fatal. A **facultative parasite** is an organism which may exist in a free-living state or as a commensal parasite.

Parasites that live on the outside of the host's body are referred to as **ectoparasites**, whereas those that live inside are called **endoparasites**. Arthropods such as mites, ticks, and lice are examples of ectoparasites. Parasitic protozoa and helminths are examples of endoparasites. Parasite may also be called **permanent** or **intermittent** ones according to the duration of parasitism, or they may be accidental or opportunistic by chance or condition available.

When a parasite enters or attaches to the body of a species of host different from its normal one, it is called an **accidental**, or **incidental parasite**. For instance, it is common for nematodes, normally parasitic in insects, to live for a short time in the intestines of birds or for a rodent flea to bite a dog or human. Accidental parasites usually do not survive in the wrong host, but in some cases they can be extremely pathogenic. Parasitism is usually the result of a long, shared evolutionary history between parasite and host species. Accidental parasitism puts both host and parasite into environmental conditions to which neither is well adapted; it is not surprising that the result may be serious harm to either or both participants.

Some parasites live their entire adult lives within or on their hosts and may be called

permanent parasites, whereas a **temporary**, or **intermittent parasite**, such as a mosquito or bedbug, only feeds on the host and then leaves. Temporary parasites are often referred to as micropredators, in recognition of the fact that they usually "prey" on several different hosts (or the same host at several discrete times).

Host

In parasitism, **host** supplies the parasite with nourishment and shelter, it is the injured partner. The host, in comparison to parasite is relatively larger in size. Parasitologists differentiate among various types of hosts according to the role the host plays in the life cycle of the parasite.

A definitive (final) host is one that harbors the adult or the sexually reproductive stage of a parasite. Human being, for instance, is the definitive host for schistosomes. Sexual reproduction has not been clearly shown in some parasites—such as amebas and trypanosomes—and in these cases we arbitrarily consider the definitive host the one most important to humans.

An **intermediate host** is one that harbors the larval or the asexually reproductive stage of a parasite, according to priority they are classified into first intermediate host, second intermediate host, third intermediate host and so on.

Definitive hosts are often but not necessarily vertebrates; the malarial parasites, or *Plasmodium* spp., reach sexual maturity and undergo fertilization in mosquitoes, which are therefore by definition the definitive hosts, while vertebrates are the intermediate hosts.

Reservoir hosts are the vertebrate hosts which harbor the same species of parasite at the same stage as a human host. They are an important source of infection in epidemiology.

In a broad sense, any animal that harbors an infection that can be transmitted to humans is called a reservoir host, even if the animal is a normal host of the parasite. Examples are rats and wild carnivores with *Trichinella spiralis*, dogs with *Leishmania* spp.

Zoonosis refers to any disease of animals that can be transmitted to man.

A vertebrate animal other than a human that is normally infected with a parasite which can also infect humans is called a reservoir host, even if the animal is a normal host of the parasite; it is a reservoir for a zoonotic infection of humans. Thus, the reservoir host, by definition, shares the same stage of the parasite with humans. Often, the reservoir host tolerates the parasitic infection better than the human host does.

A Paratenic host or transport host is an abnormal host in which some parasitic larvae can survive but can not develop into adults. If the larvae have a chance to enter their appropriate hosts, they can continue to develop into adults there. Paratenic hosts may bridge an ecological gap between the intermediate and definitive hosts. For example, when *Paragonimus westermani* invades and lives in a wild boar, it can not grow up and hence keeps its larva state. However, if the boar meat containing the larva is ingested by a dog, the larva will develop into an adult in the dog. The wild boar is a paratenic host for *P. westermani*.

Vector

Some parasitic infections may be carried from one host to another by means of arthropod **vectors.** A vector may also be a host if development of the parasite takes place within the body. In this instance the vector plays a role of host.

Carrier: A person who harbors parasite has no clinical symptoms and signs; it is an important source of infection in epidemiology.

Parasite Life History

Life Cycle is the whole biological process of growth, development and reproduction of a parasite, which proceeds in one or more different hosts depending on the species of parasites.

Infective Stage is a stage when a parasite can invade human body and continue to live in it.

Infective Route is the specific entrance through which the parasite invades the human body.

Infective Mode means how the parasite invades human body, such as the cercariae of the blood fluke actively penetrate the skin of a swimming man and the infective ascaris eggs are swallowed by man.

Direct and indirect life cycles

The life cycle of a parasite can be divided into two types. The one in which the parasite only needs one host to complete its life cycle is called **direct type** (**monoxenic life cycles**). That is the parasites produce infective stages that can directly infect another susceptible definitive host individual. This type of life cycle is simple without an intermediate host, such as the life cycle of *Ascaris lumbricoids*. Some species of protozoa and many helminthes have complex life cycle, with two and sometimes more hosts, definitive host(s) and intermediate host(s). Examples are plasmodium in protozoa and lymphatic filaria in helminth. This type of life cycle is **indirect type** (**heteroxenic life cycles**). Those parasites utilize a number of intermediate hosts or vectors in their transmission between definitive hosts. Almost all species in Trematoda, Cestoda, Acanthocephala and a few of nematodes belong to this type of life cycle.

In the life cycles of some parasites, there are regular alternations of sexual and asexual reproductions; this phenomenon is called **alternation of generation**, such as the life cycle of *Plasmodium vivax*.

Chapter 2 Host-Parasite Interactions and Immune Responses

The relationships between parasites and hosts are complex. Living organisms are constantly exposed to microbes. Nevertheless a disease as an outcome of the pathogen attack remains an exception rather than a rule, and most species are remarkably resistant to infectious agents. In some cases, pathogens invade more than one host to complete their complex life cycle. To warrant a successful transmission from one host to another, parasites have developed a number of strategies and tricks, many of which rely on the passive or active participation of the host. Inside their hosts, the parasites change looks and coats and invade a diverse set of cells and tissues, some for a transient passage, whereas others to establish a long-term infection. The past decade has shown an explosion in the field of host-parasite interactions. The rapid progress was made possible by the availability of sequence information and bioinformatics and the development of a series of functional assays. These efforts firmly established an intricate crosstalk between the interacting organisms.

The factors that determine the initiation, development and outcome of an infection involve a series of complex and shifting interactions between the invading organism and the host, which can vary with different infecting organisms. These interactions include the following: (1) The organism's ability to breach host barriers and to evade destruction by innate local and tissue host defenses; (2) The organism's biochemical tactics to replicate, to spread, to establish infection and to cause disease; (3) The parasite's ability to transmit to a new susceptible host; (4) The body's innate and adaptive immunological ability to control and eliminate the invading pathogens.

A major barrier to fit or adapt to the host's environment by parasites is the immune response. The presence of the parasite stimulates the host trying to destroy the parasite. In order to survive in the host, parasites must have some means of avoiding this reaction.

In any real case of parasitic relationship, some kind of balance must be achieved between the host and the parasite. The host must adapt the parasite to survive long enough for its reproduction and removing its progeny, since death to the host means death to the parasite.

The outcome of a parasitic infection is highly variable. It may be subclinical latent infection (or carrier) or overt clinical disease.

The characteristics of parasitic diseases mainly include host specificity, chronic infection, larva migrans, polyparasitism, parasitic zoonosis and opportunistic parasitism.

Pathogenesis of the parasitic diseases is a dynamic process and depends on the complex interaction of a variety of host and parasite factors. The host factors include nutritional stage of the host, immune response to a parasitic infection, immune status of the host, the presence or absence of the co-existing disease or other physiological conditions and the age and level of the immunity at the time of infection. The parasite factors include the site of attachment of the parasite, the size of the parasite, the number of invading parasites, the strain, the growth, the development and multiplication of parasites inside the human body, and their metabolic products.

Effects of the parasite on the host are complex. The parasite can cause damage or disease in humans in various ways, including: (1) nutrition robbing; (2) mechanical damage; (3) toxic effects; (4) allergic reactions or hypersensitivity.

In human beings there is a complete immune system. When parasites invade into the body, the defense from non-specific innate immunity works firstly and the acquired immunity develops later. In order to escape the host defense mechanism, parasites develop many ways to fit the environment of parasitism.

Parasites have evolved enough to evade the natural and the acquired defenses of the host immune responses.

Host immune responses to parasites

Immune responses can be innate (nonadaptive) or acquired (adaptive).

A general feature of many parasitic infections by protozoa or helminths is their chronicity and the capacity of parasites to withstand or to evade destruction by specific immune responses of the vertebrate host.

Innate immunity

Innate immunity is a resistance that is pre-existing and is not acquired through contact with a nonself (foreign) entity known as an antigen. It is nonspecific and includes barriers to infectious agents—e. g. , skin and mucous membranes, phagocytic cells, inflammatory mediators, and complement components. It may vary with age and with hormonal or metabolic activity.

The skin and the linings of the respiratory, gastrointestinal, and urogenital tract present formidable physical and chemical barriers to infective organisms and represent a first line of defense. These barriers provide a natural resistance, also called innate immunity, to infection, but they are not perfect. Protozoan and helminthic parasites, have evolved in such a way that they either are able to penetrate the body's barriers directly or are transmitted by insect bites.

In the body the alternative pathway of complement activation provides defense mechanism against many parasites.

Another defense is provided by macrophages and neutrophilic leukocytes, which play a major role in all stages of host defense. These cells by means of their CR3-

receptors are able to recognize microbial substances and thus ingest the parasites. In addition, Toll-like receptors (TLRs) have been defined as important transmembrane receptors that confer a certain degree of specificity to the cells of innate immune system. TLRs have been implicated in recognition of every known category of pathogen that causes infectious disease. TLRs can recognize minute concentrations of microbial components and orchestrate an early defense, largely dependent on the MyD88-dependent activation of NF-κB, which will trigger microbiostatic/microbicidal effector mechanisms and lead to the production of proinflammatory cytokines thereby also shaping the adaptive immune response. Once parasites have survived the innate immune response, the acquired immunity comes into effect.

Acquired immunity

Acquired immunity, which occurs after exposure to an antigen (e. g. , an infectious agent) is specific and is mediated by either antibody or lymphoid cells. It can be passive or active.

Passive immunity is transmitted by antibodies or lymphocytes preformed in another host. The main advantage of passive immunization with preformed antibodies is the prompt availability of a number of antibodies; disadvantages are the short life span of these antibodies and possible hypersensitivity reactions if antibodies (immunoglobulins) from another species are administered.

Active immunity is induced after contact with foreign antigens (e. g. , microorganisms or their products). This contact may consist of clinical or subclinical infection, immunization with live or killed infectious agents or their antigens, exposure to microbial products (e. g. , toxins, toxoids), or transplantation of foreign cells. In all these instances the host actively produces antibodies, and lymphoid cells acquire the ability to respond to the antigens. Advantages of active immunity include long-term resistance (based on the memory of prior contact with antigen and the capacity to respond faster and to a greater extent on subsequent contact with the same antigen); disadvantages include the slow onset of resistance and the need for prolonged or repeated contact with the antigen.

Acquired immunity is mediated by the humoral and cellular immune system, in which the B-lymphocytes are mediators of the humoral responses. Upon direct recognition of the parasites, i. e. , antigen, they produce antibodies of different isotypes, which are specific for the antigen. A remarkable difference between bone-marrow-derived B and thymus-derived T cells is the inability of T cells to recognize antigens directly as B cells do. T cells, on the other hand, need adequate presentation of antigens mostly by major histocompatibility complex (MHC) molecules expressed on antigen-presenting cells (APCs), such as dendritic cells, Langerhans cells, macrophages, B cells, and vascular endothelial cells. The T cells are distinguished according to their T cell receptor (TCR) and accessory molecules. The TCR is composed of an α and β chain or a γ and δ chain. Accessory molecules are the CD4 or the CD8 marker.

Antigen presentation

Several classes of molecules are encoded in MHC gene complex, of which the MHC class Ⅰ and class Ⅱ molecules are central to antigen presentation. MHC genes are organized in a gene complex of about 3.5mb on chromosome 6 in man. Association of antigen with MHC molecules occurs inside the antigen-presenting cell and processing of foreign antigen to peptide fragments is an essential prerequisite for successful association and presentation. The complex of the MHC molecule and antigen peptide is transported to the cell surface and presented to T cells. MHC class Ⅰ and class Ⅱ molecules can be subdivided into classical and nonclassical MHC molecules. Classical class I molecules are encoded in man by the HLA-A, -B, and -C genes. These highly polymorphic molecules present processed peptides to $CD8^{+}$ T cells. Nonclassical class Ⅰ molecules are much less polymorphic and are encoded by HLA-E, -F, and -G. Their function in man is still ill defined. The great polymorphism of genes coding for MHC molecules allows man to bind and present a vast diversity of different peptides produced by the many parasite pathogens, to a large T cell repertoire, resulting in highly specific immune response.

T cell mediated responses

In man, the T cell population in the periphery amounts to more than 10^{12} cells, of which more than 90% carry the α/β T cell receptor (TCR) and less than 10% the g/d receptor. The TCR associates with the variable region of the MHC-molecule which carries the antigenic peptide and the CD4 or CD8 molecules bound to the constant regions of the MHC molecules. The $CD4^{+}$ T cells according to their cytokine secretion pattern have been subdivided into the Th1 and Th2 family, Th1 cells producing IL-2 and IFN-γ, cytokines that serve as stimuli of T cells or macrophages respectively, and Th2 cells producing IL-4, IL-5, and IL-10, which act as true helper cells for B cells. The Th1 cells, via IFN-γ, seem to act as classical cells of delayed type of hypersensitivity, i. e., of cell-mediated immunity, for instance in the tuberculin reaction. Thus, they are of prime importance in the control of intracellular microorganisms such as toxoplasma, leishmania, mycobacteria, and others.

By virtue of their IFN-γ production Th1 cells also downregulate Th2 cells. The Th2 cells, on the other hand represent the classical T helper cells, which are involved in the allergic reaction and in humoral immune responses. IL-4 is central to IgE production and IL-5 to IgA production and IL-10 downregulates Th1 cells. The subdivision of $CD4^{+}$ T cells in Th1 and Th2 cells should, however, not be taken too strictly because during a developing immune response, T cells producing both Th1 and Th2 cytokines are found, and Th1 and Th2 cells might well coexist in the tissue. Differentiation of Th0 cells into Th1 or Th2 is driven by cytokines produced by different cells of the immune system. IL-12 is the major player in the Th1 pathway and IL-4 driving the Th2 cells.

Besides $CD4^+$ T cells, $CD8^+$ cells are involved in immune reactions to most if not all intracellular parasites including plasmodia, toxoplasma, and leishmania. $CD8^+$ cells function by their capacity to act as cytolytic killer cells as well as producers of cytokines such as IFN-γ, etc. $CD8^+$ T cells lyse infected target cells by cell-to-cell contact subsequent to the recognition of the target peptide that is presented by class I molecules. Target cell lysis is mediated by 2 separate mechanisms. The first mechanism involves the secretion of perforins and granzymes by the killer cells, which both lead to osmotic lysis of the target cells. The second mechanism requires the cross-linking of the Fas-ligand and the cytolytic $CD8^+$ cells with the Fas-antigen on the target cells with subsequent chromatin condensation, DNA fragmentation, and cell rupture. This mechanism induces apoptosis, also known as programmed cell death, in the target cells. Cytolytic activity is most prominent in $CD8^+$ T cells, however also some $CD4^+$ T-cells have been shown to act as killer cells as in the case of *Toxoplasma gondii*-infected macrophages.

Another type of T cells involved in the regulation of antiparasitic immunity are regulatory T cells (T_{reg}). Several types have been described based on their origin, generation, and mechanism of action, with 2 main subsets identified: "natural" $Foxp3^+$ $CD4^+CD25^+$ T_{reg}, which develop in the thymus and regulate self-reactive T cells in the periphery, and "inducible" T_{reg} (e. g., Tr1 or Th3 cells), which can develop in the periphery from conventional $CD4^+$ T cells. Both types of T_{reg}, by virtue of their capacity to control the intensity of effector responses, have been shown to play a major role in the control of various parasitic infections.

Specific points of immune responses to helminths

Worms such as filaria, ascaris, and schistosomes induce high levels of specific IgE antibodies and eosinophilia. This characteristic response pattern is caused by the particular ability of helminths to preferentially stimulate the Th2 subset of $CD4^+$ cells, which secretes the cytokines IL-4 and IL-5, IL-4 involved in the production of IgE antibodies and IL-5 acting as a growth factor for eosinophils. In vitro studies suggest that helminths opsonized with specific IgE antibodies are lysed by eosinophils that carry Fc receptors specific for IgE, the toxic product contained in the major basic protein of the eosinophils granules.

Strategies of evasion mechanisms by parasites

The capacity of parasites to survive and to persist in their hosts is a result of coevolutionary events that enable the parasites to evade immune effector mechanisms. Most parasites have developed multiple evasion strategies to circumvent both innate and acquired defense mechanisms of the host. These include:

(1) Intracellular location and seclusion of parasite (e. g. , *Plasmodium*, *Toxoplasma*, *leishmania*)

The intracellular habitat of some protozoan parasites protects them from the direct effects of the host's immune response. By concealing the parasite antigens, this strategy also delays detection by the immune system.

Many protozoan parasites grow and divide within host cells. For example, *Plasmodium* parasites grow first in hepatocytes and then in red blood cells. *Leishmania* and *Toxoplasma* organisms are capable of growing in macrophages; one genus of parasitic protozoa, *Theileria*, not only multiplies in lymphocytes but appears even to stimulate the multiplication of the infected lymphocytes. Although some parasites, such as *Plasmodium*, are restricted to a limited number of host cell types, others, such as *Toxoplasma*, appear to be able to grow and divide in a variety of different host cells. An intracellular refuge may protect a parasite from the harmful or lethal effects of antibody or cellular defense mechanisms.

(2) Antigenic shedding (e. g. , *Entamoeba*, *Toxoplasma*, *Fasciola*, *Trichinella*)

(3) Antigenic variation (e. g. , *Trypanosoma*, *Giardia*)

Three major groups of parasitic protozoa are known to be able to change the antigenic properties of their surface coat. The African trypanosomes can completely replace the antigens in their glycocalyx each time the host exhibits a new humoral response. It has been estimated that African trypanosomes have approximately 1,000 different genes coding for surface antigens. These genes are located on various chromosomes. Considerably less information is available on the phenomenon of antigenic variation in malaria or babesiosis. However, antigen variation could be a major problem in reference to the development of a blood stage (merozoite) vaccine for malaria. Finally, antigenic variation has been observed in *Giardia lamblia*. Antigenic variation has been suggested to assist *Giardia* in escaping the host's immune response.

(4) Antigenic mimicry or masking (e. g. , *Trypanosoma*, *Schistosoma*)

Various species of trypanosomes have host immunoglobulins associated with their cell surfaces. There are several reports that these antibodies are not bound to the trypanosomes through their variable regions, but presumably through the Fc portion of their molecule. These antibodies may mask the parasite—that is, prevent immune recognition by the host. Mimicry, in which the parasite has the genetic information to synthesize antigens identical to those of its host, has been demonstrated in some parasites.

(5) Modification of host immune responses. This is done by inactivation of complement (e. g. , *Taenia*), immune suppression (e. g. , *Plasmodium*, *leishmania*, *Toxoplasma*, *Wuchereria*, *Brugi*), activation of lymphocytes (e. g. , *Trypanosoma brucei*, *Schistosoma* species), modified leucocyte function (e. g. , *Fasciola hepatica*)

and immune complex (e. g., *Leishmania*, *Trypanasoma brucei*, *Toxoplasma*, *Plasmodium*).

Chapter 3 Control of Parasitic Diseases and Current Status in China

The epidemic of parasitic diseases must have three basic conditions, e. g., source of infection, route of transmission and susceptible population. The ways of transmission include food, soil, air, water, arthropods and direct contact. The common portals of entry include skin, mouth, insect bite, contact and placenta.

The epidemic and transmission of parasitic diseases are affected by biological factor, natural factor and social factor. The epidemiological feature of them is endemic, seasonal and natural focal epidemic.

Prevention of parasitic disease depends on its interception. Control includes checking the possibilities of dissemination of infection and epidemics, reducing and maintaining a low level of parasitic infections in the human population, and protecting susceptible population.

Control methods can be aimed at controlling and eradicating the disease at its reservoir and source of infection. It can be achieved by the follows:

Chemotherapy and isolation. It is useful to prevent the spread of infection and eliminate the reservoir and source of infection. Immuno-prophylaxis. It is carried out by artificial immunization such as vaccines but has not been possible for most of the parasitic diseases. Pilot studies of the vaccine have been carried in the field of falciparum malaria and a few other infections. There is also control of infection in animal reservoir for zoonotic prophylaxis.

Many kinds of human behavior can influence the epidemiology and the control of parasitic diseases, probably many more kinds than we appreciate at present. Some forms of behavior are highly disease-specific in their epidemiological impact; others can affect transmission of a considerable variety of parasitic and infectious agents.

Current status of human parasitic diseases in China

From 2001 to 2004, a national survey of the prevalence of parasitic diseases was carried out in China's mainland sponsored by the Ministry of Health of China, involving stratified, random, and mass sampling. The data of that survey revealed two major trends in the epidemiology of parasitic diseases in China. First, the prevalence of the intestinal parasites such as *Entamoeba histolytica*, *Fasciolopsis buski* and soil-transmitted helminths declined markedly, in comparison with the data from the first national survey conducted in 1990. In 2003, the prevalence of hookworms, *Ascaris* and *Trichuris* has reduced by 60.72%, 71.29% and 73.60%, respectively, and the number of people infected by soil-transmitted nematodes has declined from 536 million in 1990 to 129 million in 2003, of which 39. 3, 85. 93, and 29. 09 million represent infections with hookworms, *A. lumbricoides* and *T. trichiura*, respectively. However, soil-transmitted helminthes in China is still unacceptably high in comparison with economically developed countries, such as Japan and South Korea.

In a remarkable contrast, the prevalence of food-transmitted parasitic diseases (e. g. , trichinellosis, clonorchiasis, paragonimiasis, cysticercosis, and echinococcosis), has increased significantly. The most striking example is clonorchiasis, for which the national average prevalence has increased by 75% when compared with the results of the first national survey, with an estimated 12. 49 million people (0. 58%) being infected in 2003, compared with 4. 7 million (0. 36%) in 1990. The prevalence of *Taenia* has increased by 52. 49%, nationwide, with Sichuan and Tibet having the highest increase of 98% and 97%, respectively.

Sixty years ago, China had about 31 million cases of lymphatic filariasis and about 330 million people were at risk of infection. By the year 1994, all of the 864 endemic counties/cities in 15 provinces/autonomous regions/municipalities (P/A/M) had achieved the criteria for effective control of filariasis (taking village as a reckoning unit, the microfilaria rate was less than 1%), and filariasis was almost eliminated in the whole country. Elimination of infection sources has been adopted as a major intervention measure in filariasis control. Because diethylcarbamazine (DEC) was safe and effective for treating microfilaremia cases, mass treatment was taken for the whole population, and inhabitants above 5 years with or without microfilaremia were all subjected to DEC therapy. In severe endemic areas, DEC was evenly mixed with table salt and supplied to inhabitants. The strategies used to interrupt the spread of lymphatic filariasis in China were recognized by the World Health Organization (WHO) and recommended to other countries.

Demographics of the distribution features of parasitic diseases in China

The geographical distribution of parasitic infections in China has some distinct features. For example, tapeworm infections are correlated to the hypsography. The land falls from west to east in China. The Qinghai Tibet Plateau in southwest of China is 4000m above sea level (on average), and taeniasis saginata, echinococcosis and alveococcosis are most common in these areas. From the Qinghai-Tibet Plateau to the Greater Higgnan Mountains in northeast of China, most plateaus and basins are between 1000 and 2000m, and the altitude of the central and east regions is commonly below 500m. Taeniasis solium and cysticercosis are common in these regions, whereas they are seldom detected in Qinghai-Tibet Plateau .

The distribution of soil-transmitted helminthiasis varies with the temperature zones and humidities. The highest infection rates of *A. lumbricoides*, *T. trichiura*, and hookworms are detected in both tropical and subtropical zones.

The latest national survey showed that the prevalence of most parasites was higher in women and children . The highest prevalence for soil-transmitted helminthiasis was found in the age groups of 5-9 years and 10-14 years.

Emerging parasitic diseases in China

A total of 25 helminth species was recorded in the last nationwide survey, including eight nematodes, 12 trematodes, and five tapeworms. Among these helminths, human infection with *Metorchis orientalis* and *Echinostoma aegypti* were detected in Fujian province, which was the first report in the world. Human infection with *Haplorchis taichui* in Guangxi was noted the first time in China, before which we only had animal infection with this parasite.

A total of 63 parasite species have been documented in China between 1950 and 2006, which cause emerging parasitic diseases. Some of them are related to the change of lifestyle to eat raw or undercooked fish and meat, the pursuit of eating exotic and delicate foods, and the increase of large transient population.

Cryptosporidiosis is one of the emerging parasitic zoonoses in China, which is considered by the "WHO Neglected Diseases Initiative" as an important infectious disease. *C. hominis* is the causative agent for human cryptosporidiosis in China, the first case of cryptosporidiosis occurred in Nanjing in 1987, and, subsequently, many cases were reported from more than ten provinces. The prevalence of cryptosporidiosis in diarrhea patients ranged between 1.4% and 13.3%, and was most commonly found in children. A recent survey of cryptosporidiosis revealed a prevalence of 2.96% in children with diarrhea, and the children of 1-4 year old had the highest prevalence of 5.45%.

Re-emerging parasitic diseases in China

During 1950s-1960s, due to poor conditions for health care, about 70 million people suffered from malaria, schistosomiasis and filariasis in China. In 1956, the State Council instructed to fight schistosomiasis, malaria, leishmaniasis, filariasis and hookworm diseases, and a number of important parasitic diseases have been controlled or eradicated in the past 50 years. However, factors interfering with parasitic diseases still exist in China (such as the influence of Climate Warming and the South-North Water Diversion Project which may transform the environment), schistosomiasis, malaria, and some food-borne parasitic diseases re-emerged in recent years.

Schistosomiasis

Although significant progress has been made in the control and prevention of human schistosomiasis (caused by *Schistosoma japonicum*) since the 1950s, schistosomiasis is still listed as China's most important parasitic disease, and remains endemic in seven southern Provinces of China, in line with the distribution of the intermediate host snail

Oncomelania hupensis. In 1989, the transformation of agriculture production modes made it more difficult to annihilate snails, and, in some areas, many acute outbreaks (a certain number of cases in a certain time period) occurred. In 1989, about 54 million people were at risk of infection, and the number of infections was about 1.5 million.

Given the high prevalence and severe consequences of schistosomiasis, a national campaign for control of this disease was officially launched in 1991, with partial financial support by a loan from the World Bank. In the 1990s, morbidity control was the backbone of disease control, helped by the administration of praziquantel, which had been introduced for large-scale use in the previous decade, coupled with health education. By the end of 1995, the number of infected people was significantly decreased from 1,638,000 in 1989 to 865,000 in 1995, and the snail habitat area was much reduced.

In 2002, the State Council undertook to strengthen schistosomiasis control. By the end of 2006, schistosomiasis was still endemic in 448 counties, of which 271 reached the status of transmission interruption, 72 counties reached the status of transmission control where the prevalence was at a very low level. Jiangsu, Anhui, Jiangxi, Hubei, Hunan (five provinces along the Yangtze River) and Sichuan, Yunnan (two mountainous provinces in southwestern China) provinces had not yet reached the standard of epidemic control.

In 2006, the number of schistosomiasis cases was 671,265, including 207 acute cases. The total area of snail habitats decreased from 14 billion m^2 in the early 1950s to 3.8 billion m^2 in 2006. Up to 2007, counted at the county level, Sichuan province has reached the control standards, and presently, there are a total of 90 counties (cities, districts) where schistosomiasis remains endemic, distributed in five provinces (Hunan, Hubei, Jiangxi, Anhui, and Jiangsu) in lake districts and Yunnan province in the mountainous area.

In the 1960s and 1970s, eradication of snails was considered as the focal point of schistosomiasis control campaign, despite the concerns that the molluscicides might lead to environmental pollution. Since the 1980s, the use of praziquantel for mass chemotherapy has become the chief means to control schistosomiasis. In 2004, the State Council established two targets for the National Schistosomiasis Control Program. First, by 2008, the goal was to reduce the rate of prevalence in humans in all counties in which *S. japonicum* is endemic to less than 5%, including 110 counties that had a prevalence exceeding 5%. Second, by 2015, the program aimed to reduce the prevalence in humans to less than 1%. To reach these targets, the Ministry of Health recognized an urgent need to develop a new schistosomiasis control strategy for China. A comprehensively integrated approach should be taken to tackle schistosomiasis in the new era, and the focus should be the elimination of infection sources in major endemic regions. This strengthened national control program has been implemented effectively since 2005, significantly reduced the acute infections.

Malaria

The most common type of malaria in China is caused by *Plasmodium vivax*. Quartan malaria caused by *P. malariae* is very rare, which was sporadic in 1950s. Since 1982, however, there were increased reports of transfusion-induced quartan malaria in several provinces such as Guangdong and Hubei.

Over the past 50 years, the Chinese government has made consistent efforts to control and prevent malaria, and has made great achievements. In 1984, the incidence of malaria dropped to 100 cases per 100,000 population; however, since 2001, the incidence has risen slightly. As the number of transient people increases, local outbreaks of malaria occurred in some regions where malaria disappeared previously. In 2006, a total of 64,178 malaria cases and 52,082 suspected cases with 38 deaths within suspected cases were reported in 917 counties of 23 P/A/M, and the annual incidence was 5 cases per 100,000 people. In 2007, 50,148 malaria cases and 83,551 suspected cases with 18 deaths were reported in 1182 counties of 23 P/A/M, and the annual incidence was 3.9 cases per 100,000 people.

Yunnan and Hainan provinces still face a severe situation of malaria endemicity because of the spread of *P. falciparum* (and imported cases of malaria in 25 border counties in Yunnan province). According to the data from the national malaria survey in 2006, the number of fatal malaria cases in Yunnan province was 32, which was still the greatest in China, accounting for 84.2% of the total fatal malaria cases in China (32/38), and the proportion of imported subtertian malaria from abroad accounted for 60.4% of these. So the malaria cases abroad still have a significant impact on malaria prevalence in China.

However, with regard to the malaria situation in Hainan province, the prevalence was 4.65 cases per 10,000 people in 2006, which has dropped markedly, 14.8% less than the previous year. All of the subtertian malaria cases came from indigenous infections, without fatal cases. This indicates that the "Global Fund Program" has achieved significant results in Hainan province.

Leishmaniasis

Visceral leishmaniasis (Kala-azar) caused by *Leishmania donovani* is one of the important parasitic diseases in China. It was once prevalent in rural areas of the north of the Yangtze River, such as Shandong, Jiangsu, Henan and Hubei provinces which were epidemic areas at one time with high prevalence. As a result of effective measures (such as annihilating sandflies and killing infected dogs) taken to control leishmaniasis, this disease was eliminated almost completely in China between 1958-1960. The number of patients with Kala-azar decreased from 530,000 in 1951 to 10,000 in 1959, and the prevalence rate was 0. 49/100,000-0. 16/100,000 during 1959 to 1968, and only a few sporadic cases occurred.

However, sporadic and imported cases have been reported in six Northern provinces. In the national survey in 2004, there were 85 cases in Xinjiang, six cases in Sichuan, and five cases in Gansu, and 80 cases out of these 96 (i. e., 83%) occurred in the age group of 0-19 years. The occurrence of Kala-azar is beginning to rise as a result of ecological changes. There were more than 300 cases of visceral leishmaniasis reported in the whole country every year, and about half of these cases came from Kashi city in Xinjiang province.

Food-borne parasitic diseases

Over the past 20 years, with the increase of income and living standard, as well as the pursuit of eating exotic and delicate foods, food-borne parasitic diseases have become one of the main factors which affect national food safety and people's health. The fastest growing food-borne parasitic diseases in China include clonorchiasis, angiostrongyliasis, echinococcosis, trichinellosis and cysticercosis.

Clonorchiasis caused by *Clonorchis sinensis* is mainly distributed in Asian countries, with an estimated 35 million infected people worldwide. In China, clonorchiasis is endemic in 27 P/A/M, and is listed by the Ministry of Health as one of the most important parasitic diseases.

Angiostrongylus cantonensis, the causative agent for angiostrongyliasis, was first discovered in rat lung in Guangzhou in 1933. Since 1984, about 400 angiostrongyliasis cases have been reported in China, these occurred mainly between 1979 and 2008.

Echinococcosis caused by *Echinococcus granulosus* and *E. multilocularis* is considered as the most severe parasitic disease in the seven western provinces or autonomous regions (Xinjiang, Ningxia, Gansu, Qinghai, Sichuan, Tibet and Inner Mongolia) in China. Nationwide, there were about 380,000 cases of echinococcosis and about 50 million were at risk of infection.

In China, human trichinellosis is caused by *Trichinella spiralis* and *T. nativa*. The first trichinellosis case was found in Tibet in 1964, and the disease is epidemic in a number of provinces, and about 20 millions people were infected. In the 1980s, when the food market in China was first opened, many outbreaks of trichinellosis occurred as a result of an inadequate and incomplete system of detection and quarantine. Since the 1990s, because the governmental departments have strengthened the detection and quarantine of food, the prevention of trichinellosis has become more effective, but in areas where minor nationalities live (in China, the Han people take up about 92% of the total population of the country, leaving about 8% for the other 55 nationalities, and these minorities live mainly in northwest and southwest of China), a number of outbreaks of trichinellosis occurred, mainly due to the lifestyle of eating raw or undercooked meat.

Although pork is the main source of infection, the meat of herbivores could also become the source of infection for trichinellosis, and several outbreaks caused by eating roast mutton or instant-boiled mutton happened during 1979 to 1999.

Human cysticercosis caused by the larval stage of *Taenia solium* occurred in 29 P/A/M, and about 7 million people were infected. Like trichinellosis, some minor nationalities prefer to eat raw pork and hence are at high risk of cysticercosis.

Perspectives for control

The major trends in parasitic diseases in China are as follows. First, biohelminths will take the place of geohelminthes to become the focus for future control programs against helminthiasis. Second, the prevalence of food-borne parasitic zoonoses has increased significantly. In the recent national survey, prevalence of *T. solium* and *C. sinensis* increased by 52. 49% and 75% respectively, over the survey in 1990. In contrast, the prevalence of soil-transmitted hookworm, *Ascaris*, and *Trichuris* has dropped significantly. Finally, the control focus on parasitic diseases is moving from the southeast coastal area to Western China. To cope with the new trends of parasitic diseases, in 2006, the Ministry of Health established the "Prevention and Control Programs for National Important Parasitic Diseases between 2006 and 2015", which include the publicity and education of scientific knowledge for the prevention and control of parasitic diseases, in addition to the implementation of different prevention and control measures against different parasitic diseases.

In China, the distribution of water resource is extremely uneven. South China is rich in water, accounting for about 80% of China's water resource, yet about 65% of arable land is in north China. Hence, the South-North Water Diversion Project was implemented in order to improve the water-shortage situation in the north, mainly to provide water for the North China Plain and Jiaodong Peninsular Region. This project was designed with three routes, the west route, the middle route and the east route. According to the plan, the three routes will transfer water to north China from upper, middle and lower reaches of the Yangtze River, respectively.

There is continued concern regarding the potential impact of this project on transmission of diseases, including schistosomiasis. The disease transmission will be mainly through the Lixia River basin in Jiangsu Province, Chaohu areas of Anhui Province in the east route, and Sihu areas of Hubei Province in the middle route. The snail transmission northward will be affected both by this project and by global warming. As a result, the endemic areas of schistosomiasis will probably extend to the Hongzehu and Chaohu areas in the future, which could cause great damage to socio-economic development.

Furthermore, in order to control emerging and re-emerging parasitic diseases, techniques for detection, surveillance and infection source-tracking must be further improved.

Concluding remarks

With the significant advancement in China's socio-economic conditions in the last three decades, major infectious diseases caused by virus and bacteria have been under well control, so have been the infections caused by soil-transmitted helminthes. However, due to the complicacy and difficulty encountered in the control of helminthiasis caused by biohelminths (such as *S. japonicum*) because of the involvement of intermediate hosts in their development, biohelminths will remain the focus of current and future national control programs in China. Also, with the increasing public awareness and concern of food safety, food-borne parasitic zoonoses have received increasing attention of the central and local governments, and have been listed as the important human diseases to be controlled in the near future by the Ministry of Health. Although facing many challenges such as the detrimental impact of global warming and ecological changes on the transmission of parasitic diseases, and problems (such as the uneven economic development between cities and rural regions, between the east and west of China), parasitic diseases will be well under control in the near future in China.

(He Shenyi)

Part II Medical Helminthology

Medical helminthology is the study of parasitic worms and their effect on their hosts. Parasitic helminthes are categorized into four groups: nematodes (roundworms), trematodes (flukes), cestodes (tapeworms) and acanthocephales (thorny-headed worms, or spiny-headed worms).

Chapter 4 Nematoda

Section 1 Introduction to Nematoda

The nematodes (roundworms) belong to the class Nematoda. There are more than 15,000 known species of nematodes, most of them are free living and widely distributed in water and soil (e. g., *Caenorhabditis elegans*). The parasitic nematodes live in plants, mollusks, annelids, arthropods, and vertebrates. Many nematodes have a free-living stage and some are even able to lead either a parasitic or a free-living existence. Some of the parasitic nematodes are of great importance because they are abundant and widespread, frequently occur as endoparasites infecting a wide variety of invertebrate as well as vertebrate hosts, and often have a serious impact on human health. Medical (or human) nematodes that infect humans have more than 10 species, including *Ascaris lumbricoides*, hookworm, filaria and *Trichinella*, etc.

Morphology

Adult

Nematodes have an intestinal tract and a large body cavity without an epithelial lining. They have elongate, cylindrical, often filiform, smooth, non-segmented body that usually tapers to a pointed posterior and to a rounded anterior end, resembling a tiny thread in many cases, and this is the origin of the group's name. The word "nematode" comes from a Greek word "*nema*" that means "thread". Parasitic nematodes vary widely in size according to species. While some are microscopic and others may reach more than one meter in length, most are between 1mm and 15cm long. The adult nematode is bilaterally symmetrical. It is usually flesh-colored or colorless, and varies from translucent (smaller nematodes) to opaque (larger nematodes) when examined alive. It is not uncommon for some to absorb colored matter from surrounding host tissues or fluids. Sexual dimorphism (dioecism-sexes are separate) is evident: at the curved, posterior end of the male are a copulatory organ and other specialized organs, males are also usually smaller than females.

The basic body design is a tube within a tube, the outer tube (the body wall) and the underlying muscles, and the inner tube (the digestive tract) (Figure 4-1-1). A true body cavity (coelom) is lacking, instead, nematodes have a pseudocoelom (pseudocoel) formed directly from the cavity of the blastula (rather than as a result of the division or folding of mesoderm) without a cellular lining or peritoneum. The small cavity of the pseudocoel lies between two tubes, being mostly filled with an intestine and oviducts or testes. The circulation of nutrients in pseudocoelom, instead of vascular system in nematodes, is assisted by body locomotion. The nematodes have primitive nervous and excretory systems and highly developed reproductive systems.

(1) **Body wall**

The body wall is composed of three layers: an outer cuticle (epidermis or integument), a thin hypodermis, and musculature. The cuticle has a noncellular, chemically complex structure that is strong, flexible (elastic) and covers the body surface of nematodes. The cuticle is secreted by and covers a layer of epidermal cells. In many nematodes, the cuticle is naturally colorless and partly translucent, but in some nematodes, they may have longitudinal and circular fine striated cuticles, which may bear sensory papillae, bosses, spines, bristles, and ridges on them. The anterior end may be equipped with hooks, teeth, plates, setae, and papillae for the purpose of abrasion, attachment and sensory response. The posterior end may posses papillae, spicules and a bursa which is a flap-like extension of the cuticle on the posterior end of some species of male nematodes, and is used to grasp the female during copulation. The cuticle in some nematodes has longitudinal ridges called alae. Some of these specialized structures are sensory, and some in locomotion; their arrangement and position are of taxonomic importance.

The cuticle not only covers the entire surface, but also lines the buccal cavity, esophagus (pharynx), rectum, cloaca, vagina, and excretory pore. The present of enzymes in the cuticle indicates that it is metabolically active, not an inert covering. The cuticle is periodically shed during the life of a nematode as it grows, usually four times before reaching the adult stage.

Beneath the basal lamina lies the thin cellular or syncytia hypodermis. The major function of the hypodermis is to secrete the cuticle. The hypodermis protrudes into the pseudocoelom to form four longitudinal cords: a dorsal, a ventral, and two lateral cords which may be seen on the surface as lateral lines. These partially divide the pseudocoel into quadrants. The lateral cords are the largest and contain the primary excretory canals when these are present, while the dorsal and ventral contain longitudinal nerve trunks.

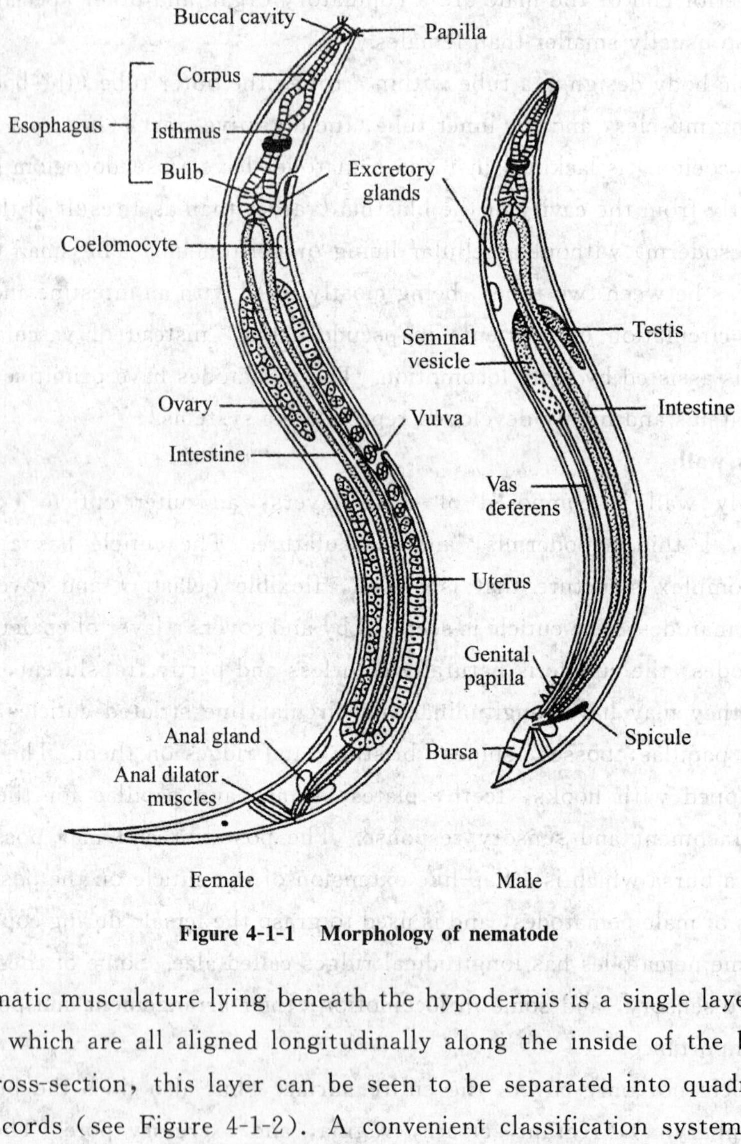

Figure 4-1-1 Morphology of nematode

The somatic musculature lying beneath the hypodermis is a single layer of smooth muscle cells which are all aligned longitudinally along the inside of the body. When viewed in cross-section, this layer can be seen to be separated into quadrants by the hypodermal cords (see Figure 4-1-2). A convenient classification system to describe muscle cell arrangement has been devised based on the number of rows of muscle cells per quadrant. According to this system, an arrangement of multiple, longitudinal rows of muscle cells in each quadrant is termed polymyarian; one with no more than two rows of cells is designated holomyarian; and one with two to five rows is called meromyarian. Each muscle cell comprises a contractile portion containing myofibrils and a non-contractile portion, in which are found the various organelles, such as nucleus, mitochondria, ribosomes, and endoplasmic reticulum, as well as stores of glycogen and lipid. Sensory processes usually extend from the non-contractile portion of each cell to the longitudinal nerve trunks. The somatic musculature connects to the cuticle by fibers that originate in the contractile portion of each cell, pass through the basal lamina, and attach the endocuticle. Nematodes move by contraction of the longitudinal muscles. Because their internal pressure is high, this causes the body to flex rather than flatten, so the nematodes can only bend their bodies from side to side.

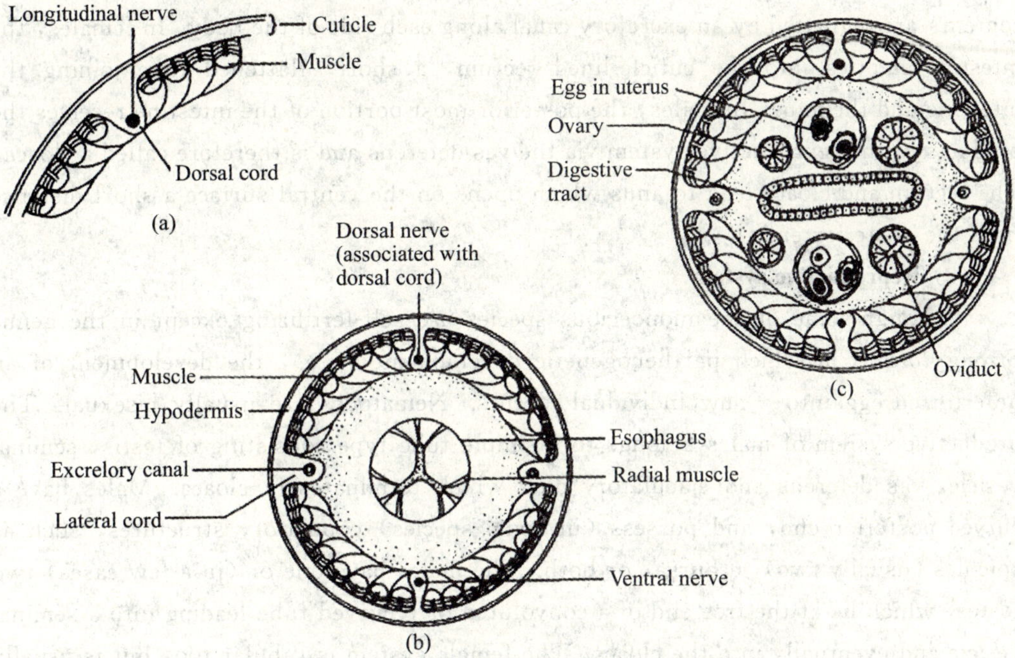

Figure 4-1-2 Morphology of cross section of nematode

(a) Portion of the dorsal body wall showing the relationship of the dorsal cord to the cuticle.

(b) Cross section through the esophageal region.

(c) Cross section through the midgut region.

(2) **Digestive system**

The digestive tract of nematodes is a simple tube extending from the mouth to the anus. It consists of mouth, buccal cavity, esophagus, intestine (its major regions being foregut, midgut, and hindgut), rectum (females) or cloaca (males), and anus. The mouth, which is surrounded by lips bearing sensory papillae (bristles), is either a simple opening of a buccal cavity leading directly to the esophagus, or a buccal capsule with thick walls, curved teeth, or cutting plates. The esophagus, a conspicuous feature of nematodes, is a muscular structure that pumps food into the intestine; it differs in shape in different species. The structure of the esophagus varies within the class Nematoda, but its similarity among members of each taxon makes it an important taxonomic feature. It may be completely muscular or completely glandular, or the anterior half may be glandular and the posterior half muscular. Esophageal action is often enhanced by one or more muscular enlargements called bulbs. The glandular portion ranges from a few unicellular glands to large, prominent glands lying along the esophagus. The intestine is a simple straight tube lined with a single layer of columnar cells possessing prominent microvilli on their luminal surface. The intestine is non-muscular, the food being moved posteriorly by the muscular activity of the foregut and overall body movements. Nutrients and waste are distributed in the body cavity, whose contents are regulated by an excretory canal along each side of the body. In females, the intestine empties into the cuticle-lined rectum, a short, flattened tube joining the intestine and the anus. In males, the posterior-most portion of the intestine receives the products of the reproductive system via the vas deferens and is therefore called a cloaca. The rectum and cloaca lead to anus which opens on the ventral surface a short distance from the posterior end.

(3) **Reproductive system**

Although some of the monoecious species are self-fertilizing except in the genus *Strongyloides*, in which parthenogenetic development (i. e., the development of an unfertilized egg into a new individual) occurs. Nematodes are usually bisexual. The productive system of males belongs to a simple tube type consisting of testis, seminal vesicle, vas deferens and ejaculatory duct which terminates in cloaca. Males have a curved posterior end, and possess (in some species) copulatory structures, such as spicules (usually two), a bursa, or both. The males have one or (in a few cases) two testes, which lie at the free end of a convoluted or recurved tube leading into a seminal vesicle and eventually into the cloaca. The female system is tubular too, but is usually didelphic (i. e., equipped with two cylindrical varies and uteri). Each ovary is continuous, with an oviduct and tubular uterus. The two uteri join to form the vagina, which in turn opens to the exterior through the vulva. Fertilization takes place when males use special copulatory spines to open the females' reproductive tracts and inject sperm into them. The sperm are unique in that they lack flagella and move by pseudopodia, like amoebas. Development of fertilized eggs is usually direct.

(4) **Excretory system**

The excretory system of nematodes, when present, is unique. In most nematodes, it consists of two long excretory ducts running inside the lateral cords. At the anterior end, these ducts are interconnected by a short horizontal tube with the shape of the capital letter H, U or U inverted, and open in the mid ventral region as an excretory sinus. It has not been shown conclusively that this system serves as the primary vehicle for excretion. Indeed, there is strong evidence that the digestive tract is the principal excretory organ and that the system described above is chiefly osmoregulatory, with merely ancillary excretory and secretory functions.

(5) **Nervous system**

There are two major nerve centers in nematodes. One, the circumesophageal commissure, or nerve ring, surrounds the esophagus. Associated with the commissure are various ganglia from which longitudinal nerves emanate. The anterior longitudinal nerves innervate the anterior sense organs, such as oral papillae and amphids. The posterior longitudinal nerves, embedded in the dorsal and ventral hypodermal cords, innervate organs in the posterior regions of the body. The ventral longitudinal nerve is the largest nerve in the nematode body. It passes posteriorly as a chain of ganglia. The most posterior chain branches and continues dorsally from the hypodermal cord into the pseudocoelom, where it encircles the rectum to form the second nerve center, the rectal commissure. Peripheral nerves branch from the main longitudinal trunks and supply sensory organs, such as the phasmids, in the cuticle.

Parasitic nematodes possess both mechanoreceptors and chemoreceptors. Located around the mouth are papillae of two main types: labial papillae on the lips surrounding the mouth and cephalic papillae behind the lips (see Figure 4-1-3). Papillae are mechanoreceptors and are innervated by papillary nerves derived from the circumesophageal commissure. Other papillae may be found at different levels of the nematode body. For example, caudal papillae, observed in many male nematodes, aid in copulation. Amphids are chemoreceptors located in shallow, anterior depressions or pits at the same level of the body as the cephalic papillae. The sensory endings are modified cilia innervated by amphidial nerves that are also associated with circumesophageal commissure. Phasmids comprise another set of chemoreceptors that appears near the posterior end of many parasitic species as a pair of cuticle-lined organs.

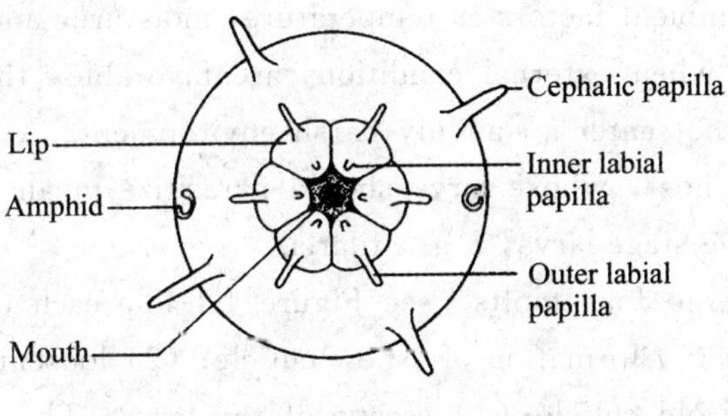

Figure 4-1-3 Labial and cephalic papillae

In face view of nematode showing relationship of mouth, lips, amphids, and papillae.

Eggs

The egg shell of parasitic nematodes ordinarily consists of three enveloping layers enclosing an embryo. During copulation, the sperm is transferred into the vulva of the female. The sperm enters the ovum and a fertilization membrane (the first layer) is secreted by the oocyte, but it is difficult to identify the layer under an optical microscope. This fertilization membrane gradually thickens to form the chitinous shell (the second layer) which is located in middle layer. It consists of chitin and protein and can resist the mechanic pressure. The second membrane below the shell makes the egg impervious to essentially all substances except carbon dioxide and oxygen. The inner membrane, the lipid layer (the third layer, or named as ascaroside layer), is formed by the zygote. In some species, an additional proteinaceous membrane is secreted as the egg passes down the uterus by the uterine wall and is deposited outside the shell. The layer may be rough-textured (*Ascaris*) or smooth (*Trichuris*).

Most nematodes that are parasitic in humans lay eggs that contain either an uncleaved zygote, a group of blastomeres, or a completely formed larva. Some nematodes, such as the filariae and *Trichinella spiralis*, produce larvae that are deposited in host tissues.

Life Cycle

Hatching and molting

The developmental process in nematodes involves egg, larval, and adult stages.

Eggs of parasitic nematodes may hatch either within the host or in the external environment. The eggs of many nematodes hatch only after ingestion by a host, in which case host carbon dioxide tension, salts, pH, and temperature may act as hatching stimuli. These conditions stimulate the enclosed larva to initiate the secretion of enzymes to partially digest the enveloping membranes, such as *Ascaris*. When hatching of some eggs (e. g., hookworm eggs) occurs in the external environment, the first-stage larva usually emerges. The process is controlled partly by the maturity of the larva and partly by such ambient factors as temperature, moisture, and oxygen tension. An egg will hatch only when external conditions are favorable, thus ensuring that the emerging larva does not enter an unduly harsh environment. A few of nematodes lay larva directly in the host, whose larva should parasitize in an intermediate host for developing to infective-stage larva, e. g., filaria.

Nematodes undergo four molts (see Figure 4-1-4), each of which involves the following four steps: (1) formation of a new cuticle; (2) loosening of the old cuticle; (3) rupturing of the old cuticle; (4) escape of the larva. The sequence of events is controlled by exsheathing fluid secreted by the larva. This fluid digests the cuticle at specific sites on the inner surface, causing it to loosen. The larva's ability to form a new cuticle in the hypodermis before shedding the old one allows the nematode to develop continuously between molts; however, growth occurs most rapidly just after molting.

In some nematodes, there is a lag phase at some stage of development, during which the nematodes are able to suspend completely their life processes temporarily when conditions become unfavorable; in these resistant states they can survive extreme dryness, heat, or coldness, and then return to life cycle when favorable conditions return. This phenomenon is thought to be an adaptation that allows the larva to withstand adverse environmental conditions while awaiting access to a new host. Renewal of the life cycle following such interruptions depends on stimuli that accompany events such as penetration of the host's skin or being swallowed by the host. This is known as hypobiosis (or cryptobiosis). In some species, hypobiosis may occur in the definitive host.

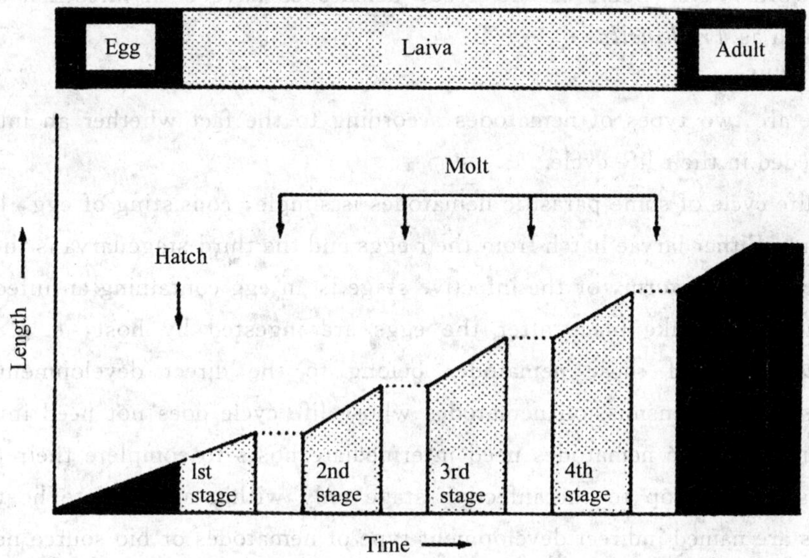

Figure 4-1-4 Stages in the development of nematodes

Larval stages preceding each of the four molts in the life cycle of parasitic nematodes are generally referred to, respectively, as first, second, third, and fourth stage (i. e. , L1, L2, L3, L4). The first-stage larva is the stage prior to the first molt. The larvae after the first molt are called second-stage larvae, and so on. The nematode formed at the fifth stage is the adult. However, various other designations are also used for specific nematode larval forms. The first-stage larvae of such parasite species as *Strongyloides* and hookworms are called rhabditiform larvae. After molting twice, the rhabditiform larvae normally retain the remnants of their last cuticle and become ensheathed, third-stage or filariform larvae which is usually the stage infective to the definitive host. The prelarvae or advanced embryos of filarial nematodes such as *Wuchereria bancrofti* are known as microfilariae. This larva is generally found in circulating blood, and is usually surrounded by a thin, cuticular sheath.

Parasitic sites of adults in the host

The adult worm of nematodes parasitize in digestive tract or blood and tissue of the host. The worms that reside in intestine are called intestinal nematodes, the worms inhabit in blood or tissue are called blood and tissue nematodes.

Intestinal nematodes of importance to man are *Ascaris lumbricoides* (roundworm), *Trichuris trichiura* (whipworm), *Enterobius vermicularis* (pinworm), *Strongyloides stercoralis*, *Ancylostoma duodenale* and *Necator americanus* (hookworms) and *Dracunculus medinensis*. *E. vermicularis* and *T. trichiura* are exclusively intestinal parasites. The major blood and tissue nematodes of man are *Trichinella* and filaria. The latter includes *Wuchereria bancrofti*, *Brugia malayi*, *Onchocerca volvulus*, and *Loa loa* (eye worm), etc. Some of the tissue nematodes have both intestinal and tissue phases, such as *Trichinella*.

Type of life cycle

There are two types of nematodes according to the fact whether an intermediate host is needed in their life cycle.

The life cycle of some parasitic nematodes is simple, consisting of egg, larva, and adult worm. Either larvae hatch from their eggs and the third-stage larva is the infective stage, such as hookworm, or the infective stage is an egg containing an infective larva and hatching will take place after the eggs are ingested by host, e. g., *Ascaris lumbricoides*. All of these nematodes belong to the direct development type of nematodes or soil-transmission nematodes whose life cycle does not need intermediate hosts. Some parasitic nematodes need intermediate hosts to complete their life cycle, and the larvae develop to the infective stage only within appropriate hosts. These nematodes are named indirect development type of nematodes or bio-source nematodes, such as filaria.

Physiology

Parasitic nematodes derive much of their energy from the metabolism of glucose. Glycogen serve is stored primarily in the hypodermis, the intestine, the non-contractile parts of the muscles, and parts of the reproductive system. It is difficult to establish with certainty whether adult intestinal nematodes are exclusively aerobic or anaerobic in their usage of carbohydrate, or whether free-living larvae are invariably aerobic. Experimental data strongly suggests the importance of determining not only whether each species uses oxygen, but also the manner in which it is utilized. For instance, intestinal nematodes belonging to the genus *Ascaris* can use oxygen if available; however, it serves only as a terminal electron acceptor in a system independent of an electron transport system or a functional Krebs' cycle. On the other hand, both larvae and adults of *Trichinella spiralis* have a functional TCA cycle and an electron transport system with oxygen being the final electron acceptor. Thus, the former organism generates ATP by means of substrate-level phosphorylation, whereas the latter organisms do so primarily through oxidative phosphorylation. The eggs and first- and second-stage larvae of *Ascaris* spp. exhibit aerobic metabolism with a functional Krebs's cycle. The optimal larval development in most species that have been studied is dependent on relatively high concentrations of oxygen.

Pathogenesis

Unlike protozoan parasites, most of adult helminthes are incapable of increasing their numbers in the definitive host. Hence, the severity of the damage caused by nematodes is related to the following factors: species of nematodes, worm burden, development stage, parasitic site, and physiological condition or immunological response of the host.

Adult nematodes cause the damage to humans by mechanical disruption and toxicity, and the changes may include erosion, bleeding, inflammation and proliferation of tissue.

The major pathogenic effects of nematodes larvae appear to be the invasion and the subsequent migration in the tissue of the host. The larvae of *Ascaris* and hookworms require the lung migratory phase to complete their life cycles. Allergic or anaphylactic reaction occurred during larval migration plays a primary role in the pathogenesis. For example, the hookworm larvae can cause dermatitis, pulmonary inflammatory response, or the transient pneumonia (Loeffler's syndrome).

Intestinal nematodes infections slant the host immune response toward a Th2-type profile leading to IgE production, mast cell activation, mucus secretion, and ultimately parasite clearance in some cases.

Classification

The common human nematodes belong to class Nematoda, which is divided into subclass Phasmidea and subclass Aphasmidea according to the presence or absence of the phasmid (see Table 4-1-1).

The common features of morphology and life cycle in class Nematoda are as following: bilaterally symmetrical unsegmented pseudocoelomates; body generally elongate, cylindrical, covered by cuticle; mouth terminal surrounded by lips; sexes separate; anterior body characteristically with 16 setiform or papilliform sensory organs and two amphids (chemoreceptors); digestive tract complete, with subterminal anus; excretory system, when present, empties through anterior, ventromedian pore; body musculature limited to longitudinal oriented muscles; no respiratory or circulatory systems; eggs with determinate cleavage, oviparous or ovoviviparous; stages in life cycle are egg, four larval stages, and adult.

Table 4-1-1 **Classification of important medical nematodes**

Subclass	Order	Family	Genus	Species
Phasmidea	Rhabditata	Strongyloididae	*Strongyloides*	*S. stercoralis*
		Rhabditidae	*Rhabditella*	*R. axei*
	Strongylata	Ancylostomatidae	*Ancylostoma*	*A. duodenale*
			Necator	*N. americanus*
		Trichostrongylidae	*Trichostrongylus*	*T. orientalis*
		Angiostrongylidae	*Angiostrongylus*	*A. cantonensis*
	Ascaridata	Ascaridae	*Ascaris*	*A. lumbricoides*
	Oxyurata	Oxyuridae	*Enterobius*	*E. vermicularis*
	Spirurida	Gnathostomatidae	*Gnathostoma*	*G. spinigerum*
		Gongylonematidae	*Gongylonema*	*G. pulchrum*
		Thelaziidae	*Thelazia*	*T. callipaeda*
	Filariata	Dipetalonematidae	*Wuchereria*	*W. bancrofti*
			Brugia	*B. malayi*
	Camallanata	Dracunculidae	*Dracunculus*	*D. medinensis*
Aphasmidea	Trichurata	Trichinellidae	*Trichinella*	*T. spiralis*
		Trichuridae	*Trichuris*	*T. trichiura*
		Capillariidae	*Capillaria*	*C. hepatica*

(Wang Zhongquan and Cui Jing)

Section 2 *Ascaris lumbricoides*

Infections with *Ascaris* have been recognized since antiquity. The first description of the parasite in the modern age was probably made by Edward Tyson (1683), who distinguished it from the common earthworm. Linnaeus gave the organism its current name in 1758 and the pig worm, *Ascaris suum*, was described by Goeze (1782). The life cycle of the disease was finally discovered in Japan in 1922 when Shimesu Koino, a researcher, infected both a volunteer and himself, and then traced the progress of the disease.

Ascaris lumbricoides is a member of the superfamily Ascaridoidea. The Ascaridoidea possess a mouth that has three conspicuous lips. Males have one or two copulatory spicules but no bursa copulatrix and usually no caudal alae. This family includes a number of human parasites that are pathogenic in their adult stage, e. g., *Ascaris lumbricoides*, or in their larval stages, e. g., *Toxocara canis* and *Anisakis*. *Ascaris suum* is the most closely related member of the genus and is a roundworm endemic to pigs. Experimental human infections with *A. suum* suggest that the parasite is unable to pass the L4 stage and thus does not cause an infection in man.

Morphology

Adult

These species are characterized by having three prominent lips, each with a dentigerous ridge, and no interlabia or alae. Lateral hypodermal cords are visible with the naked eye.

The adult *Ascaris lumbricoides* is a long whitish pink cylindrical worm, tapering at both ends, curving ventrally in the male.

Females are 20cm to 49cm long and 3mm to 6mm wide. The vulva is about one-third the body length from the anterior end. The ovaries are extensive, and the uteri may contain up to 27 million eggs at a time.

Males are much smaller, slightly more than half of the size of females. They are 15cm to 31cm long and 2mm to 4mm at greatest width. The posterior end is curved ventrally, and the tail is bluntly pointed. Spicules are simple, nearly equal, and they measure 2. 0mm to 3. 5mm long(see Figure 4-2-1).

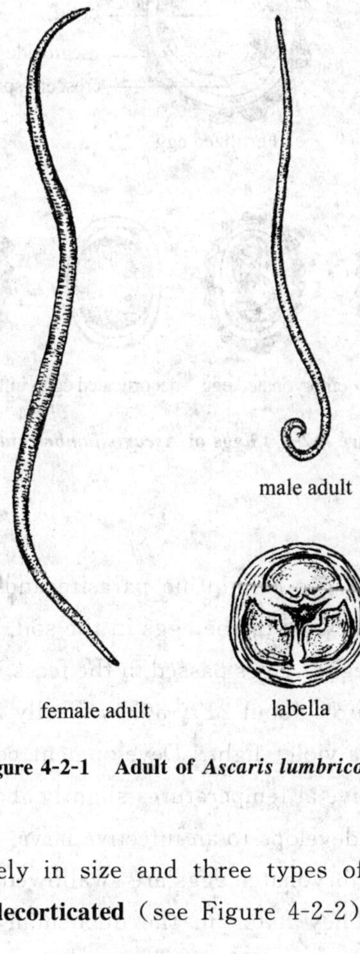

Figure 4-2-1 Adult of *Ascaris lumbricoides*

Eggs

Ascaris eggs vary widely in size and three types of eggs may appear in feces, **fertilized, unfertilized** and **decorticated** (see Figure 4-2-2). Fertilized eggs are oval to round, 45μm to 75μm long by 35μm to 50μm wide, with a thick, lumpy outer shell (mammillated, uterine, or proteinaceous layer) that is contributed by the uterine wall. When eggs are passed in the feces, the mammillated layer is bile-stained golden brown. Embryos are usually uncleaved when laid and passed in the feces. The thick external mammillated layer may disappear, giving a decorticated appearance, and can be confused with eggs from hookworms or other worms. A female before insemination or one in early stages of oviposition commonly deposits unfertilized eggs. The unfertilized eggs are longer and narrower than fertilized ones, measuring 88μm to 94μm long by 39μm to 44μm wide. The internal structure of the egg is poorly differentiated. Female worms produce up to 240,000 eggs/day. The egg shell is made up of four layers: an outer mucopolysaccharide layer, a vitelline layer, a protein and chitin layer, and an inner selectively permeable layer consisting of an unsaponifiable lipid ascaroside.

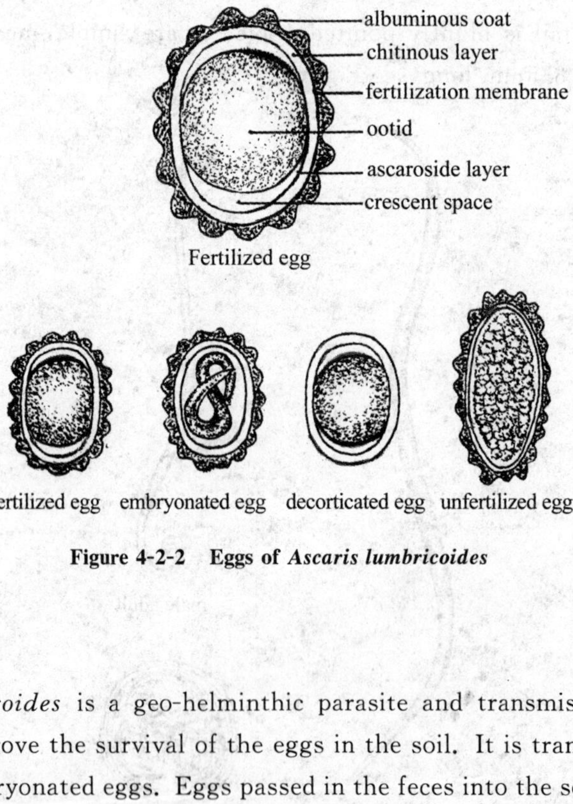

Figure 4-2-2 Eggs of *Ascaris lumbricoides*

Life Cycle

Ascaris lumbricoides is a geo-helminthic parasite and transmission is favored by conditions that improve the survival of the eggs in the soil. It is transmitted to humans by ingestion of embryonated eggs. Eggs passed in the feces into the soil develop over 10-25 days, at optimal temperatures about 21℃-30℃, ideally in moist soil conditions with oxygen and shaded from ultra-violet light. Development ceases at temperatures below 15.5℃, and eggs cannot survive at temperatures slightly above 38℃. The embryo molts at least once in the shell and develops to an infective larva.

Infection occurs when embryonated eggs are swallowed with contaminated food and water (see Figure 4-2-3). They hatch in the duodenum, where they penetrate the mucosa and submucosa and enter lymphatics or venules. After passing through the right heart, they enter the pulmonary circulation and break out of capillaries into the air spaces. Many worms get lost during this migration and accumulate in almost every organ of the body, causing acute tissue reactions.

While in the lungs, larvae molt twice during a period of about 10 days, to a length of 1.4mm to 1.8mm. They then move up the respiratory tree and trachea to the pharynx, epiglottis where they are swallowed or are coughed up. Many larvae make this last step of their migration before molting to the fourth stage. Fourth-stage larvae are resistant to gastric juices environment and pass through the stomach to the small intestine, where they mature. Within 60 to 65 days of being swallowed, they begin producing eggs. The adults live for about a year and are subsequently passed in the feces.

In endemic areas environmental contamination can be severe, and in dry windy conditions the eggs can become airborne and be ingested.

Eggs containing infective larva may remain viable in the soil for two years or longer.

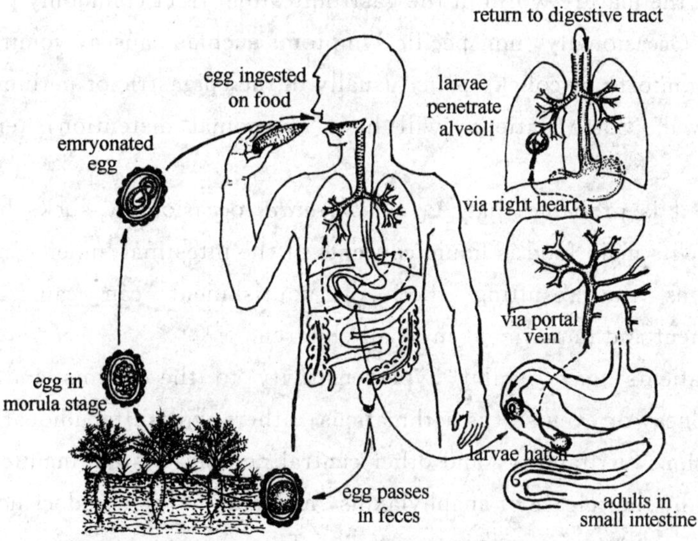

Figure 4-2-3 Life cycle of *Ascaris lumbricoides*

Pathogenesis and Clinical Manifestation

Pathogenesis from migrating larva

Little damage is caused by the penetration of intestinal mucosa by newly hatched worms. Larvae that become lost and wander and die in anomalous locations, such as spleen, liver, lymph nodes, or brain, often elicit an inflammatory response. Transplacental migration into a developing fetus is also known. Allergy and immunopathology of ascariasis are reported.

When larvae break out of lung capillaries into the respiratory system, they cause a small hemorrhage at each site. Heavy infections will cause small pools of blood to accumulate, which then will initiate edema with resultant clogging of air spaces.

Accumulations of white blood cells and dead epithelium add to the congestion, which is known as *Ascaris* pneumonitis (Loeffler's syndrome). Loeffler's syndrome is usually unsuspected clinically and rarely diagnosed.

Thus, in heavy infections 5 to 6 days after ingesting infective eggs, patients may develop a fever of 37.5℃-40℃ with chills, dyspnea, paroxysmal coughing, and hemoptysis, which may worsen during the following week. These symptoms may persist for 7 to 10 days, after which the patient improves and becomes asymptomatic after 3 weeks.

If examined, the sputum may show numerous eosinophils, Charcot-Leyden crystals, and Ascaris larvae, which may also be found in gastric washings. There may be a high blood eosinophilia during this larval stage of the disease. Symptoms in occasional patients may be quite severe, even leading to death in rare cases.

Pathogenesis from adult worm

In adults, the mature worm in the gastrointestinal tract commonly produces few or no symptoms. Occasionally, nonspecific symptoms such as nausea, vomiting, anorexia, abdominal discomfort, or colicky pain, usually in the epigastric or periumbilical region, will be observed. Some patients will have abdominal distention, tenderness, and constipation.

Although it is probable that *A. lumbricoides* occasionally sucks blood from the intestinal wall, its main food is liquid contents of the intestinal lumen. In moderate and heavy infections the resulting theft of nourishment can cause malnutrition, underdevelopment and impairment in small children.

A few patients may exhibit hypersensitivity to the worms and present with urticaria, dyspnea, or even status asthmaticus; others will suffer idiopathic epilepsy or febrile convulsions, irritability, and other central nervous system manifestations which may be caused by the release of anaphylaxins, neurotoxins, and endocrinotoxins present in adult ascarids ("Ascaris encephalopathy"). The eosinophil count may be normal or only slightly elevated during the phase of intestinal ascariasis.

Complications of ascariasis

Wandering adult worms cause various conditions, some serious, some bizarre, all unpleasant.

The frequent and severe complication of ascariasis is partial or complete intestinal obstruction caused by a heavy infection; this is seen much more commonly in children than adults especially during a febrile infection or after therapy with anthelmintics. The most common site of obstruction is at or near the ileocecal region. There are case reports of 1,063 and over 2,000 worms in individual children.

Ascaris worms can enter the bile duct, pancreatic duct, appendix, etc., and cause biliary or hepatic, pancreatic, and appendix ascariasis or ascariasis granulomas. The most common complication is biliary ascariasis. The symptoms usually include right upper abdominal pain, which is characterized by a sudden onset, and a very strong intensity. Vomiting with bile-stained gastric contents frequently coexists with the pain. A typical sign is the pain at the pressure point just below the xiphoid process. Penetration of the intestine or appendix is not uncommon. The resulting peritonitis is usually quickly fatal.

Ascaris worms may crawl into the eustachian tubes and middle ears, causing extensive damage; or they may simply exit through the nose or mouth, causing a predictable consternation.

Epidemiology

Ascariasis affects a large portion of the world population. Many estimate that over 1.5 billion people are infected today, mostly in areas of poor sanitation. In some tropical areas with sufficient poverty, infection approaches 100%.

Ascariasis is commonly present in China; national surveys from 2001 to 2004 showed mean prevalence of 12.72%, with an estimated 87.93 million people infected in the population.

The resistance of *Ascaris* eggs to chemicals is almost legendary. They can be embryonate successfully in 2% formalin, in potassium dichromate, in 50% solutions of hydrochloric, nitric, acetic, and sulfuric acid, and among other similar inhospitable substances. This extraordinary chemical resistance is a result of the lipid layer of the eggshell, which contains ascarosides.

Ascaris eggs kept for 10 years in soil can still infect people.

Contamination, then, is the typical means of infection. Children are the most likely to become infected by eating dirt or placing soiled fingers and toys in their mouths. In regions in which night soil is used as fertilizer, uncooked vegetables become important vectors of *A. lumbricoides* eggs.

Cockroaches can carry and disseminate *A. lumbricoides* eggs. Even windborne dust can carry eggs when conditions permit.

Diagnosis

The diagnosis of ascariasis depends on the identification of the adult worms passed through the rectum or from some other body orifice, or by identifying the eggs of *A. lumbricoides* in the stool, vomitus, sputum, or small bowel aspirate. Occasionally eggs, larvae, or adult worms may be identified in tissue sections. Once the fertile females within the gut begin to release eggs, the diagnosis of ascariasis can usually be made by direct fecal smears. However, concentration techniques using centrifugation may facilitate diagnosis. The radiological appearance of the worms in the gastrointestinal or biliary tracts is highly characteristic. Diagnosis during the stage of larval migration is difficult, although occasionally larvae may be found in the sputum or gastric contents.

Prevention and Control

Albendazole is the drug of choice. Albendazole binds to tubulin in the worm's intestinal cells and body wall muscles; it blocks microtubule growth and glucose intake within the helminthes thereby causing death. Side effects can include diarrhea and some abdominal pain that passes usually within a few days. No efficient treatment of migrating larvae has been discovered.

Mebendazole also works in much the same way with many of the same side effects as Albendazole.

Nitazoxanide appears to be effective against a variety of helminthes, including *A. lumbricoides*. Ivermectin is effective against *A. lumbricoides*.

Surgical intervention is needed with severe complications of ascariasis.

To prevent the spread of Ascaris as well as many other helminthes, both education and chemotherapy must play major roles. The drug treatment with Albendazole has already been covered, however, on the larger scale, education about sanitation and public works must expand. Because Ascariasis is spread through contaminated topsoil, higher levels of hygiene can stop the spread of the disease. Even better, communities can move areas of "waste" away from food and water supply chains, thereby eliminating accidental contamination of food and water.

Better infrastructure also will enable better public health control of the disease. With better infrastructure, a single dose of Albendazole can be provided to each school child every few months, helping to reduce the amount of infected persons. If each child were educated about the disease, and grew up taking Albendazole in high-risk areas, the disease burden could be significantly reduced.

(He Shenyi)

Section 3 *Trichuris trichiura*

Trichuris trichiura, or named whipworm, has a worldwide distribution but is more common in tropic areas and in regions where sanitation is poor. The worm parasitizes mainly in ileocecal junction of humans and causes trichuriasis.

Morphology

The adult worm is whip-shape. The long thin anterior part of the body forms the lash, which takes anterior three fifths of the whole body. The thick posterior portion is stock. The buccal capsule is simple. The pharyngeal canal is minuteness, and the first half of pharyngeal canal is muscular substance, the post part is glandule. It is surrounded by the rhabdite constituted by the rhabdocytes secreting antigen. The expanded posterior part of the worm contains intestine and reproductive organs. The male worm is from 30mm to 45mm long, and its caudal part is tightly curled to ventral aspect appearing twist. The tail of male has a single copulatory spicule, and on the outside of which there is a telescopic spicule sheath. The female worm is longer and bigger than the male, it is about 35mm to 50mm long. The vulva of female is near the junction of the esophagus and the intestine. The end of the female body is blunt round and has an anus (see Figure 4-3-1).

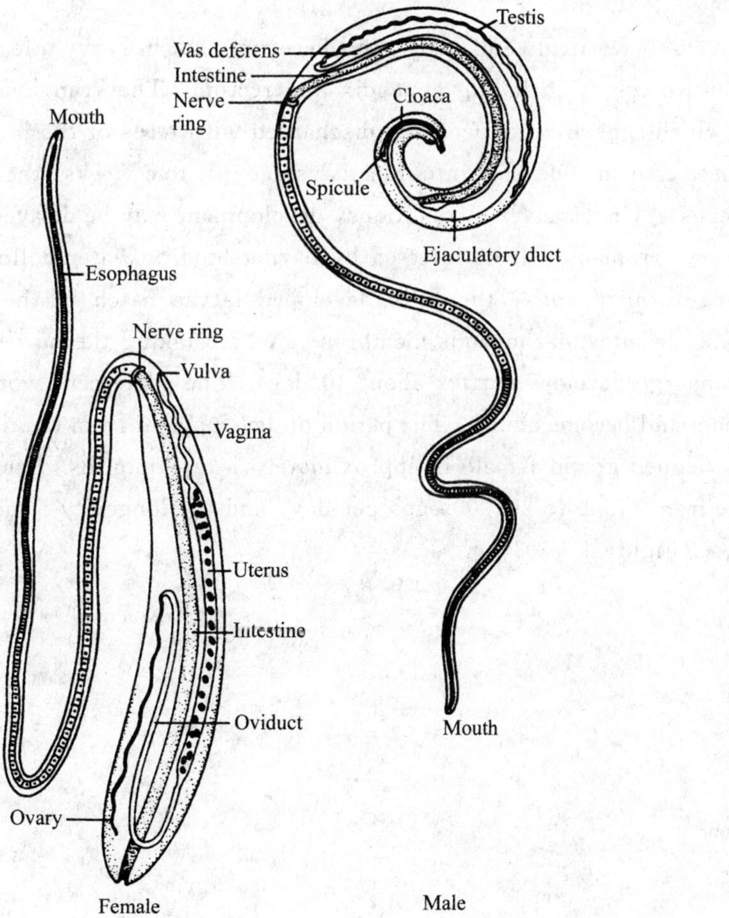

Figure 4-3-1 Adult of *Trichuris trichiura*

The egg is typically barrel shaped, about 50-54μm in length, and 22-23μm in width. The egg is stained by bile pigments. The shell of the egg is thick, and the inner part is fat layer, the middle part is chitin and the outer part is albumen film. The egg contains translucent polar plugs and an uncleaved zygote at oviposition when the egg is discharged from the human body (see Figure 4-3-2).

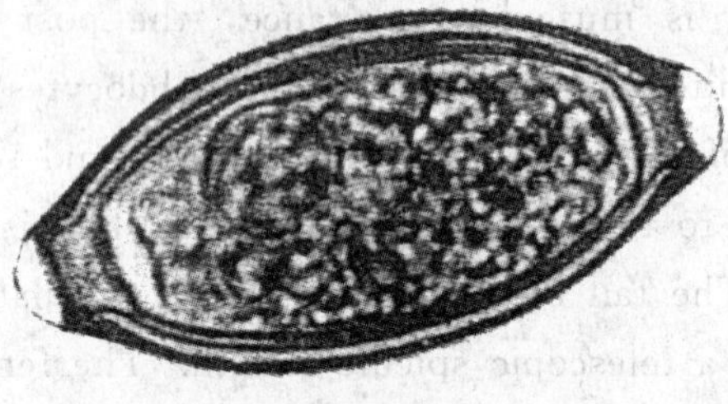

Figure 4-3-2 Egg of *Trichuris trichiura*

Life Cycle

The adult worms live primarily in the cecum, but in heavy infections, can be found in the entire colon, including appendix and rectum. They can live for several years, during which eggs are produced and discharged with feces of the host. In moist, damp soil, these eggs may develop into infective stage in 3 to 5 weeks (there are mature larvae in the eggs). Under adverse conditions, development may be delayed several months or even years. Humans will be infected by having food or water polluted by those eggs. After ingestion of eggs, the fully developed larvae hatch in the jejunum and then penetrate the intestinal mucous membrane. Where taking the nutrition (blood), these larvae undergo development for about 10 days. The adolescent worms then move into the cecum and become adults. The period of development from the time of ingestion to a fully developed gravid female is approximately 1 to 3 months. Each female worm can produce from 3,000 to 20,000 eggs per day, and the longevity of adult is about 3 to 5 years (see Figure 4-3-3).

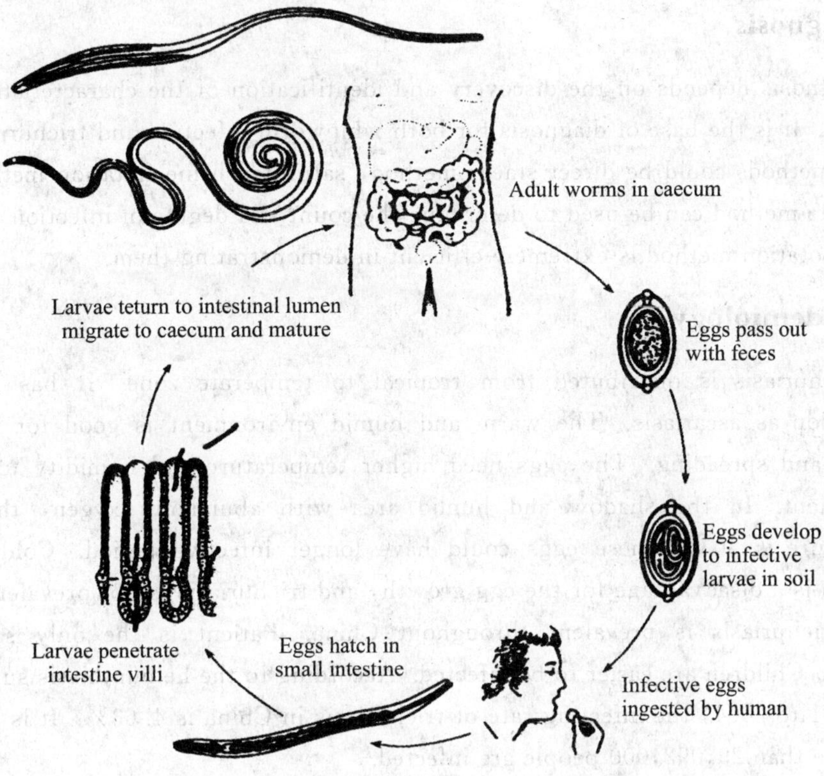

Figure 4-3-3 Life cycle of *Trichuris trichiura*

Pathogenesis and Clinical Manifestation

The anterior ends of the worms interlaced in mucosa, submucous and muscle layer of ileocecal junction, apparently produce little damage to the host unless present in large numbers. These worms damage the organs and tissues by the protease, and lead to inflammation of the intestinal wall. Congestion, edema and hemorrhage may be seen in some heavy infections. The obvious hyperplasia of intestinal wall may be visible in a few patients. The worms take the blood and interstitial fluid of the host as food. Chronic blood loss may be seen in some heavy infections.

Light whipworm infections are usually asymptomatic. Heavier infections may be characterized by abdominal pain and distention, bloody or mucoid diarrhea, tenesmus, weight loss, and weakness. Prolapse of the rectum is occasionally seen, usually in children with heavy infections of malnutrition and bacteria infection of intestines. Worms may be visible on the prolapsed, edematous rectum. Urticaria, edema, moderate eosinophilia, anemia may be seen in heavy infections.

Diagnosis

Diagnosis depends on the discovery and identification of the characteristic eggs in the feces. It is the base of diagnosis for both whipworm infection and trichuriasis. The general methods could be direct smear method, saturated brine flotation method, etc. Kato-Katz method can be used to determine the count and degree of infection. The zinc sulfate flotation method is extremely efficient in demonstrating them.

Epidemiology

Trichuriasis is distributed from tropical to temperate zone. It has the same distribution as ascariasis. The warm and humid environment is good for the eggs' growing and spreading. The eggs need higher temperature and humidity to grow in environment. In the shadow and humid area with abundant oxygen, the proper temperature is 30℃, these eggs could have longer infective period. Cold and dry condition is a disadvantage for the egg growth, and trichuriasis is not prevalent in such area. Trichuriasis is prevalent throughout China. Patient is the only sources of infection. Children are easier to be infected. According to the helminthiasis survey done from 2001 to 2004, the infecting rate of trichuriasis in China is 4.63%. It is estimated that more than 29,092,000 people are infected.

Prevention and Control

The prevention of trichuriasis is much the same as ascariasis. Emphasis should be put on individual hygiene and environment sanitation, as well as protecting the drinking water and enhancing management of feces. Mebendazole is presently the drug of choice for treating trichuriasis. Albendazole is also known to be effective.

(Cui Yu)

Section 4 *Enterobius vermicularis*

Enterobius vermicularis, commonly known as pinworm, threadworm, seatworm, is perhaps one of the most common helminthic infections worldwide. Pinworm has the broadest geographic range of any helminth. It is commonly found in school-aged children, though it is seen in adults as well. The organism was first identified in 1758 by Karl Linnaeus, who named it *Oxyuris vermicularis*. There are two species recognized currently: *E. vermicularis* and a more recently identified *E. gregorii*, although some authors have cast doubt on the validity of this species.

Morphology

Adult

The worms are small, white, and threadlike, with the larger female measures 8-13mm in length by 0. 3-0. 5mm in diameter. The tail is sharply pointed and the vulva opens mid-ventrally just in front of the middle third of the body. The anterior end tapers and is flanked on each side by cuticular extensions called "alae". The esophagus terminates in a prominent muscular bulb. In gravid females the uteri are distended and the entire body is packed with eggs. The male is only about one-of third to one-half of the size of a female and measures 2-5mm in length by 0. 1-0. 2mm in diameter and has a single conspicuous copulatory spicule (see Figure 4-4-1).

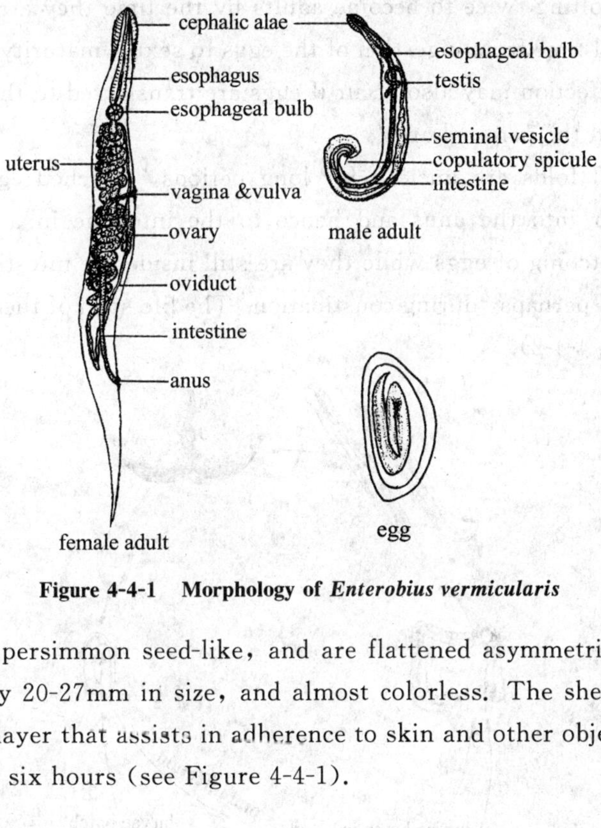

Figure 4-4-1 Morphology of *Enterobius vermicularis*

The eggs are persimmon seed-like, and are flattened asymmetrically on one side, ovoid, 50-54mm by 20-27mm in size, and almost colorless. The shell is thick with an outer albuminous layer that assists in adherence to skin and other objects. The eggs can be embryonated in six hours (see Figure 4-4-1).

Life Cycle

Adult worms inhabit the caecum, appendix and the adjacent portions of the ascending colon, but they commonly wander throughout the gastrointestinal tract from the stomach to the anus. They attach themselves to the mucosa where they presumably feed on epithelial cells and bacteria. Gravid females begin migrating within the lumen of the intestine, commonly passing out of the anus nocturnally onto the perianal and perineal skin. As they crawl about, both within the bowel and on the outer skin, they leave a trail of eggs. One worm may deposit from 4,600 to 17,000 eggs. Females die soon after oviposition, and males die soon after copulation. Consequently, it is usual to find many more females than males within a host.

When laid, each egg contains a partially developed larva, which can develop to infectivity within six hours at body temperature. Shelled larvae are resistant to putrefaction and disinfectants but succumb to dehydration in dry air within a day.

Reinfection occurs by two routes. Most often the eggs, containing larvae, are ingested via person-to-person transmission through the handling of contaminated surfaces (such as clothing, linen, curtains, and carpeting), or airborne eggs may be inhaled and swallowed, and they hatch in the duodenum. They slowly move down the small intestine, molting twice to become adults by the time they arrive at the ileocecal junction. The total time from ingestion of the eggs to sexual maturity of the worms is 15 to 43 days. Self-infection may also occur if eggs are transferred to the mouth by fingers that have scratched the perianal area.

If the perianal folds are unclean for long periods, attached eggs may hatch and larvae may wander into the anus and hence to the intestine in a process known as retroinfection. Hatching of eggs while they are still inside the intestine apparently does not occur, except, perhaps, during constipation. The life span of the adults is about one month (see Figure 4-4-2).

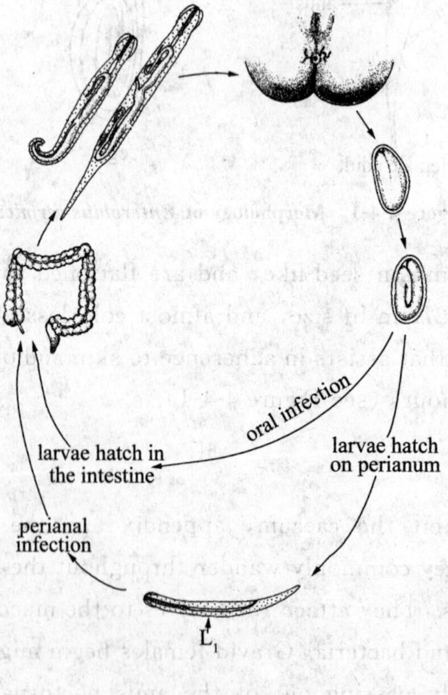

Figure 4-4-2 Life cycle of *Enterobius vermicularis*

Pathogenesis and Clinical Manifestation

About one third of infections are completely asymptomatic, and, in many more, clinical symptoms are negligible.

Pathogenesis has two aspects: damage caused by worms within the intestine and damage resulting from egg deposition around the anus.

By far the most common clinical sign of pinworm infection is perianal or perineal itching, and the itching is usually the most severe at night. This is caused by the migration of female pinworms to the anus to lay eggs, and scratching leads to finger contamination and subsequently the spread of eggs to others. The scratching may also excoriate the skin and lead to secondary bacterial infections. Other symptoms, which are due to heavy pinworm infection in children, include nervousness, restlessness, irritability, loss of appetite, nightmares, insomnia, bed wetting, grinding of the teeth, perianal pain, nausea, and vomiting.

However, pinworm infection is not always harmless, as it has been implicated in causing appendicitis, intestinal obstruction, intestinal perforation, enterocolitis, and eosinophilic ileocolitis.

Extra-intestinal infections are also possible, and while most involve the female genital tract, infection of other sites has been documented, including the lungs, breast, liver, and spleen. These extra-intestinal infections may lead to pruritis vulvae, urinary tract infections, postmenopausal bleeding, epididymitis, pelvic mass and unilateral salpingitis, among others. The dead parasites and eggs deposited in ectopic sites can also be responsible for the formation of granulomas and abscesses.

Cases have been reported of gravid female worms wandering up the vagina, uterus, where it may ascend through oviducts to the coelom, to become encased by granulomatous tissue in the peritoneum. They have been known to become encapsulated within an ovarian follicle. The pinworms may pass through intact intestinal wall to produce pelvic peritoneal granulomata.

Diagnosis

The diagnosis can be made by finding eggs or worms on or in the patient. Ordinary fecal examinations are usually unproductive because few eggs are deposited within the intestine and passed in feces. Heavy infections can be discovered by examining the perianus closely under bright light, during the night or early morning. Wandering worms can be seen easily. When adults cannot be found, eggs often can be, as they are left behind in the perianal folds. The most common means of diagnosing pinworm infection is via the "Scotch tape" test, where a clear adhesive cellophane tape is applied to the anal area early in the morning before bathing or defecation. The tape is then reversed and stuck to a microscope slide for observation under a microscope for the presence of pinworm eggs. If a drop of xylene or toluene is placed on the slide before the tape, it will dissolve the glue on the tape and clear away bubbles, simplifying the search for the characteristic, flat-sided eggs. These eggs may also be stained blue with lactophenol cotton blue, which aids in detection and identification. The sensitivity of this test when performed for three consecutive mornings is 90%. Anal swabs (paddles coated with adhesive material) may also be used. Commercial systems to facilitate specimen collection are available.

Epidemiology

E. vermicularis is a cosmopolitan parasite with particularly high prevalence in countries with a temperate climate. It has the widest distribution of any parasitic helminth. Children, especially of early school-age, are most vulnerable to pinworm infection. It has become the most common intestinal parasite seen in a primary care setting, regardless of factors such as race, socioeconomic status, and culture. As such, pinworm serves as an exception to the general rule that intestinal parasites are uncommon in affluent societies. White people seem more susceptible than black people to pinworms.

In China, enterobiasis is found in all provinces with an average infection rate of 23.61% in children. Prevalence in children in certain communities has been found to be as high as 71% in Jiangsu and Fujian.

Humans are the only natural host of pinworms. Although *Enterobius* spp. has been reported from other primates, there currently is no confirmed pinworm reservoir. Infections occur in one of four ways: (1) retroinfection, when hatched larvae migrate back into the large intestine; (2) self-infection, when the patient is reinfected by hand-to-mouth transmission; (3) cross-infection, when infective eggs are ingested, either with contaminated food or from fingers that have been in contact with contaminated surface or body parts from infected humans; (4) inhalation of airborne eggs. Humans can inhale and subsequently swallow airborne eggs, or the eggs may remain in the nose until they hatch. This, together with nose picking, accounts for the occasional case of pinworm in the nose. In household with heavily infected individuals, infective eggs have been found in samples of dust taken from chairs, tabletops, dresser tops, floors, baseboards, etc. In a survey to determine the distribution of airborne pollen in public places, pinworm eggs were found in theaters, not only on arm rests and baseboards but also on chandeliers high above the seats.

Contrary to popular belief, pinworms cannot be transmitted by dogs and cats because these animals are free of pinworms. But they can, of course, pick up eggs from their environment on their fur and serve as a source of infection for a human who affectionately nuzzles them. The eggs remain viable in cool, moist conditions for up to a week.

Prevention and Control

Benzimidazoles, such as mebendazole and albendazole, are active. Piperazine and pyrantel can also be used. It is usually necessary to treat the whole family to prevent re-infection, and a second dose 1 month after the first is often used.

Although diagnosis and cure of enterobiasis are easy, the management of pinworm infection can be very difficult, with patients re-attending with re-infection on several occasions. In practice, preventing reinfection is more difficult. Personal hygiene is the most important. Completely sterilizing the household is a difficult activity. Nevertheless, at the time of treatment, all bed linens, towels, and the like should be washed in hot water, and the household should be cleaned as well as possible to lower the prevalence of infective eggs in the environment. If all people in a household are undergoing chemotherapy while reasonable care is being taken to avoid reinfection, the family infection can be eradicated.

(He Shenyi)

Section 5 Hookworms (*Ancylostoma duodenale* and *Necator americanus*)

Hookworms include two organisms, *Ancylostoma duodenale* (*A. duodenale*) and *Necator americanus* (*N. americanus*). Hookworm infections are found in moist, warm areas and are responsible for much human disease. Although there are distinct morphologic differences between the two most common human hookworms (adult worms), the diagnostic stage (egg) is essentially identical for both.

Morphology

The adults of both species are pinkish-white in color when living. The head is often curved in a direction opposite to that of the body. The adult females measure about 9 to 12mm long by 0.25 to 0.5mm wide. The adult males are typically smaller, measuring 7 to 11mm long by 0.4 to 0.5mm wide. The posterior end in male is expanded to form a copulatory bursa.

The adult *Ancylostoma* worm tends to be larger than the *Necator* worm. Adult worms are rarely seen, since they remain firmly attached to the intestinal mucosa by means of well-developed mouth parts. The differences in the structure of the buccal capsule distinguish the adults of *A. duodenale* and *N. americanus* (two pair of teeth in *A. duodenale* and a pair of cutting plates in *N. americanus*) (see Figure 4-5-1).

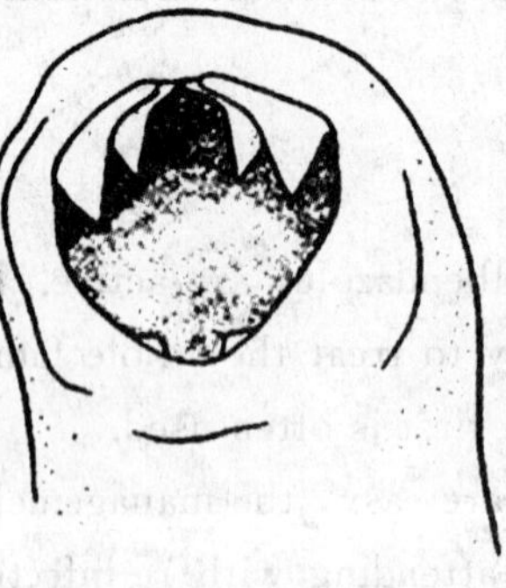

Teeth in *A. duodenale*

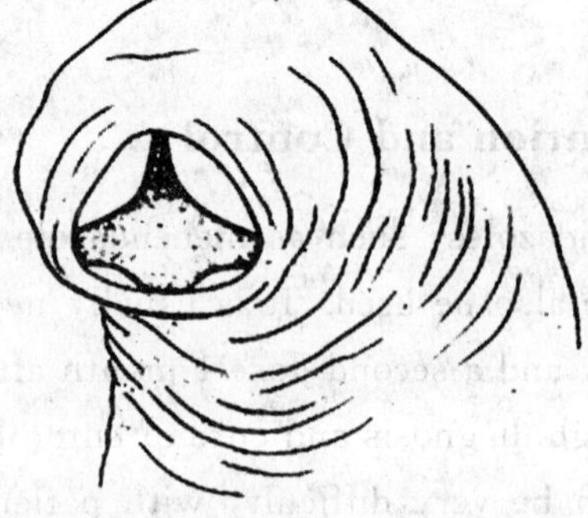

Cutting plates in *N. americanus*

Figure 4-5-1 Buccal capsule of hookworms

The eggs of both species are essentially alike. The only difference between the eggs of *A. duodenale* and those of *N. americanus* is size. The average *A. duodenale* egg ranges from 55 to 60μm in length, whereas *N. americanus* egg is about 60 to 75μm long. The eggs are usually in the early cleavage stage when passed in the stool (see Figure 4-5-2). However, if the stool samples have been kept at room temperature for several hours, particularly in moist and warm conditions, eggs in feces may reveal many cells in the stage of cleavage, even a developing larva. They are oval with broadly rounded ends and approximately 60μm long by 40μm wide. They characteristically have a clear space between the developing embryo and the thin, clear, colorless eggshell.

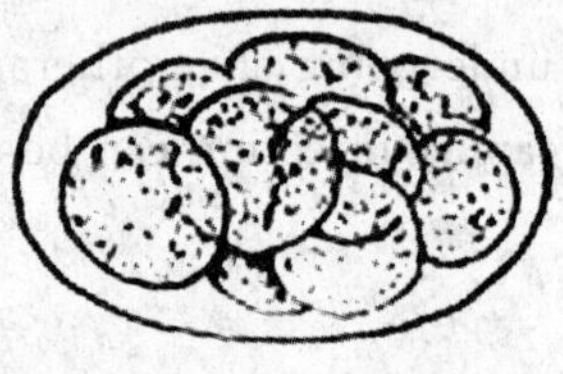

Figure 4-5-2 Egg of hookworm

Life Cycle

The life cycles of two hookworms are identical. The adults of hookworms inhabit the small intestine and attach to the intestinal mucosa firmly by their buccal teeth. The eggs are passed in feces and reaching the soil. Egg survival and larval development are favored in moist, shady, warm soil, where rhabditiform larvae hatch from the eggs within 1 to 2 days. The newly hatched rhabditform larva is about 270μm by 15μm. The rhabditiform larvae move actively in the surface layers of soil, and feed on bacteria. It ranges from 540μm by 15μm and forms a long buccal cavity in the fifth day. The rhabditiform larvae molt to become the infective filariform larvae within 5 to 8 days. The filariform has a shorter esophagus and a distinct pointed tail. The filariform larvae may remain viable in the soil for several weeks.

Infection in humans is acquired through skin penetration of filariform larvae from the soil (see Figure 4-5-3). During skin penetration, hookworm hyaluronidase activity has been confirmed and can facilitate the passage of the infective larvae through the epidermis and dermis during larval migration. After skin penetration, the larvae are carried by the venules or lymphatics to the right heart and then to the lungs. Larvae break into the alveoli, migrate via the bronchi until they reach the trachea and pharynx, and are then swallowed and brought to the small intestine, where they reside and mature to adulthood. If mature filariform larvae of *A. duodenale* are swallowed, they can develop into mature worms in the intestine without migrating through the lung. The adults attach to the mucosa of the small intestine by their teeth or cutting plates. The resulting adults multiply in the small intestine. The adults lay 10,000 to 20,000 eggs per day. Many of the eggs are passed into the outside environment via the feces. The females begin to deposit eggs about 5 months after the initial infection, although the permanent period may be 6 to 10 months. The adults may survive 2 to 14 years in human body.

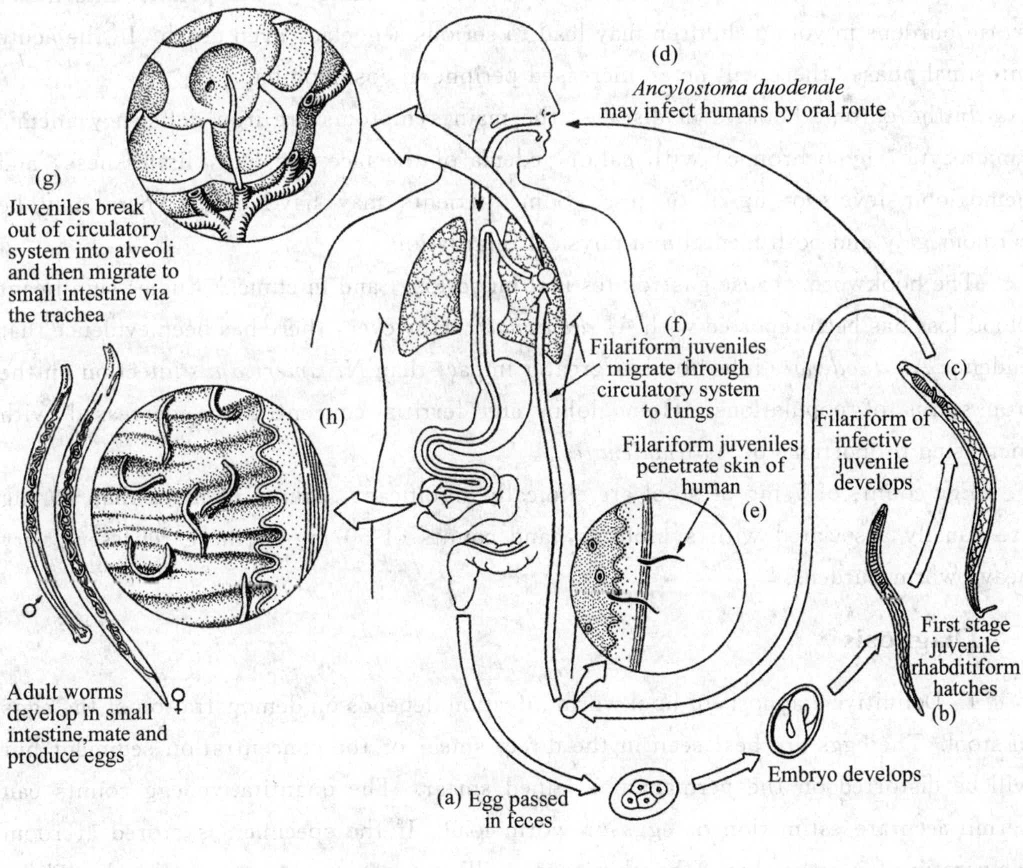

Figure 4-5-3 Life cycle of hookworm

Pathogenesis and Clinical Manifestation

Initial symptoms after larval penetration of the skin often depend on the number of larvae involved. There may be minimal to severe pruritus and possible secondary infection if the lesions become vesicular and are opened by scratching. The development of vesicle from the erythematous popular rash is called ground itch.

Any pneumonitis due to migrating larvae depends on the number of larvae present. These larvae do not cause the same level of sensitization seen with *Ascaris* or *Strongyloides* infection.

Symptoms associated with the intestinal phase of the infection are caused by: (1) damage of the intestinal phase of the intestinal tissue by the adult worm buccal teeth;(2) blood loss by direct ingestion of blood by the worms and continued blood loss from the original attachment site, possibly as a result of anticoagulant secreted by the worm.

People with acute hookworm disease may have fatigue, nausea, vomiting, abdominal pain, diarrhea with black to red stools, weakness, and pallor. The heavy worm burdens in young children may lead to serious sequelae, even death. In the acute intestinal phase, there will be an increased peripheral eosinophilia.

In the chronic hookworm disease, the main symptoms are iron deficiency anemia (microcytic, hypochromic) with pallor, edema of the face and feet, listlessness, and hemoglobin levels of 5g/dl or less. Some patients may have pica. There may be cardiomegaly and both mental and physical retardation.

The hookworms cause gastrointestinal blood loss, and in clinical studies significant blood loss has been reported with *A. duodenale*. However, there has been evidence that endemic *A. duodenale* infection has greater impact than *N. americanus* infection on the iron status of populations. Hemoglobin and ferritin concentrations decreased with increasing proportions of *A. duodenale*.

Egg counts of 5/mg of stool are clinically significant, counts of more than 20/mg are usually associated with symptoms, and counts of 50/mg or more represent very heavy worm burdens.

Diagnosis

1. Definitive diagnosis of hookworm infection depends on demonstration of the eggs in stool. The eggs are best seen in the direct smear or the concentration sediment but will be distorted on the permanent attained smear. The quantitative egg counts can permit accurate estimation of eggs or worm load. If the specimen is stored at room temperature for more than 24h, the larvae will continue to mature and hatch. These larvae must be differentiated from *Strongyloides* larvae.

2. Examining stools for eggs by the Kato-Katz method. The larvae may be cultivated by fecal culture in a test tube (a modified Harada-Mori nematode larval culture method). There was an 81. 8% agreement between the two methods for the detection of hookworm infection.

3. Recovery and examination of the buccal capsule is necessary to determine the specific hookworm species (*A. duodenale* or *N. americanus*).

Epidemiology

Hookworm infection is found worldwide between the latitudes of 45°N and 30°S. Transmission required deposition of egg-containing feces on shady, well-drained soil; the frequency of hookworm infection is high in warm areas where the inhabitants practice poor sanitation habits, especially with regard to proper fecal treatment and disposal. *A. duodenale* is found primarily in southern Europe, the north coast of Africa, northern India, Northern China, and Japan. *N. americanus* is found throughout the Southern United States, the Caribbean, Central America, Northern South America, Central and Southern Africa, Eastern and Southern Asia (China and India), Melanesia, and Polynesia.

Several factors influence hookworm prevalence: infection in the human population, defecation onto the soil, acceptable environmental conditions, and human contact with the infective larvae in the soil. Environmental conditions include temperature, rainfall pattern, and the presence of open, sandy soil.

Prevention and Control

There are three effective anthelmintic agents, including mebendazole, pyrantel pamoate, and albendazole.

On the other hand, anemia must be corrected. When it is mild or moderate, iron replacement is adequate. Adequate nutrition can prevent and overcome disease symptoms but not the infection itself. Apparently, adequate absorption of iron and nutrients is not possible in heavy infections, even with extensive dietary supplements. More severe anemia may require blood transfusion.

Hookworm prevention is similar to that of *Ascaris*. Sanitary disposal of feces is the primary means of infection control. An overall prevention approach also requires educational programs. Personal protection of persons entering known endemic areas, and prompt treatment of infected persons are such measures targeted at breaking the life cycle of hookworm. The wearing of shoes and the use of soil sterilization has not proven to be practical.

(Cheng Yanbin)

Section 6　Filariae

Filariae are slender, thread-like nematodes which inhabit the lymphatics, subcutaneous tissues, deep connective tissue, peritoneal and thoracic cavity. There are eight species of filariae infecting human beings. Three of them are more important in medicine, *Wuchereria Bancroft*, *Brugia malayi* cause lymphatic filariasis, and *Onchocerca volvulus* causes onchocerciasis (river blindness). The other five species are *Brugia timori*, *Loa loa*, *Dipetalonema perstans*, *D. streptocerca*, and *M. ozzardi*. All of filariae produce larval form known as microfilariae which appear in the circulating blood or tissue fluids. *W. bancrofti* and *B. malayi* are prevalent in China. However, the patients with onchocerciasis and loasis are found in China in recent years, these cases worked in Africa (see Table 4-6-1).

Table 4-6-1　The filarial infections of humans

Species	Site of inhabitation	Vector	Pathogenesis	Distribution
W. bancrofti	lymphatic tissues	mosquito	lymphatic damage	worldwide
Brugia malayi	lymphatic tissues	mosquito	lymphatic damage	Asian
Brugia timori	lymphatic tissues	mosquito	lymphatic damage	Island of Timor
Onchocerca volvulus	subcutaneous; eye	black fly	blindness, dermatitis	Africa
Loa loa	subcutaneous	deer fly	skin swellings	Africa
D. streptocerca	skin, subcutaneous	midge	dermatitis	Africa
Dipetalonema perstans	thoracic and abdominal cavities	midge	indefinite	Middle and South America
Mansonella ozzardi	peritoneal cavity	midge	indefinite	South America

Wuchereria bancrofti and *Brugia malayi*

The microfilariae of *W. bancrofti* were first described by Demarquay in 1863 and the adult worms in 1877 by Cobbold. Manson, in 1878, completed the description of the life cycle by showing that mosquitoes acted as intermediate hosts for the parasite. In China, Manson first reported that there was elephantiasis of the scrotum in Xiamen of Fujian province in 1872. He described microfilariae, their sheaths and a female adult of *W. bancrofti* in 1876. A case of brugia filariasis that came from Wenzhou, Zhejiang province, was first reported by Feng Lanzhou in Xiamen in 1933.

W. bancrofti is strictly a human pathogen and is distributed in tropical and subtropical areas. It is prevalent in Asia, Africa, South America and some islands in the Pacific Ocean. *B. malayi* infects a number of wild and domestic animals besides human and is restricted to South-East Asia. Mosquitoes are vectors for both parasites. Lymphatic Filariasis puts at risk more than a billion people in more than 80 countries.

Over 120 million have already been affected by it, and over 40 million of them are seriously incapacitated and disfigured by the disease. One-third of the people infected with the disease live in India, one third are in Africa and most of the remainder are in South Asia, the Pacific and the Americas. In tropical and subtropical areas where lymphatic filariasis is well-established, the prevalence of infection is continuing to increase. A primary cause of this increase is the rapid and unplanned growth of cities, which creates numerous breeding sites for the mosquitoes that transmit the disease.

Morphology

The adults of *W. bancrofti* and *B. malayi* are cream-white, thread-like worms that lie coiled in the lymphatic vessels, male and female together, for the duration of their decade-long lifespan. The head is slightly expanded and surmounted by two rings of small papillae. The adult female worms of *W. bancrofti* range in size from 80 to 100mm in length by 0.24 to 0.3mm in diameter, while the adult males usually measure 40mm in length by 0.1mm in diameter. The male is provided with two copulatory spicules. *B. malayi* adults are approximately half these sizes. Female worms measure 43 to 55mm in length by 0.13 to 0.17mm in width, and males measure 13 to 23mm in length by 0.07 to 0.08mm in widths. The female worms are ovoviviparous, and their larvae are called microfilariae. As the embryonated eggs migrate to the genital pore they gradually become elongated micromifilariae with sheaths. The anterior part of a micromifilaria is blunt and the posterior end is pointed. A large number of nuclei seen in the body are arranged in a column from the head to the posterior. A nerve ring without nuclei is found in the anterior 1/5 of the body. The morphological differences between bancroftian and malayan microfilariae are following (see Table 4-6-2 and Figure 4-6-1).

Table 4-6-2 Differentiation of bancroftian and malayan microfilariae

Species	bancroftian microfilariae	malayan microfilariae
Size	Larger (244-296μm × 5.3-7μm)	Smaller (177-230μm × 5-6μm)
Appearance	Graceful, sweeping curves	Irregular, stiff curves
Cephalic space	Shorter	Longer
	Length to width equals 1 : 1 or 1 : 2	Length to width equals 2 : 1
Body nuclei	Equal sized, clearly defined, countable	Unequal sized, coalescing, uncountable
Terminal nuclei	No	Two

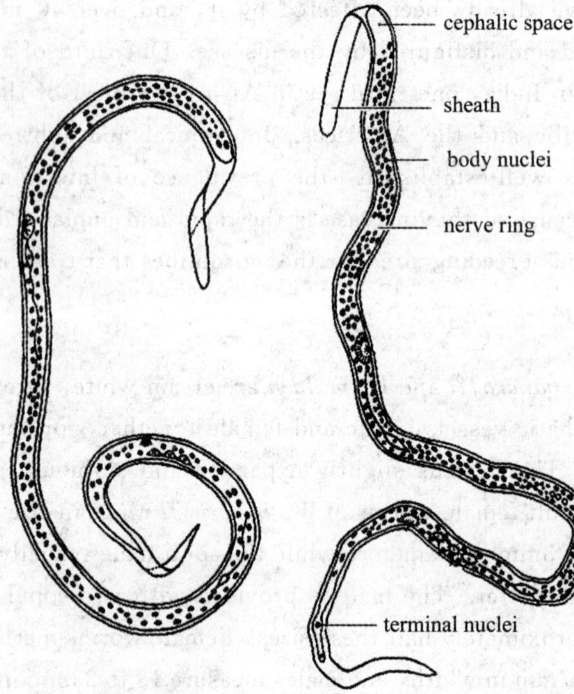

Figure 4-6-1 Microfilaria of *W. bancrofti* and *B. malayi*

Life Cycle

The characteristics of life cycle in filariae:

(1) They inhabit tissue (tissue parasites) instead of the intestinal tract.

(2) They are viviparous, producing microfilariae instead of eggs.

(3) They are biohelminths, with the intermediate host in their life cycle.

The life cycles of *W. bancrofti* and *B. malayi* are similar, adults live intertwinedly with each other in the major lymphatic ducts near lymph glands. Gravid females produce microfilariae which find their way to form the lymphatic circulation into the bloodstream. The filariae are transmitted by mosquitoes.

In mosquitoes: Upon biting an infected person, the mosquito takes the microfilariae into its stomach with the blood meal. The microfilariae take off their sheaths and penetrate the stomach wall and migrate to the thoracic muscles. During the next 1 to 2 weeks, the larvae undergo two molts, and the microfilariae develop into the sausage (Larva 1), pre-infective (Larva 2) and infective stage (Larva 3 or filariform larvae). When the next blood meal is taken, they escape from the proboscis into the skin through the puncture wound left by the mosquito and infect the new host. The process of bancroftian in mosquito larva takes bout 10-14 days, while malayan larva spends 6-6. 5

days.

In human body: The infective larvae invade skin through the bitten wound, and migrate to lymphatics within 16 hours and then migrate to the 1st intervening lymph nodes. They develop in the perinodular sinuses and molt on 9-10th day after infection. The second molting takes place 35-40 days after infection. They then leave the node and migrate retrograde to the lymphatic close to the node, where they develop into the adults. The adults dwell in various human tissues where they can live for several years. The shortest time taken by *B. malayi* to produce microfilariae in peripheral blood is 75 days (average 80-100 days). The adult worms are known to live for 10-15 years.

In most *W. bancrofti* and *B. malayi* infections, the density of microfilariae in the peripheral blood during daytime is very low, and usually undetectable. The number of microfilariae gradually increase from evening to midnight, and reach the greatest density between 10 p. m. and 2 a. m. This phenomenon is called as the **nocturnal periodicity** of microfilariae. The microfilariae accumulate in the pulmonary vessels during the day. At night, in response to changes in oxygen tension, they spill out into the peripheral circulation, where they are found in greatest numbers. Microfilariae circulate in peripheral blood once each day. Periodicity has an important epidemiologic consequence, because it determines the species of mosquito to serve as the vector and the intermediate host. Mosquito is the essential vector and the intermediate host.

Although the adult stages of *W. bancrofti* and *B. malayi* live within the lymphatic vessels of human, their living location has some difference. *W. bancrofti* parasitizes in the superficial and deep lymphatic systems, while *B. malayi* parasitizes in the shallow lymphatic system only. *W. bancrofti* usually parasitizes in the genitourinary lymphatic system, while *B. malayi* does mainly in the lymphatics of limbs. The difference in parasitic sites between the two species of filariae could produce clinical manifestations at different parts of human body (see Figure 4-6-2).

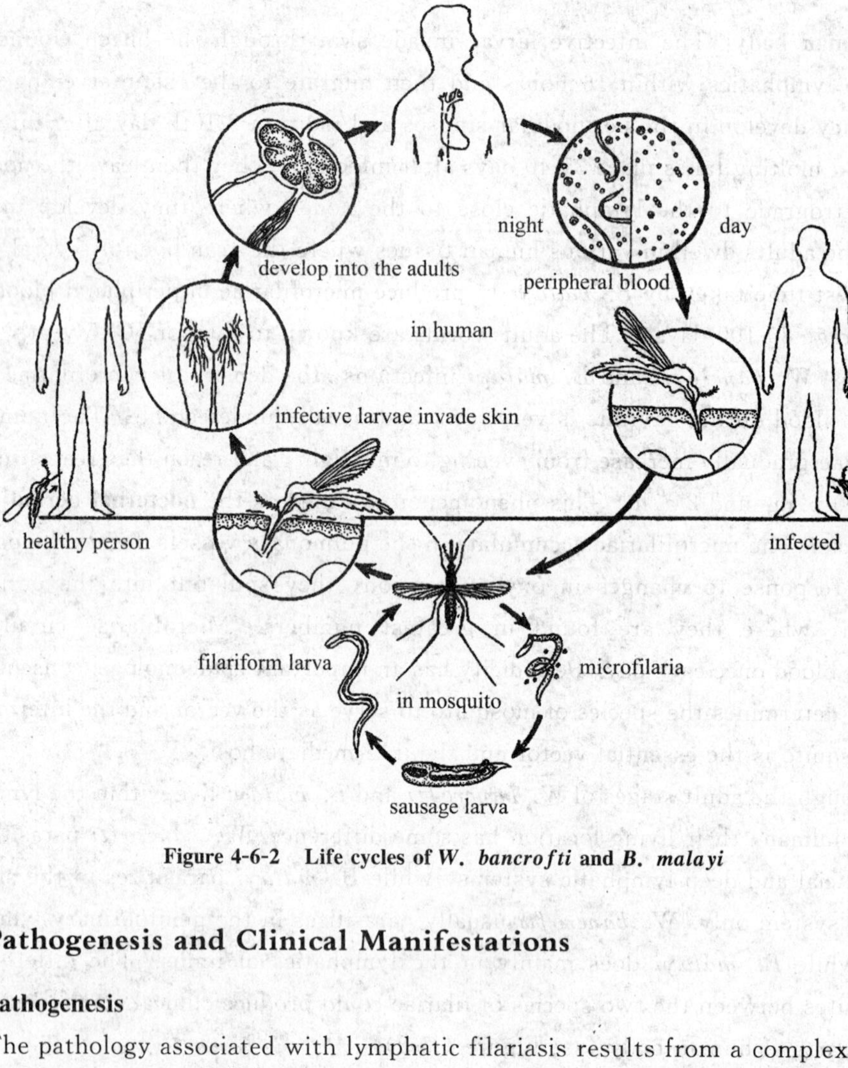

Figure 4-6-2 Life cycles of *W. bancrofti* and *B. malayi*

Pathogenesis and Clinical Manifestations

Pathogenesis

The pathology associated with lymphatic filariasis results from a complex interplay of the pathogenic potential of the parasite, the immune response of the host, and complicating bacterial and fungal infections. Pathologic changes are confined primarily to the lymphatic system, and are the result of the immune responses to adult worms and not to the microfilariae. Adult worms living in the lymph nodes and larger lymphatic vessels evoke the inflammatory response and proliferation. The clinical course is broadly divided into asymptomatic microfilaremia, acute adenolymphangitis, and chronic irreversible lymphedema and obstruction.

Microfilaremia refers to that microfilariae can be detected in peripheral circulation of a case who has no clinical manifestations.

In acute phase, three acute syndromes have been described in filariasis, as follows:

Filarial fever often begins with a chill and is followed by a high body temperature, 40℃-41℃, lasting for 1 to 2 days, which accompanies with or without lymphangitis and lymphadenitis. The fever often happens after being tired, and is accompanied with headache, muscle pains, sweating and anorexia, and other systemic manifestations.

Lymphadenitis refers to the sudden onset of febrile painful enlargement of lymph node. Lymphangitis is characterized by a retrograde progress, distinguishing it from bacterial lymphadenitis. Lymphadenitis is not always accompanied by lymphangitis, but lymphangitis appears generally together with lymphadenitis. Erysipelas-like dermatitis is a type of superficial lymphangitis. In cases with bancroftian filariasis, the lymphatic vessels of the testicle, epididymis, and spermatic cord are frequently involved, producing a painful orchitis, epididymitis, and funiculitis; inflamed retroperitoneal vessels may simulate acute abdomen. Lymphadenitis, urticaria, and eosinophilia are early findings. Symptoms usually abate within one week, but recurrences are possible.

Chronic manifestations

Lymphedema and elephantiasis: The lymphedema and elephantiasis are common signs observed both in bancroftian and brugian filariasis. Elephantiasis results from repeated infection and attacks, permanent lymphatic obstruction developing in the involved areas and the course of disease over a decade. Elephantiasis due to bancroftian filariasis affects the four limbs, external genital organs, thighs, and breasts. In brugian filariasis, elephantiasis is limited in the limbs, and leg elephantiasis seldom expands beyond the knee level. The elephantiasis in the upper limbs is rare and mostly restricted below the elbow joint. Due to the lowering of blood circulation of affected legs and remarkably reduced immunity, the elephantiasis legs are easily infected with bacteria or fungi.

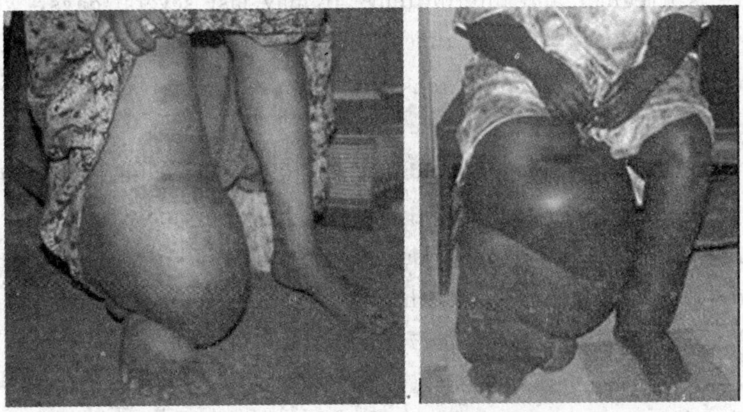

Figure 4-6-3 Lymphedema and elephantiasis of legs

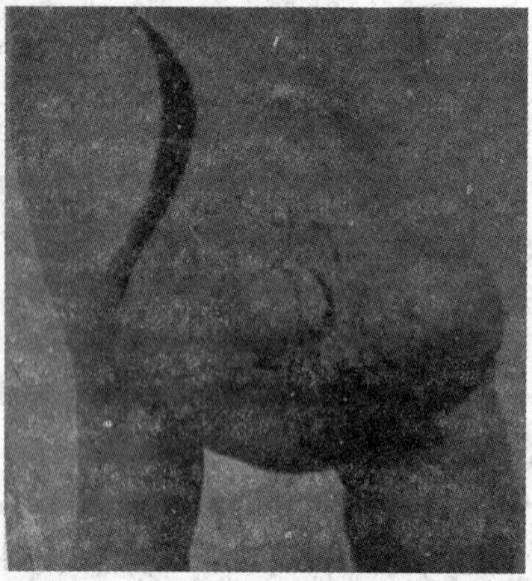

Figure 4-6-4 Elephantiasis of scrotum

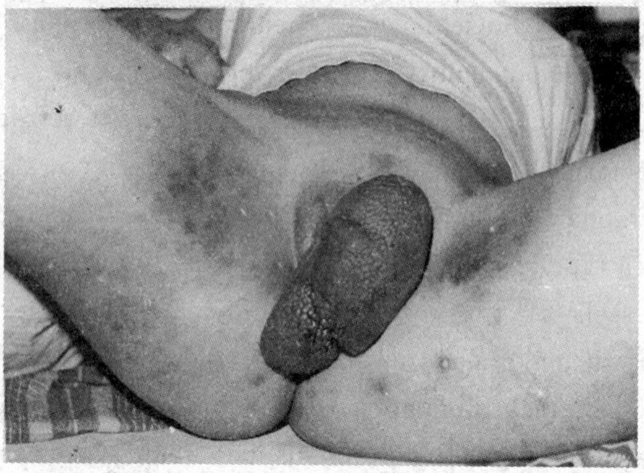

Figure 4-6-5 Elephantiasis of labium

Hydrocoele: The worst symptoms of the chronic disease generally appear in adults, and in men more often than in women. In endemic communities, some 10-50% of men suffer from genital damage, especially hydrocoele (fluid-filled balloon-like enlargement of the sacs around the testes) and elephantiasis of penis and scrotum. Even though found only with *W. bancrofti* infections, hydrocoele is one of the most common clinical manifestation of lymphatic filariasis. There is no tenderness. The transillumination test is positive. Microfilariae can be found in hydrocele fluid sometimes.

Chyluria: Chyluria (chylous urine) is the main symptom of bancroftian filariasis, which results from the lymphatic rupture of renal pelvis. The urine is cloudy milklike. Its appearance is irregular and intermittent. It may last several days, weeks or even months. There are several factors that will trigger chyluria recurrence, as chyluria appeared after overwork, mental tension, sadness, annoyance, anger, and diet features, etc.

Tropical pulmonary eosinophilia syndrome (TPE): Presenting symptoms include a paroxysmal dry cough, wheezing, dyspnea, anorexia, malaise, and weight loss. Symptoms of TPE are usually due to the inflammatory response to the infection. Characteristically, peripheral blood eosinophilia and military shadows on chest radiography are observed. TPE is usually related to *W. bancrofti* or *B. malayi* infection.

The other clinical manifestation of filariasis are filarial pericarditis, filarial granuloma in spleen or other parts, filariasis in eyes, and so on.

Diagnosis

Filariasis is usually diagnosed by identifying microfilariae on a Giemsa or Wright-stained thick blood film. Blood must be drawn at night (from 10 p. m. to 2 a. m.), since the microfilaria circulate at night (nocturnal periodicity). Eosinophilia is a frequent concomitant of all filarial syndromes, but only when the levels are extremely high (as in tropical eosinophilia) are they diagnostically helpful. Otherwise microfilariae can be found in hydrocele, chyluria and acetic or pleural fluid. If specimen collection proves difficult at night, the patient may be challenged with the antifilarial agent diethylcarbamazine (DEC). This drug stimulates the migration of the microfilariae from the pulmonary to the systemic circulation and enhances the possibility of their recovery. If the microfilaremia is scant, the specimen may be concentrated by millipore membrane before examination.

Filarial infection generates significant inflammatory immune responses that participate in the development of symptomatic lymphatic obstruction. Increased levels of immunoglobulin E (IgE) and immunoglobulin G4 (IgG4) secondary to antigenic (from dead worms) stimulation of Th2-type immune response have been demonstrated.

Serological diagnosis: Many lymphatic filariasis patients are amicrofilaraemic, and because no serologic test other than that detecting circulating filarial antigen (CFA) is specific. The new development of a very sensitive, specific, and simple immunochromatographic card test (ICT) to detect circulating parasite antigens without the need for laboratory facilities and using only finger-prick blood droplets taken anytime of the day, has completely transformed the approach to diagnosis. With this, it will now be possible both to improve our understanding of where the infection actually occurs and to monitor more easily the effectiveness of treatment and control programmes. Circulating filarial antigen (CFA) detection should now be regarded as the "golden standard" for diagnosing *Wuchereria bancrofti* infections. Antigen detection may thus prove to be a specific indicator of active disease. The specificity of these assays is near complete, and the sensitivity is greater than that achieved by the earlier parasite-detection assays.

Antibody detection: A number of serologic tests have been employed for the diagnosis of microfilaremic disease, but until recently they have lacked adequate sensitivity and specificity.

X-rays and ultrasound diagnosis: The conventional X-rays are rarely helpful in diagnosing lymphatic filarial infection, except in the case of tropical eosinophilia where the picture can be variable but characteristically includes interstitial thickening and diffuse nodular mottling in the lung fields. Ultrasound examination of the lymphatics (especially the scrotal lymphatics in men, and the breast and retroperitoneal lymphatics in women) can reveal rapidly moving ("dancing") adult worms, and lymphoscintigraphy, though not diagnostic of filarial infection, can identify lymphatic functional and gross anatomical abnormalities.

Identification of adult worms: In situations of lymphadenopathy with or without accompanying the inflammation of nodes or lymphatic vessels, biopsy can often detect adult worms, but this approach is rarely used as a diagnostic procedure.

Epidemiology

Geographical distribution and vectors: Lymphatic filariasis is primarily distributed in Asia and other tropical areas. Lymphatic filariasis currently infects about 120 million individuals in Africa, Latin America, the Pacific Islands, and Asia; One-third of the infected individuals live in Africa, one third in India, and most of the remainder in South Asia, the Pacific Region and the Americas. India, Nigeria, Bangladesh, Indonesia, Democratic Republic of Congo, the Philippines and Madagascar are among the most endemic countries. *W. bancrofti*, transmitted primarily by mosquitoes of the genera of *Culex* and *Anopheles*, is the more cosmopolitan of the two species; it is found in patchy distribution throughout the poorly sanitated, densely crowded urban areas of all three continents. *B. malayi*, is mainly transmitted by mosquitoes of the genus of *Anopheles*, while *Aedes* and *Mansonia* are the vecters in coastal areas of Asia and the South Pacific. Humans are the only vertebrate hosts for *Wuchereria*. Humans are the only known vertebrate hosts for most strains of *B. malayi* and *W. bancrofti*. There are reports that some kinds of cat and monkey can be naturally infected by *B. malayi*. In the eastern Indonesian archipelago, a closely related species, *B. timori*, is transmitted by night-feeding *Anopheles mosquitoes*.

Source of infection: The persons with microfilarae in peripheral blood are the source of infection. The patients with chronic manifestations (e. g., elephantiasis, hydrocele, chylous urine) are not important for transmission since they are usually amicrofilaremic.

Filariasis in China: Filariasis was distributed in 16 provinces, autonomous regions (municipalities) to the south of Yellow River, including 864 counties or cities. Of these, 461 counties, cities had bancroftian filariasis, 222 had brugian filariasis, and 181 had two kinds of filariasis. Out of the 16 endemic provinces, autonomous regions, Shandong, Hainan had bancroftian filariasis only, and the other 13 provinces, autonomous regions two kinds of filariasis. *C. pallens* (*Culex pipiens pallens*) and *C. quinquefasciatus* (*Culex pipiens quinquefasciatus*) are two geographical subspecies of *C. pipiens*. *C. pallens* is the principal vector transmitting bancroftian filariasis in areas to the north of 32° north latitude. *C. quinquefasciatus* is the principal vector transmitting bancroftian filariasis in areas to the south of 32° north latitude. The main vectors for transmitting brugian filariasis are *A. sinensis* and *A. anthropophagus*.

Based on the situation of lymphatic filariasis and surveillance schedule, the 10th Five-Year Work Plan for Parasitic Disease Control issued by the Ministry of Health (MOH) proposed the goal to eliminate lymphatic filariasis in the whole China by the year 2005. In 2002, a cross-sectional parasitological survey was carried out in 869 administrative villages in 180 counties. An entomological survey was also done in 208 sites. The survey results showed that only one microfilaremia case was found in 488,679 persons examined by blood smear, and that no new infected case was found. In addition, there was no filarial larvae found in 58,339 mosquitoes dissected. Up to the end of 2002, 11 P/A/M had reached the Chinese criteria for elimination of lymphatic filariasis within 16 endemic P/A/M, and a total of 828 out of 864 endemic counties had met the criteria. Another 2 provinces, Henan and Shandong had also reached the criteria in 2004.

Prevention and Control

Lymphatic filariasis is a major cause of disability, psychosocial and economic reductions in life opportunities, and a major burden on direct health and hospital resources especially through the costs for surgical intervention. Diethylcarbamazine (DEC, hetrazan) is the drug of choice for treatment of lymphatic filariasis. It eliminates the microfilariae from the blood and kills or injures the adult worms, resulting in long-term suppression of the infection or parasitological cure. It is recommended that the dosage is 6 mg/kg per day for 12 days in bancroftian filariasis and for 6 days in brugian filariasis. Ivermectin has also been registered for treatment of filariasis, and albendazole was shown to have additional antifilarial effects. Frequently the dying microfilariae stimulate an allergic reaction in the host. This response is occasionally severe, requiring the use of antihistamines and corticosteroids.

DEC-fortified table salt (3 : 1000) is sold in endemic areas. People take this salt over 6 months, resulting in an elimination or great reduction of microfilariae in the blood stream, for treating and preventing filariasis. This method has hardly side effects, which is Chinese invention and makes a great contribution to filariasis control in China.

While it is important to try to cure the infection itself, management of the consequences of that infection (particularly the lymphoedema, elephantiasis and hydrocoeles) is what is often of greatest concern to the patient. Interestingly, with respect to hydrocoele it has now been shown repeatedly that treatment of infection in communities with either intermittent (monthly, 6-monthly, yearly) drug administration or the steady use of DEC-fortified table (cooking) salt, leads to clinical improvement with decreases in both hydrocoele size and prevalence. Similarly, it is not uncommon to find early lymphoedema regressing completely after treatment of an affected patient with DEC. In more chronic states, those larger hydrocoele that do not regress spontaneously or after treatment must be subjected to surgical procedures.

Non-invasive management of chyluria relies on nutritional support, especially substitution of fat-rich foods by high protein, high fluid diets supplemented. "Correction" of the lymphatic defect can be effected through surgery, but even the sclerosing effects of lymphangiography or, often, time alone can lead to the cessation of the lymphatic leakage into the renal pelvis collecting system and the urine.

The tissue changes of elephantiasis are often irreversible, but the enlargement of the extremities may be ameliorated with pressure bandages or plastic surgery according to the traditional measures. Recently, the management regimens of elephantiasis recommended by World Health Organization (WHO) should include the following: (1) twice-daily washing of the affected parts with soap and water; (2) raising the affected limb at night; (3) regularly exercising the affected limb to promote lymph flow; (4) keeping the nails clean; (5) wearing shoes; (6) use of antiseptic or antibiotic creams to treat small wounds or abrasions.

These same intensive local hygiene efforts and antibiotic ointments can also decrease the frequency of recurrent infection episodes in patients with elephantiasis of the penis or scrotum, but, unfortunately, principles of management have not yet been developed for successfully reversing the anatomic distortions caused by the infection.

Filarial infection can be acquired only from vector-borne infective larvae. Therefore, prevention of infection can be achieved either by decreasing contact between humans and vectors or by decreasing the amount of infection the vector can acquire, by treating the human host. Transmission can also be reduced by avoiding mosquito bites in endemic areas (e. g., through use of personal repellents, bed-nets, or insecticide-impregnated bed-nets). Mosquito vectors often breed in polluted urban waters (such as blocked drains and sewers), so good sanitation and environmental management to minimize mosquito breeding places can play a major role in reducing the risk of the disease.

More recently, the extremely effective treatment strategy is now based on annual, single-dose, 2-drug-regimens of ivermectin plus albendazole in countries that are co-endemic for onchocerciasis, and of DEC plus albendazole in all other countries. At present, the World Health Organization is utilizing the strategy of yearly mass treatment to all "at risk" population to eliminate lymphatic filariasis as a public health problem by decreasing microfilariae in the population, thereby interrupting transmission and preventing infection.

Onchocerca volvulus

Onchocerciasis or river blindness, produced by the skin filaria *O. volvulus*, is characterized by subcutaneous nodules, thickened pruritic skin, and blindness.

Morphology and Life Cycle

Humans are the only definitive hosts, while black flies (*Simulium*) are the intermediate hosts. The 40 to 60cm thread-like female adults lie, together with their diminutive male partners, in coiled masses within deep fibrous subcutaneous tissue nodules. The female gives birth to more than 2,000 microfilariae each day of her 15-year lifespan. These progeny lose their sheaths soon after leaving the uterus, exit from the fibrous capsule, and migrate for up to 2 years in the subcutaneous tissues, skin, and eye. Ultimately they die or are ingested by black flies of the genus *Simulium*, which breed along the banks of turbulent, fast-moving streams. After transformation into filariform larvae, they are transmitted to another human host. There they molt repeatedly over 6 to 12 months before reaching adulthood and becoming encapsulated.

Pathogenesis and Clinical Manifestation

The subcutaneous nodules that harbor the adult worms can be located anywhere on the body, generally over bony prominences. Subcutaneous nodules may be multiple with hypersensitivity reaction to microfilariae. In Mexico and Guatemala, where the fly vector typically bites the upper part of the body, they are concentrated on the head; in South America and Africa, they are found primarily on the trunk and legs. Although nodules may number in the hundreds, most infected individuals are less than 10. They are firm, freely movable, and measure 1 to 3cm in diameter. Unless the nodule is located over a joint, pain and tenderness are unusual. Of greater consequence to the patient are the side effects of the presence of microfilariae in the tissues. An immediate hypersensitivity reaction to antigens released by dead or dying parasites results in acute and chronic inflammatory reaction. In the skin, this reaction is manifested as a papular or erysipelas-like rash with severe itching. In time, the skin thickens and becomes lichenified. As subepidermal elastic tissue is lost, wrinkles and large skin folds or hanging groins are formed. In parts of Africa, fibrosing obstructive lymphadenitis may result in elephantiasis. Invasion of the eye, however, causes the most devastating lesions. Punctate keratitis, iritis, and chorioretinitis can lead to a decrease in visual acuity and, sometimes, total blindness. In Central America, eye lesions may be seen in up to 30% of infected patients. In certain communities in West Africa, 85% of the population has ocular lesions and 50% of the adult male population is blind.

Diagnosis

The diagnosis is made by demonstrating the microfilariae in a thin skin snips taken from an involved area. When the eye is involved, the organism may sometimes be seen in the anterior chamber with the help of a slit lamp.

Epidemiology

Onchocerciasis occurs in 38 countries worldwide, including areas of Africa, South America, and the Middle East. More than 123 million people live in endemic areas, and an estimated 18 million people are currently infected. Of those infected, about 270,000 are blind, and an additional 500,000 have severe visual impairment. The original source of this disease is African black people. The disease still persists on the high slopes of the

Sierra, where coffee plantations lie along the rapidly flowing streams that serve as breeding places for *Simulium* species.

Prevention and Control

Traditionally, DEC has been used to kill the microfilariae. Treatment may cause hypersensitivity reactions. Treatment was begun with very small doses to prevent rapid parasite destruction and the allergic consequences. This consideration was particularly important when the eye was involved; a treatment-induced inflammatory reaction can damage it further. A new microfilaremic agent, ivermectin, has been demonstrated to be more effective than DEC and does not appear to induce the severe allergic manifestations seen with the latter agent. Re-treatment over a period of several years is necessary, because it does not kill the adult worm, no satisfactory methods of control have yet been developed. Application of insecticides to the vector's breeding waters must be sustained for decades to disrupt transmission permanently. With the introduction of ivermectin, mass treatment or chemoprophylaxis is now possible.

Several onchocerciasis control programs provide onchocerciasis control in 38 endemic countries in the world (OCP—Onchocerciasis Control Program—initial area of vector control; APOC—African Program for Onchocerciasis Control—World Bank and WHO supported ivermectin distribution; OEPA—Onchocerciasis Elimination Program for the Americas—ivermectin distribution in Latin America).

Loa loa

Loiasis is a filarial disease of West Africa produced by the eye worm, *Loa loa*. In Zhejiang, Guangdong and Shanghai of China, loasis was found in more than 30 returnee from Africa. The cases with loasis were also reported in the students who studied in Africa. The long-lived adults migrate continuously through the subcutaneous tissues of humans. During migration, they produce localized areas of allergic inflammation termed Calabar swellings. These egg-sized lesions persist for 2 to 3 days and may be accompanied by fever, itching, urticaria, and pain. At times, the adult worms may cross the eye subconjunctivally, producing intense tearing, pain, and alarm.

The female produces sheathed microfilariae, which are found in the bloodstream during daytime hours. Deer flies of the genus *Chrysops* serve as vectors.

The diagnosis is made by recovering the adult worm from the eye or by isolating the characteristic microfilariae from the blood or Calabar swellings. Eosinophilia is constant. DEC destroys both adults and microfilariae, but must be administered cautiously to avoid marked allergic reactions. Albendazole slowly decreases microfilarial levels without producing allergic reactions, possibly by preferential action on the adult worms.

(Cui Jing and Wang Zhongquan)

Section 7 *Strongyloides stercoralis*

Strongyloides stercoralis is also called as intestinal roundworm. Attached to Nematode, it belongs to facultative parasite. Its life cycle is complicated, and can be divided into two phases. One is free-living generation and the other is parasitic generation. The adult worm parasitizes in the small intestine of human or other hosts, such as dog and cat. It could lead to the ulcer of the small intestine and colon. The larva could also invade into the brain, liver or kidney of human body causing suffusion damage of the organs and tissues.

Morphology

The parasitic female is small, approximately 2. 2mm long and 0. 4mm wide. The worm is transparent and has short buccal capsule. There are 4 small lip flaps around the apertura oralis. The esophagus pharyngeal canal is longer, extending one-third the body length. The vulva lies in the posterior third of the body; and the uteri are divergent and contain few eggs at a time. Each female could lay 30 to 40 embryo eggs. In free-living generation, the females and males are about 1. 0mm to 2. 0-2. 5mm, respectively. The uteri of a free-living female contain far more eggs than those of parasitic counterpart. The freeing female is also somewhat larger and has a vulva situated in the midsection of its body (see Figure 4-7-1).

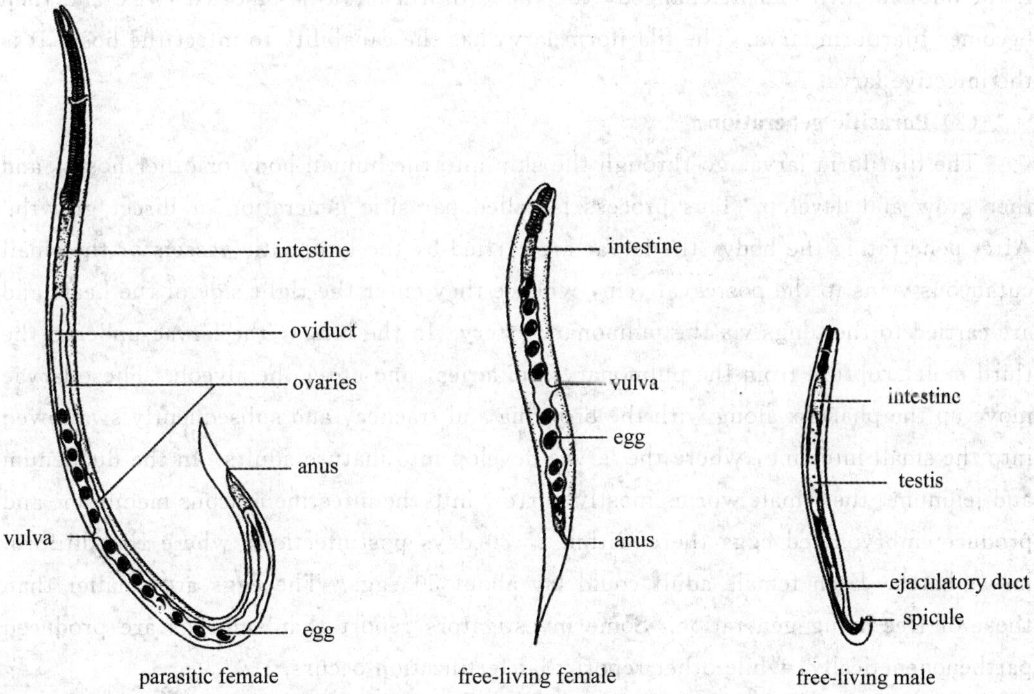

Figure 4-7-1 Adult of *Strongyloides stercoralis*

The larva is divided into 2 periods, one is rhabditiform larva and the other is filariaform larva. The rhabditiform larvae are the first-period larvae, which are produced by females parasitizing in intestinal mucous membrane of hosts. These larvae could be found in feces, and it is about 0. 2 to 0. 5mm long. The filariform larva is infective period. It is tenuity with short mouth and long pharynx. It can pass through the skin to invade the human body.

The egg is like the egg of hookworm, round and transparent, and measures 50 to 70μm by 30 to 40μm. The shell of egg is thin with embryo. When the eggs are laid, rhabditiform larvae hatch out and move to the intestine of the host, then they are discharged into surroundings with feces of the host. Eggs are seldom found in feces.

Life Cycle

The life cycle of S. *stercoralis* can be divided into three phases: free-living generation, parasitic generation and autoinfection.

(1) **Free-living generation**

The adult lays eggs in the warm and humid soil. After several hours, these eggs hatch in the soil, where the liberated larvae feed actively on organic debris, pass through four molts, and develop into sexually mature adults in 36 to 38 hours. The male and female mate, and then lay eggs. When the outside environment is proper, the life cycle of the free-living generation could have several times. It is called indirect growth. If the outside environment changed, the rhabditiform larva has molted twice and then becomes filariform larva. The filariform larva has the capability to infect the host. It is the infective larva.

(2) **Parasitic generation**

The filariform larvae go through the skin into the human body or other hosts, and then grow and develop. This process is called parasitic generation or direct growth. After penetrating the body, the larvae are carried by the lymphatic vessels or the small cutaneous veins to the postcaval vein, whence they enter the right side of the heart and are carried to the lungs via the pulmonary artery. In the lungs, the larvae undergo the third molt, rupture from the pulmonary capillaries, and enter the alveoli. These larvae move up the pharynx along with the bronchia and trachea, and subsequently swallowed into the small intestine, where the larvae develop into mature adults. In the duodenum and jejunum, the female worms mostly burrow into the intestine mucous membrane and produce embryonated eggs there within 25-30 days postinfection, where rhabditiform larvae hatch. Each female adult could lay about 50 eggs. The eggs are smaller than those of free-living generation. Some investigators report that embryos are produced parthenogenetically, while other report that fertilization occurs.

The rhabditiform larva overshoots from the mucous membrane of intestine, and is discharged out with the feces. The rhabditiform larva has two kinds of growing ways. One undergoes a molt in the surrounding and develops into the infective filariform larva. It lives in the soil and finds ways to go through the skin and parasitizes in the host. The other way is to grow to be male and female in free-living generation in surrounding, and live independently.

(3) **Autoinfection**

S. stercoralis, when parasitizes in the human body, has autoinfection. The autoinfection has 3 types: ① parasitic generation: the eggs hatch out rhabditiform larva in intestinal mucous membrane and then go to the blood circle to continue growing. ② free-living generation: rhabditiform larva has two edysis and grows to be filariform larva, and then goes into the blood system. ③ autoinfection: filariform larvae are discharged with the feces, then reinvade human body through the skin around the anus (see Figure 4-7-2).

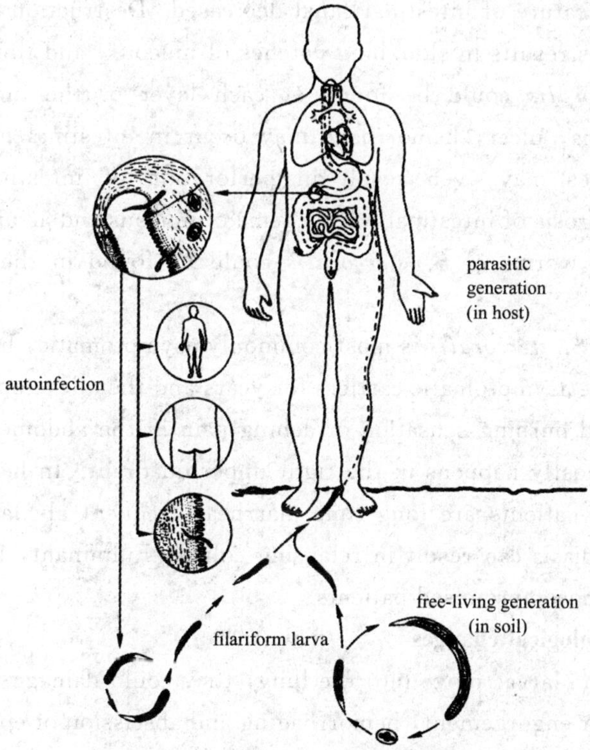

Figure 4-7-2 Life cycle of *Strongyloides stercoralis*

Pathogenesis and Clinical Manifestation

Most infections are light with no clinical symptoms. However, heavy infections can produce different pathologic changes and symptoms, when worms parasitize in different part of the human body.

(1) **Pathological changes around the anus**

When filariform larvae enter into human body through the skin around the anus, the patient may feel pricking pain and pruritus, and the edema, line or girdle-shaped urticaria may be seen in focus of infection. Because the larvae move fast in the skin, urticaria occurs very quickly. It is reported that one patient's urticaria spread quickly at the speed of 10-12cm/h.

(2) **Intestinal pathological changes**

The pathological changes by S. *stercoralis* are divided into light, medium and heavy infections in intestinal canal. The catarrh enteritis, congestion, bleeding point and abscess of intestine mucous may be seen in light infections. We may observe eosinophils and monocytes under the optical microscope, and there are worms existing in intestinal gland. In medium infections, the edematous enteritis, hyperplasia, and edema may be seen, and the duplicature of intestinal canal decreased. Destruction of tissues by adult worms and juveniles results in sloughing patches of mucous, and fibrotic changes. The worms of S. *stercoralis* could be found at each layer of the intestines. In heavy infections, anabrosis, ulcer, hemorrhage may occur in intestinal mucous membrane, pathological changes may even result in perforation of intestine. Under optical microscope, the fibrosis of intestinal wall, edema of mucous and atrophy of muscle layer may be seen. The worms of S. *stercoralis* could be found in the entire incrassated intestine wall.

Infection with S. *stercoralis* is most commonly asymptomatic, but cases are known in which hosts were asymptomatic carriers for years and then developed serious disease. An intense localized burning sensation or aching pain in the abdomen is usually felt at this time, which mostly happens in the right upper quadrant. In heavy infections, the main symptoms of patients are long time diarrhea, frequent alv laxat, liquid stools. Chronic strongyloidiasis can result in relapsing colitis. Fulminant, fatal hyperinfection can occur in immunocompromised patients.

(3) **Other pathological changes**

When filariform larvae move into the lung, they could damage the capillary vessel and lead to vascular engorgement, hemorrhaging and abscission of epithelium, therefore the larvae in the exudation could been found. If the larvae parasitize in the lung long enough to develop into mature adults, the abscesses of lung could occur. Besides, filariform larvae migrate into other organs, such as endocardium, liver, ovary, lymphonodi mesenterici and brain, etc. , and form granuloma.

Diagnosis

Diagnosis depends on the discovery and identification of the characteristic rhabditiform larva and filariform larva in the feces of patients. It is the surest means of diagnosis for this disease. The general methods could be direct smear method. If there is no larvae in the feces, other methods like Bering separation or modified aldehyde-ether mixing centrifugal method may be adopted. If the rhabditiform larva and filariform larva were discovered in the feces discharged within 24h, we could say it is autoinfection. Sometimes eggs also could be found in the feces of a diarrhea patient. If the examination of patient's feces is negative, the gastric juice, duodenum juice or sputum should also be checked. The immunological assay may be adopted to assist the diagnosis, such as using ELISA to check the differential antibody in sera, and the positive rate may be up to 94.4%. These methods are highly sensitive and specific.

The clinical manifestations for this disease are complicated, and the course of disease is very long, so it is easy to make misdiagnosis. The identification of this disease should be differentiated from other diseases. When bloody purulent stool and liquid stools appear in the patient's feces, it must be distinguished from bacillary dysentery, amebic dysentery and ulcerative colitis. When abdominal pain occurs, the appreciation of this disease should be made with gastric ulcer, duodenal ulcer and acute cholecystitis.

Prevention and Control

S. stercoralis is mainly distributed in tropical and subtropical zone. This disease is seldom in temperate and cold zone, and it is sporadic case. There are many reports of this disease overseas. According to the investigation of the worms in 1995, all infections are distributed in 26 provinces in China. The rate of average infection is up to 0.122%, it is estimated that there are 1,510,000 infections.

The filariform larvae enter into human body through the skin. The patients and carriers are the main sources for the disease. The spreading factor of *S. stercoralis* is much the same as that of hookworm diseases, and therefore the prevention of this disease is the same as hookworm disease. Prevention requires the sanitary disposal of human excrement, protection of skin from contact with contaminated soil, and appropriate treatment in cases of autoinfection. Screening for *S. fuelleborni* in pregnant woman and for *S. stercoralis* in patients who are candidates for immunosuppressive therapy should be followed by treatment where infection is present.

No entirely satisfactory drug for strongyloidiasis is currently available. Thiabendazole and albendazole are recommended. Ivermectin shows considerable promise. Therapy should be repeated after a week because of difficulty in confirming cure.

(Cui Yu)

Section 8 *Trichinella spiralis*

Trichinella spiralisis [(Owen, 1835) Railliet, 1895] is the smallest human nematode and a biohelminth. It exhibits an unusual life cycle. The adult and juvenile (larva) live in the same host, but the juvenile has to change its host to complete life cycle. They cause trichinosis, a zoonosis, which is spread by the law of the jungle (the weak are the prey of the strong). This disease is widespread and clinically important throughout the world. Human infections result from eating raw meat.

Over the last decade, the application of molecular and biochemical methods in conjunction with experimental studies on biology have resulted in the identification of eight *Trichinella* species, (*T. spiralis*, *T. nativa*, *T. britovi*, *T. pseudospiralis*, *T. murrelli*, *T. nelsoni*, *T. papuae*, and *T. zimbabwensis*), which have distinct epidemiological and geographical distributions. All of eight Trichinella species parasitize humans and a wide variety of carnivorous mammals. While *T. spiralis* is the most important of these parasites in most parts of the world, being cosmopolitan in distribution and of high pathogenicity, the other species are of more regional importance. *T. nativa* is prevalent in sylvatic carnivores in arctic and subarctic areas, it has also been detected in wild boars. The main biological characteristic of this species is the ability of larvae to survive in frozen(−18℃) muscle of carnivores for up to 5 years. *T. britovi* infections could be less severe than those caused by *T. spiralis* and could be due to the fact that *T. britovi* females are less prolific. *T. murrelli* seems to be more likely to provoke skin reactions and less likely to cause facial oedema. *T. pseudospirali*, which is non-encapsulated, seems to provoke signs and symptoms that last longer. There are at least two species of *Trichinella* in China: *T. spiralis*, which appears in pigs and dogs, probably in most parts of China and *T. nativa*, which is has been found in dogs in northeastern China. In this section, this discussion focuses on *T. spiralis*.

Morphology

The males measure 1.4-1.6mm long and are more slender at the anterior than at the posterior end. The anus can be found in the terminal and they have a large copulatory pseudobursa on each side (Figure 4-8-1). The copulatory spicule is absent. Females are about twice the size of males, also tapering toward the anterior end. The vulva is located near the middle of the esophagus, which is about a third of the length of the body. The single uterus is filled with developing eggs in its posterior portion, whereas the anterior portion contains fully developed juveniles(larvae). The stichosome consists of a row of 50-55 discoid cells called stichocytes and surrounds the posterior part of the esophagus. The structure and function of this organ have been investigated. These stichocytes can secrete digestive materials entering the esophagus, which have strong antigenicity resulting in immunopathologic reaction (see Figure 4-8-1). The juvenile also has the same number of stichocytes as the adult.

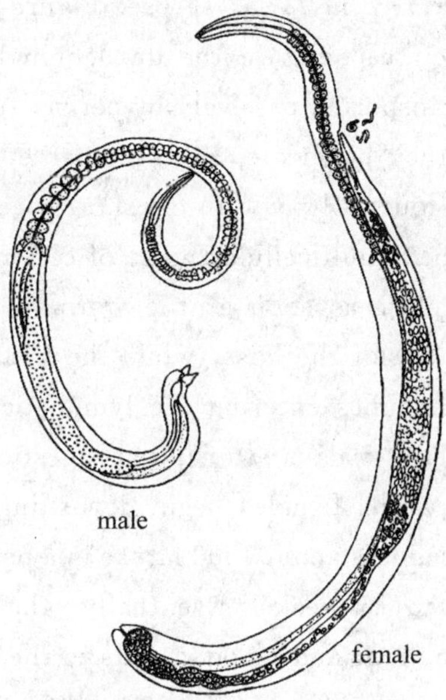

Figure 4-8-1 Male and female adult worms of *Trichinella spiralis*

The newborn larvae are 80 to 120μm long and 5 or 6μm in diameter. After reaching skeletal muscles they are encapsulated in a cyst. Although one worm per cyst is most common, up to seven have been observed in a single cyst. The size of the fusiform cyst is about 0. 25-0. 5mm by 0. 21-0. 42mm (see Figure 4-8-2).

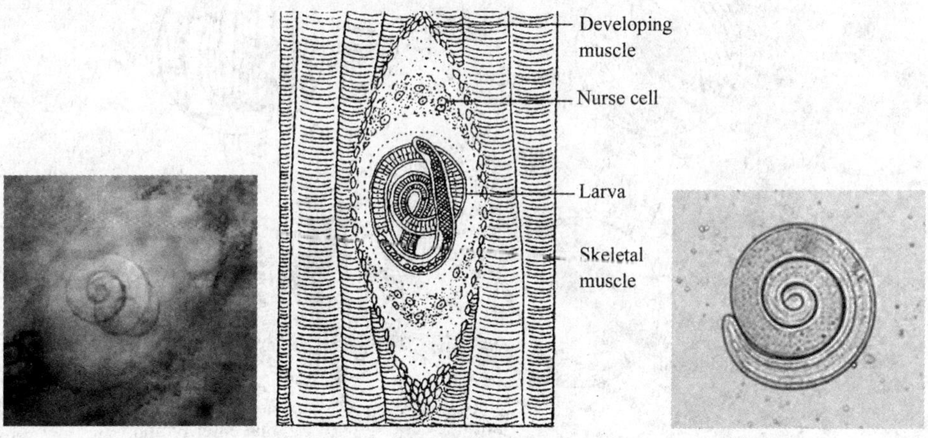

Figure 4-8-2 *T. spiralis* larvae encapsulated in skeletal muscle

(a) The encapsulated larva; (b) Schematic representation of encapsulated larva; (c) The living larva freed from muscle by pepsin-HCl digestion.

Life Cycle

Infection is initiated by the consumption of raw or undercooked pork or other meat containing the encapsulated *Trichinella* larvae (see Figure 4-8-3). Once ingested, the larvae are released from their capsules in the duodenum by the action of the host's digestive enzymes and are transported passively by peristalsis to the upper two-thirds of the small intestine. There they penetrate the columnar epithelium at the base of the villus and, after undergoing four molts within the short space of 24 to 30 hours, become adult worms which live in intra-multicellular niche of columnar epithelium of intestinal mucosa. Mating may take place as soon as the worms sexually mature. Soon after copulation, the male passes out of the host, while the female burrows deeper into the mucosa and submucosa, sometimes entering the lymphatic ducts to be carried to the mesenteric lymph nodes. About 5 days after initial ingestion of the infective larvae by the host, the adult ovoviviparous females begin depositing the newborn larvae. It is estimated that one female produces about 1500 larvae in a period of 5 to 10 days, and the birthing can continue for 4 to 16 weeks. Eventually, the female dies. The newborn larvae are carried by the lymphatic and blood vessels to the right side of the heart.

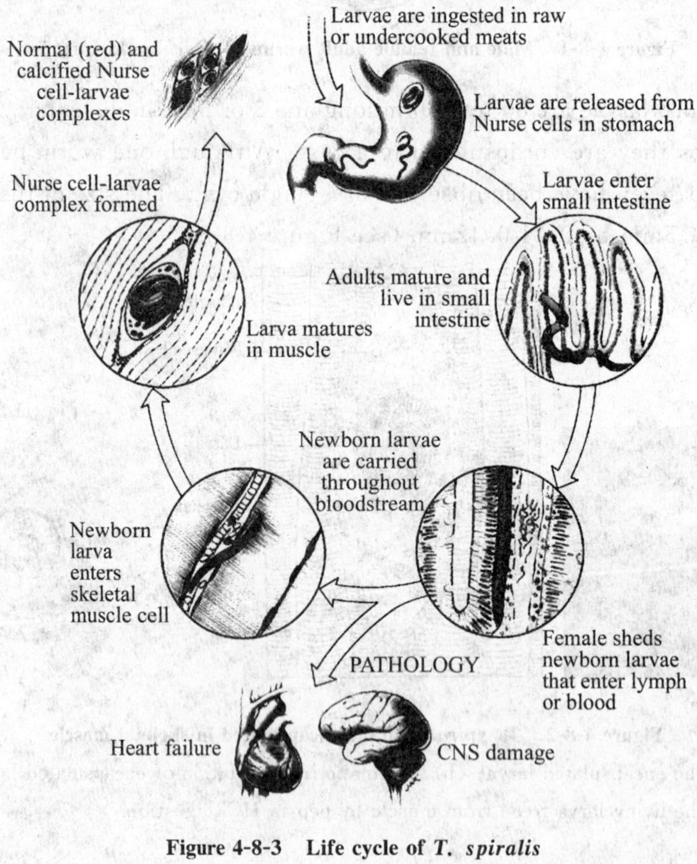

Figure 4-8-3 Life cycle of *T. spiralis*

From the heart, the larvae enter the peripheral circulation and are distributed throughout the body. It is only in skeletal muscles that larvae develop into the infective stage. Penetration of muscle cells and establishment as intracellular parasites within myofibers occur about 6 days after initial infection. Degeneration and inflammatory changes occur in the parasitized contractile fibers. The myofilaments disappear, mitochondria degenerate, the smooth endoplasmic reticulum increases, and the nuclei enlarge, forming a complex surrounding the larva. Shortly thereafter, collagen is produced by neighboring fibroblasts. The skeletal muscle cell invaded by the larva is a modified, viable cell. It was named the Nurse cell (see Figure 4-8-4) because it functions to recruit nutrients for the growth and maintenance of the larvae. On about the 17th day, the larva begins to coil in a spiral, absorbs nutrients from the host muscle sarcoplasm and gradually becomes surrounded by a sheath derived from the muscle fiber. A network of capillaries eventually surrounding the Nurse cell-larva complex (see Figure 4-8-5), probably afford additional nourishment to the growing larva. Growth is rapid, the larva reaching a length of about 1mm in approximately 8 weeks. Encapsulation begins at about the 21st day as the larva is gradually enveloped by a double, ellipsoidal capsule (0. 25 to 0. 5 mm long) of host origin. The outer capsule membrane is derived from the sarcolemma, while the inner membrane is a combination of degenerative myofibers and other cells such as fibroblasts. Capsule formation is complete in about 3 months. The muscles invaded most frequently include the extraocular muscles of the eyes, jaws, larynx, tongue, the deltoid, pectoral, and intercostal muscles, the diaphragm, and the gastrocnemius.

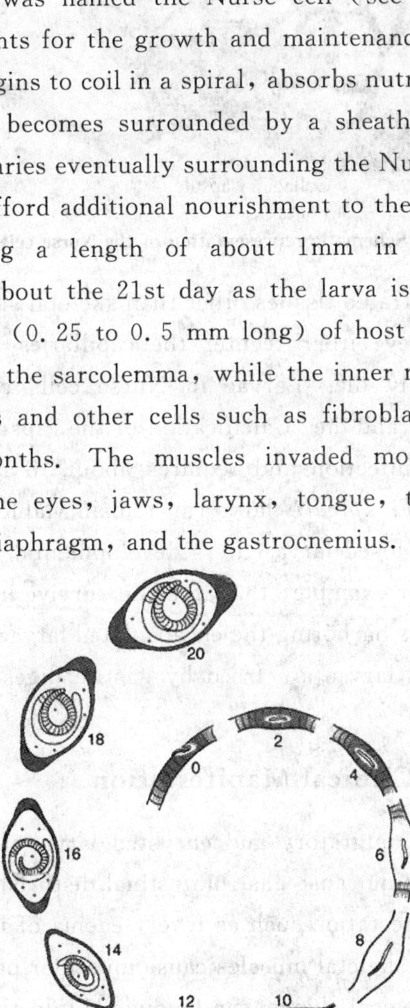

Figure 4-8-4 The course of Nurse cell and capsule formation
(The numbers in the figure represent the days on which the larva invades muscle fiber.)

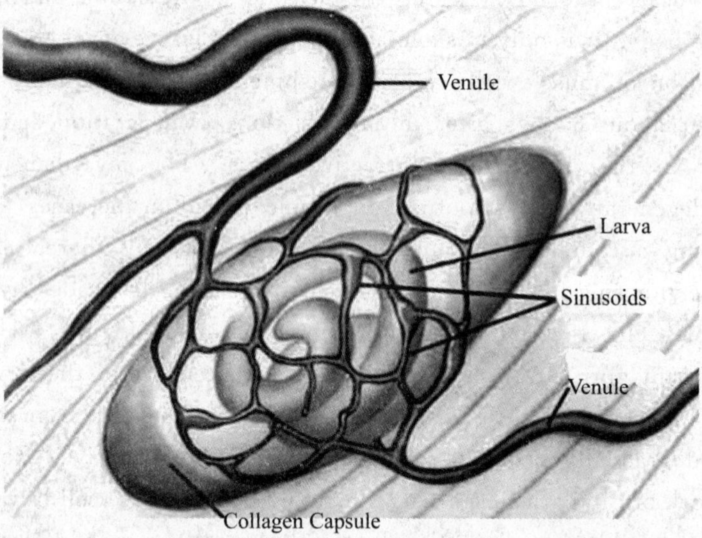

Figure 4-8-5 Schematic representation of the Nurse cell-larva complex

Larvae that have penetrated tissues other than skeletal striated muscle fail to induce Nurse cell formation. They either reenter the capillaries or become surrounded by granulomas, and eventually die. Larvae in Nurse cells can survive for years but eventually become calcified and die. Calcification of the capsule wall may begin as early as 6 months after initial infection and requires about 18 months for completion. If calcification is delayed, a *T. spiralis* larva can remain viable for several years. During capsule formation, the enclosed larva enters developmental arrest, a state in which it can survive indefinitely, for example, the larva can survive in the human host for up to 30 years. When the muscles harboring the encapsulated larvae are eaten by a carnivorous mammal, the encapsulated larvae are freed by gastric digestion and reinitiate the life cycle.

Pathogenesis and Clinical Manifestation

Adult worm and both migratory and encysted larvae are pathogenic: (1) Adult worms present in the intestine cause gastrointestinal disturbances; (2) Migrating larvae cause various allergic manifestation such as fever, edema of the face, eosinophilia, and (3) Encysted larvae in the skeletal muscles cause muscular pain.

The process of pathological change can be divided into three phases.

Invade phase: The phase occur within the first week after ingestion of infected meat, during the intestinal phase; this phase is associated with the development of larvae develop into adult. Because of the invading of larvae and adult worms, the wall of intestine is damaged. Microscopic ulceration, mucosal hyperemia, localized edema, punctate hemorrhages, and intestinal inflammation are main pathological changes.

Gastrointestinal signs and symptoms may be the first evidence of infection, including fever, nausea, vomiting, abdominal discomfort, diarrhea, etc. This period usually terminates with facial edema and fever 5 to 7 days after the first symptoms.

Migratory phase: This phase, beginning about 7 to 9 days after exposure, is associated with the migrating larvae which penetrate capillaries, reach muscles and initiate a strong inflammatory response. The juveniles damage blood vessels, resulting in localized edema, particularly in the face and hands. Wandering juveniles may also cause pneumonia, pleurisy, encephalitis, meningitis, nephritis, deafness, peritonitis, brain or eye damage, and subconjunctival or sublingual hemorrhage. Death resulting from myocarditis may occur at this stage.

After the juveniles reach striated muscles, they cause a intense muscle pain, difficulty in breathing or swallowing, swelling of masseter muscles, weakening of pulse and blood pressure, and heart damage. Eosinophilia is common. Death is usually caused by heart failure, respiratory complications, toxemia, or kidney malfunction.

Encysted phase: The formation of cyst result in the stimulation of larvae and tissue reparation. With encystation, the inflammation disappears gradually, the clinical manifestation becomes light, but the muscular pain can still last for months.

Diagnosis

Experienced doctors can suspect trichinosis depending on symptoms, signs and history of eating raw meat. Routine examination rarely detect juveniles in feces, blood or other secretions. A definitive diagnosis of trichinellosis can be made by finding larvae in a biopsy of skeletal muscle, but detection rate only reaches 50%. Xenodiagnosis, feeding suspected remainder of meat to laboratory rats, may be employed. Several immunodiagnostic techniques, indirect fluorescent antibody test (IFAT) and enzyme-linked immunosorbent assay (ELISA), can be used but those are for reference only.

Epidemiology

Trichinellosis is cosmopolitan in its distribution and is widespread in carnivores. The transmission of trichinellosis can be classified into two kinds: sylvatic cycle and domestic cycle. The sylvatic cycle is that which occurs in nature among carnivores with cannibalistic and scavenger behavior. The term "domestic cycle" refers to the transmission pattern occurring among humans, rats and pigs. Domestic pigs generally acquire trichinellosis by eating uncooked pork scraps from other infected pigs or ingesting garbage (i. e., garbage-fed pigs).

Human trichinellosis has been documented in 55 (27. 8%) countries of the 198 countries of the world. Human beings acquire the *Trichinella* infection mainly by ingesting the raw or improperly prepared pork products. Its prevalence is high in

Europe, Mexico, Central and South America, and Asia. There have even been epidemics in Japan, Thailand and China. 3,000-5,000 cases occurred only in European Union during 1990-2004.

It has been considered that the domestic pig is the most important element of the domestic cycle of trichinellosis. Swine trichinellosis in China was mainly transmitted by feeding pigs with uncooked pork scraps. Swine trichinellosis has been reported in 26 provinces, autonomous regions, or municipalities of China. The prevalence rate in swine varied from 0.12 % to 34.2 % in 5 provinces (Liaoning, Heilongjiang, Hubei, Henan, and Yunnan) during 1980-1998. At present, *Trichinella* infected pigs are predominately from the small farms of suburbs where pigs are fed on swill from the restaurants and from some mountainous areas where pigs are raised outdoors. Pigs were sometimes slaughtered clandestinely at home in rural and mountainous areas without veterinary inspection. The prevalence of *Trichinella* infection in pork sold at the market was from 0.52 % to 3.66 % in China during 1999-2004. Pork was the predominant source of outbreaks of human trichinellosis in China, 525 (95.8%) out of 548 outbreaks were caused by eating pork. At present, the endemic foci of trichinellosis is mainly located in the southwestern, the central and northeastern China. From 2000 to 2004, 17 outbreaks of human trichinellosis, with 828 cases and 11 deaths, were recorded in 8 P/A of China. All of 11 deaths occurred in the southwestern China, where the ethnic groups have the habit of eating raw meat. Out of 17 outbreaks, 13 (76.47%) outbreaks were caused by eating raw or poorly cooked pork, 2 (11.77%) outbreaks caused by eating raw dog meat and 2 (11.77%) outbreaks caused by eating game meat (wild boar and bear), suggesting the increasing significance of dog and game meat as source of infection for human trichinellosis.

The dumpling with raw pork or mutton filling is one kind of favorite Chinese foods, however, when the dumplings are too large or undercooked, the central portion is often undercooked. In addition, some Chinese have the habit of tasting the raw meat filling for dumplings before they are prepared. Scalded mutton (i.e., slices of mutton boiled for 1-3 min) is also a source of infection in China. If the slices of meat were too thick and the time of scald was insufficient, the temperature in the centre of meat would not be sufficient to kill the larvae. Other several foods readily cause human trichinellosis in the southwestern China (e.g., Yunnan province). These foods and preparation methods include: (1) skin-dry raw: roast pig leg cooked until the skin color changes to yellow, but the meat under the skin is still raw; (2) cross bridge rice noodle: sausage is prepared with raw pork, mixed with noodles and cooked just long enough so the noodles are ready to eat; (3) red raw: raw blood is mixed with raw pork; (4) chopped raw: pork is broken into small pieces; (5) acidic meat: raw pork is fermented; (6) white prosper: the raw fat of pork.

Another important mode of *T. spiralis* infection in human in China is that knife and tableware for cooked food and raw meat are not separated. Most of households have one set of tableware, one knife and one chopping board, used both for cooked and raw food.

The high incidence season of trichinellosis in winter in China was believed to be the result of eating dumpling, roasted or scalded meat during the winter. The reverse is true for the southern hemisphere (e. g., Argentina and Chile), where the incidence rises in the winter period of June-August. The increased consumption of game meat, the increased number of farms breeding wild animals for sport hunting, and the increased number of wild boar populations (following reductions in human rural populations) represent increased risks.

Prevention and Control

Prevention

(1) **Development of industrialized pig farms**: In order to eradicate swine trichinellosis, the industrialized pig farms should be founded. The control of *Trichinella* infection in domestic pigs could be restricted to those raised by traditional pig-rearing practices. An epidemiological survey carried out in Nanyang area of Henan province in 2000 showed the prevalence of swine trichinellosis was 0.1033% (26/25,178) in pigs reared in large industrialized farms where commercial grain or granule forage was used, while the prevalence was 22.7642% (28/123) in pigs raised in small piggeries in the suburbs of Nanyang city where the garbage or swill from the restaurants or hotels were used. All pigs should be raised in industrialized farms and all swill should be heated so that the *Trichinella* larvae contained in the swill can be completely killed.

(2) **Inspection of meat**: It is clear from the experience that the mandatory inspection of pork is highly effective for the control of trichinellosis.

(3) **Healthy education**: The most effective preventive measure of trichinellosis is educating the consumers not to eat raw or undercooked meat. The consumer should cook the meat to an internal temperature of at least 70℃. The meat may be frozen at −15℃ for 20 days, or −23℃ for 10 days, or −30℃ for 6 days, if the meat is less than 6 inches thick.

Treatment

The medical treatment includes anthelmintics (albendazole or mebendazole) and glucocorti-costeroids. The treatment goal for the very early infection phase is to limit muscle invasion by larvae; when this has already occurred the goal is to reduce muscle damage, which is responsible for the major clinical manifestations. To eliminate larvae from the gastrointestinal lumen, thus preventing muscle invasion and the development of trichinellosis, anthelmintics should be used at the enteral stage, that is, less than 1 week after infection. However, this is rarely possible and treatment is usually begun during the beginning of their development in muscle cells. Since it has not been clearly confirmed how long the adult females survive and produce newborn larvae in the human intestine, it is recommended that anthelmintics should be administrated to all patients with trichinellosis during the 4-6 weeks after infection. The later the treatment is prescribed, the higher the probability that the infected person will harbor viable larvae in their muscles for years, with possible persistent myalgia. Mebendazole was shown to prevent the occurrence of clinical disease when given to people 48h after the consumption of meat highly infected with *Trichinella* larvae. Therapeutic plasma levels of the drug should be maintained for an extended period, rather than high levels for short periods. The success of treatment is evident from clinical improvement of the patient's symptomatology.

The principal anthelmintics used for trichinellosis are albendazole (Zentel) and mebendazole (Vermox). Albendazole and mebendazole halt the production of new larvae, but in severe infection, the destruction of tissue larvae may provoke a hazardous hypersensitivity response in the host. Pyrantel has been proposed for children and pregnant women.

Albendazole is the drug of choice for the treatment of trichinellosis in China. The dosage for adults and children over the age of 2 years is 15-20 mg/(kg・day), two times daily for 7 days.

Mebendazole is commonly used in Europe and Africa. It is usually administered at a daily dose of 5mg/kg but higher doses [up to 20-25 mg/(kg・day)] are recommended in some countries. This drug should be taken for 10-15 days. When the larvae are already encapsulated in muscles, mebendazole is not able to kill the encapsulated larvae.

In severely symptomatic infections, glucocorticosteroids are beneficial, may alleviate the general symptoms of the disease, and may at times be lifesaving. They must always be used in combination with anthelmintics and never alone, since they could prolong the intestinal phase of the infection and increase the larval burden by delaying the expulsion of worms from the intestine. It is showed that steroids used in combination with mebendazole would significantly shorten the duration of fever, but they could also provoke a prolonged eosinophilia resulting from a delayed encapsulation process of the muscle larvae. The most commonly used glucocorticosteroid is prednisolone, which is available in tables of 1 or 5 mg and is administered at 30-60 mg/day in multiple doses for 10-14 days.

The prognosis of patients with trichinellosis is usually good with the exceptions of the rare, heavily infected cases. The mortality of symptomatic patients is 1%, rising to 10% if the central nervous system is involved.

(Wang Zhongquan and Cui Jing)

Section 9 Other Human Nematodes

Thelazia callipaeda

Thelazia callipaeda mainly parasitizes in the conjunctival sac and lacrimal ducts of dogs or cats. It is also found in human eyes, and may cause thelaziasis. This parasite was first discovered in human bodies in Beijing and Fujian in 1917. Up to now more than 380 cases of human thelaziasis have been reported in China. This parasite is commonly found in Asia, so it is also named as Eastern Eye Parasite.

Morphology

The adult of *T. callipaeda* is elongated and light pinkish in color when parasitizing in the conjunctiva sac of human or animal eyes. After leaving the human or animal body, the adult turns to be translucent creamy white. Except the head and the tail, there are tiny cross veins on the surface of the whole body, and the edge of the cross veins are sharp with hackle. The head is bluntly rounded, without lips, possessing horny buccal capsule, and surrounded by two rings of papillae. Below the buccal capsule is the columniform oesophagus. The male measures 4.5 to 15mm long by 0.25 to 0.75mm wide, with its tail curving ventrally to the belly. There are two copulatory spines different in length and shape stretched out of the cloaca. The female is larger, 6.2 to 20.0mm long by 0.3 to 0.85mm wide. The anus is quite near the tail, and the vulva is at the anterior end in front of the connection of esophagus and intestinal tract (see Figure 4-9-1).

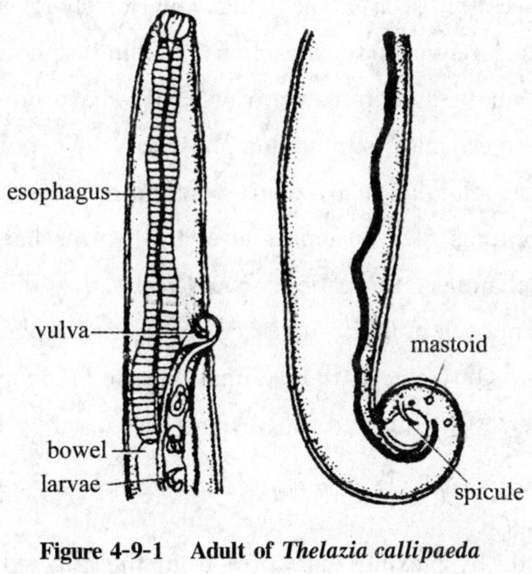

Figure 4-9-1 Adult of *Thelazia callipaeda*

The egg is nearly round with a thin and transparent shell, measuring about 54 to 60μm by 34 to 37μm. In the egg near the vulva, there are coiled larvae. The shell gradually becomes thinner and turns to be a sheath. The larva is hatched out by ovoviviparous pattern, measuring

350 to 414μm long by 13 to19μm wide.

Life Cycle

To complete the life cycle, it has to grow in the intermediate host and the final host. The intermediate host is *Amiota variegate*. The final host is cat, dog or other mammals.

The adults mainly parasitize in the conjunctival sac and lacrimal duct of dogs or cats, occasionally in human eyes. It is also reported that they have been found in rabbits, rats, horses, monkeys, raccoon dogs, silvery foxes and wild foxes. The larvae are produced by females in the final hosts' eye sockets. They are eaten with eye secretion by *Amiota variegate*, and become vesicle bursa through the flies' middle intestines into the wall of blood cavity. The larvae grow in the bursa till the sausage stage, then molt once to become pre-infective stage, and then transform into infective stage after molt twice within 2 to 4 weeks. The infective larvae go through the bursa wall but still stay in the blood cavity and then move into the head. When *Amiota variegate* again eat other hosts' eye secretion, these infective larvae move into the eye conjunctiva sac of the hosts through the mouth part of the *Amiota variegate*. After they grow to be mature, males and females mate. As the result of the experiments, the infective larvae live in proper temperature (about 24℃ to 30℃), after more than 1 to 2 months, the females begin to produce larvae and then complete their life cycle. The adult commonly live for more than 2 years.

Pathogenesis and Clinical Manifestation

The adults parasitize in human conjunctiva sac of eyes, mostly seen on the external canthus of upper vault, secondly seen in the ocular anterior chamber or lacrimal ductule. The patients could appear as foreign body sensation, tickling, photophobia, more secretion, ophthalmalgia, etc. The above symptoms are caused by sharp cross veins and horny buccal capsule of the larvae, the mechanical stimulation and injury by copulatory spines of males, and also including the chemical stimulation by their secretion and excretion. But it will cause no visual disorder. The symptoms may disappear after the worms have been taken out. If they parasitize in the anterior chamber, the patients could feel a threadlike shadow floating, ciliary congestion, turbidity of aqueous humor, increasement of intraocular pressure, enlargement of pupil, and diminution of vision, etc. If the lacrimal ductule is involved, the lacrimal punctum may evaginate. A single eye was infected in the most cases, rarely both eyes are involved.

Diagnosis

The diagnosis is made by picking the worm from the affected part and identifying with microscope.

Prevention and Control

Thelaziasis is distributed in the Far East areas of former Soviet Union in Asia, Korea, Japan, the Philippines, India, Thailand, Burma and China. In China, it has been reported that there are such cases in 24 provinces, cities and municipalities. Normally it is emanation, but it also spreads in some certain areas. Human infections have not much to do with gender or age; they just depend on the chance of infection. The infections are mostly seen in infants, but they are also seen in adult persons. The disease often occurs in suburban areas in summer and autumn, normally after the reproduction of the *Amiota variegate*. According to a survey, infant dogs in Anhui province were infected with the worm. The epidemic season of the disease is from May to October, among which June and September are the peak time.

Dogs, cats and humans infected by *T. callipaeda* are the main sources of this disease. The dogs and cats as pets live closely with humans. In order to prevent it from infecting humans, it is better to make a diagnosis and give treatment of the pets in time. 1% decicaine solution or 1% Levamisole solution could be used to drip eyes, and then take the worm out of eyes with tweezers.

The flies are the intermediate host of the parasite. The flies firstly take the parasite from the eyes of an infected animal and then transfer it to other animals or humans, so we should manage and prevent the animal hosts, clean the environment and eliminate flies. For humans, personal sanitation practices should especially focus on the cleaning of children's eye region. All of the above practices are to prevent the spreading of the disease. The main treatment is to extirpate the worms. The symptoms could disappear soon after proper treatments. 0.5% to 2% decicaine could be used to drip the eyes 3 times, and then take the worms out with tweezers or wet tampon, at last drip the antibiotic drug and smear eye ointment. It is common that there are several worms parasitizing in a host, and it is uneasy to take them out for one time, so it is better to enhance the prevention.

(Cui Yu)

Trichostrongylus orientalis

Trichostrongylus orientalis parasitizes in the stomach and small intestine of many animals such as sheep, camels or horses and so on. It can also be found in humans.

Morphology

The adult of *T. orientalis* is slender, colorless and transparent. The transverse striation of cuticle is not obvious. The buccal capsule is not prominent. It is followed by a pharyngeal canal. The male measures 4.3 to 5.5mm by 0.072 to 0.079mm. It possesses a copulatory bursa equipped with a pair of short and stout copulatory spines at the posterior end, at the end of which there is a hooklet. The female measures 5. 5 to 6. 5mm by 0. 07mm. Its posterior end is conical. The vulva is situated at the posterior one sixth of the body. The uterus contains 5 to 16 eggs.

The ovum is ovoid, colorless and transparent. It measures 80 to 100μm by 40 to 47μm. It is slightly longer than an egg of hookworm. Its longitudinal diameter is generally twice longer than the transverse diameter. One end is rounded and the other end is relatively pointed. One side is raised than the other side. The shell is thinner. There is space at both ends of the egg especially at the pointed end. Ovum cell has already split into 10 to 20 in eggs in fresh feces (see Figure 4-9-2).

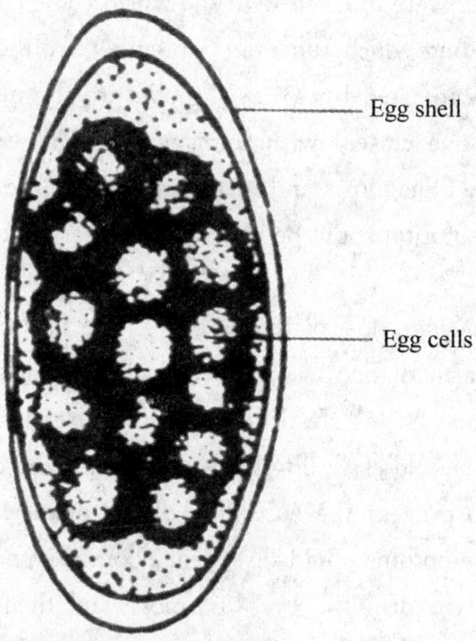

Figure 4-9-2 Egg of *Trichostrongylus orientalis*

Life Cycle

T. orientalis needs a single host to complete the life cycle. The adults parasitize mainly in the stomach and small intestine of sheep, camels, horses, cattle, donkeys and other herbivorous animals. It may also live in human small intestine. The eggs are discharged with the hosts' feces and develop in soil. The larvae hatch and develop to infective larvae after molt twice. Humans acquire the infection by swallowing raw vegetables contaminated with the infective larvae. The larvae molt for the third time in the intestinal lumen and then invade into small intestinal mucosa. Several days later, larvae molt for the fourth time after releasing from the mucosa, then drill the mucosa with their anterior end and develop into adults.

Pathogenesis and Clinical Manifestation

The pathogenic changes caused by this parasite are not obvious. The symptom of abdominal pain is slightly serious than that caused by hookworm. Eosinophilia is commonly less than 10%. Anemia and toxic responses caused by the parasites' metabolic products appear in the severe cases. It is difficult to distinguish which symptoms are caused by this parasite other than hookworm, because hosts are often mixedly infected with this worm and hookworm at the same time.

Diagnosis

The diagnosis is generally confirmed by finding the characteristic eggs in the patients' feces. Attention should be paid to differentiate them from hookworm eggs.

Prevention and Control

Trichostrongylus orientalis mainly distribute in the suburban area. It has been found in 18 provinces (cities, autonomous regions) in China. The principles of treatment and prevention are similar to those of hookworm disease.

(Cui Yu)

Gongylonema pulchrum

Gongylonema pulchrum mainly parasitizes in the mucous and submucous membrane of oral cavity and esophagus in mammals (especially in the ruminants), sometimes it also parasitizes in human body and causes gongylonemiasis.

Morphology

The adult worm is slender like a thread, and presenting white in color. The male which parasitizes in ruminants measures 21. 5 to 62mm by 0. 1 to 0. 36mm and the female measures 32 to 150mm by 0. 2 to 0. 53mm. The adult worm that inhabits in human is smaller. It is reported in China that the male is 21. 00 to 30. 68mm in length by 0. 16 to 0. 23mm in width and the female is 32 to 68. 8mm by 0. 2 to 0. 37mm. There are fine transverse striations on the surface of the body. There is a mouth in the middle of the anterior end, which is infundibulate in shape. The mouth is small and there are leaf-like lips around the mouth. There are 8 small mastoid processes and one collar on the lips and outside the lips respectively, and there is one amphid on both the right and the left of the collar. There are festoon-like ecderon processes at the anterior part of the body, which are in line, and are unequal in size and different in numbers. There is one cervcial papilla separately at each side of the anterior end, behind which there is a segment of lateral wing (alae). The male tail has apparently a tail wing, which is asymmetry. There are pairs of mastoid processes behind or in the front of anus. The male adult has two copulatory spines, and the left one is thinner and longer than the right one. The posterior end of the female is asymmetry, blunt and pyramidal in shape, curving a little to the ventral aspect. The vulva is situated just in front of the anus. The uterus is big and contains a lot of eggs.

The egg is oval-shape, and the two ends are blunt round. Its size is 50 to 70μm by 25 to 42μm. The shell of egg is thick and transparent, the surface of which is smooth and glossy. There is a larva in each egg (see Figure 4-9-3).

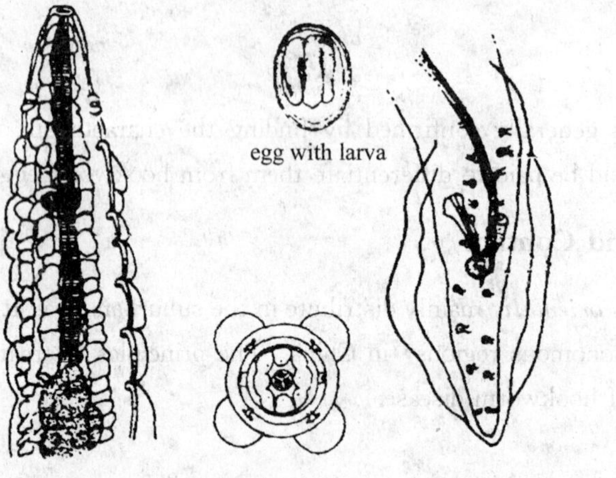

Figure 4-9-3 Morphology of *Gongylonema pulchrum*

Life Cycle

The final host and the intermediate host of *Gongylonema pulchrum* are extensive. The naturally infected final hosts are buffalo, scalper, sheep, goat, horse, donkey, mule, pack animal such as ruminants, and other animals such as pig, porcupine, monkey, dog, mouse and bear. Cattle, sheep and pig are the specified hosts, but human could be the final host occasionally. The intermediate hosts relative to human infection are chafer and roach. There are some patients who like eating mantis, grasshopper, longicorn, katydid and bean bug, which are presumed that they also may be the intermediate hosts. The adult worms inhabit the submucosa of the mouth and the esophagus of the final host. The eggs could go into the digestive tract through broken mucous membrane and were discharged with the feces. If eggs had been eaten by the intermediate host, larvae hatched in the digestive tract of the insect, and then went through into the haemocoel, exuviated twice and grew to be infective larvae. The final hosts take infective larvae by mistake. The larvae hatch and invade the mucous membrane of stomach or duodenum, and then move to the mucous membrane of esophagus, pharynx and mouth. They grow to be adult worms after 60 days. The number of parasites in human body is 1 to 10, sometimes up to 16.

The adult worms inhabit in the mucous and submucous membrane of oral cavity, nose and esophagus in humans. It is also reported that they are found in the nasal cavity and below nasolabial groove. The eggs have ever been found in biopsy of the esophagus and bloody sputum. The egg is discharged with the feces of the final host, and is swallowed by the intermediate host. The first period larva hatches out in the esophagus, goes through the digestive canal into the coelom of human body. The adults can survive about 1 year in the human body, and the longer time could be more than 5 years.

Pathogenesis and Clinical Manifestation

Gongylonema pulchrum could move freely between the mucosa and submucosa of oral cavity and esophagus when it parasitizes in the human body. So its parasitizing position is unstable. The worm could produce damage such as small bleb and swell on the site of infection, and could cause squirm and anaesthesia feelings for the movement of the worm. The damage even could lead to hoarseness. The focus of infection could appear itch, swelling and pain. Mucous membrane presents blain and blood blister. The patient could feel swallow difficulty when worm parasitizes in the mucous membrane of esophagus. The eosinophile granulocyte increased, sometimes could be up to 20%. If the worms parasitize in the vagina mucous membrane, most patients may appear leucorrhea, itch or squirm and anaesthesia feelings for the movement of the worms. Some patients could show up disordered fear. The symptoms could disappear soon after removing the worms.

Diagnosis

The first diagnosis could be made based on the disease history and the mouth symptoms. If the patient tells he has sometimes feeling of creeping in the mouth, the doctor could make a definite diagnosis for this disease through extirpating the worms from diseased region, and then check it under the microscope. In the saliva and feces of infected person, it could hardly find the eggs, so it has less meaning to detect eggs for diagnosing.

Prevention and Control

In 1850, Leidy first found such infected case in Philadelphia, USA. Since then, such cases happened all over the world including Italy, Germany, USA and former Soviet Union, and all together there are much more than 10 countries. In China, since the first case found in Henan in 1955, now there are more than 80 cases found in 26 provinces.

Infection of human body has relation with the food and drinks, such as having raw or half cooked infected insects or infected water. For example, it was reported the infected cases caused by eating baked or fried grasshoppers, mantis and beetles in Shandong. In Shanxi, some children like to eat burnt chafer. Based on the experiment, the larva could live through the winter in the beetles. After the intermediate host died, infective larva was released into water or soil and to contaminate water and vegetables. If human take them by mistake, infection of humans will occur.

The main treatment is to remove the worms. The symptoms could disappear soon after proper treatments. The main prevention is to keep individual sanitation well, not to drink untreated water or eat insects like beetle, grasshopper, roach and so on.

(Cui Yu)

Angiostrongylus cantonensis

No metastrongyle is considered to be a normal inhabitant of humans. However, two species found in rodents cause disease: *Angiostrongylus cantonensis* and *A. costaricensis*, found in the Eastern and Western Hemispheres, respectively. Both of these nematodes are parasites of the arterial system, rather than the lungs, and the problems of pathogenesis for humans result to an extent from these parasites being in an abnormal host.

Angiostrongylus cantonensis causes angiostrongylosis, eosinophilic meningitis, meningitis, or tropical eosinophilia in humans.

Morphology

The female worms are 18 to 33mm long by 0. 28 to 0. 5mm wide with the vulva about 0. 25mm from the posterior end. Males are 15 to 22mm by 0. 25 to 0. 35mm and have subequal spicules that are 490 and 1200μm long. Both sexes feed on blood and therefore have a red intestine around which the reproductive system winds; this gives a barber-pole appearance also noted in such worms as *Haemonchus*(see Figure 4-9-4).

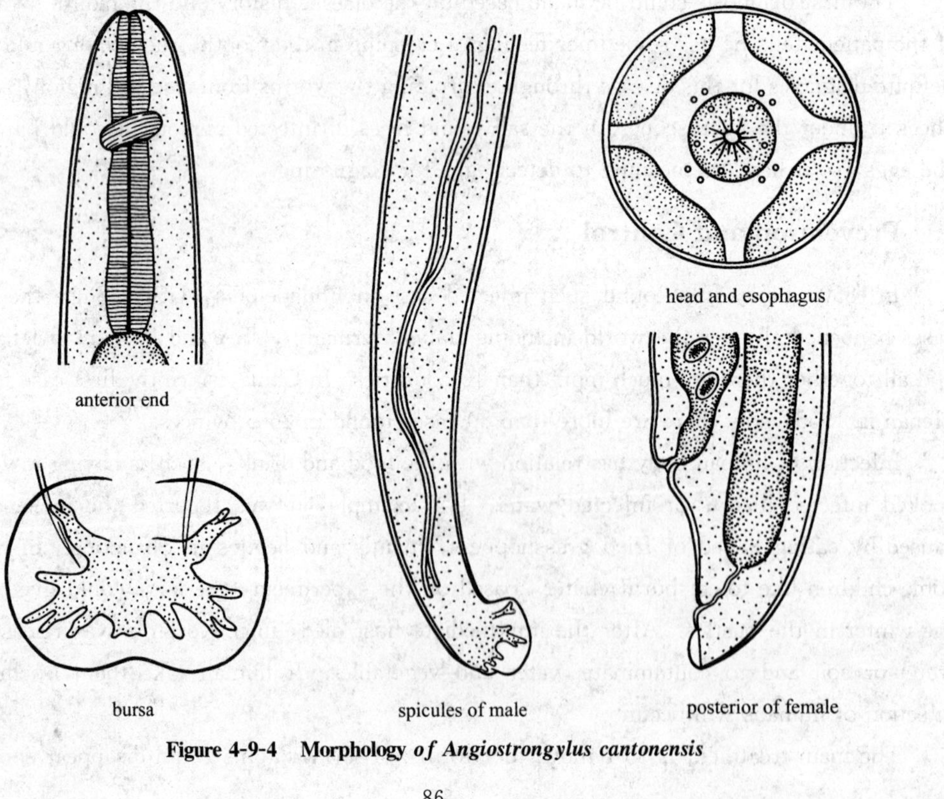

Figure 4-9-4 Morphology *of Angiostrongylus cantonensis*

Life Cycle

The life cycle described here is that which occurs in the normal rat host, and in the invertebrate hosts. As is true with many other metastrongyles, the L_3 S are ensheathed in the cast cuticles of the two previous stages. The L_3 S are eaten by rats and within a day reach the central nervous system via the circulatory system. The early adult stage is reached in 11 to 13 days after infection, and migration then begins. The worms move to the meninges covering the brain and remain between the layers (subarachnoid space) for about two weeks. They then move to the venous system and are carried through the heart to the pulmonary arteries, where they remain and begin laying eggs. The unembryonated eggs are carried with the arterial blood to the capillaries in the alveoli of the lung, where they lodge. The L_1 S hatch, break out of the alveoli, pass up the respiratory tree and are swallowed; the prepatent period is 42 to 45 days, with larvae appearing in the feces at that time (see Figure 4-9-5).

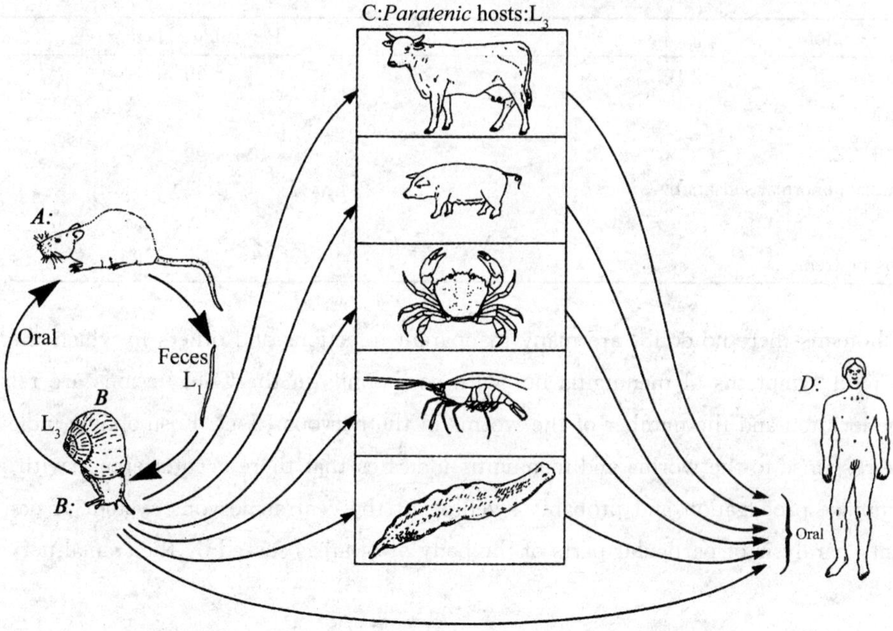

Figure 4-9-5 Life cycle of *Angiostrongylus cantonensis*

The first intermediate host is a snail or slug, usually a terrestrial one. The host range is quite broad, but development takes place more readily in some species than in others. The L_1 S penetrate the foot of the mollusk and reach the L, in about 18 days at 21℃ to 25℃.

Having reached the infective stage, the L3 can reach the definitive host by one of the following means:

(1) The gastropod can be eaten.

(2) The L_3 S can escape from the gastropod and be eaten with food or with water.

(3) A transport host can be infected by either of these routes and then it, in turn, may be

eaten by the definitive host. The most important transport hosts seem to be freshwater crustacea such as prawns and crab, and land planaria. The most frequent mode of infection in wild rats is not known.

The life cycle in humans seems to be the same as that in the rat except for the final site. In humans the worms remain in the brain, lying either between the meninges or migrating through the brain tissue itself.

Pathogenesis

Frequently, but not invariably, *A. cantonensis* has a low degree of pathogenesis in the rat. On the other hand, in humans there is a full range of effects including severe damage to the central nervous system leading to death.

Table 4-9-1 Clinical Signs and Symptoms of Eosinophilic Meningitis and Presumably Infection with *A. cantonensis*

Sign or Symptom	Percentage Having
Headache	90
Stiff neck	56
Vomiting	56
Paresthesia(abnormal sensation)	54
Fever	41
Paralysis or tremors	9

In humans there no doubt are many inapparent infections and others in which there may be only mild symptoms of meningitis but with eosinophils in the CSF. Lesions are related to both the location and the number of the worms in the nervous tissue. Eosinophilia indicates an immune response to the worms and meningitis indicates that there is interference with normal nerve impulse propagation and probably swelling of the central nervous system. If damage is sufficient, paralysis of particular parts of the body or of areas served by the cranial nerves may result.

Diagnosis

Diagnosis is difficult in humans; in the other hosts, a postmortem examination may be done to find the worms in the pulmonary arteries. Unless the person has died, the diagnosis of *A. cantonensis* infection is indirect and is based on the following:

(1) Clinical signs and symptoms(see Table 4-9-1);

(2) Food habits and a history of having eaten a likely source of larvae about two weeks previously;

(3) The presence of eosinophils in the cerebrospinal fluid(CSF);

(4) Evidence of antibody production;

(5) Finding worms in the CSF(rare; only two in stances are on record).

There are many causes of meningitis; therefore both a skilled diagnostician and a laboratory capable of isolating and identifying various infectious agents are required to determine whether bacterial, viral, or other parasitic agents may be the cause of the disease. Skin and serological testing can indicate whether a nematode may be involved in producing antibody. A further narrowing of the possible causes of meningitis comes from questioning of the patient. In an enzootic area, the typical symptoms coupled with suggestive laboratory tests and food habits consistent with becoming infected provide a good indication of infection with *A. cantonsis*. Other infections with which *A. cantonensis* can be confused are *Taenia solium* cysticerci, *Paragonimus westermani* and *Gnathostoma spinigerum*. Many other infectious or noninfectious processes may also be associated with an increase in eosinophils.

Epidemiology and Control

Since eosinophilic meningitis is usually a sporadic infection in small numbers of persons at any one time, control programs have not been developed. At the public health level, there are three approaches that might be considered:

(1) Treatment of infected individuals;

(2) Changing food habits to avoid infection;

(3) Rat control.

Anthelmintics along with anti-inflammatory drugs have been used with some success in treating laboratory animals. However, reservations have been expressed on the desirability of treatment. The concern is that a worm migrating through the brain tissue clearly causes damage, but a dead worm becomes a foreign body against which a strong inflammatory reaction is directed. The result is a large granuloma, which itself causes damage. Although some cases are on record in which persons have died from the infection, most recover completely without specific therapy. This is clear in cases where the treatment may be worse than the disease. The physician's cardinal principle pertains: first, do no harm.

The food habits of people in various localities or their ethnic derivation determine whether infection is likely to occur. In this case, food preferences are the key.

Among certain peoples of the Pacific islands, foods such as tiaro on Tahiti or keloguen on Guam consist principally of grated coconut mixed with the juice from ground or crushed freshwater prawns. On some of the Pacific islands. 5% to 10% of freshwater prawns have been found to be infected, mostly with two or three larvae of *A. cantonensis*; in one instance more than 3,000 larvae were found in a single prawn.

The predilection of Europeans and North Americans for green salads leads to infection. Terrestrial gastropods, and planaria secondarily, shed infective larvae onto plants in the field and the larvae are then eaten with the salad. In some enzootic areas, eosinophilic meningitis occurs in visitors and not in the natives where the latter do not eat leafy salads.

Since the definitive host range is relatively narrow, rat control might be worthwhile, but in general rats are not restricted to areas of human habitation. Control is therefore likely to be unproductive. Drinking untreated surface water is also a hazard since larvae escape from the intermediate host or from planaria and may be transmitted if this happens in small streams.

At the public health level, probably the best that can be done is to monitor the extent of the infection in the intermediate and transport hosts and make available information on the consequences and likelihood of infection. The responsibility then falls on the individual on whether to avoid infection or not.

(Chen Xiaoguang)

Gnathostoma spinigerum

Gnathostoma spp. are distributed in some areas of the world. In the United States, *G. procyonis* is common in the stomach of raccoons and opossum, *G. spinigerum* infects a wide variety of carnivores in Asia. *G. doloresi* is common in pigs in Asia. Although *Gnathostoma* have 20 or so species, only *G. spinigerum* is considered to be medically important. This parasite is normally found in dogs and cats, and Thailand has the most infections, both in humans and in reservoir hosts. Areas of endemicity include Japan, China, the Philippines, and other areas in the Far East. *G. spinigerum* harbours in animals and human body, and lead to gnathostomiasis. Up to now, 34 cases of gnathostomiasis have been reported in China. Although the entire life cycle is not fully understood, a patient was reported eating raw brook trout about 2 months before the onset of the creeping eruption.

Morphology

The adult worms are stout and pink in life, and about 25 to 54mm (females) and 11 to 25mm (males) long. The swollen head bulb is covered with four circles of stout spines. The anterior half of the worm is covered with leaflike or toothed spines, followed by a bare portion. The posterior tip of the body has numerous tiny cuticular spines (see Figure 4-9-6).

Eggs are oval in shape, $65\mu m$ to $70\mu m$ by $38\mu m$ to $40\mu m$ in size, and have a polar cap at only one end, and contain 1 to 2 embryo cells. Eggs are unembryonated when laid.

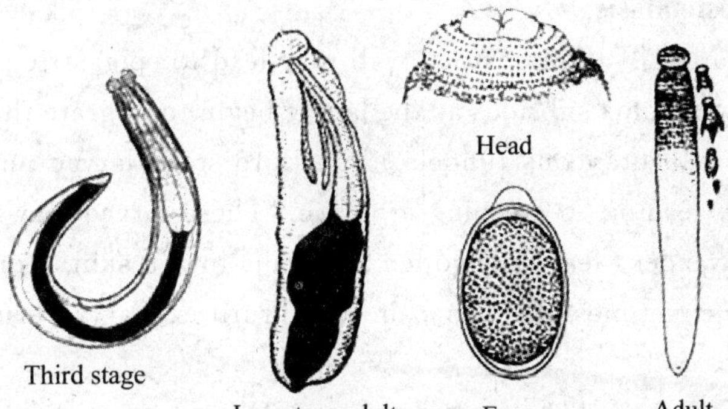

Figure 4-9-6 Morphology of adult, larva and egg of *G. spinigerum*

Life Cycle

The definitive host include cats, dogs, and some wild carnivores, and the first intermediate host are copepods, the second intermediate host are fish, amphibians, reptiles, birds, and mammals. The adult worm lies coiled in a rumor-like mass in the stomach wall of the definitive hosts. Eggs are extruded from the stomach lesions and are passed out with the feces. These eggs complete embryonation and hatch in 10 to 12 days at 27℃ to 31℃ after reaching water, releasing fist-stage larvae. The larvae are then ingested by copepods, where they penetrate into the hemocoel and develop into second-stage larvae within about 2 weeks. Second-stage larvae already have a swollen head bulb covered with 4 transverse rows of spines. When an infected copepod is then ingested by any of the many second intermediate hosts, the second-stage larvae penetrate the intestine of and migrate to muscle or connective tissue, where they molt to the third stage. The third-stage larvae encyst in tissues. The third-stage larvae are infective to the definitive hosts. Once the intermediate host is ingested by the definitive host, the parasites become localized in the stomach wall, where they mature in 2 to 12 months.

Human infections are required by the ingestion of raw or poorly cooked or pickled freshwater fish, chicken and other birds, frogs, or snakes. Human infection may occur from ingestion of copepods containing the advanced third-stage larvae or by actual skin penetration of larvae from handling infected meat.

Pathogenesis and Clinical Manifestations

In the human body, the larvae do not mature into adults in the wall of the stomach but may migrate throughout the body. The disease is usually seen in two very different clinical forms, larval gnathostomiasis (cutaneous larvae migrans) or eosinophilic myeloencephalitis (eosinophilic gnathostomiasis).

Larval Gnathostomiasis

Larval penetration of the intestinal wall may lead to epigastric pain, vomiting, and anorexia. These symptoms subsides as the larvae begin to migrate through the tissues in deep cutaneous or subcutaneous tunnels. The third-stage larvae migrate to superficial layers of the skin, leading to creeping eruption. These larvae may become dormant in the skin, or may wander, leaving swollen red trails in the skin. Sometimes the lesions are painless, and sometimes there is pain and pruritus. Larvae erupt out of the skin spontaneously.

These swellings probably result from the allergic response of the host to the presence of the worms, and an eosinophilia of 35% to 80% occurs in patients with cutaneous gnathostomiasis.

Eosinophilic Gnathostomiasis

However, erratic migration may take them into an eye, the brain, or the spinal cord, with serious results that even may cause death. The larval migration occurs along a peripheral nerve, into the spinal cord, and then into the brain. Symptoms include pain, paralysis, seizures, coma, and death. In areas of endemic infection, cerebral hemorrhage in a younger individual should indicate possible infection with *Gnathostoma* spp. Ocular invasion probably occurs via the optic nerve.

Diagnosis

Diagnosis depends on the recovery and accurate identification of the worm. Newer serologic methods may also be helpful. An intradermal test has been employed with success. Gnathostomiasis should be suspected in an endemic area when a localized edema is accompanied with eosinophilia.

Epidemiology

Most human infections result from a raw poorly cooked fish, domestic ducks, and chickens or paratenic hosts containing the third-stage larvae. In Japan, it is most often fish, whereas in Thailand, domestic ducks and chickens are probably the most important vectors. However, any amphibian, reptile, or bird may harbour larvae and contribute an infection if eaten raw. Untreated groundwater is also a potential problem and source of transmission because it can contain infected copepods. Once the life cycle is established in an area, potential infection can become a serious public health issue.

Prevention and Control

The only effective therapy is surgical incision of the lesion and removal of the worm. Chemotherapy is not effective against gnathostomiasis. In general, albendazole has also been recommended as an adjunct to surgical removal.

Prevention is the best means of controlling gnathostomiasis. Cooling or boiling by any means will kill the worms. In epidemic regions, the fish should be well frozen before preparation, or marine fish should be used. The most effective preventive measure of gnathostomiasis is educating the consumer not to eat raw or undercooked freshwater fish, chicken and other birds, frogs, or snakes.

(Cheng Yanbin)

Rhabditis axei

The worm belongs to the free-living nematodes, and is common in soil, foul water, decaying fruit, and so on. The adult of *Rhabditis axei* commonly parasitizes in the lungs of toads and frogs, sometimes may invade the digestive system and urinary system of human being, and cause rhabditelliasis axei.

The adult is a slender and cylindrical worm. At the anterior and posterior end of their esophagus have two prominent bulbs. The male adult is about 1.2mm in length, but the female adult is about 1.55mm. The uterus contains 4-6 eggs. The egg is similar to that of hookworm, but it is smaller.

The worm has very curious life cycles. The parasitic adult is a protandrous hermaphrodite. Sperms are produced in an early male phase and stored in a seminal receptacle. Then the gonad produces functional ova that are fertilized by the stored sperms. Resulting shelled zygotes pass up the trachea of the host and then are swallowed. The juveniles hatch in the intestine of the frog, and first-stage juveniles which are called as rhabditiform accumulate in the cloacae to be voided with feces. The rhabditiform feeds on bacteria and other inhabitants of humus soil, and develop to become infective stage which is referred to as filariform. The filariform juveniles undergo developmental arrest unless they penetrate the skin of a toad or frog. After penetration they lodge in various tissues; those that reach the lungs mature into hermaphroditic adults, whereas the rest apparently expire.

However, the juveniles may enter into the urinary duct of human body through contacting with the infected water for swimming or fishing, and cause the damage to human body. When it invade the urinary system, the patient shows fever, lumbodynia, urethrorrhagia, frequent micturition and urodynia, even edema of lower limbs or scrotum, chyluria, albuminuria, and pyuria. If the juveniles invade the digestive duct, the symptoms of abdominal pain, diarrhea and constipation may occur. Detecting the worms or eggs in feces or in urine sediment may confirm this disease.

Rhabditis axei distribute in Japan, Mexico, Israel, and other countries. 144 case of rhabditelliasis axei were reported in China from 1950-1996, and mainly distribute in Hunan, Guizhou, Hainan, and other 15 provinces. In 125 cases of all, the worms were found in feces, but in 19 cases, worms in urine.

Mebendazole, Albendazole and Levamisole are very effective for treatment.

(Si Kaiwei)

Dracunculus medinensis

Dracunculus medinensis has been known since antiquity, particularly in Middle East and Africa. During the Egyptian, Greek and Roman periods, human have known the clinical syndrome. The contemporary term, guinea worm disease, derives its name from a European explorer who named the disease for the geographic area in which it was found, along the western African coast. The staff of Aesculapius removed the adult worm by slowly winding it around a stick. Up to now, people have known that the adult harbours in the tissues of mammalian and human body, and results in dracunculiasis.

Morphology

Dracunculus medinensis is one of the largest nematodes. The females measure up to 1m in length by 2mm in width, and contain coiled uteri filled with rhabditiform larvae. The male is much smaller and does not exceed 40mm long. The male has a curved tail (1 to several cycles) with two unequal spicules. The mouth is small and triangular. The esophagus has a large glandular portion that protrudes and lies alongside the thin muscular portion. In the female the gravid uterus has an anterior and a posterior branch, each of which is filled with numerous of embryos (see Figure 4-9-7).

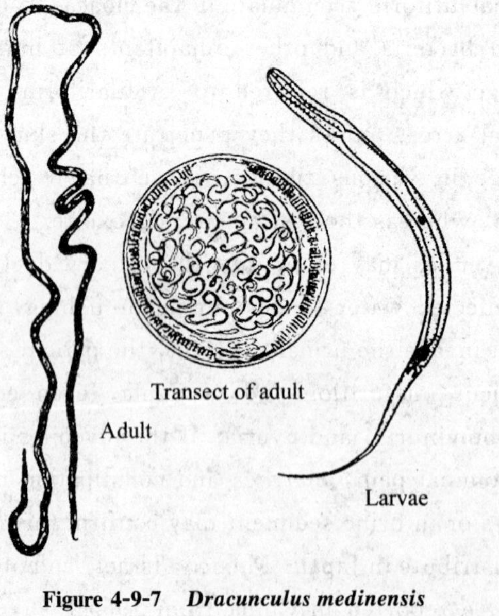

Figure 4-9-7 *Dracunculus medinensis*

Life Cycle

Human infection is acquired from ingestion of infected copepods (*Cyclops*, water fleas). *Dracunculus medinensis* is ovoviviparous. The worms mature in the deep connective tissues of host, and the gravid females filled with rhabditiform larvae in uterus migrate to the subcutaneous tissues. Maturation takes approximately 1 year. At this stage, the female migrates to the skin and the papule is formed in the dermis, usually by the ankles or feet. The papule changes into a blister in the skin of the host. The blister eventually ruptures, forming an exit for the larvae, which trickle out onto the surface of the skin. Sometimes, on contact with freshwater, a portion of the uterus prolapses through the worm's body wall, bursts open, and discharges thousands of larvae into the water. This may happen several times until all of the larvae are discharged. As portions of the uterus empty, they disintegrate, and adjacent portions move into the ulcer. Eventually all of the worms is "used up" and the wound heals.

The first-stage larvae must enter water directly to survive. The larvae are then ingested by an appropriate species of *Cyclops* in water. Development takes about 8 days before the larvae are infective for humans. The released larvae penetrate into the hemocoel, especially dorsally to the gut, or the loose connection tissue where they develop into the third-stage larvae (infective larvae). The possibility also exists that paratenic hosts, such as tadpoles or frogs, are important means of transporting infective larvae of *Dracunculus medinensis* up the food chain, thus facilitating transmission to the definitive hosts.

Pathogenesis and Clinical Manifestations

After ingestion of an infected copepod, the larvae penetrate into the deep connective tissues and mature. Once the gravid female begins to migrate to the skin, female worms elicit an allergic reaction caused by the release of metabolic waste into the host, and there may be some erythema tenderness and localized edema in the area. Subsequently, the patient may exhibit some systemic reactions, including an urticarial rash, intense pruritus, nausea, vomiting, diarrhea, or asthmatic attacks. Rapidly this becomes a blister. Local itching accompanies blister formation, with an intense burning pain. Feet and legs are most often affected. Symptoms usually subside when ruptures of the blister discharge the larvae and worm metabolites.

If the worms are removed or are expelled, healing usually occurs with no problems. If the worm is damaged or broken during removal, there may be an intense inflammatory reaction with possible cellulites along the worm's migratory tract. If secondary infection occurs or worms do not emerge, they begin to release antigens, and cause serious sequelae, including arthritis, synovitis, and other symptoms.

Some cases are complicated by bacterial infection of ulcer. Bacterial infection can become very serious if bacteria are drawn under the skin and lead to abscesses.

Diagnosis

The appearance of an itchy, red papule that rapidly transforms into a blister is the first strong symptom of dracunculiasis. Infected lesion must be distinguished from carbuncles, deep cellulites, focal myositis or periostitis, or even rheumatism. After the blister ruptures, larvae can be obtained by placing cold water on the wound; when mounted on a slide, they can be observed actively moving about by a low-power microscope. Diagnosis can be confirmed at the time the cutaneous lesion forms, with subsequent appearance of the adult worm.

Treatment

The worms have been removed by slowly being wound around a stick for treatment since antiquity. This approach works well unless the worm is accidentally broken and secondary infection occurs. An alternate treatment is removal of the complete worm by surgery. Surgery is best performed before ulcers develop and consequent bacterial contamination occurs when worms can be removed much more easily and quickly.

Four drugs have been used for the treatment of dracunculiasis: niridazole, thiabendazole, metronidazole, and mebendazole. The evidence for their effectiveness is dubious, and the action seems to involve suppression of inflammation rather than any specific effect on the adult worms.

Epidemiology and Prevention

Dracunculiasis transmission depends on the following factors: (1) the water must contain *Cyclops* spp., (2) the skins of the infected humans must directly contact with the water, and (3) use of this water for drinking. There is circumstantial evidence that infection can be acquired by eating a fish paratenic host. In many parts of the world, certain types of water sources (e. g., step wells in India, covered cisterns in Iran, and ponds in Ghana) provide all of these transmission requirements.

The target date for eradication of guinea worm infection of 1995 had been set by the World Health Organization and accepted by the United Nations Children's Found and the United Nations Development Program. The only two countries in Asia where infections are still endemic are India and Pakistan, and significant reductions have been achieved to date. Africa remains the largest and most difficult area to handle. In China, up to the present, only a case in human was reported in 1995.

The disease can be eliminated within 1 to 2 years by provision of safe drinking water.

(Cheng Yanbin)

Anisakis

Anisakid nematodes include a number of anisakidae in Ascaridata that normally infect the stomach and intestines of various marine fishes, birds, and such fish-eating mammals as dolphins, whales, seals, and porpoises. The larvae of certain *Anisakis* may invade the wall of gastro-intestine and cause human anisakiasis (Herring worm disease) with acute abdomen as major clinical manifestation.

The species causing human anisakiasis are *A. simplex*, *A. typical*, *A. physeteris*, *Pseudoterranova decipiens*, *Contracaccum* spp. and *Hysterothylacium* spp. Among them, *A. simplex* is more popular.

Morphology

Adults live mainly in the paunch of dolphins with a length of 65mm and a diameter of 2mm. It has three lips on the head like other ascarids, among which the dorsal lip is larger than the others. The excretory pore is open between the two subventral lips.

The larva is easily visible, being 12. 5-30mm or longer in body length and long fusiform in appearance. In a left lateral view of the anterior part and the tail end, we can find characteristics important for identification. It has a boring tooth on the ventral side of the mouth located on the head end. The glandular part of the esophagus at its end is specifically called ventriculus, which is followed by the midgut, rectum and anus. At the tail end there is a mucron. The excretory tube starting here proceeds forward to be open at the excretory pore immediately behind the boring tooth. The features around both ends of the body stated above can be found by scanning electron micrograph.

Life Cycle

Adult anisakids parasitize in the gastrointestinal tract of a wide variety of animals, but those of medical importance locate in the stomach of marine mammals (seals, sea lions, whales, and dolphins).

Fertilized eggs, passed in the feces of the mammalian host, hatch to liberate larvae swallowed by marine crustaceans. In these animals the larvae grow and molt, and if then eaten by fish or squid, the contained third-stage larvae are released to penetrate into the muscles or body cavity of that host. The squid or fish acts as a transport, in which the larvae do not molt to become adults. When fish and squid holding such larvae are eaten by some large-size fish, larvae again become encysted in the new host at the same stage of development as before. In this way, fish at the top of the food chain may become severely infected. When these hosts are eaten by the final hosts-marine mammals, the larvae grow into adult worms. Humans are infected by eating marine fish and squid either raw or insufficiently cooked. The larvae are unable to complete their development and attempt once again to adapt to a paratenic host (see Figure 4-9-8).

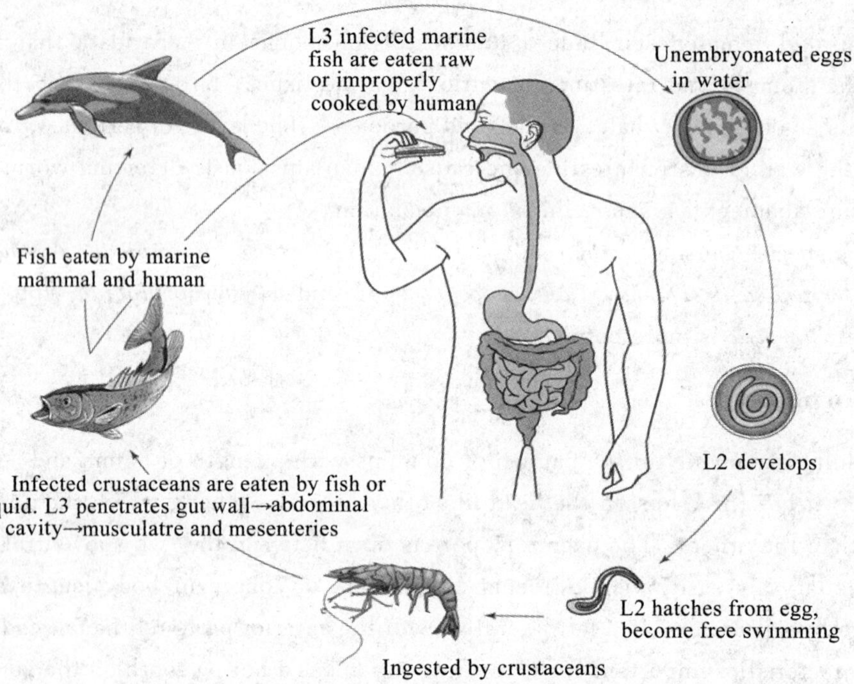

Figure 4-9-8　Life cycle of Anisakids

Pathogenesis and Clinical Manifestation

After swallowed by humans together with marine fish or squid, the advanced third-stage larvae invade the stomach walls and the intestinal walls. Some of them invade the abdominal cavity through the walls of the digestive tract. The worm induces infiltration of eosinophiles and lymphocytes, then connective tissue proliferation, finally granuloma formation. Therefore, such granulomas are observed as small tumors on the stomach walls. In a sectioned specimen, a section of the worm can be found in the center of the granuloma. Invasion of the stomach walls is more common than that of the intestinal walls, the ileum being involved most frequently in the latter. With the development of fiber endoscope it is easy to observe a live worm invading the stomach walls, usually accompanied by edema and hyperemia or slight bleeding in the surrounding mucosa.

The anisakiasis most commonly involves the stomach and may be characterized by the abrupt onset. Epigastric pain is invariably noted, which starts 1-12 (mostly 3-8) hours after eating the infested fish. When the intestines are involved, the onset of symptoms is delayed compared with gastric anisakiasis, which includes severe pains and sometimes vomiting or diarrhea, with signs of peritoneal irritation and incomplete ileus of the small intestine, frequently misdiagnosed as ileus, intestinal perforation, appendicitis, etc. Perforation of the bowel has been reported, with the finding of an anisakid larva in an inflammatory omental mass. On the other hand, pains might be so mild that the patient would be left untreated, which could later result in ileus.

Pains, usually associated with nausea and vomiting, are repeated periodically that frequently require analgesics. In cases with mild pains and left untreated, the infection proceeds to a chronic stage and is notice by tumor formation.

Diagnosis

A history of consuming raw fish shortly before the onset of symptoms should suggest the possibility of anisakiasis. Definitive diagnosis rests upon the demonstration of worms obtained by gastroscopy, at surgery, or vomited by the patient. The worm itself can be seen and removed using a pair of forceps for biopsy. If larvae are well preserved, they may be cleared in glycerin and identified by the structure of the digestive tract.

Epidemiology

It is widespread in seas all over the world, since its major final host is various dolphins as well as other toothed whales. The prevalence of larval anisakids in fish depends in turn on the prevalence of marine mammals, which is high in the North Sea, in Japanese and Alaskan coastal waters, and is increasing along the Pacific cost of North America.

Treatment

The best treatment is to remove the worms by gastroscopy as early as possible. If too late for doing this, anti-inflammatory therapy should be tried. Albendazole, 400mg twice daily for 21 days, has been reported to successfully treat a patient with anisakiasis. For prophylaxis, eating raw marine fish and squid should be avoided. Sashimi and other uncooked seafoods are both unsafe. The worms are killed immediately at 70℃, or gradually at −20℃, which must be taken into account.

(Wang Meilian and Luo Enjie)

Capillaria hepatica

Capillaria hepatica [(Bancroft, 1893) Travassos, 1919] primarily infests rodents and is rarely found in humans. Till date only 37 cases have been reported worldwide out of which two are from India.

Morphology

The male, about 24-37mm in length, is a little smaller and shorter than the female measuring 53-78mm long. Capillarids eggs differ from whipworm eggs by the following features: the shell wall has stripe; the eggs are slightly irregular in shape; the color is light amber and the plugs are less prominent.

Life Cycle

Capillaria hepatica is zoonotic nematode, primarily found in the liver of the rats. Human beings are accidental hosts. The unembryonated eggs of *Capillaria hepatica* are found in the liver of the first host and reach the intestine of the second host when the first host is eaten by a predator, or undergoes natural decomposition after death, whereby these eggs are released in the soil. They become embryonated in the soil and on ingestion by the second host by feco-oral contamination, or geophagy, reach the intestine of the second host. Here they migrate via the walls of intestines and through the portal vein, reach the liver where they grow into adult forms.

Pathology

Hepatic capillariasis (*C. hepatica*) clinical manifestations are usually that of an acute or subacute hepatitis. Eosinophilia and massive hepatomegaly may develop. Anemia is frequently observed and so is hypergammaglobulinemia, common parasite of rodents; causes hepatic capillariasis (*Capillaria hepatica* infection, liver-worm infection); rare disease of liver (adult hepatitis); also acts as occasional cause of visceral larva migrans. It may be fatal.

Diagnosis

The specific diagnosis of *C. hepatica* infection is based on demonstrating the adult worms and/or eggs in liver tissue at biopsy or necropsy, but serological testing by indirect immunofluorescence assay is also recommended for diagnostic and screening purpose. Identification of *C. hepatica* eggs in the stool is a spurious finding, which does not result from infection of the human host, but from ingestion by that host of livers from infected animals.

Epidemiology and Prevention

So far in the world literature only 37 cases of this disease have been reported, out of which 16 have been children. Two cases have been reported from India so far. Pica is an important presenting complaint, and this explains why this parasite infects the younger especially those between 1 and 5 years of age (94%). Treatment of choice is thiabendazole for 3 months. Alternative drugs include albendazole, and possibly ivermectin. Steroids are sometimes used to reduce hepatic inflammation. Prognosis depends on severity of infestation. With massive destruction of liver tissue, hepatic failure and death ensue if liver transplant is not available.

Dioctophyma renale

Dioctophyma renale [(Goeze, 1782) Stiles, 1901] has been reported from various countries and is known as the largest parasitic nematode of domesticated animals. The predilection site of this nematode is the kidney parenchyma, but it is also found in the abdominal cavity, subcutaneous tissues, stomach, mammary gland and other organs. Its larvae have also been reported from human subcutaneous tissues. The worm has a blood-red color; the male measures up to 35cm by 0.3-0.4cm and female up to 103cm by 0.5-1.2cm. Its size and predilection sites are sufficient for identification. Females are oviparous; the eggs are passed in the urine and are ingested by the annelid intermediate host. The final host (fish-eating carnivores such as foxes, minks and dogs as abnormal hosts) is infected by the ingestion of an intermediate host or a paratenic host. In the final host, the infective larvae migrate through the intestine wall, develop in the body cavity and penetrate the kidney. The prepatent period has been considered to be up to 2 years, though without certainty.

Specialist reported that usually only one kidney is affected in domesticated animals and there may be up to four worms in a kidney. It was reported that a total of 26 specimens were recovered from various locations in a dog from Brazil. The mature worm in the kidney destroys the kidney parenchyma. If it is located in the abdominal cavity, it causes chronic peritonitis, adhesions and damage on the surface of the liver. No clinical signs are usually seen but in some cases, depending on the localization of the worm, dysuria, haematuria and lumbar pain can be observed. The eggs of the nematode can be seen in the urine if the worm is located in the kidney. For treatment, the worm is surgically removed from confirmed cases.

(Li Wei)

Chapter 5 Trematoda

Section 1 Introduction to Trematodes

Trematodes, or flukes, are parasitic flatworms with unique life cycles involving sexual reproduction in mammalian and other vertebrate definitive hosts and asexual reproduction in snail intermediate hosts. Important species causing trematodiasis belong to Trematoda of Platyhelminthes. The majority of these species belong to Order Digenea which we call digenetic trematode. The digenetic flukes constitute the flukes of the intestinal tract, liver, lungs and blood in human beings. Some of the trematodes have been or are still the greatest disaster to the world or to some countries, such as three species of blood flukes.

Morphology

The structure of helminthes is very complex, and each has a unique form. It is very important to know the morphological characteristics of them in order to distinguish a species and also to diagnose diseases. Although members of Schistosomatidae in Trematoda are sexually dimorphic, the others are all hermaphroditic, which complicates the body structure(see Figure 5-1-1).

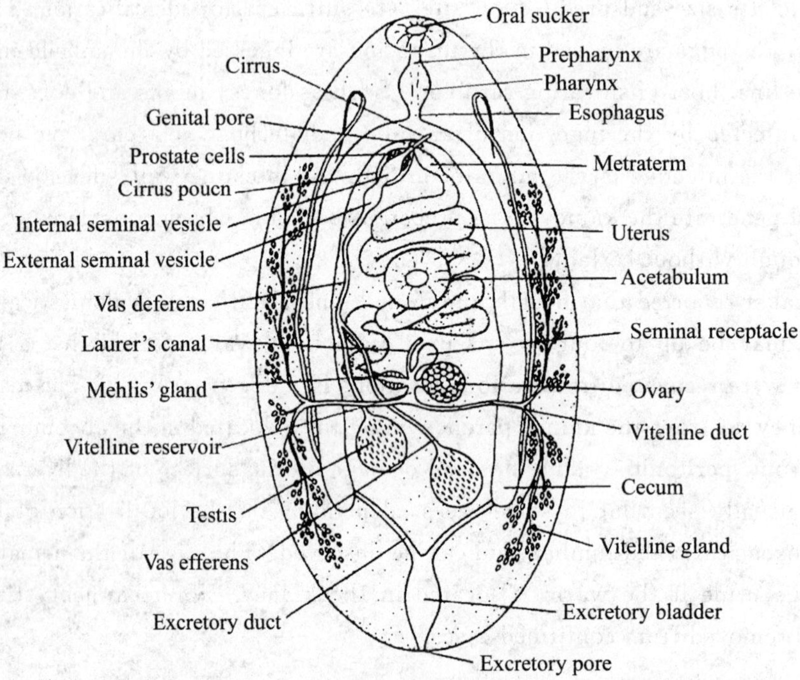

Figure 5-1-1 Morphology of Digenetic Trematodes

Adult

Most of trematodes are hermaphroditic, leaf-flat and unsegmented worms except schistosomas which are cylindrical and unisexual. Size varies from less than 1mm to several centimeters. Body surface is covered with a smooth cuticle or with spines on the surface, which is specific in species.

Tegument: The body of trematode is covered by a noncellular cuticle called tegument. In light microscope, it is a homogeneous layer 7-16μm thick, and shows affinity for basic dyes. It may be partially or completely covered with spines, tubercles or ridges. Under electron microscopy, the tegument shows two zones—an outer zone thrown into fold to form microvilli and an inner zone containing mitochondria endoplasmic reticulum and glycogen granules.

The tegument plays an important role in absorption of carbohydrates. It may also serve for excretion of excessive mucous and other metabolites.

Motile organs: There are two muscular suckers on the abdominal side. Oral sucker situated near the frontal end is also called the anterior sucker, and the ventral sucker the posterior sucker. Cuticular spines are relatively long and thick on the anterior half of the body. Those enable the fluke to move in the host body and to attach to the parasitic site. Size and location of suckers, and shape and growing pattern of the cuticular spines are very useful in identifying species.

Digestive system: The digestive system of trematodes is incomplete. It begins at the mouth in the center of the oral sucker and passes through the pharynx, esophagus, and intestine which divide into two branches to terminate at the blind end and there is no anus in fluke.

Excretory system: The excretory system is of protonephritic type and collecting tubules are lined by ciliated flame cells which excrete waste products into the ducts terminating in a posterior excretory pore.

Male reproductive organs: They contain a pair of testes, vas efferens, common vas deferens, cirrus sac or pouch in which lie seminal vesicle, prostate glands, and the protrusible cirrus. Sperms produced in the testes are collected in the seminal vesicle via the vas efferens and vas deferens and are ejected via the ejaculatory duct, around which there is a prostate gland covered by a cirrus sac. Some genital pores are common to male and female organs, and others open separately.

Female reproductive organs: They consist of single ovary, a short oviduct that opens in a minute chamber called ootype, Mehlis' gland, common vitelline duct, the duct from seminal receptacles, uterus, attached to ootype by convoluted tube, terminal part of uterus opens into genital atrium which in most species is the common chamber into which the cirrus organ also opens, and genital pore.

Nervous system: The central nervous system is near the pharynx, on both sides of the body. The left and right nerves join to become a thick nerve cord toward the posterior part of the body. Nerve fibers from the cord run throughout the body and are particularly dense at both suckers that move continually. Sensory papillae and sensory hairs exist at the ends of the nerve fibers.

Egg

Trematode eggs are ovoid, shelled egg containing vitelline substance, the embryo, ancillary membranes, and other materials. The eggs vary in length from under 30μm to as much as 175μm, depending on the species. They are transparent and generally brown or yellow-brown. The majority are equipped at one end with a lid-like structure, the operculum, an "escape hatch" through which the larva (miracidium) eventually will emerge. An operculum is absent in the eggshell of human blood flukes. In many species the egg contains a fully developed miracidium, which is covered with cilia when they are passed in the feces.

Life Cycle

Development of digenetic trematode must go through the alternation of sexual generation and asexual generation. The asexual generation occurs generally at intermediate host (snail) and the sexual generation at final host (vertebrate) (see Figure 5-1-2).

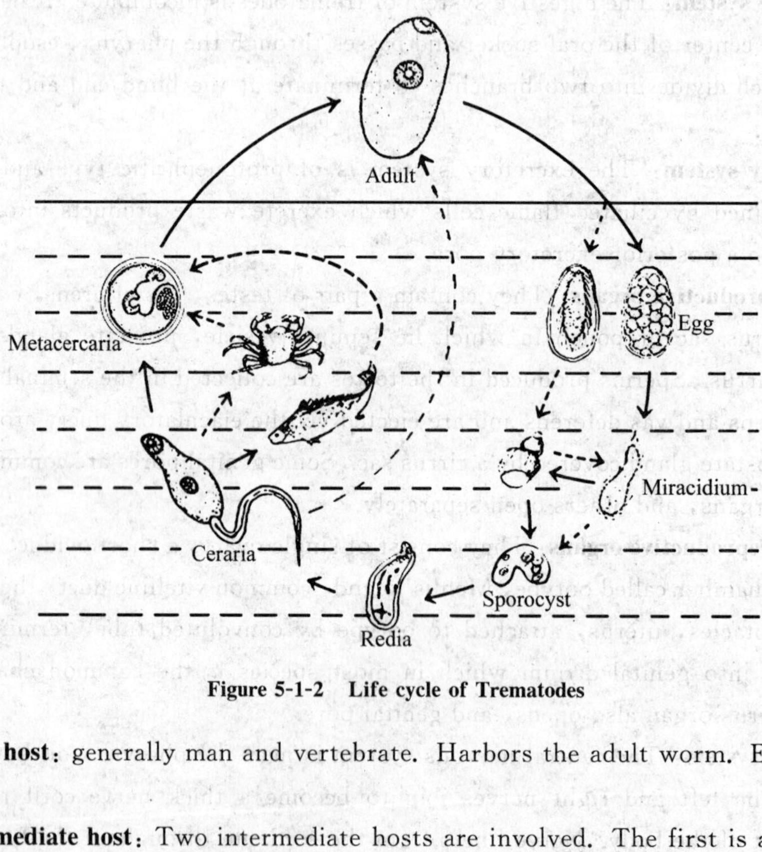

Figure 5-1-2 Life cycle of Trematodes

Final host: generally man and vertebrate. Harbors the adult worm. Eggs excreted in feces.

Intermediate host: Two intermediate hosts are involved. The first is a fresh water snail or mollusk for larval development and second intermediate host required for encystment in some trematodes may be a fresh water fish or crab or water plant, depending on the species of flukes.

When eggs egested in feces or sputum come in contact with water, the cleavage begins. Completed larvae are called miracidia, which swim in the water after putting off the operculum. The miracidium penetrates into its appropriate species of snail and develop into sporocyst which changes into a redia and finally cercaria. A multitude of cercariae is produced by just one miracidium.

The cercariae formed gradually are shed from the snail into the water, and then swim actively with their long tails. When the cercaria comes into a suitable second intermediate host, it encysts either on water-plants or in another intermediate host, a fresh water fish or a crab and becomes metacercariae, which is big, resistant and strongly infectious. *Schistosomatidae* has no metacercaria stage, and a cercaria in the water directly invades the final host percutaneously and then becomes an adult.

Man is infected either by drinking contaminated water or ingestion of metacercairae form in insufficiently cooked or pickled fish or crab, depending on the species, with the exception of *Schistosomatidae* which infects cutaneously by free cercariae.

The metacercairae excyst in the intestine and the young worms proceed to their sites of localization to grow into adult worms, become sexually mature and repeat the life cycle.

Classification of Trematodes

Classification of familiar digenetic flukes parasitizing human in China are shown in Table 5-1-1.

Table 5-1-1 Classification of familiar digenetic flukes parasitizing human in China

Order	Family	Genus	Species	Parasitizing sites
Digenea	Opisthorchiidae	Clonorchis	*C. sinensis*	Bile duct
	Heterophyidae	Heterophyes	*H. heterophyes*	Intestine
	Fasciolidae	Fasciolopsis	*F. buski*	Intestine
		Fasciola	*F. hepati*	Bile duct
	Paragonimidae	Paragonimus	*P. westermani*	Lung
		Pagumogonimus	*P. skrjabini*	Subcutaneous
	Schistosomatidae	Schistosoma	*S. japonicum*	tissue
	Echinostomatidae	Echinochasmus	*E. japonicus*	Portal vein
				Intestine

(Wang Meilian and Luo Enjie)

Section 2 The Liver Flukes

Several trematodes are parasites of the biliary passages of humans. Three genera of quite dissimilar trematodes, *Clonorchis*, *Opisthorchis*, and *Dicrocoelium*, are parasites of the biliary passage of humans. They are relatively elongate and narrow-bodied worms, which tend to localize in the smaller branches of the biliary tree. Only in heavy infections are these worms found in the common bile duct or gallbladder. Fasciola, a much larger worm, is confined by its size to the larger passages.

These worms all produce hyperplastic changes in the epithelium of the bile ducts and fibrosis around them. Massive infection by any of these worms may lead to biliary cirrhosis with all its associated manifestations.

The eggs of the opisthorchid flukes are very similar in appearance to those of the heterophyids, while those of fasciola closely resemble both fasciolopsis and the echinostomes. If eggs of one of these forms are found in the stool, and a differential diagnosis between hepatic and intestinal infection cannot be made on clinical grounds, examination of bile obtained by duodenal drainage will provide the correct answer. If one is successful in obtaining uncontaminated bile, and eggs are found in this material, they must have been produced by worms in the liver or gallbladder.

Clonorchis sinensis

Clonorchis sinensis, the Chinese liver fluke, belongs to the family *Opisthorchiidae*, genus *Clonorchis*. It was first discovered in the bile passages of died body of a Chinese carpenter in Calcutta, an India harbor city, in 1875. This worm was named *Clonorchis sinensis* because its testes were deeply branched. Not long after other infections were reported in Hong Kong and Japan. In China this worm was found in Hongkong, Wuhan, Shanghai and Guangdong province in 1908. Nowadays, clonorchiasis was reported in various districts all over the country, except in Gansu province, Xinjiang and Inner Mongolian autonomous regions. Our archaeologists found this worm in a body from a tomb dating from the second century B. C. in Jiangling, Hubei province.

Today it is known that the "Chinese liver fluke" is widely distributed in China (including Taiwan), Korea, Japan, Thailand, Kampuchea and Vietnam. It is also called Oriental liver fluke, and has been estimated to infect at least 19 million people, which causes untold economic loss. Human infection results from eating raw or half-cooked fresh-water fish, such as fish slice on congee. Fish may be eaten raw, pickled, smoked, or dried. People outside the Orient may become infected when they visit Orient or by eating infected fish imported from endemic areas. Dogs and cats are the most important reservoir hosts.

Morphology

The adult worm resides in the bile ducts of the human host and varies in size from 12 to 25mm long and from 3 to 5mm wide. The body is tapered anteriorly, while the posterior end is somewhat blunt. It is dorsoventrally flattened and looks like a sunflower seed. The oral sucker is at the top and the poorly developed ventral sucker lies about one-fifth the body length from the anterior end, just behind the common genital pore. The esophagus divides into two caeca which extend to the posterior region of the body. The excretory bladder is long and pouch-like, opening at the posterior end.

The reproductive system is hermaphroditic. The male reproductive organs consist of two large, deeply branched testes in tandem in the posterior third of the body. Two vas deferens from the testes unite to form a seminal vesicle leading to the genital pore in front of the ventral sucker, without penis. A small ovary with three lobes is situated two-thirds of the way from the anterior end. Just behind the ovary there are a seminal receptacle, ootype surrounded by Mehlis' gland and Laurer's canal on the oviduct. A loosely coiled uterus filled with eggs extends from the ootype to the genital pore. The vitelline glands are in the lateral fields (see Figure 5-2-1).

The eggs measure 29μm by 17μm, being the smallest of the helminth eggs. They are yellow-brown in color and operculated, with a ridge or collar at the base of the operculum, like "shoulder" as lateral view. There is also a characteristic knob at the abopercular end of the shell. When the egg is passed in feces, it contains a developed miracidium. The egg looks slightly like a sesame seed under the low power and a watermelon seed under the high power (see Figure 5-2-1).

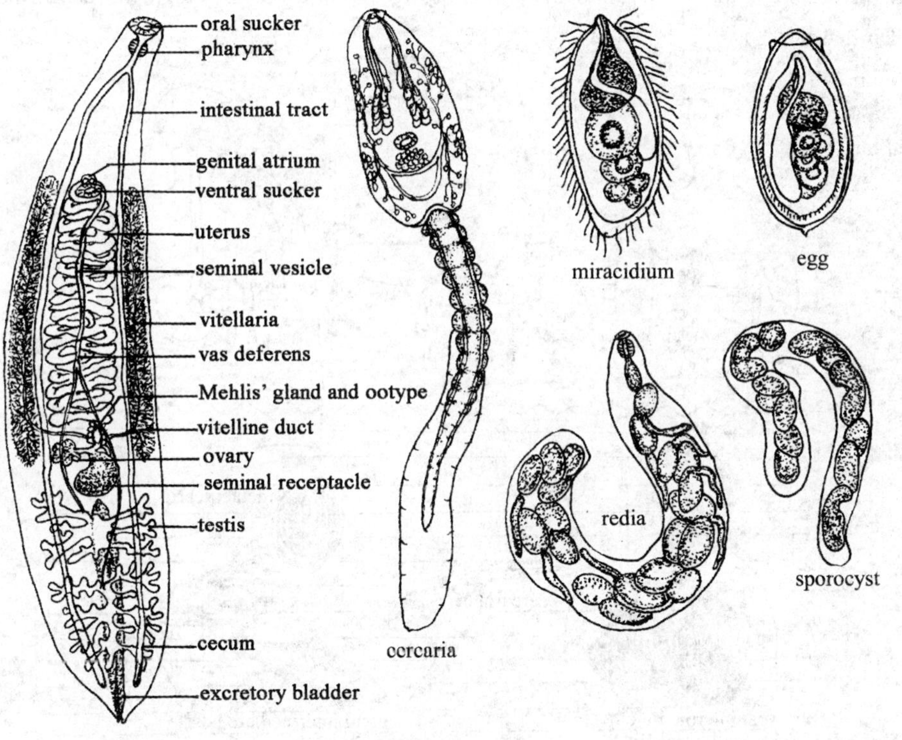

Figure 5-2-1 Morphology of *Clonorchis sinensis*

Life Cycle

Adult worms live in the bile ducts of the liver, where they deposit eggs. In more massive infections they occupy most of the bile passages and may even be found in the gallbladder and pancreatic duct. The eggs pass into the duodenum, and then are discharged in feces. The eggs get into fresh water and are ingested by suitable snails, the first intermediate host (Bithynia, Alocinma, Parafossarulus) by chance. The miracidium hatches and penetrates the intestinal wall of the snail and moves through the hemocoel to the digestive gland, where it metamorphoses into a sporocyst. The sporocyst gives rise to rediae, which erupt from the sporocyst and, in turn, produce cercariae. In order to survive, the free-swimming cercariae that emerge from the snail must penetrate the skin, gills, fins, or muscles of a freshwater fish host within 24-48 hours. Each cercaria burrows into one of these tissues, loses its tail, and encysts as a metacercaria. A wide variety of fish species belonging to the family Cyprinidae serve as second intermediate hosts. Humans become infected by eating raw or poorly cooked fish (including steamed, smoked, or pickled fish). The metacercaria excysts in the duodenum and migrates up the common bile duct to the biliary ducts, feeding continually on the contents of the ducts. The worm reaches sexual maturity about a month after excystation and has been known to live up to 25 years in the human host (see Figure 5-2-2).

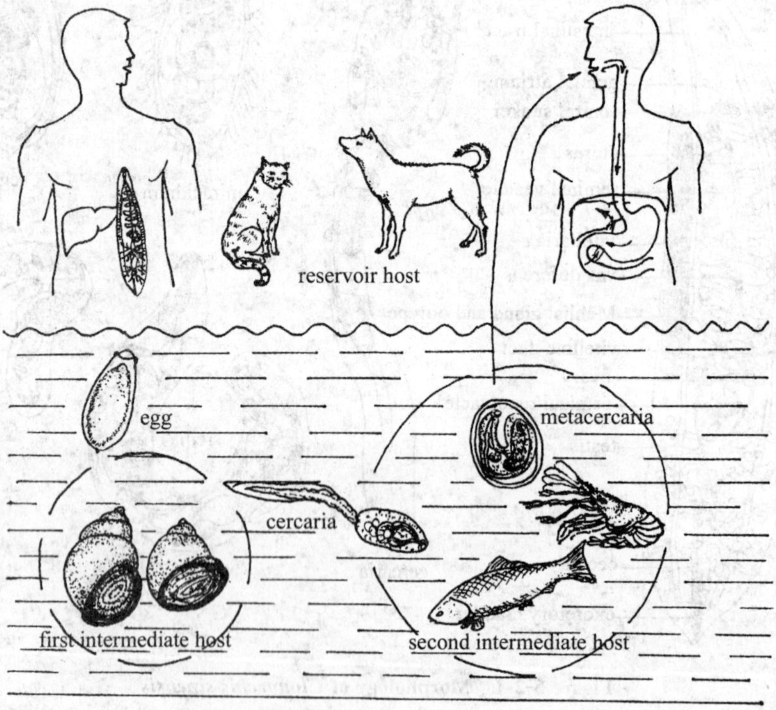

Figure 5-2-2 Life cycle of *Clonorchis sinensis*

Pathogenesis and Clinical Manifestation

The basic pathogenesis of *Clonorchis sinensis* infection is erosion of the epithelium lining the bile ducts. The ultimate effect depends mainly on the intensity and duration of infection, and, fortunately, worm burdens are usually small. The mean intensity of infection in most endemic areas is 20 to 200 flukes, but infection of 1,000 is not rare and as many as 21,000 have been removed at a single autopsy. The adult worms live in bile ducts with most of them being in small hepatic ducts. The mechanical and chemical factors coming from the worms' bodies and antigenic materials result in chronic inflammation, defoliation and proliferative reactions in biliary epithelia. These lead to gradual thickening and occlusion of the ducts (fibrosis in bile ducts). Pockets form in the walls of bile ducts, and complete perforation into surrounding parenchyma may occur. Infiltrating eggs become surrounded by connective tissues, thereby interfering with liver function. The eggs and sometimes remains of flukes may become nuclei of gallstones, and bacterial infections may also take place. So the symptoms and signs of cholegitis, cholecystitis and cholelithiasis appear. Heavy worm burdens—the result of repeated infection over a period of years—may result in a degree of functional impairment of the liver; this impairment is secondary to localized biliary obstruction and is at times aggravated by intrahepatic stone formation, cholangitis, and the formation of multiple liver abscesses. Cholecystitis and cholelithiasis may be the result of invasion of the gallbladder by these worms, which have also been considered to cause acute pancreatitis.

As a great number of bile ducts are blocked, the pressure in the bile ducts is raised to the extent that the bile secretion is stopped. The bile is stored increasingly in hepatic cells and diffuses among the cells. This may result in the degeneration of local cells. If the obstruction of the bile passages cannot be removed, necrosis of the cells ensues. Jaundice is in a small percentage of cases and is probably caused by bile retention when duct are obstructed. After the fibrosis of liver tissue, the liver gets hard and green, and biliary cirrhosis occurs. Then liver function failure and portal vein hypertension become obvious. In children's cases with high infection, the physical and mental growths are retarded. Ascites nearly always occurs in severe advanced cases. Cancer of the liver is more prevalent in endemic areas than elsewhere, and its relationship to clonorchiasis should be investigated.

Light infections, which are the rule, are generally asymptomatic. Heavier infections, if acquired over an extended period of time, seldom cause symptoms. The ingestion of large numbers of metacercariae over a short period of time may produce symptomatic early infections. The acute phase lasts less than a month and may be characterized by fever, diarrhea, epigastric pain, anorexia, enlargement and tenderness of the liver, and sometimes jaundice. There may be leukocytosis, and eosinophilia is generally present. Eggs appear in the feces about a month after infection takes place, and the acute symptoms subside. Once this has happened, persons not subject to repeated reinfection generally do not have any recognizable symptoms from a chronic low-grade infection. Many of those persons without effective treatment still harbored an asymptomatic infection 20 years later. In light infections, prognosis is good even without treatment because tissue invasion is not involved.

In general cases, loss of appetite, anorexy for oily food (fear of greasy food), fullness in abdomen, diarrhea, physical weakness, hepatomegaly and hepatic pain may appear.

In severe cases, icterus and weight loss may be present. The symptoms like systemic toxemia including fever, vertigo, mental depression, palpitation of the heart.

Cirrhosis is probably a rare complication. Advanced cases manifest portal-hypertension syndrome—emaciation, ascites, abdominal varicosity, icterus, hepatomegaly, splenomegaly and anemia. Patients may die of upper digestive tract bleeding, secondary infection and hepatic coma.

The cancer arising from the hyperplastic bile duct mucosa in persons chronically infected with C. *sinensis* have long been considered to be related to the infection.

Diagnosis

Clinical examination is warranted whenever there are liver pain and enlargement, anorexia, diarrhea and icterus. The liver abnormalities just described, experience of eating raw freshwater fish and residing in endemic areas should suggest clonorchiasis, but care must be taken to exclude other hepatic and biliary diseases. The confirmative diagnosis is based on the recovery of the characteristic eggs in the feces or by biliary drainage (duodenal aspiration). Eggs must be differentiated from others of Opisthorchis.

The eggs are so small that they easily missed during microscopic examination of a direct fecal smear. Concentration methods that are effective, include: (1) alkali digestive method, (2) water sedimentation method, (3) inverted precipitation method.

The flotation method is not satisfactory. The immunological tests are for reference only, including: (1) intradermal tests, (2) indirect haemagglutination test (IHA), (3) enzyme-linked immunosorbent assay (ELISA).

Prevention and Control

The drug of choice is praziquantel, with cure rates in the neighborhood of 100 percent when administered at 25mg/kg three times daily for 2 days. Alternate drugs include bithionol and hexachloroparaxylol.

Albendazole, thiabendazole and mebendazole seem equally effective when given at 10mg/kg twice daily for 7 days. These drugs have minimal toxicity.

Epidemiology

Clonorchiasis is found in Far East. In China it is prevalent in 23 provinces, municipality directly under the Central government, autonomic regions and special administrative region. The prevalence may range from an average of 1% to 30%. It is more prevalent in Guangdong, Liaoning, Jilin and Heilongjiang province. Local prevalence reaches 12.3% in Korea and 13.7% in Vietnam.

Reservoir hosts that are wild or domestic fish-eating mammals, including cats, dogs, tigers, foxes, badgers, and mink, play a significant role in maintaining Oriental fluke populations in endemic areas. The high incidence of mammalian infection, the increase in freshwater fish farming in the Orient, and the practice of eating raw fish have made clonorchiasis a serious problem. The spread of the disease is closely related to human habits such as making a meal of raw fish slices on congee, and oriental aquaculture ponds are commonly fertilized with human excrement to enhance the growth of vegetation, which gives chance of the eggs getting into the water.

(Yuan Fangshu, He Shenyi and Guo Shuling)

Section 3 *Fasciolopsis buski*

Fasciolopsiasis was first noted by Busk in 1843, when worms were detected in the duodenum of a deceased East Indian sailor. *Fasciolopsis buski* is the largest digenean infecting humans, reaching a size of 75mm long and 20mm wide and has also been known as the giant intestinal fluke.

Morphology

Adult

The living worm is yellowish pink. After died, the worm becomes pale. The adult worm measures 20-75mm in length, 8 to 20mm in width, and 0.5 to 3mm in thickness. It has two suckers. The oral sucker is located at the anterior part of the body. The ventral sucker is larger, funnel in shape, which is close to the oral sucker. The mouth is located at the middle part of the oral sucker, followed by a pharynx, a short esophagus. The digestive tract divides into two branches, which are along two laterals of the body to the end. Two testes are

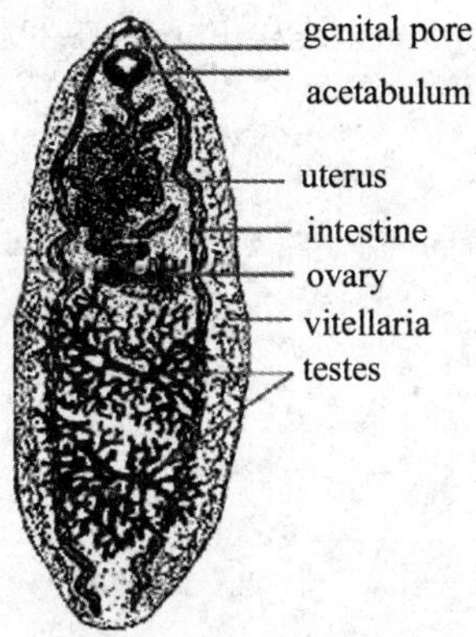

Figure 5-3-1 Adult of *Fasciolopsis buski*

highly-branched in tandem, which occupy almost the posterior two-thirds of the body. The branched ovary lies in the middle of the body to the right of the midline. The convoluted uterus, filled with eggs, opens into the genital atrium(see Figure 5-3-1).

Egg

It is the largest among all human helminthic eggs. The eggs are ellipsoidal in shape, and light yellow-brown in color. They measure about 130-140μm by 80-85μm, with the operculum found at the more pointed end of the transparent eggshell. When passed in the feces, containing a embryonic cell and some yolk cells in the egg (see Figure 5-3-2).

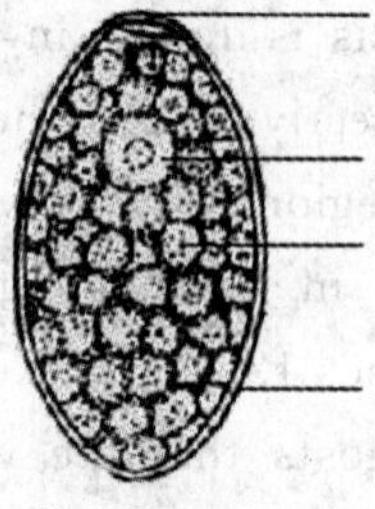

Figure 5-3-2 Egg of *Fasciolopsis buski*

Life Cycle

Adult worms inhabit the duodenal and jejunal regions of the small intestine and are attached by the suckers to the mucosal epithelium. Each deposits about 25,000 eggs daily. The eggs are expelled in feces and must reach fresh water in order to continue the cycle. Depending on the temperature, the eggs become embryonated within 3-7 weeks in the water, then the mature miracidium hatches from the egg. After locating and penetrating a planorbid snail of the genus Segmentina or Hippeutis, the miracidia metamorphose into sporocysts, which subsequently give rise to two sequential redial generations and finally develop to cercariae. The cercariae are released from the snail and encyst as metacercariae on aquatic plants such as water caltrops, water chestnuts, and water bamboo. Humans become infected by ingesting the raw or undercooked plants containing the metacercariae. The metacercariae excyst, attach to the duodenal or jejunal mucosa, and develop into adult worms within 3 months. The adults have a life span of about one year(see Figure 5-3-3).

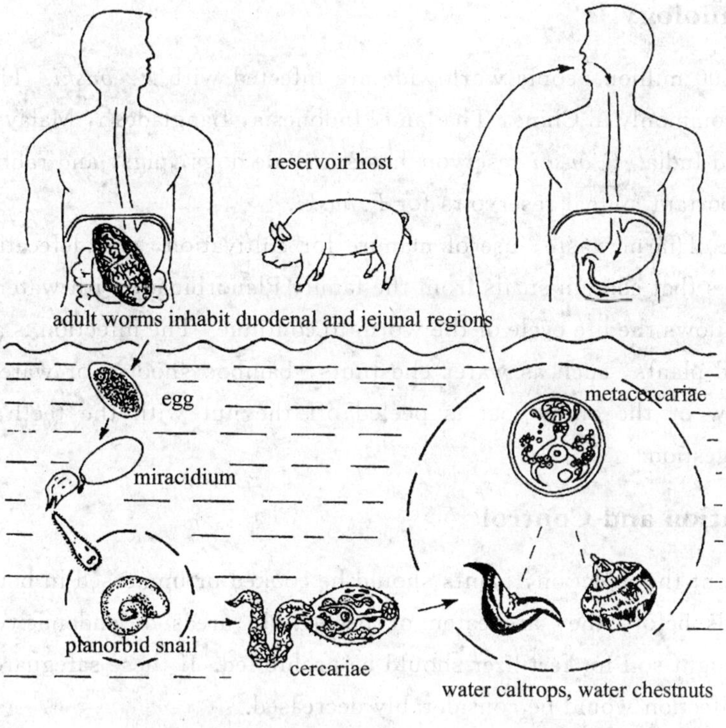

Figure 5-3-3 Life cycle of *Fasciolopsis buski*

Pathogenesis and Clinical Manifestation

The worms inhabit small intestine and feed actively not only on the host's intestinal contents but also on the superficial mucosa. Most infections are light and asymptomatic. In heavier infections, the worms may be found in the stomach and most of the intestinal tract, causing inflammation, ulceration, hemorrhage and abscesses at the sites of attachment. Diarrhea, nausea, and intestinal pain are common, especially in the morning hours. The stools are profuse and yellow-green and contain increased amounts of undigested food, suggesting a malabsorption process. The reaction of toxic or allergic worm metabolites can produce general edema, ascites, eosinophilia and leukocytosis. The large numbers of the worms may also lead to intestinal obstruction or acute ileus. The disease can be fatal, depending on the worm burden.

Diagnosis

The diagnosis is suggested by the clinical manifestations in endemic areas and is confirmed by detecting the eggs in the stool. Microscopic identification of eggs, or more rarely of the adult flukes, in the stool or vomitus is the basis of specific diagnosis.

Epidemiology

Nearly 100 million people worldwide are infected with *F. buski*. The infection is found most commonly in China, Thailand, Indonesia, Bangladesh, Malaysia, Pakistan, Cambodia and India. *F. buski* reservoir hosts include dogs, pigs, and rabbits. Hogs are the most important animal reservoirs for *F. buski*.

Drainage of farm waste, use of manure for cultivation, and defecation in or near ponds or lakes that contain snails from the family Planorbidae, with water plants acting as vectors, allows the life cycle of the worm to continue. The infection is acquired when these infested plants, such as water chestnuts, bamboo shoots, or water caltrops are consumed raw or the outer coat is peeled off the nut with the teeth, resulting in accidental ingestion.

Prevention and Control

To prevent the infection, plants should be cooked or immersed in boiling water for a few seconds before they are eaten or peeled. In areas of endemicity, the use of unsterilized night soil for fertilizer should be prohibited. If these safeguards were used, the risk of infection would be considerably decreased.

Praziquantel is the drug of choice.

(Liu Peimei)

Section 4 *Paragonimus* spp.

There are more than 50 species of *Paragonimus* that infect a wide variety of animals, and among which, 28 species are found in China. The adult worms of the genus *Paragonimus* are found in the lungs, and also called "lung fluke". Those flukes are widely spreaded among humans and mammals in the world and cause an important zoonosis-paragonimiasis. The main species of *Paragonimus* in humans are *Paragonimus westermani* and *Pagumogonimus skrjabini*.

Paragonimus westermani

The most common of *Paragonimus* spp. is the Oriental lung fluke, *Paragonimus westermani*. *Paragonimus westermani* causes inflammatory lung diseases in several Asian countries of Korea, Japan, China, Far-east of Russia, the Philippines, Malaysia, Indonesia, and India.

Morphology

Living adult worms are pinkish-brown in color and bean-shaped (7.5 to 12mm in length,

3. 5 to 5. 0mm in width, and 3. 5 to 5. 0mm in thickness). Its tegument is covered in many small spines. Adults have 2 muscular suckers, an oral sucker situated anteriorly and a ventral sucker at mid-body on the ventral surface. The bifurcated gut is not branched. For the sexual organs, the testes are lobed, and are parallel in the posterior portion of the body, whilst the ovary is also lobed, and is located above the testis, usually on the right hand side of the body, opposite a tightly coiled uterus. The vitellaria are located laterally, running from the anterior to the posterior of the parasite. The worm's name, Paragonimus, refers to as the parallel of the reproductive organs.

The egg is broadly ovoid with a distinct relatively flattened operculum, golden brown in color, measuring 80-118μm to 48-60μm, and containing a germ cell and many yolk cells when ova deposited. The shell varies in thickness, thickened at the non-operculate end. The maximum width is near the operculum than the equator of the eggs (see Figure 5-4-1).

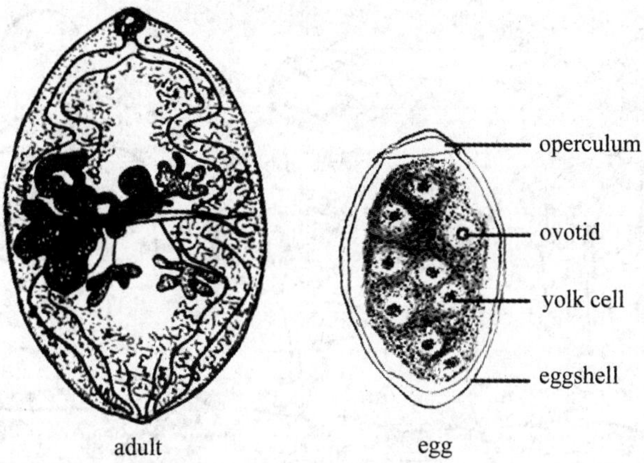

Figure 5-4-1 Adult worm and egg of *Paragonimus westermani*

Life Cycle

Paragonimus require three hosts to complete their life cycle.

Definitive host: Man and many other carnivorous animals (dog, cats, tiger, lcopard).

First intermediate host: Fresh water snail of the genus Melania.

Second intermediate host: Fresh water crab or crayfish.

In appropriate final host, the adult parasites normally live in the cystic cavities of the lungs, which always rupture or lead into the bronchia, though ectopic parasites found in other locations are also frequently seen. Unembryonated eggs are laid by the parasites, and are passed either directly in the sputum, or may be swallowed then passed in the faeces. The miracidium develops over 3 weeks at 30℃, then hatches in water to infect the snail intermediate host by penetration. These snail hosts belong to a number of genera depending on the geographical location of the parasite, but the principle host is species of the genus *Semisulcospira*. The parasite undergoes a series of asexual developments from sporocyst, two generations of redia, then finally the cercaria. Morphologically these cercaria are unusual having only a small tail, a spiny tegument and a stylet. They, which can survive up to 48 hours, do not swim to find their next host, but either crawl in a leech-like manner or are carried by currents in the water. Once the cercaria locate the second intermediate host, they penetrate in the gills, muscles and viscera of them, and encyst as metacercaria, where they are infective after 6 weeks. Infection of the definitive hosts takes place by eating raw or undercooked fresh-water crustaceans. The metacercariae excyst and adolescariae penetrate through the gut wall into the peritoneal cavity, from where they migrate through the diaphragm into the thoracic cavity and into the lungs. The migration through the body takes 2-3 weeks, becoming mature parasites in 2-3 months and living up to 20 years (see Figure 5-4-2).

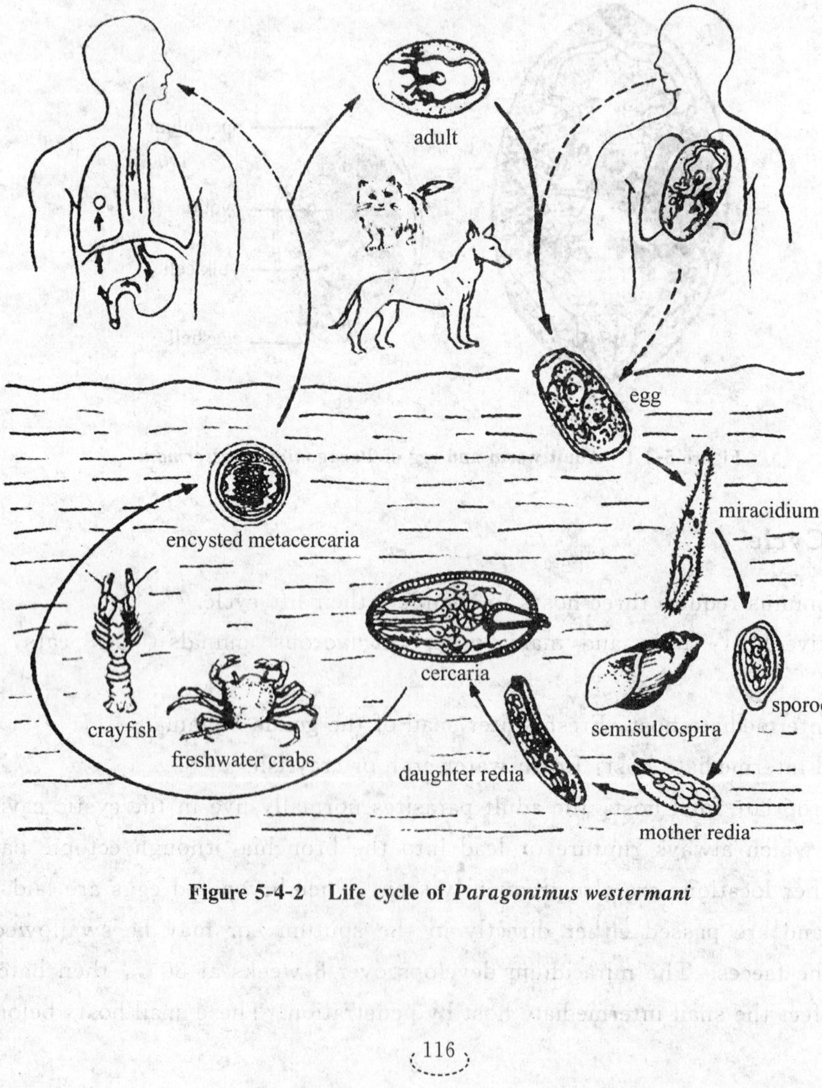

Figure 5-4-2 Life cycle of *Paragonimus westermani*

Pathogenesis

Pathogenic effects result from migratory phase of juveniles as well as from adults migrate in the tissue and organs. The metabolite and secretion of juveniles and adults also can cause anaphylatoxis. The disease process can be divided into two stages:

Acute stage: During larval migratory phase, once the larvae penetrate through the mucosa of the intestinal wall and reach the peritoneal cavity, they begin to migrate through organs and tissue, inducing the formation of localized hemorrhagic or purulent tunnels and leucocytic infiltration.

Chronic stage: As the worm settle down in the lungs, more pronounced tissue reaction occur, which can be divided into three phases:

(1)**Abscess stage**: In the lung, the worm's migration leads to the damage of tissue and hemorrhage. A cyst with thin wall is formed by leukocytic infiltration around the worm and fibrous tissue. In the cyst, there are numerous neutrophils and eosinophils. On chest radiograms, infiltrative shadows with edge blurry may be recognized in the majority of cases.

(2)**Cystic stage**: Following the exudative inflammation, around the worms a large number of cells infiltrate, die and liquate, and the fibrous granulation tissue of the wall proliferate, making the cystic wall thicker and nodule-like construction formed. On X-ray, the nodule-shadows with distinct border may be observed. The cyst is filled with many eggs, Charcot-Leyden crystals and metabolites including brown breakdown product of hemoglobin excreted from the mouth of the worm. When the communication the cyst with a bronchiolar branch occur, these contents may appear in the sputum, which becomes blood tinged and dark (so-called rusty sputum), and then in the feces.

(3)**Fibrous scar stage**: If the worms die or escape, the cystic contents are expelled or absorbed and the cysts gradually shrink. The granulation tissue eventually is replaced by fibrous scar tissue.

When the worms settle down in the peritoneal cavity or other sites outside the lungs, the worm cysts are similar to pulmonic cysts. More dangerous, however, is an intracranial invasion of the worm itself, which may be fatal to the host.

Clinical Manifestation

About 20% of patients with paragonimiasis are asymptomatic. Abdominal pain, diarrhea, and urticaria occur during the acute phase, which corresponds to the period of invasion and migration of immature flukes. These initial symptoms are followed a few days later by fever, cough, dyspnea, chest pain, malaise, and sweats. The acute phase usually persists several weeks. During the chronic phase, manifestations may be pulmonary or extrapulmonary. Chronic pulmonary symptoms consist of dry cough followed by a cough productive of tenacious and rusty or golden sputum. Pulmonary symptoms begin approximately 6 months after infection and are often mistaken for symptoms of tuberculosis (TB). If not treated, the symptoms can last several years. Ectopic paragonimiasis results in granulomatous lesions in the organs other than the lung. The most commonly affected tissues include spleen, kidney, brain, intestinal wall, peritoneum, mesenteric lymph nodes, muscle, testis/ovary, subcutaneous tissues, spinal cord. Migrating subcutaneous lesions can also be developed. The most serious illness is cerebral paragonimiasis, which is associated with several neurological symptoms. Migrating worms frequently invoke subacute hematoma. Chronic cerebral paragonimiasis, which results from calcifying granuloma, is mainly manifested by partial seizure, headache, and homonymous hemianopia. Predilection sites of the cerebral involvement include temporal, occipital, and parietal lobes.

Diagnosis

Diagnosis is based on microscopic demonstration of eggs in stool or sputum, but these are not present until 2 to 3 months after infection. Intradermal test is also available in large-scale based screening but not good for individual patient due to its low specificity. Enzyme-linked immunosorbent assay (ELISA) and immunoblot are reliable in detecting specific IgG antibodies. In case of cerebral paragonimiasis, CSF tests are highly recommended. Radiologic examination by high resolution chest CT provide definitive clue for paragonimiasis. Brain CT/MRI are also highly diagnostic either in active or in chronic calcified neuroparagonimiasis.

Epidemiology

P. westermani is distributed worldwide in foci, but is particularly prevalent in the coastal regions of Africa, South America, Far East including Japan, Korea, China, South East Asia and Papua New Guinea. In China, paragonimiasis is endemic in 23 provinces except Tibet, Xinjiang, Inner Mongolia, Qinghai, and Ningxia. The prevalence is related to the consumption of uncooked fresh water crabs and cray fish. Many wild carnivores (wild bores, pigs, foxes, cats, dogs, and monkeys) serve as reservoirs of metacercariae.

Human infections occur from ingestion of flesh or juice of insufficiently cooked, or pickled crab or cray fish that contains *Paragonimus* metacercariae. The practice of maintaining raw crab in brine, wine, or vinegar is usually ineffectual in killing metacecariae. In China, shrimps have also been found to be infected. Infection can also occur by ingesting metacercarie from fingers contaminated during food preparation.

Prevention and Control

Human infection is closely related with eating habits of foods. In many endemic regions, people acquire the infection by eating raw/undercooked freshwater crustaceans. Raw boar meat harboring excysted metacercariae are also infective.

Praziquantel is a drug of choice to treat paragonimiasis with more than 95% efficiency. Praziquantel is definitely effective in early stage of active cerebral paragonimiasis. Bithionol is an alternative drug for treatment of this disease. Triclabendazole is also effective. In the cases of chronic calcified cerebral paragonimiasis, surgical removal is recommended.

Pagumogonimus skrjabini

It was found by Chen (1959) and named in commemoration of the Russian parasitologist. Reported cases of its infection are so far limited to China. The adult is characterized by a long, slender, spindle-shaped body, with its posterior half being markedly tapered and its ventral sucker being situated anteriorly. The ovary and testis are well-branched and small for the size of the body. The surface of the body is covered with singly spaced cuticular spines (see Figure 5-4-3). The eggs measure 71.0×48.0μm on the average and the eggshell is generally of uniform thickness. The life cycle is identical with those of other lung flukes. Final hosts are Paguma larvata, cats, dogs and possibly weasels. Snail hosts are *Tricula gushuiensis* and *Akiyoshia orientalis*; crab hosts are *Sinopotamon denticulatum* and *S. yaanensis*. Human infection is effected by ingestion of raw or improperly cooked crabs such as "drunken crabs". It was due to its characteristic clinical features that this paragonimiasis attracted the attention of Szechuan doctors: frequent pleural effusion and eosinophilia, infrequent ectopic parasitism—most commonly in the subcutaneous tissues and sometimes even in the eyeball, and rather rare detection of eggs in the sputum. Thus, as the adult of *P. skrjabini* requires the exchange of sperm. Pathology, diagnosis and treatment are the same as for the other paragonimiasis.

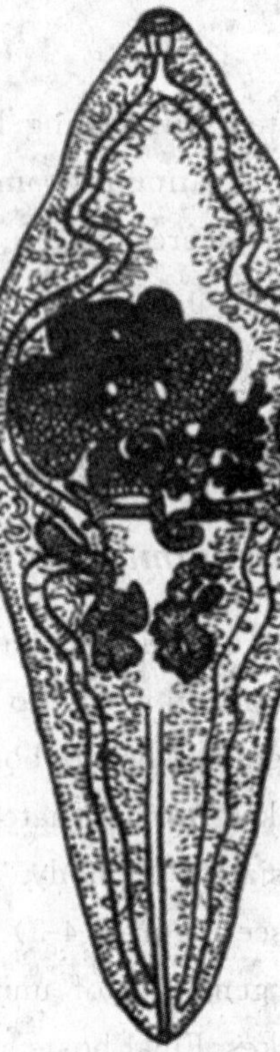

Figure 5-4-3 Adult worm of *Pagumogonimus skrjabini*

(Shi Junyan and Luo Enjie)

Section 5 Blood flukes

Three species of schistosomes that parasitize humans are of major importance: *Schistosoma mansoni*, *S. japonicum*, and *S. haematobium*. Less common are *Schistosoma intercalatum* in Africa and *Schistosoma mekongi* in the Mekong Basin. Otherwise, many birds' and mammals' schistosomes are the common dermatitis-producer.

Unlike other flukes, adult worms are diecious (gonochorism), and the two sexes are dissimilar in appearance. Female worms are long (12 to 26mm) and slender, with a body almost circular in cross section and 0.3mm or less in diameter. Male worms are 6 to 22mm long, and although the body is flattened behind the ventral sucker, it looks cylindrical, as it is characteristically incurved ventrally to form a gynecophoral canal in which the female reposes. Adult schistosomes reside in mesenteric veins that drain the intestine (*S. mansoni* and *S. japonicum*) or in vesicular veins serving the urinary bladder (*S. haematobium*). In single-sex infection, the sexual organs of female worms are undeveloped, leading to the hypothesis that one or more male factors are essential for complete maturation of the female. The pregnant females deposite eggs in smaller venules. Eggs are not operculated, and the most important pathogenic agent that causes delayed hypersensitivity leading to impairment of involved organs. Schistosomes have only one snail intermediate host and their infective stage is the cercaria swimming in water. Human gets infection by the cercaria penetrating the skin.

Schistosomiasis is often know as "bilharziasis" after German parasitologist Theodor Bilharz, working in Egypt, discovered one of the parasites (*Schistosoma haematobium*) responsible for urinary schistosomiasis in 1852. However, there are recorded accounts of the disease dating from pharaonic times. Schistosome eggs have been recovered from both Egyptian mummies. This disease is widely prevalent in Nile Valley. In 1904, in Hubei province of China, a Japanese professor Katsurada recognized this worm and named it *Schistosoma japonicum*. Chinese archaeologists found this worm in bodies from tombs dating from the second century B. C. respectively in Jiangling, Hubei Province and Changsha, Hunan Province. *Schistosomiasis mansoni* occurs over extensive areas of Africa and in the Arabian Peninsula. A consequence of the African slave trade was the establishment of S. *mansoni* in the South America. Schistosomiasis is one of the Six Major Tropical Diseases to which WHO pays great attention.

Human infections by these flukes number in excess of 250 million worldwide, and in spite of efforts to control this disease, the level of incidence has shown no significant decrease. In China alone, a recent estimate indicated at least 15 million cases of schistosomiasis japonica, representing the single most serious disease in that country. Egypt has one of the most heavily infected populations in the world, since not only is S. *haematobium* endemic to that country, but S. *mansoni* also occurs with great frequency. Among the inhabitants of some endemic areas of the Nile Valley, the infection rate exceeds 80%. Other areas of high incidence include tropical and subtropical Africa, parts of South America, and several of the Caribbean islands.

Schistosoma japonicum

The Oriental blood fluke S. *japonicum* is confined to the Far East, where it occurs in parts of China (including Taiwan), Japan, the Philippines, and Indonesia (Sulawesi). Unlike S. *mansoni*, which rarely infects other animals, S. *japonicum* is found in virtually all mammals exposed to infected water. In 1904, in China, a Japaneses professor Katsurada recognized a fluke which lived in human body and other mammals, and differentiated from S. *haematobium*, so that named it *Schistosoma japonicum*. Chinese archaeologists found this worm in a body from a tomb dating from the second century B. C. in Jiangling, Hubei province. Only this schistosomiasis has been found in China, which is one of the five major parasitic diseases of China. It is prevalent in 12 provinces, municipalities directly under the Central government, and autonomic regions along the Yangtze River and in the south of Yangtze. These are the main regions for producing rice and fish in China, where this disease seriously harms the health of the people who work in rice fields, fish and play in fresh water. Before 1949, there were 20 million patients suffering from schistosomiasis japonica. A recent estimate indicated at least 15 million cases, representing the single most serious disease in that country, and 100 million people exposing to the danger of infection. Chairman Mao's poem "Farewell God to the Plague", vividly described the tragic scene of endemic areas in old China. As a result of concerted control measures for 50 years, the incidence in China has been somewhat reduced. Today, in order to eradicate this disease, we still have much to do.

Morphology

Unlike other flukes, adult worms are diecious (gonochorism), elongate and cylindrical in shape, and gray white in color but females much darker. Two sexes are dissimilar in appearance.

Male worms are thick and short measuring 10 to 20mm by 0.5 to 0.55mm in size. The oral sucker is on top, just anterior to the ventral sucker. Although the body is flattened behind the ventral sucker, it looks cylindrical, as it is characteristically incurved ventrally to form a gynecophoral canal in which the female reposes (see Figure 5-5-1). The mouth opens in the oral sucker. The esophagus is separated into two branches, which converge and fuse at the mid part of the body, then continue as a single cecum to the posterior end. Seven testes are situated one after another behind the ventral sucker. Each testis has a delicate vas efferens which combines to form a vas deferens. The latter dilates to become the seminal vesicle, which opens ventrally through the genital pore just behind the ventral sucker (Figure 5-5-1).

Female worms are longer and more slender than males and measure 12 to 26mm by 0.1 to 0.3mm in size. Their digestive tracts are similar to those of the males. The vitellaria surrounding the cecum are in the posterior part of the body. The unbranched and oval ovary lies in the mid-portion of the body. The uterus lies in the anterior part of the body and opens into the genital pore just behind the ventral sucker. It contains 50 to 300 eggs, which are arranged in single row (Figure 5-5-1).

The mature eggs are oval in shape and slightly yellow in color. They measure 74 to 106μm by 55 to 80μm. The thin shell does not have an operculum but has a minute lateral spine. It is difficult to see egg structure as the host's necrotic tissue adheres to it. When they are discharged in feces, a miracidium is present in the shell (Figure 5-5-1).

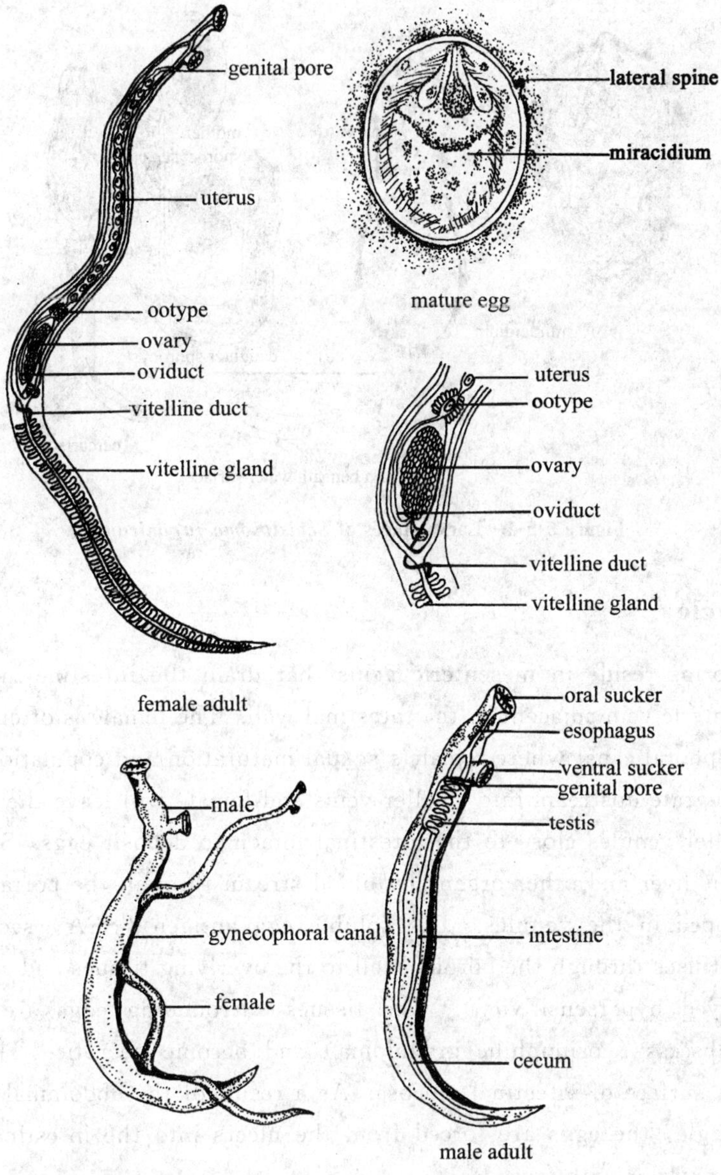

Figure 5-5-1 Adults and egg of *Schistosoma japonicum*

The cercaria swims in fresh water. It is composed of three parts, body, tail stem and tail fork. The body measures 100 to 160μm, tail stem 140 to 160μm, tail fork 50 to 75μm. It has 5 pairs of penetrating glands in the posterior part of the body. The oral sucker is slightly large than the ventral sucker (see Figure 5-5-2).

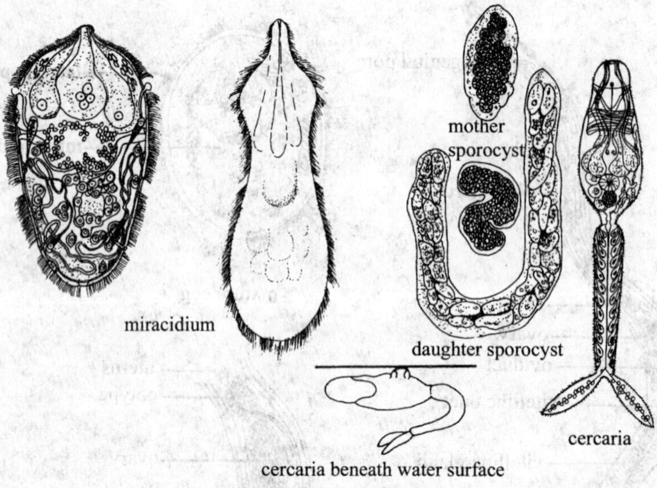

Figure 5-5-2 Larva stages of *Schistosoma japonicum*

Life Cycle

Adult worms reside in mesenteric veins that drain the intestine, mainly in the inferior mesenteric vein adjacent to the intestinal wall. The female is often found in the male's gynecophoral canal where female's sexual maturation and copulation take place. The worms migrate upstream into smaller veins and female will leave the gynecophoral canal for smaller venules close to the intestinal lumen to deposit eggs. Some eggs are carried into the liver and other organs by blood stream through the portal vein. Many eggs are trapped in the venules. The soluble egg antigen (SEA) secreted by the miracidium diffuses through the porous shell to the overlying tissues and cause localized allergy (delayed hypersensitivity). The tissues surrounding eggs are replaced by eosinophilic abscess (eosinophilic granuloma) and become necrotic. The ulcers are formed on the surface of intestinal mucosa. As a result of the abdominal pressure and intestinal wriggle, the eggs are forced from the ulcers into the intestinal lumen and passed to the exterior with feces.

Upon eggs reaching fresh water, the miracidia hatch in 6 hours at 20℃-30℃. To survive, the free-swimming miracidium (see Figure 5-5-3) must penetrate an Oncomelania snail, the intermediate host, within a few hours. In the snail it undergoes a process of asexual reproduction, including mother sporocyst, daughter sporocyst and cercaria stages. Then many cercariae escape from the snail host into the water. The cercariae alternately swim to the surface of the water and then sink slowly to the bottom, or they may adhere to the surface film and come to rest while they await contact with their next host, continuing in this way for 1 to 3 days. As appropriate definitive hosts, such as human or buffalo, contact with the water contaminated by cercariae, cercariae actively adhere to the hosts' skin by means of both its muscular suckers and then penetrate the skin under the help of the secretions from their penetrating glands. They require only half an hour or less to completely penetrate the epidermis and then disappear through the skin surface in 10 to 30 seconds. The penetration is accompanied by a vigorous wiggling, together with exhaustion of the products of penetrating glands. The tail is cast off in this process. Within 24 hours they develop into schistosomulum (adolescent), as they are now called, and then enter the peripheral circulation or lymphatic, and are swept off to the right heart. Schistosomules appear in pulmonary capillaries by the third day after penetration. A week to 10 days late, they move through the pulmonary vein to the left side of the heart and then into the systemic circulation. They reach the liver via the mesenteric arteries, capillaries and hepatoportal vein or liver artery. After undergoing a period of about 3 weeks of development in liver sinusoids, the young worms migrate upstream to the branches of mesenteric vein, where the females begin to reside in the males' gynecophoral canal. They reach sexual maturity and mate after penetration 40 days. Males with females enclosed in their gynecophoral canals then migrate against the portal flow to venules at the definitive sites. The pregnant female migrates alone to smaller venules close to the intestinal lumen before depositing eggs. The development in human body takes about 4 to 5 weeks (see Figure 5-5-3).

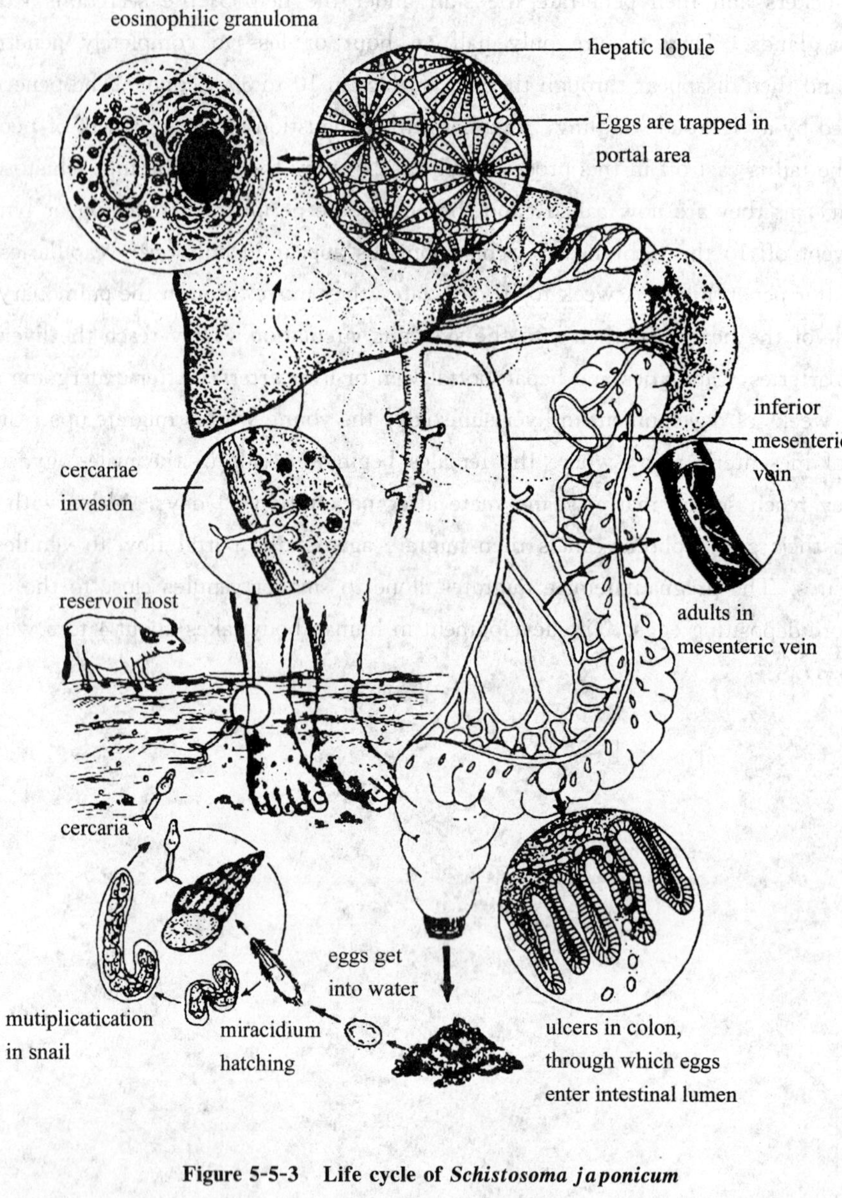

Figure 5-5-3 Life cycle of *Schistosoma japonicum*

Pathogenesis and Clinical Manifestation

The pathogenic mechanism of schistosomes differs somewhat according to the species of the fluke involved, mainly because of the preferred site of each.

Due to cercaria and schistosomulum: When human or bird schistosome cercariae repeatedly penetrate human skin, an anaphylaxis (allergy I) takes place. Local schistosomal dermatitis manifests petechiae and rashes with itching and burning sensation. The blood to lung migration of schistosomulums causes the same hypersensitivity as pneumonitis, hepatitis and urticaria. These may be very mild and may pass unnoticed, or there may be generalized malaise, fever, cough, hemoptysis, vague intestinal complaints and so forth.

Due to adult: The mechanical and toxic effects of adults and their metabolites, excreta and secretions cause mesenteric phlebitis, hepatitis, eosinophilia and abdominal pain. Some immunocomplex causes nephritis (allergy III).

Due to egg: the most serious damage is done by eggs. Many eggs are trapped in the venules. The soluble egg antigen (SEA) secreted by the miracidium diffuse through the porous shell to the overlying tissues and cause local antibody dependent cell mediated cytotoxicity (ADCC, allergy II) and delayed hypersensitivity (allergy IV). The tissues surrounding eggs are replaced by eosinophilic abscess (eosinophilic granuloma) and fibroplastic infiltration. These finally become necrotic and fibrous nodules or pseudotubercles (fibrosis or cirrhosis). The involved tissues include the colon, where ulcers are formed, and the liver. As eggs lodged in the intralobular veins in front of the hepatic sinusoids, the pathologic change occurs there. An apparent portal hypertension and slightly functional loss are the pathophysiological characteristic of this interstitium liver cirrhosis. In severe cases, several years later, the portal hypertension, splenomegaly, anemia, decrease in albumin level and ascites ensue. The cirrhosis will impair the blood flow to the liver via the portal vein, and the collateral circulations have to be established so that the esophageal and abdominal wall varicosities follow. Lungs, spinal and brain may also be involved because the there are anastomoses between the portal vein, vena cava and spinal vein. The damage to the central nerve system may cause paralysis. There is no enough evidence to prove that the eggs induce liver cancer (see Figure 5-5-3).

Symptoms

Incubation period, prior to the onset of symptoms may vary from several days to 2 month. The first symptom of schistosomiasis is localized dermatitis, often appearing after cercariae penetrate the skin. The characteristic itching and local rashes usually disappear after 4 days. Following skinpenetration, the symptoms of human schistosomiasis appear in four phases.

Migration phase, 4 to 10 weeks after infection, is characterized by toxic reactions and pulmonary congestion (pneumonitis) accompanied by fever, manifesting dry cough, distension of abdomen, lumbar and back pain, diarrhea, and urticaria. These phenomena are caused by the migration of adolescents.

Acute stage is considerably longer, lasting 2 months to several years. Characteristic symptoms, such as bloody stools with chill, fever and malaise, are caused by the passage of eggs through the intestinal wall. The Patients pass stool 5 to 10 times a day with blood, pus, mucus and massive eggs. Then these symptoms gradually subside.

Chronic stage lasts several years to 20 years. The patients experience fatigue, loss of weight and their general condition and work ability gradually deteriorate. Child patients may manifest the retardation of both physical and mental growth and loss of interest. The spleen and liver may be enlarged and anemia may result. In women of childbearing age there may be amenorrhea, sterility and abortion. In endemic areas, the reinfection is common. There are excessive eggs and scar tissue formation in the involved organs of the patients, which impedes the normal functioning of involved organs.

In terminal stage, patient may manifest all symptoms and signs of portal vein hypertension syndrome and liver function failure. The patient is very emaciated from the long illness, with a big abdomen distended by a great deal of ascites. Anemia is very serious. The patients may die of nutritional exhaustion, hepatic coma, and complications such as secondary infection and upper digestive tract bleeding.

Diagnosis

The patients' experience of being born and having been in endemic areas, and symptoms and signs are for reference, but the surest means of diagnosis is finding and identifying characteristic eggs in excreta or in tissue biopsies, particularly rectal biopsies. In chronic cases in which very few if any eggs are passed, biopsies can be used advantageously. The stool examination can be performed by direct smear or sedimentation and miracidium hatching technique. The direct fecal smear is suitable for the stool with blood and pus from the patients in acute stage. The concentration methods, such as water sedimentation and nylon net filter, are used for the stool from patients in chronic stage, who pass a few eggs.

Immunodiagnostic tests are for reference only, however, false positive or false negative results from these tests should be confirmed by identification of eggs, because false positives sometimes result from concomitant infections with other parasites or exposure to various animal schistosome cercariae. The following methods can be used, e.g., (1) intradermal test, (2) Cercarien Hüllen Reaction (CHR), (3) circumoval precipitation test (COP), (4) indirect haemagglutination test (IHA), (5) immunofluorescent test (IF), (6) enzyme-linked immunosorbent assay (ELISA), (7) circulating antigen detection(CAgD).

Immunity

Immunity to human schistosomiasis is not totally understood. It is known that animals experimentally infected with schistosomes normally infective to humans develop immunity to these parasites. The life span of adult schistosomes in the human host can be more than 30 years. As noted earlier, during much of their life time the worms are prolific egg producers, and this output over such a long period elicits a wide range of immune responses, both humoral and cell-mediated. In fact, such responses can be correlated with various parasitic stages in the human host. The first, or skin-penetration stage, is characterized by a reaction to the penetrating cercaria's surface coat and penetration gland secretions, both released into the host's tissues. During the second, or early development stage, there is a response caused by the tegumental changes in the migrating schistosmulum. The third, or adult worm and egg stages, precipitates a response to immunogens released from the adult worm's intestine, tegument, and excretory system. The reaction to eggs is in response to immunogens released from either migrating or trapped eggs. The immunogens are macromolecules that diffuse through micropores in the eggshell. While some of these macromolecules facilitate migration of the eggs through the tissues, they also elicit a granulomatous response to eggs trapped in the tissues, causing pronounced pathological changes.

If worms produce immunogens to which the host responds, how do the worms evade this response? Although there is not yet a complete answer to this question, several significant factors provide clues. Perhaps the most remarkable of these is the ability of the worm to acquire host antigens on its surface. These antigens afford protection by disguising the worm's surface so that it escapes detection by the host immune mediators. Antigen acquisition apparently begins during the early schistosomule stage and may be associated with the initiation of feeding on host blood. Logically, therefore, an effective vaccine should be a living vaccine or must target the larval stage before such protection is attained.

Epidemiology

The Oriental blood fluke (*Schistosoma japonicum*) is confined to the Far East, where it occurs in parts of China (including Taiwan), Japan, the Philippines, Indonesia (Sulawesi), Thailand , Laos, Kampuchea, and Vietnam. In China it is prevalent in 12 provinces, municipalities directly under the Central Government, autonomic regions along the Yangtze River Valley and in the south of Yangtze. These are the main regions for producing rice and fish in China, where this disease seriously harms the health of the people who work in water as rice farmer, fishing man or play in fresh water and causes great economic loss. A recent estimate indicated at least 15 million cases, representing the single most serious disease in that country, and 100 million people exposing to the danger of infection.

The geographical distribution of schistosomiasis is limited by existence of Oncomelania snails. The Oncomelania are amphibious. They measure 10mm or less in length and 3-4mm in width. They live in warm (annual temperature over 0℃) and rainy (annual rainfall over 750mm) regions where grass and vegetation grow along canal, stream and river or by pool and lake. The old custom of defecating in or near the water in which people play, swim, fishing and wash clothes, is an important factor for the spread of this disease.

In endemic areas, animal reservoir hosts help to maintain the infection although human infections are not common. Buffalo, cattle, dogs, pigs, rodents, and other mammals are appropriate hosts. Rodents and buffalo are the most dangerous source of infection. Generally, adult and young men have a higher incidence than women because they more frequently expose to the water contaminated by cercariae.

Prevention and Control

The chemotherapeutic agent recommended for all species of human schistosomes is praziquantel. By disrupting the integrity of the schistosome tegument, this drug apparently exposes otherwise inaccessible antigens as targets for host antibodies. It is effective and safe. Other useful drugs are hexachloroparaxylol. These drugs frequently result in side effects such as vomiting, headache, cramps, dizziness, rash, etc.

It is difficult to prevent people from schistosomiasis because of the wild and domestic reservoir hosts. The eradication of sail hosts and changing of unhealthy habit are not easy. No reliable prophylactic regimen is presently available other than the observance of proper hygiene and sanitation procedures, avoidance of cercaria-infested waters, and prevention of water contamination by human excreta.

According to the World Health Organization, the key to eventual schistosomiasis control lies in a four-pronged attack: population-based chemotherapy, with repeated drug administration to infected individuals; use of molluscicides; introduction of biological controls, such as carnivorous snails and fish; and education of the population to control night soil, avoid coming into direct contact with water contaminated by cercariae; realize modernization of agriculture and fishing and control reservoir hosts.

(Yuan Fangshu, Guo Shuling and He Shenyi)

Other *Schistosoma* spp.

In addition to S. *japonicum*, five other species of schistosomes can infect humans. They are S. *mansoni*, S. *haematobium*, S. *intercalatum*, S. *mekongi* and S. *malayensis* respectively. They are generally similar to S. *japonicum*, and may also give rise to heavy infections, pathology and serious disease. The comparisons of six human species in detail are listed in Table 5-5-1.

Table 5-5-1 The comparison of six human schistosome

Item		*S. japonicum*	*S. mansoni*	*S. haematobium*	*S. intercalatum*	*S. mekongi*	*S. malayensis*
Location of adult in host		Mesenteric veins	Mesenteric veins	Vesical plexus	Mesenteric veins	Mesenteric veins	Mesenteric veins
Size (mm)	Female	20-25× 0. 1-0. 3	7-17× 0. 25	16-20×0. 25	11-26×0. 25	12×0. 23	9. 16×0. 21
	Male	12-20× 0. 5-0. 55	6-14× 0. 8-1. 1	10-15× 0. 75-1. 0	11-14× 0. 3-0. 5	6. 48-11. 3 ×0. 41	6. 82×0. 32
Tegumental tubercles	Female	Absent	Fine	Fine	Fine	Absent	Absent
	Male	Absent	Coarse	Fine	Fine	Absent	Absent
Length of post gut cecum		Medium	Very long	Short	Short	Medium	Medium
Uterus	Length	Short	Very short	Long	Long	Short	Short
	Position in body	Front half	Front half	Front two thirds	Front two thirds	Front half	Front half
	No. of eggs	50-300	1-2	10-100	5-60	10+	Many
Position of ovary in body		Middle half	Front third	Rear half	Rear half	Rear third	Middle half
Position of vitellaria		Posterior quarter of body	Few follicles, Posterior to ovary	Few follicles, Posterior to ovary	Few follicles, posterior to ovary	posterior five eighth of body	posterior half to two third of body
Eggs/female (day)		3500	100-300	20-300	150-400	?	?
No. of testes		6-8	2-14	4-5	4-6	7	6-8
Egg	Shape	Round	Ovoid	Ovoid	Ovoid	Round	Round
	Size (μm)	89×67	140×61	150×62	176×61	45 × 40	67×54
	Spine	Lateral	Lateral	Terminal	Terminal	Lateral	Lateral
	normally passed in	Feces	Feces	Urine	Feces (and Urine)	Feces	Feces
	Size of deposit in body	Normally in colon and liver	Normally in colon and liver	Urogenital system	Normally in colon and liver	Normally in colon and liver	Normally in colon and liver
Site of pathological changes		Mainly in liver and bowel wall	Mainly in liver and bowel wall	Urinary bladder and genital system	Mainly in liver and bowel wall	Mainly in liver and bowel wall	Mainly in liver and bowel wall
Type of disease		Intestinal schistosomiasis	Intestinal schistosomiasis	Urinary schistosomiasis	Intestinal schistosomiasis	Intestinal schistosomiasis	Intestinal schistosomiasis
Intermediate host		*Oncomelania*	*Biomphalaria*	*Bulinus*	*Bulinus*	*Neotricula*	*Robertsiella*

Reservoir host	Wide range of domestic and wild animals	Primates, field mouse, etc.	Primates, sheep, pigs, Nile rat, etc.	Primates, sheep, rodents	Primates, carnivores	Primates, rodents
Distribution	Asia (China, Japan, Philippines and Indonesia)	Africa, Latin America, West Indian archipelago	Africa, West Asia, Portugal	Africa (Cameroon, Congo, Gabon, Chad and Zaire)	Southeast Asia (Cambodia, Laos and Thailand)	Southeast Asia (Malaysia)

S. *intercalatum* is morphologically indistinguishable from S. *mattheei*, a natural schistosome of African ruminants. However, S. *mattheei* apparently can merely infect primates in the presence of a coinfection with S. *mansoni* or S. *haematobium*. In Southeast Asia, careful examinations of morphology, biology, and molecular analysis have supported recognition of S. *mekongi* and S. *malayensis* as distinct from S. *japonicum*, which they closely resemble and are arranged in a group, i. e., S. *japonicum* group (rounded, minutely-spined, or spineless eggs). Species in the S. *japonicum* group use snails of the class *Prosobranchia* as intermediate hosts and other species of *Schistosoma* use snails of the class *Pulmonata*.

Humans can also be infected by nonhuman schistosomes, such as bird and mammal schistosomes. Although many die in the skin, others may progress to various levels of development. Especially if hybrid pairing appears in mixed infections, the parasites sometimes even reach maturity. Such zoonotic infections do not, generally, cause severe disease although they may produce minor pathology. However, the results of immunodiagnostic tests can be confused. Especially for antibodies, immune responses can be triggered and cause cross-reactions. It has also been suggested that the severity of normal human schistosome infections might be ameliorated by provoking heterologous immunity. Ingesting animals infected with nonhuman schistosomes, especially their livers, may lead to exotic schistosome eggs being found by parasitological stool examinations, causing spurious reports of human infections with these species. The intermediate host snails of human schistosomes can also transmit nonhuman schistosomes. This complicates transmission studies because the different cercariae are difficult to distinguish under field conditions.

Schistosome Cercarial Dermatitis ("Swimmer's Itch")

Several species of bird and livestock schistosomes in the genus *Schistosoma* cause a severe rash but cannot complete the life cycle and tend to die without migrating or maturing when their cercariae penetrate the skin of human, an unsuitable host. It is cercarial dermatitis. It is called swimmer's itch in swamp of USA and Canada, and paddy-field dermatitis in the planting rice areas of China. It is distributed in Jilin,

Liaoning, Jiangsu, Fujian, Guangdong, Hunan, Sichuan, and other provinces and Shanghai Municipality.

A lot of species of bird and livestock schistosomes are distributed throughout the world and can cause cercarial dermatitis when their cercariae attack anyone on whose skin the organisms land. In China, the genera *Trichobilharzia* and *Ornithobilharzia* are the guilty parties. Several species of the genus *Trichobilharzia* are *T. paoi*, *T. jianensis*, *T. ocellate*, *T. gigantica*, *T. zongshani*, etc. The genus *Ornithobilharzia* are *O. turkenstanica*, *O. cheni*, etc. *Lymnea* is their intermediate host. Duck, cattle and goat are their definitive host, respectively.

For the most part the skin reaction is a product of sensitization, with repeated infections causing increasingly severe reactions. The human's defense responses can rapidly kill cercaria when it penetrates the skin and is unable to complete its migration or maturing. Simultaneously, the cercariae release allergens that cause pruritic papular skin rash and, typically, a pus-filled pimple. The toxic reaction may also be general, with an itching rash produced over much of the body. It is immediate and delayed hypersensitivity reaction. Their usefulness is limited.

(Dong Huifen)

Section 6 Other Flukes

Fasciola hepatica

Fasciola hepatica (Linn, 1758) is a trematode that infects sheep and cattle, human infection is sporadic. It is commonly called the sheep liver fluke and one of the largest flukes of the world. It has been known as an important parasite of sheep and cattle for hundreds of years, although it is rare in humans in most countries. It has been the subject of many scientific investigations and is probably the best known of any trematode species because of its size and economic importance. The first published record of it is that of Jean de Brie in 1379.

Morphology

Although the shape varies somewhat, *F. hepatica* is rather willowy, leaf-like shaped with pointed posteriorly and wide anteriorly (see Figure 5-6-1). The marked widening of the body at the base of the so-called cephalic cone or oral cone gives the worm the appearance of having shoulders. The combination of a cephalic cone and "shoulders" is an immediate means of identification.

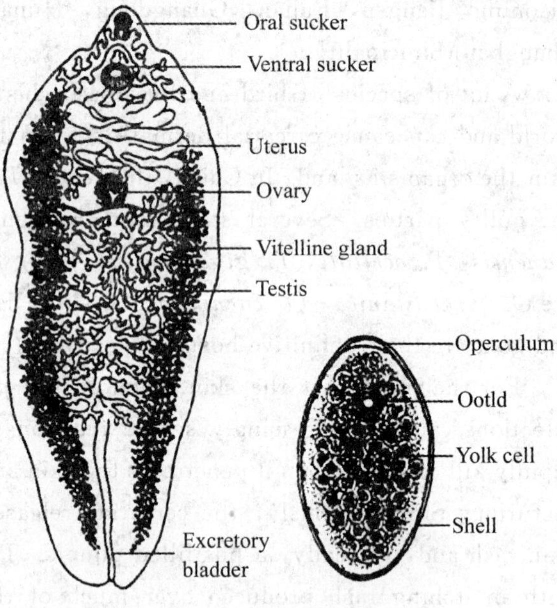

Figure 5-6-1 Morphology of *Fasciola hepatica*

Adults measure 20 to 50mm by 8 to 13mm in size. The small but powerful oral sucker is located at the end of a cone-shaped projection at the anterior end. The acetabulum is somewhat larger than the oral sucker and is quite anterior, at about the level of the shoulders. The intestinal ceca are highly branched and extend to near the posterior end of the body. The large and greatly branched testes are arranged in tandem behind the ovary. The ovary is smaller and branched, lies on the right side, shortly behind the acetabulum. The short uterus coils between the ovary and the preacetabular cirrus pouch. The vitelline follicles fill most of the lateral body. They are extensive and become confluent behind the testes.

The eggs are elongated-oval, ranging in size of 130 to 150μm by 63 to 90μm, with a thin shell and a small operculum. They are light yellow-brown, a fertilized ovum inside, which is surrounded with many vitelline-cells.

Life Cycle

Adult *F. hepatica*, a hermaphroditic liver fluke, lives in the bile ducts of the liver of many kinds of mammals, especially ruminants. Humans are occasionally infected. The flukes feed on the lining of the biliary ducts and produces large numbers of eggs every day for many years. Their eggs are passed out of the liver with the bile and into the lumen of the small intestine, from which they leave the body to the environment in the feces. If they fall into fresh water, the eggs will complete their development into ciliated miracidia and hatch in 9 to 10 days during warm weather. Their development will be retarded in the colder water. On hatching, the miracidium has about 24 hours in which to find a suitable intermediate host, which in our country is mainly *Galba truncatula*. Upon contact with host snails, the miracidia penetrate them and undergo several developmental stages (sporocysts, mother rediae, daughter rediae, and cercariae). Cercariae begin emerging five to seven weeks after infection. Then they are released from the snail host and encyst as metacercariae on aquatic plants. When the definitive host eats metacercariae encysted on these raw vegetations or in water, juvenile flukes excyst in the small intestine. They immediately penetrate through the intestinal wall into the peritoneal cavity, and creep over the viscera until contacting the liver capsule. Then they burrow into the hepatic tissues and wander about for almost two months, feeding and growing and finally entering bile ducts. The flukes become sexually mature in another month and begin producing eggs. Adult flukes can live as long as 11 years in sheep, 1 year in cattle, and 12 years in human (see Figure 5-6-2).

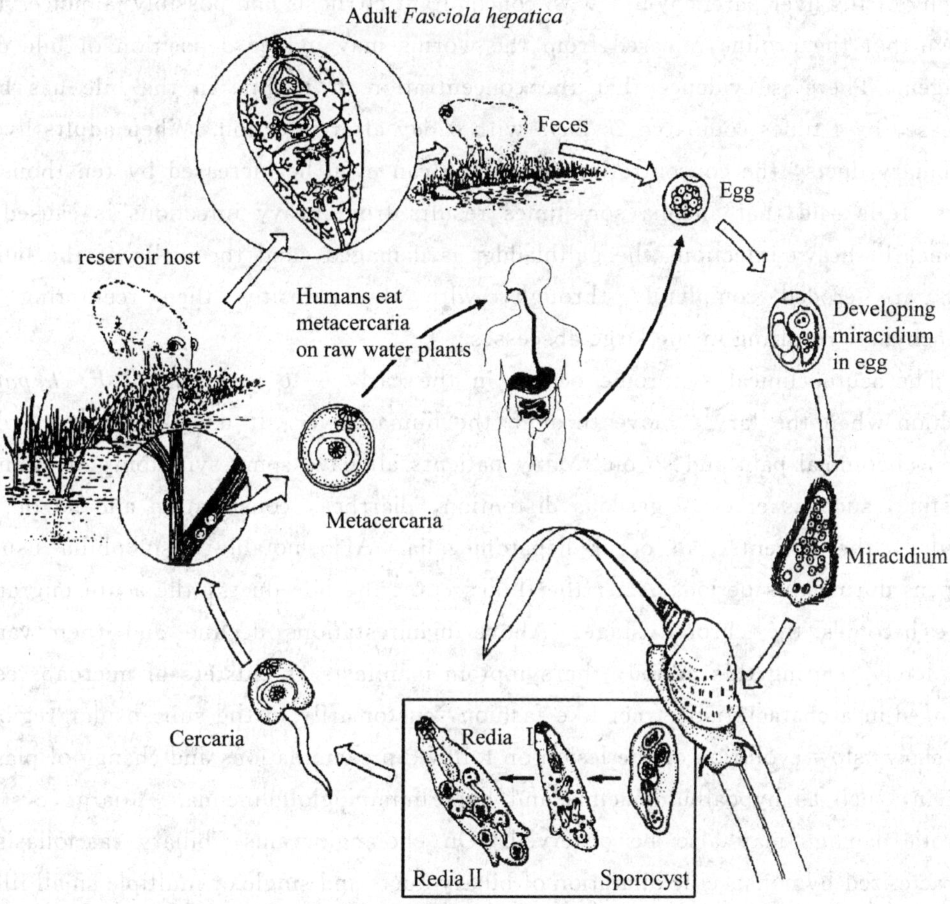

Figure 5-6-2 Life cycle of *Fasciola hepatica*

Pathogenesis and Clinical Manifestation

Pathological consequences of *F. hepatica* infection concern mainly with the numbers of the juveniles penetrating the intestinal wall and the biliary tract surrounding the liver. The damages may result from the migration of juveniles. In the liver parenchyma, the flukes commonly cause inflammation and localized destruction of liver cells. Once in the biliary ducts, they may finally produce several hepatobiliary diseases including cholangitis, hepatitis, hepatomegaly, anaemia, obstructive jaundice, and so on. It is caused by the mechanical irritation of the worms and the irritation of chemical excretions/secretions (ES) released from the worms. The basic pathogenesis is inflammation, edema and erosion of the epithelium lining the bile ducts. The worms induce proliferation of epithelial cells, desquamation of the biliary duct epithelium, bile duct hyperplasia, periductal fibrosis and inflammation. Thus thickened, the ducts can handle less bile and are less responsive to the needs of the liver. Back pressure results in atrophy of the liver parenchyma, with concomitant cirrhosis and possibly jaundice. It is known that the proline released from the worms may induce deposition of bile duct collagen. There is evidence that the concentration of proline in the bile has been increased by 4 times compared 25 days with 0 day after infection. When adults live in the biliary ducts, the concentration of proline can even be increased by ten thousand times. It is said that anemia sometimes results from heavy infections is caused by proline. In heavy infections the gallbladder is damaged, and the walls of the biliary ducts are eroded completely through, with the parasites then reentering the parenchyma, resulting in the large abscesses.

The acute clinical syndrome occurs in the early 6 to 9 weeks of *F. hepatica* infection when the larvae move through the human liver. It usually appears ardent fever, abdominal pain and so on. Many patients all have some symptoms of stomach intestine, such as emesia, gaseous distention, diarrhea, constipation and so on. In addition, the patients can occur hepatomegalia. Also notable eosinophilia usually happens during this period. After the flukes enter the bile ducts, the acute migratory stage becomes the chronic stage. Above manifestations decline and then vanish completely. During this period, the symptom manifests as clusters of microabscesses arranged in a characteristic tract like fashion, customarily in the subcapsular regions, and shows slow evolution of the lesion on follow-up examinations and change of plasma protein, such as hypoalbuminaemia and hyperimmunoglobulinemia. A large cystlike necrotic damage may also be observed. On cholangiograms, biliary fascioliasis is characterized by nonspecific dilatation of biliary ducts and single or multiple small filling defects, which represent worms themselves. Sometimes, anaemia may be seen in the patients with heavy worm burdens. Furthermore, obstructive jaundice may be caused by adult *F. hepatica*. It is quite scarce to see the chronic biliary tract disease in humans but normally found in animals with particularly heavy worm burdens. Occasionally, worms are found in the biliary ducts at surgery or autopsy. Nevertheless, foci of chronic human fascioliasis have been known in rural areas of Peru.

Migrating juveniles commonly produce ulcers in ectopic locations, such as the skin, abdominal wall muscle, peritoneum, brain, lung, eye, bladder, and so on. Among them, the skin is the most frequent locations. In addition, ectopic parasitism can also occur in the pars laryngea pharynges in the areas where locals ingest raw cattle or sheep liver and bowel. The resulting respiratory blockage is called halzoun in Arabic.

Immunity

The resistance to reinfection of *F. hepatica* has been revealed in experimental animals. Adoptive and passive transfer of resistance has been finished with cells and serum. And nonliving vaccines can induce immunity. It is interesting to find that immunization with *Fasciola* antigens will induce resistance to *Schistosoma* infection and vice versa. In this model, it is defined that the antigens responsible for protective immunity are *F. hepatica* 12 kDa fatty acid binding protein and *S. mansoni* 14 kDa fatty acid binding protein respectively. Relatively little study in this area has been performed with the other flukes.

Diagnosis

Whenever liver blockage coincides with a history of raw watercress ingestion, fascioliasis should be suspected. Definitive diagnosis of infection is based on the finding of characteristic eggs of *F. hepatica* in human feces or duodenal aspirates. Never identify *Fasciola* eggs with *Fasciolopsis* eggs or *Echinochasmus* eggs. A false record can result when the patient has eaten infected livers and characteristic eggs of *F. hepatica* pass through with the feces. This false diagnosis will be unmasked by daily examination during a liver-free diet. An enzyme-linked immunosorbent assay (ELISA) test also is available, especially in acute symptomatic fascioliasis and the case of ectopic parasitizing. Early diagnosis plays an important part in avoiding irreparable damage to the liver.

Epidemiology

F. hepatica occurs worldwide in ruminants. Sheep, cattle, and rabbits are the most frequent reservoirs of infection. The worms cause significant morbidity and mortality, and enormous loss in cattle and sheep. Humans are accidental hosts who usually eat metacercariae encysted on raw aquatic plant, particularly wild watercress. Only a few hundred cases have been reported in the world literature. Human infections appear in parts of Europe, northern Africa, South America, Cuba, and other locales. Surprisingly, few cases are found in humans in the United States, although the fluke is fairly common in parts of the South and West. In China, the infections happen in 15 provinces where the cattle and sheep are usually bred. The infection rate is the highest in Gansu, and then in Hainan. They are 1.71‰ and 1.51‰, respectively. Human fascioliasis has almost always been identified during the acute stage. Occasionally, flukes are found in the biliary ducts at surgery or autopsy. Foci of chronic fascioliasis have been found in rural areas of Peru.

Prevention and Control

Several drugs, such as a halogenated phenol, bithinol, triclabendazole, rafoxanide and so on, are all effective in chemotherapy of fascioliasis, both in humans and in domestic animals. But praziquantel is ineffective against *F. hepatica*. With respect to prevention of infection, the measures are mostly the avoidance of ingestion of raw vegetation and adherence to good sanitary practices.

(Dong Huifen)

Echinostoma

A number of species of echinostomes have been reported to infect humans. Most of the species are found in oriental countries; *E. ilocanum* is the most important species. The infection was first noted by Garrison in 1907.

Morphology

Adult

Adult echinostomes, while varying greatly in size, are easily identified by the collar of spines along the dorsal and lateral sides of the head. In general appearance, The adults are less than 1cm long and 0. 2cm wide and are reddish gray. The anterior end of the adult worm has a circumoral disk with a crown of spines surrounding the oral sucker. A relatively large ventral sucker situated immediately behind the head. The ventral sucker and oral sucker are closed. The testes lie in tandem in the posterior portion of the body, the ovary is anterior to the testes, and the short uterus consists only an ascending limb terminating at the genital pore anterior to the ventral sucker. The uterus fill with a few eggs.

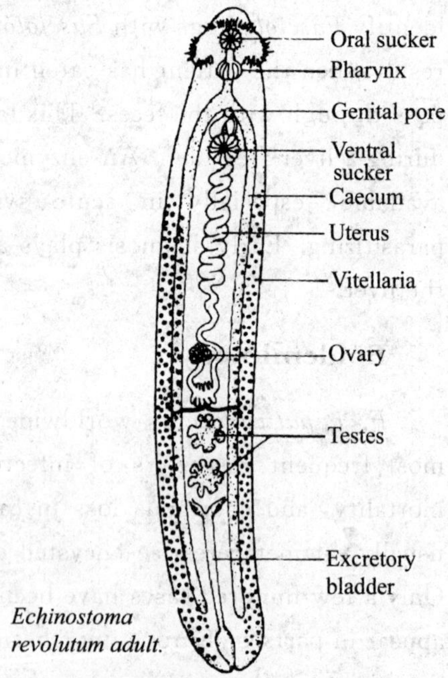

Figure 5-6-3 Adult of *Echinostoma*

Egg

The eggs measure 90 to 126μm long by 54 to 71μm wide and are oval in shape. It has operculum with thin shell. *Echinostoma trivolvis* is the prototype for echinostome species infecting humans, essential differences consisting primarily of the number and arrangement of collar spines (see Figure 5-6-3).

Life Cycle

Adult worms inhabit the upper regions of the small intestine, occasionally parasitize bile duct. The adult worms lay eggs which are passed from the definitive host with feces. The eggs must reach fresh water for the life cycle to continue. The eggs requires 2 to 5 weeks to reach maturity in the water, after which it hatches and penetrates a snail of one of the genera Lymnaea, physa, or Bithynia. Various freshwater pelecypods and gastropods serve as hosts for other echinostomes. A single sporocyst generation, two redial generations and cercariae develop in the molluscan host. The cercariae escape from daughter rediae and enter the water, then penetrate and encyst in a variety of aquatic animals including fresh water fish, batrachia or polliwog, mollusks, some of which may serve as first intermediate hosts, or, at times, on aquatic vegetation. The life cycle is completed when the definitive host ingests encysted metacercariae, which excyst and develop to sexual maturity in the small intestine.

Pathogenesis

Adult worms inhabit small intestine and their heads penetrate intestinal mucosa, causing local inflammation at the site of penetration. In severe infections, the spinose collar may cause ulceration of the intestinal mucosa. Echinostomiasis in humans is usually a minor affliction, often causing nothing more serious than diarrhea. Children sometimes experience abdominal pain, diarrhea, anemia, and/or edema.

Diagnosis

Diagnosis must be confirmed by fecal examination for eggs or adults which help identification of species. The identification of eggs from feces is facilitated by a number of distinctive features of echinostome eggs, namely, their dark brownish color and the very immature larvae, even uncleaved zygotes, which are unlike those of other intestinal trematodes. Otherwise, the diagnosis may have to be made on the basis of patient history or clinical findings.

Epidemiology

While as many as 15 species of *Echinostoma* have been reported in humans, most are incidental parasites. *Ecbinostoma trivolvis* and *E. revolutum*, for instance, are commonly parasites of birds and mammals in the United States and Europe, respectively. Human infections of *E. ilocanum* are most frequently reported from the Philippines, China, Taiwan, and Indonesia. Infection occurs when the infected second intermediate host is eaten either raw or improperly cooked. Because of the variety and number of potential intermediate and definitive hosts, it is impossible to the parasite, but human infections can be prevented if food is cooked adequately.

Heterophyid Trematoda

Heterophyid trematoda which belongs to the family Heterophyidae is one of the smallest trematodes infesting humans. The heterophyids are capable of parasitizing birds, mammals and human. Heterophyid trematoda causing human infections are *Heterophyes heterophyes* (V. Siebold, 1852), *Metagonimus yokogawai* (Katsurada, 1912), *Haplorchis pumilio* (Looss, 1899), *Haplorchis yokowai* (Katsuta, 1932), *Centrocestus formosanus* (Nishigori, 1924).

Morphology

Adult

The adult worms measure 1. 4 to 3mm in length by 0. 3 to 0. 5mm in width and are oval or pyriform in shape. The tegument of these flukes contains scalelike spines. In addition to an oral and ventral sucker, The adult worms contains a third sucker, the genital sucker, surrounding the genital pore. In *H. heterophyes*, the genital pore, situated posterolateral to the prominent ventral sucker, is surrounded by a genital sucker or gonotyl. In *M. yokagawai*, the ventral sucker and gonotyl are fused, and the complex is displaced to the left side of the body. The reproductive system is located in the posterior half of the body with the testes lying side by side; the ovary is medial, just anterior to the testes, with lateral, follicular vitelline glands restricted to the posterior third of the body. The gravid uterus loops between the long intestinal caeca, terminating at the gonotyl (see Figure 6-1-4).

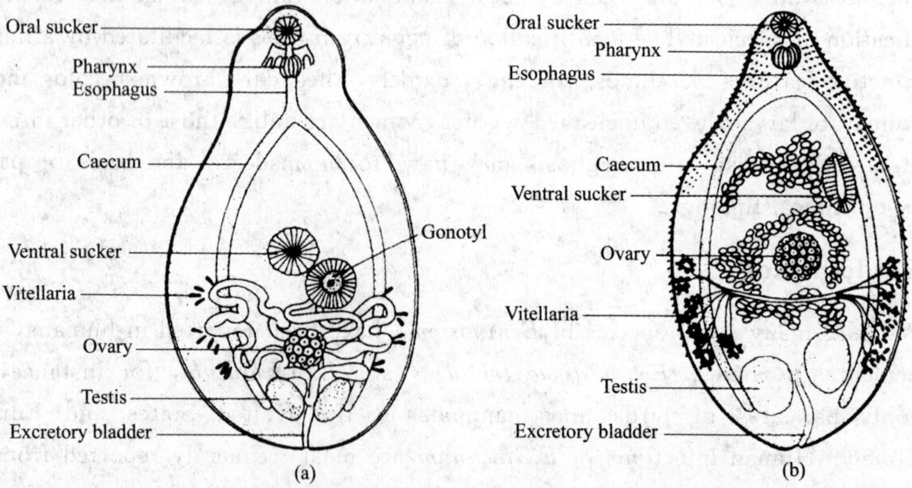

(a) *Heterophyes heterophyes* adult (b) *Metagonimus yokogawai* adult

Figure 6-1-4 Morphology of *Heterophyid trematoda*

Egg

The eggs of both species resemble those of *Clonorchis sinensis* except for their indistinct opercular shoulders and the absence of an abopercular knob. The eggs are small, brownish yellow, and operculate, and they possess prominent opercular shoulders. They measure 27 to 30μm by 15 to 17μm.

Life Cycle

The adult worms inhabit intestinal luman of birds, mammals and human, and lay embryonated eggs. The eggs are discharged into the environment via the feces and are ingested by the snail intermediate host before the miracidium hatches. A sporocyst and one or two redia generations develop in the snail before the production and release of cercariae. Daughter rediae giving rise to cercariae that escape to the external environment, penetrate the musculature of any of a number of food fishes, and encyst as metacercariae under the scales or in the flesh of freshwater fish and froggy. Humans become infected by eating raw, pickled, or poorly cooked fish or froggy containing the metacercariae. The metacercariae excyst in the intestinal tract, attach to the walls of small intestine and grow to maturity in about a week.

Pathogenesis

Following ingestion of metacercariae, the latent period is approximately 9 days. The adult worms produce little damage to the intestinal tract mucosa except for a mild inflammatory reaction. In heavy infections, the worms produce abdominal pain, mucous diarrhea, and ulceration of the intestinal wall. Eosinophilia is also common but without anemia.

Because of the small size of the eggs and the fact that the adult may attach itself deeply into the intestinal wall, the eggs may infiltrate the lymphatics or venules and then carried by the circulation to various parts of the body, where they may cause granulomatous responses in such organs as heart or brain. In the Philippines, 15% of fatal heart disease may be a result of heterophyid myocarditis. Neurologic manifestations due to adult worms or eggs in the brain have been reported.

Diagnosis

Diagnosis depends on positive identification of eggs from feces. Because the eggs of *H. heterophyes* are similar in shape and size to those of *M. yokogawai* and *C. sinensis*, differentiation must be made on the basis of patient history, clinical findings, or recovery of adult worms in the stool.

Epidemiology and Prevention

The infection is found in China, the Philippines, Tunisia, and Turkey. Human infection by *H. heterophyes* occurs in Asia, Egypt, and Hawaii, while *M. yokagawai* is the most common intestinal fluke of humans in the Far East, Spain, and the Balkan countries.

Numerous fish-eating mammals, including dogs, cats, and birds, act as reservoirs. Snails serving as the first intermediate host include pironella and Cerithidea spp. In *H. heterophyes*, this is a freshwater or brackish water snail belonging to one of the genera pirenella (in Egypt), Cerithidia (in Japan), or Tarebia (in Hawaii); *M. yokagawai* infects members of the snail genus Semisulcospira. A variety of freshwater fish can serve as the second intermediate hosts. One of the principal fishes used by *H. heterophyes* as the second intermediate host is the mullet Mugil cephalus, which can harbor several thousand metacercariae. Salmonoid fish commonly serve as second intermediate hosts for *M. yokagawai*.

Humans become infected by ingestion of pickled, uncooked or salted fish. Metacercariae can survive for up to 7 days in salted fish. The life cycle could be disrupted by improved sanitary conditions and educational information about proper sewage disposal away from ponds or lakes where the intermediate hosts reside.

(Liu Peimei)

Chapter 6 Cestodes

Section 1 Introduction to Tapeworms

The cestodes, or tapeworms, constitute a class of the phylum Platyhelminthes. The adult tapeworms found in humans all have a flat and ribbonlike body. Living worms are white or yellowish in color. The cestode body consists of an anterior attachment organ, or scolex, followed by a chain of segments, or proglottids, also known as a strobila. The strobila grows throughout the life of the tapeworm by continuous proliferation of new segments or proglottids in the region immediately posterior to the scolex. The new segments are referred to as immature because they do not yet contain fully developed internal structures. The mature segments are larger and are found near the middle of the chain, and each may contain both male and female reproductive organs. The terminal portion of the strobila contains the gravid segments, usually filled with eggs. The eggs are enclosed in the uterus, a structure that varies in shape and size in different cestode species. The form of the uterus is quite characteristic and serves as an important diagnostic feature. Terminal proglottids of some species may become detached in the intestine and pass out with the stool; some types may be too small to be seen in gross examination.

Adult tapeworms inhabit the small intestine, where they live attached to the mucosa. Tapeworms do not have a digestive system; their food is absorbed from the host's intestine. Attachment is accomplished by means of the scolex, an organ that varies in morphology from species to species. However, with the exception of *Diphyllobothrium latum*, the broad or fish tapeworm, and related species, all cestodes of humans have four muscular, cup-shaped suckers on the scolex. In addition to suckers, the scolex may have an elongate and protrusible structure, the rostellum, situated in the center of the scolex. In some species the rostellum bears hooks and is referred to as armed. While precise identification of the tapeworms of humans is usually made on the basis of eggs or proglottids, the scolex of each species is quite characteristic and is sufficient for specific diagnosis. Of greater practical importance is the recognition of the scolex in stool specimen from a patient who has received anthelmintic treatment. Therapy has been successful only when the whole worm has been expelled. Discovery of the scolex from treated patients is essential because the strobila regrows if the scolex remains in the intestine. If, for any reason, expulsion of the whole worm is uncertain, the patient should have another stool examination three or four weeks after treatment.

The cestodes parasitizing humans have complex life cycles that generally involve both a definitive and an intermediate host. Some species utilize humans only as the definitive hosts, growing to adulthood in the intestine after ingestion of the infective larvae. For some species, humans are equally acceptable as definitive or intermediate hosts. Still others, such as *Echinococcus*, utilize humans as one of their possible intermediate hosts, but never as the definitive host. In general, extraintestinal infection with the larval forms is a much more serious matter than infection with the adult tworm.

Unlike the trematodes, the eggs of which are usually operculate, human tapeworms, with few exceptions, do not have operculate eggs. Cestode eggs vary considerably in the appearance of the external shell as well as in the number and thickness of the embryonic membranes. These membranes serve as protective coverings of the embryo, which is called an oncosphere and bears six elongate hooks.

Life cycle patterns

Tapeworms that infect humans display two basic life cycle patterns, one typical of members of the order Pseudophyllidea, the other typical of members of the order Cyclophyllidea.

Pseudophyllidean pattern: In members of the order Pseudophyllidea, coracidia-containing eggs leave the host with feces. In water, the coracidium escapes from the eggshell through the operculum and swims for a brief time by means of its ciliated embryophore. Survival of the organism depends upon ingestion of the coracidium by an aquatic arthropod, the first intermediate host, within which the embryo sheds its ciliated embryophore and metamorphoses into a globular procercoid in the hemocoel. During this stage of development, the oncosphere hooks are retained, albeit nonfunctionally, in a tail-like structure called the cercomer. When the first intermediate host is ingested by a second intermediate host, usually a fish, the procercoid migrates via the peritoneal cavity to any of several parts of the body, principally the musculature, where it grows and develops into a solid, vermiform plerocercoid that manifests the beginning of strobilization and a developing adult scolex. The plerocercoid is infective to humans; when ingested, it attaches to the wall of the small intestine, where strobilization occurs. All of the aforementioned stages possess penetration glands that secrete lytic enzymes, which aid in penetration of and migration among the various host tissues and organs.

Cyclophyllidean pattern: Adapted as it is to terrestrial hosts, the cyclophyllidean hexacanth embryo, or oncosphere, lacks a ciliated embryophore and must remain passive until the egg is ingested by a vertebrate or invertebrate intermediate host. In species that normally utilize an invertebrate intermediate host (usually an arthropod), the oncosphere, upon hatching in the digestive tract, employs its six hooks and its penetration glands to enter the hemocoel, where it metamorphoses into a cysticercoid. This form is solid-bodied and possesses a fully developed acetabulate scolex. It is surrounded by several layers of cystic tissue and has a prominent cercomer equipped with hooks. The cystic layers and the cercomer are eaten away in the digestive tract of the definitive host, freeing the scolex and neck to begin strobilization.

In species that utilize vertebrate intermediate hosts, the oncosphere, after ingestion, penetrates the intestinal lining and enters a venule. It is carried by the circulating blood to any of several areas of the body, where it develops into a cysticercus with an acetabulate scolex invaginated into a fluid-filled vesicle or bladder; hence, the common name for these parasites is bladder-worm. Two other forms that follow this developmental pattern are the coenurus and the hydatid cysts. In the former, the wall of bladder develops several invaginated scolices; in the latter, secondary cysts are formed as invaginations on the walls. These second-generation cysts are called brood capsules because they in turn give rise to scolices, each of which can develop into an adult worm when ingested by a suitable definitive host.

In some tapeworms, certain immature stages—including the cysticercus, coenurus, and hydatid cyst of some cyclophyllideans and the plerocercoid of several pseudophyllideans—are capable of developing in extraintestinal tissues of humans.

Physiology

The adaptive morphology of adult tapeworms and the environment in which they dwell are probably the most significant factors influencing their physiology. Lacking a digestive tract, these worms must derive all of their nutrient molecules from the host or from their microhabitat, and such molecules must cross the tegument. The methods by which nutrients cross the tegument include active transport, facilitated diffusion, and simple diffusion. The most important nutrient molecule is glucose, which, after polymerization within the parasite, is stored as glycogen usually in the parenchyma and interstitial fluid. The only other major transported carbohydrate is galactose. The sites on the tegument over which various molecules are transported vary for carbohydrates, amino acids, and purines and pyrimidines, the last two requisite for synthesis of nucleic acids. Most adult tapeworms also absorb lipids, probably by simple diffusion.

The environment in which tapeworms reside, the small intestine, is one of very low oxygen tension, necessitating anaerobic metabolism. Some tapeworms possess a mammalian-style electron transport system, but its role in energy production is minor. Metabolic rates differ in different parts of the strobila. The neck and immature proglottids have a much higher rate of metabolism than mature and gravid proglottids, reflecting the high energy requirements for new proglottid formation and organ development. Most of the energy requirement in mature proglottids is for egg production.

In general, the common gut-dwelling adult cestodes are well adapted to the human host, induce few symptoms, and only rarely cause serious pathology. This reality belies innumerable fearsome and largely apocryphal stories of tapeworms stealing food and causing ravenous hunger (far more commonly, the appetite is depressed). Larval cestodes, however, develop in human organs or somatic tissues outside of the gut and are therefore far more pathogenic.

The adult cestodes elicit little host inflammatory or immune response in contrast to the strong responses elicited by the larval stages in tissues. Adult cestodes are often acquired by ingestion of meat from intermediate hosts. Extraintestinal infection with larvae results from ingestion of eggs of fecal origin. Diagnosis of infection with adult cestodes is based on identification of eggs and segments (proglottides) in feces. Larval infections are more difficult to assess; serology and biopsy are helpful. Control depends on sanitation, personal hygiene, and thorough cooking of meat and fish.

Treatment

In most instances, adult tapeworms have little visible effect upon their hosts except in heavy infections, which may result in anemia, weight loss, and various secondary manifestations. The treatment of choice for all tapeworms infecting the small intestine of humans is oral administration of the drug niclosamide, which disrupts proglottids and interferes with the worm's substrate-level phosphorylation, depriving the worm of required ATP. Praziquantel is an excellent broad-spectrum anthelmintic and, like niclosamide, causes disruption of proglottids. As in the case of schistosomes, additional effects of praziquantel upon tapeworms are vacuolization of the tegument and rapid paralysis of the worm's musculature. These drugs should be used cautiously in the treatment of *Taenia solium* infections, because cysticercosis can result from autoinfection by eggs released from disrupted proglottids. Five to six weeks after treatment, the patient's feces should be reexamined for the reappearance of eggs, which may indicate that the scolex was retained and developed into a "new" worm.

Section 2 *Taenia solium*

This parasite, commonly referred to as the "human pork tapeworm", is common among humans in areas where raw or inadequately cooked pork is regularly consumed.

Morphology

The adult worm: It usually measures 2-4m (sometimes up to 8m) long and contains 700-1000 proglottids. The small scolex, measuring about 1mm in diameter, is armed with two circles of 25-50 rostellar hooks. These hooks are of two sizes—long (180μm) and short (130μm)—alternating in the two circular rows.

The mature proglottid is squarish in outline and has a common genital pore situated on the lateral edge, about halfway down. The pores on successive proglottids may be on alternate sides or may be positioned unilaterally. The testes (150 to 200) are scattered throughout the medullary region of the proglottid. The ovary consists of two prominent lobes and one small, central lobe. The vitellaria are compact, as is characteristic of cyclophyllideans, and are located in the basal portion of the proglottid just posterior to the ovary. The oviduct arises at the junction of the three ovarial lobes and continues anteriad as the cul-de-sac uterine stalk. As eggs are produced, they are pushed up into the stalk, which forms lateral branches as the number of eggs increases. The number of lateral branches serves as a tool for distinguishing *T. solium* from *T. saginata*; *T. solium* has 7-13 lateral branches, while *T. saginata* has more than 13 (15 to 30) (see Figure 6-2-1).

Egg: Eggs of *T. solium* are indistinguishable from those of *T. saginata*. Eggs are spherical in shape, about 31-43μm in diameter. The oncosphere (six-hooked larva) is enclosed in a thick, radially striated coat called the embryophore, usually dark brown in color. The six-hooked larva can be easily seen in living eggs but frequently become indistinct and vague in preserved specimens. The thin, hyaline shell is usually lost by the time the egg is voided from the gravid proglottid. The radially striated coat is, however, sufficiently characteristic so that *Taenia* eggs cannot be confused with any of the other eggs of human helminthes (see Figure 6-2-1).

Cysticercus: The larval stage of *Taenia* is called a cysticercus, formerly termed Cysticercus cellulosae. The worm is semitransparent, milk white in color, elongate oval in shape, and about 6-18mm in length. The bladder is filled with fluid and on one side is seen a denser area that is the invaginated head equipped with four suckers and hooklets (see Figure 6-2-1).

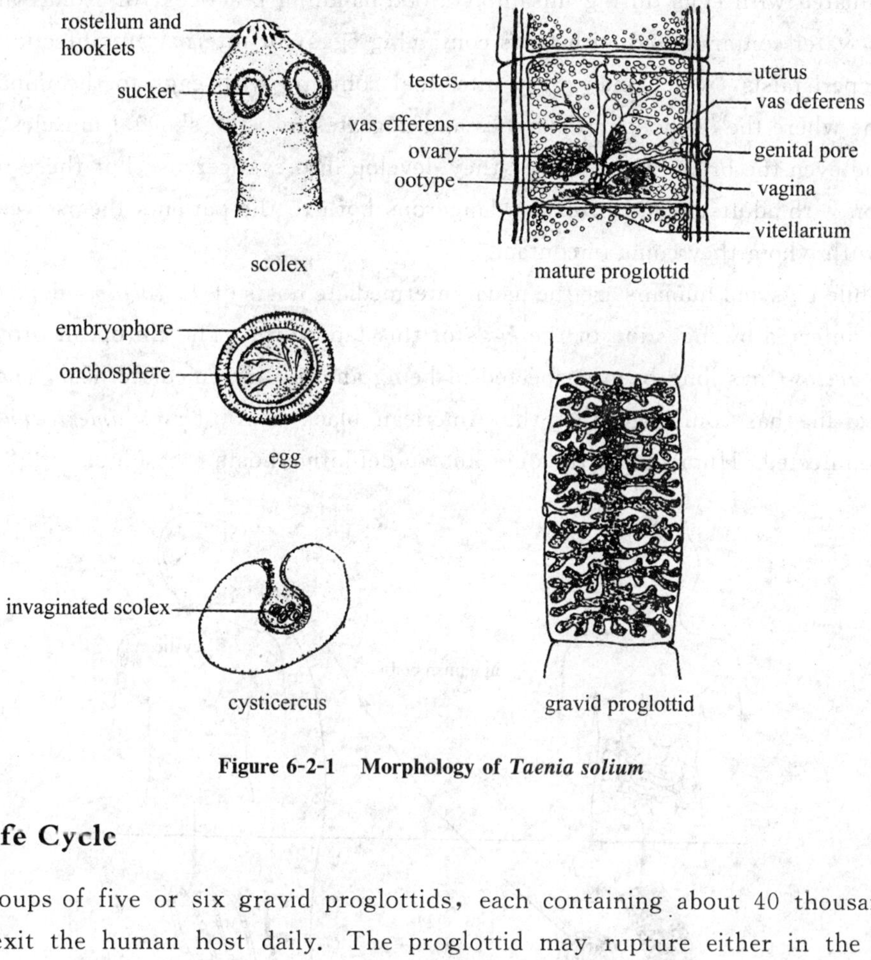

Figure 6-2-1 Morphology of *Taenia solium*

Life Cycle

Groups of five or six gravid proglottids, each containing about 40 thousands of eggs, exit the human host daily. The proglottid may rupture either in the host's intestine or after it leaves the host. When eggs are ingested by the intermediate host-pig, the liberated oncospheres, using their hooks and penetration gland secretions, penetrate the intestinal wall, enter the circulatory system, and are carried by blood stream to the heart and spread to any port of the body, but are mainly found in muscles, where they develop into cysticerci in 10 weeks. The muscles of the tongue, neck, shoulder, and buttock are most often infected. In addition, the liver, heart, brain and eyes may be parasitized. When infected or measly pork is consumed by a human, the scolex evaginates in the duodenum under the stimulation of bile. The worm attaches itself to the intestinal mucosa by hooklets and suckers; there the parasite develops to sexual maturity in 2-3 months. Humans are the only known natural definitive hosts. The adults of *T. solium* have been known to live for as long as 25 years.

Although the adult tapeworm develops in humans after the ingestion of infected meat, infection with the larval stage or cysticercus occurs after the ingestion of eggs of *Taenia solium*. This may result from hand-to-mouth autoinfection, from eating food contaminated with eggs during unsanitary food-handling practices, or from consuming food or water contaminated with faces containing eggs, or internal autoinfection due to reverse peristalsis, which may carry intestinal contents with eggs to the upper small intestine where the onchosphere hatches and migrates into the skeletal muscles, heart, eyes and even the brain. Once there, they develop into cysticercus. For these reasons, infection with adults of *T. solium* is dangerous both to the patients themselves and to those with whom they come in contact.

While pigs and humans are the usual intermediate hosts of *T. solium*, dogs can also become infected by ingestion of the eggs of this tapeworm. The European brown bear (*Ursus arctos*) has long been suspected of being another intermediate host, and recent DNA testing has confirmed that the American black bear (*Ursus americanus*) may become infected. Humans are the only known definitive hosts (see Figure 6-2-2).

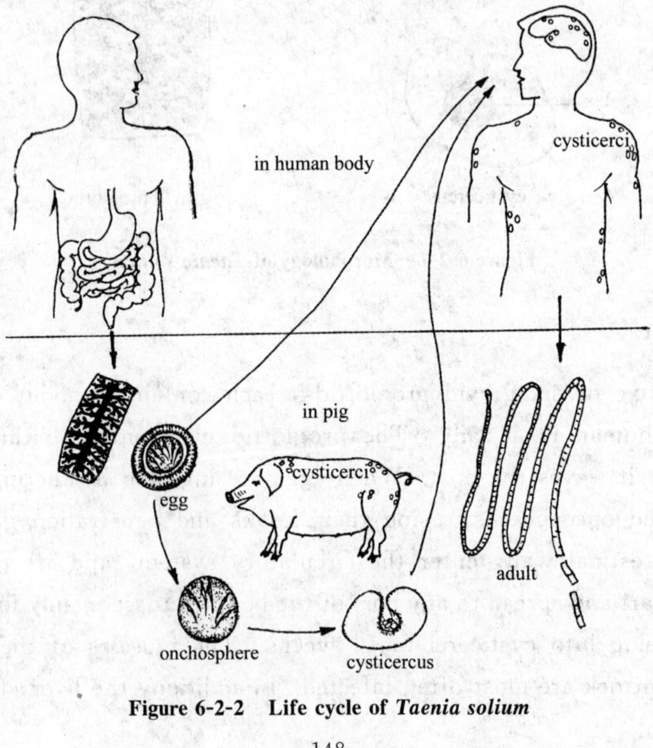

Figure 6-2-2 Life cycle of *Taenia solium*

Pathogenesis and Clinical Manifestation

Usually only a single adult tapeworm infects a human. The adult worms probably cause no symptoms in the majority of patients. Sometimes the worm may cause irritation of the mucosal lining. Vague abdominal discomfort, hunger pangs, and chronic indigestion have been reported. Moderate eosinophilia frequently occurs because of the absorption of the toxic metabolites of the worm. In infections with cysticerci, the symptoms vary with the number of larvac and the tissues invaded. The cysticerci may be found in almost any tissue in human body, but most common in the subcutaneous tissues and skeletal muscles, sometimes in the eye and brain, causing cysticercosis. Cysticercosis may be classified into 3 types according to the organs involved.

Subcutaneous type: The subcutaneous nodules are usually found in arms, legs, neck, abdomen and back. They are about several millimeters in diameter, movable and show no tenderness. Skeletal muscle encystment usually is asymptomatic but may cause muscle spasms, weakness, and muscular pseudohypertrophy with a heavy parasite burden.

Ocular type: Ocular cysts are mostly vitreous, but they may be found in subretinal locations. It may give rise to visual difficulties that fluctuate with eye position, or to a generalized decrease in visual acuity, retinal edema, hemorrhage or vasculitis, or detachment. Cysts developing along the optic tracts may give rise to visual field defects. Visualization of cysts via funduscopy may be diagnostic of the disease.

Brain type: The most dangerous symptoms are a result of encystment in the central nervous system. Clinical manifestations of neurocysticercosis (Central Nervous System Cysticercosis or cysticercosis of the brain) depend primarily on the number and location of cysticerci and the host's immune response to infection. Serious pathologic findings of neurocysticercosis can include seizures (epilepsy), obstructive hydrocephalus, meningoencephalitis, and vascular accidents. Involvement of brain parenchyma is common and leads to the most frequent presentation of seizure or headache. Extraparenchymal ventricular and subarachnoid cysts also are found. These carry a worse prognosis and often lead to obstructing hydrocephalus requiring surgical intervention. Cysticerci within the basilar cisterns or sylvian fissures may become quite large. Those within the cisterns may also cause serious vasculitis and stroke. Spinal neurocysticercosis is rare.

Diagnosis

Taeniasis

The history of eating raw or insufficiently cooked pork and discharged gravid proglottids is helpful to the diagnosis.

Stool examination reveals characteristic *Taenia* eggs by the direct fecal film or saturate brine floatation method. Because eggs of *T. solium* and *T. saginata* are morphologically indistinguishable, the species cannot be identified by the eggs. Identification of proglottids in feces is the most reliable method of diagnosis. Gravid proglottids are compressed between two slides, held against the light, and the number of the main branches of the uterus counted. *T. solium* has less than 13 on either side, *T. saginata*, more than 13 (15 to 30). The scolex may be discovered after treatment. The morphology of the scolex, particularly the rostellum, is also useful in diagnosis: *T. saginata* has no rostellum and its scolex bears no hooks, making it easily distinguishable from *T. solium*, which has an armed rostellum.

Cysticercosis

Clinical diagnosis can be made by linking symptoms, such as the late onset of epilepsy, to a history of residence in an endemic area. X-ray examination of infected muscles or central nervous system tissues may confirm diagnosis by revealing calcified cysts. Computerized tomography (CT) scans and magnetic resonance imaging (MRI) show both calcified and uncalcified cysticerci in the brain. Surgical removal of subcutaneous cysts with demonstration of the organism is diagnostic. Funduscopy can be used for diagnosis of the ocular cysticercosis. Examination of cerebrospinal fluid by ELISA is also useful in diagnosis of patients with cerebral cysticercosis.

Epidemiology

Taeniasis is a tapeworm (cestode) infection acquired by the ingestion of raw or undercooked pork of infected pigs. The infections are worldwide in distribution—approximately 50 million cases of infection world-wide annually. Incidence of infection of *T. solium* is also based on other factors such as religious inhibitions on eating pork, inspection of pork before distribution for human consumption, and high degrees of sanitation which limits exposure of the intermediate hosts (pigs) to human feces. *T. solium* is more prevalent in poorer communities where humans live in close contact with pigs and eat undercooked pork, and is very rare in Muslim countries. Pork tapeworm is endemic to many parts of the world including China, Southeast Asia, India, sub-Saharan Africa, and Latin America. Some studies suggest that the prevalence of cysticercosis in Mexico is between 3.1 and 3.9 percent. Other studies have found the seroprevalence in areas of Guatemala, Bolivia, and Peru as high as 20 percent in humans, and 37 percent in pigs. In Ethiopia, Kenya and the Democratic Republic of Congo around 10% of the population is infected, in Madagascar 16%. The frequency has decreased in developed countries owing to stricter meat inspection, better hygiene and better sanitary facilities. The distribution of cysticercosis coincides with the distribution of *T. solium*.

In Latin America, an estimated 75 million persons live in endemic areas and 400,000 people have symptomatic disease. Cysticercosis is also found to be associated with Hispanic ethnicity, immigrant status, and exposure to areas of endemicity. In the US, the disease is found in immigrants from Mexico, Central and South America. Current livestock for pigs in the U. S. do not play a role in the transmission of *Taenia solium*, and thus cysticercosis in the U. S. is an imported disease.

Prevention and Control

Taeniasis

Chinese herb medicine, pumpkin seed and areca nut are quite effective and safe for the treatment of both pork tapeworm infection and beef tapeworm infection. The chemicals, praziquantel and niclosamide are also effective for taeniasis. Before treatment with praziquantel, it is ensured that the patient of taeniasis is not infected with cysticercus in brain. The recognition of a scolex in patient's stool after the application of taeniafuge is very important. When the entire worm has been expelled, the therapy is successful, otherwise the strobila regrow if the scolex remains in the small intestine.

Cysticercosis

Surgical removal is required for the superficial and ocular cysticercosis. But this may be impossible when they are located in areas of difficult or dangerous surgical access. Praziquantel is effective for the treatment of brain and visceral cysticercosis, but for the brain cysticercosis, steroids may be started a few days before the antiparasitic, in order to avoid problems caused by swelling. If swelling and immune response are not controlled, the treatment itself can be lethal, so the medication is given in low dosages over several days and in hospital.

Section 3 *Taenia saginata*

Morphology

Taenia saginata (beef tapeworm) is the most common of the large tapeworms of humans. Morphologically, the adult worm resembles *T. solium.* It is usually 4-8m long, the strobila contains approximately 1,000-2,000 proglottids. As mentioned earlier, the scolex is unarmed, having neither hooks nor rostellum. The morphology of mature proglottids in the two species differs primarily in that *T. saginata* has a bilobed ovary and about twice as many testes as *T. solium.* In addition, as previously noted, the gravid uterus of *T. saginata* has in excess of 13 main lateral branches (Figure 6-3-1).

The biological differences between *Taenia solium* and *Taenia saginata* are shown in the following table:

Table 6-3-1　Biological Differences between *T. solium* and *T. saginata*

	T. solium	*T. saginata*
Length	2-4m	4-8m
Scolex	1mm in diameter with 4 suckers and hooklets	2mm in diameter with 4 suckers but no hooklets
Number of proglottids	700-1000	1000-2000
Mature proglottids	3 lobes of ovary	2 lobes of ovary
Gravid proglottids	7-13 uterine lateral branches on one side	15-30 uterine lateral branches on one side
Number of gravid proglottid detached	usually several segments together	usually single segment
Mode of proglottids passing out	passively expelled	actively migrate out of anus
Cysticercus	scolex with hooklets found in pig and man	without hooklets only found in cattle
Disease caused in man	taeniasis and cysticercosis	taeniasis

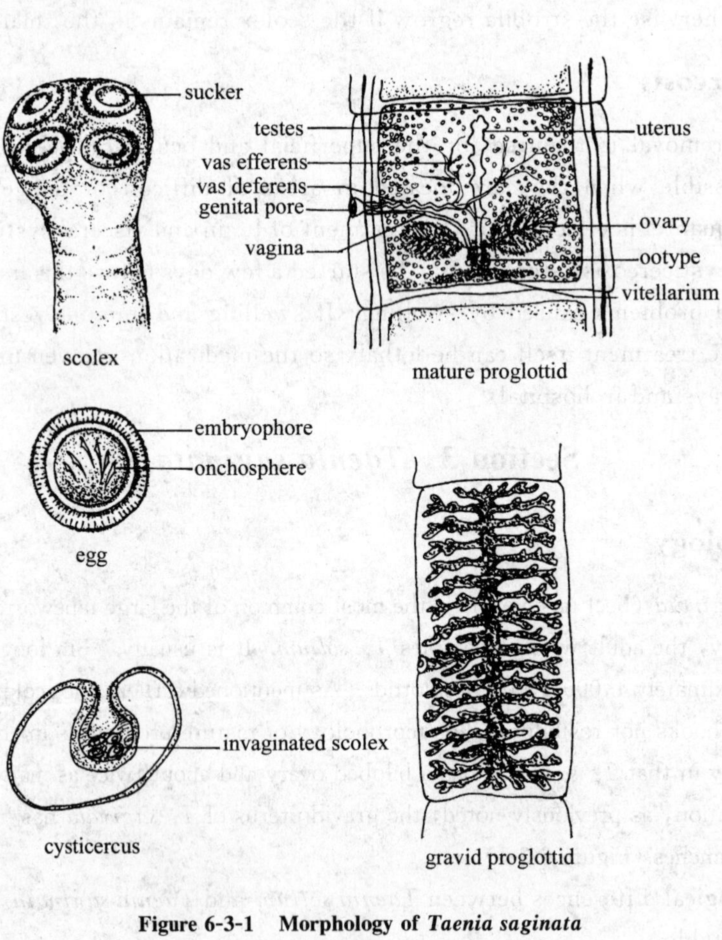

Figure 6-3-1　Morphology of *Taenia saginata*

Life Cycle

The life cycle of *T. saginata* strongly resembles that of *T. solium*. Adults of both species reside in the small intestine of humans and gravid proglottids of *T. saginata* detach singly from the strobila and pass to the outside. The eggs of *T. saginata*, indistinguishable from those of *T. solium*, are ingested by a suitable intermediate host, such as a cow or other ungulate. The liberated oncosphere penetrates the intestinal wall and is carried by the lymphatic or blood circulatory system to intramuscular connective tissue, where it develops into a cysticercus known as *Cysticercus bovis*. Humans become infected by ingesting cysticerci in beef. Following evagination of the scolex and subsequent attachment to the jejunal wall, the worm develops to sexual maturity in 8-10 weeks (see Figure 6-3-2).

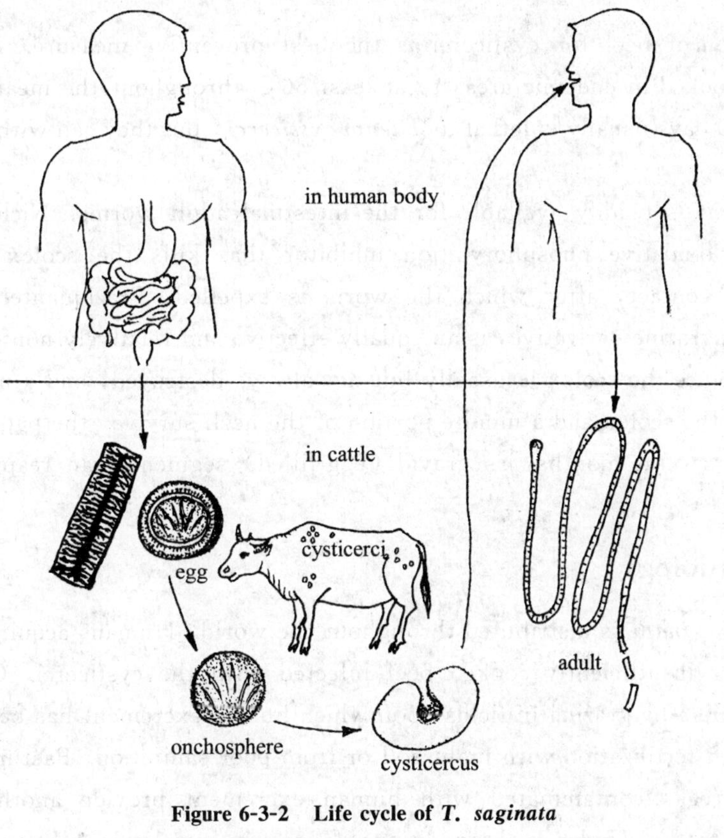

Figure 6-3-2 Life cycle of *T. saginata*

Pathogenesis and Clinical Manifestation

Saginatus taeniasis in humans is often characterized by such symptoms as abdominal pain, greatly diminished appetite, and weight loss. These symptoms are especially common in patients already debilitated by malnutrition or other illness. Moderate eosinophilia may develop. A disturbing manifestation of *T. saginata* infection is the active crawling of the muscular segments out of the anus. Unlike victims of *T. solium* infection, *T. saginata* victims rarely develop cysticercosis, and the prognosis is generally good.

Diagnosis

The diagnosis depends on the finding of eggs at the perianal region by adhesive cellophane tape technique or identifying segments. The species of *Taenia* can be identified only by the segments, because their eggs are identical. The uterus of *T. saginata* usually forms 15 to 30 branches on each side of the main uterine stem, whereas there are 7 to 13 branches in the smaller and thinner *T. solium* segment.

Prevention and Control

Inspection of beef for cysticerci is the best preventive measure. Beef must be thoroughly cooked in endemic areas to at least 56℃ throughout the meat. Freezing at −10℃ for 10 days usually is lethal to *Taenia cysticerci*, but they can withstand 70 days at 0℃.

Treatment is readily available for the intestinal adult worms. Niclosamide, is a nonabsorbed oxidative phosphorylation inhibitor that kills the scolex and anterior segments on contact, after which the worm is expelled. Praziquantel, a synthetic isoquinoline-pyrazine derivative, is an equally effective and relatively nontoxic cesticidal compound. Since the scolex is usually but not always destroyed, and a new worm can regenerate if the scolex and a minute portion of the neck survive, the patient should be observed for several months, as gravid (egg-filled) segments can reappear in 10-12 weeks.

Epidemiology

Taenia saginata is distributed throughout the world. Humans acquire infection by eating raw or insufficiently cooked beef infected with the cysticerci. Cattle acquire *Cysticercus bovis* by grazing in fields upon which human excrement has been deposited, either through fertilization with night soil or from poor sanitation. Pastures flooded by rivers and creeks contaminated with human excrement provide another source of infection for cattle. Under such conditions, eggs may remain viable for 2 months or longer. Thorough cooking of beef at 57℃ until the reddish color disappears or freezing at −10℃ for 10 days effectively destroys infective cysticerci. The beef tapeworm is comparatively rare in Indian populations, where cows are regarded with reverence and rarely eaten by humans.

Section 4 *Echinococcus granulosus*

The genus *Echinococcus* contains the smallest tapeworms in the Taeniidae. However, their juvenile forms are often huge and are capable of infecting humans, resulting in hydatidosis, a very serious disease in many parts of the world.

Echinococcus granulosus uses carnivores, particularly dogs and other canines, as definitive hosts. Many mammals may serve as intermediate hosts, but herbivorous species are most likely to become infected by eating the eggs on contaminated herbage.

Morphology

Adult

The adult lives in the small intestine of the definitive host. It measures 3mm to 6mm long and consists of a typically scolex, a short neck, and usually only three proglottids. The nonretractable rostellum bears a double crown of 28 to 50 (usually 30 to 36) hooks. The most anterior segment is immature, and the genital organs are immature. The middle one (mature segment) has fully developed reproductive organs consisting of 45-60 testes, paired irregular ovaries, and a single spherical vitelline gland. The terminal one is gravid and contains a median uterus with 12-15 or more lateral branches filled with ova(see Figure 6-4-1).

Egg

The egg cannot be differentiated from those of other taeniidae(see Figure 6-4-1).

Hydatid cyst

The larva of *Echinococcus granulosus* is called hydatid cyst. It grows slowly and requires several years for development. In hogs they are usually 4-5cm in diameter; in man, with a longer period of growth, they may reach 15-20cm. The cyst is more or less spherical in shape. It consists of a cyst wall, cystic fluid, brood capsules containing protoscolices, daughter cyst and grand daughter cyst whose structures are the same as that of the mother cyst. The cyst wall is composed of a thick outer (1-4mm), laminated, noncellular layer, also called laminated cuticle and an inner, thin, nucleated germinal layer (20-25μm). The inner layer produces the protoscolices. Protoscolices are usually produced singly into the lumen of the bladder and also within brood capsules. The latter are small cysts, containing 10 to 30 protoscolices, which usually are attached to the germinal layer by a slender stalk; they may break free and float within the hydatid fluid. Individual scolices and brood capsules may break free and sink to the bottom of the bladder, where they are known as hydatid sand. The daughter cysts are replicas in miniature of the complete hydatid. In the daughter cysts there may be small cysts called grand daughter cyst, whose structure is similar to that for daughter cysts. Cystic fluid is colorless or slightly yellowish and has a specific gravity of 1.012 and a pH of 6.7 to 7.2. It remains sterile and contains albumin, creatinine, urea, calcium, sodium chloride, phosphates, and some enzymes such as protease, lipase, and oxidase. It has antigenicity(see Figure 6-4-1).

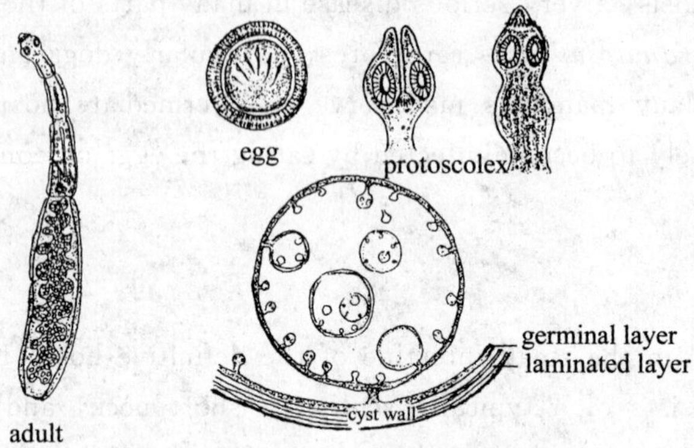

Figure 6-4-1 Morphology of *Echinococcus granulosus*

Life Cycle

Dogs acquire the infection by eating infective cysts in the tissues of herbivorous animals, such as sheep, which act as intermediate hosts. Each cyst contains many scolices. Each scolex develops into an adult in the small intestine of a dog, which acts as a definitive host. In humans, who act as intermediate rather than definitive hosts, this parasite causes hydatid cyst disease, an illness characterized by the presence of one or more cysts in a variety of tissues and organs of the body. The ripe gravid segment detaches, releasing the eggs, which are fully capable of infecting an intermediate host including humans. The eggs pass in feces, are ingested by men or other intermediate hosts. In the duodenum the oncosphere hatches and penetrates the intestinal wall into the lymphatics or mesenteric venules, and is carried by the blood stream to various parts of the body. It enters the portal vein and lodges in the liver, the first capillary filter. If it passes the liver, it reaches the lungs and other distant organs, where it develops into a hydatid cyst and the cyst increases in size, attaining a diameter of about 1mm in 1 month, 10mm in 5 months, and 20cm after several years(see Figure 6-4-2).

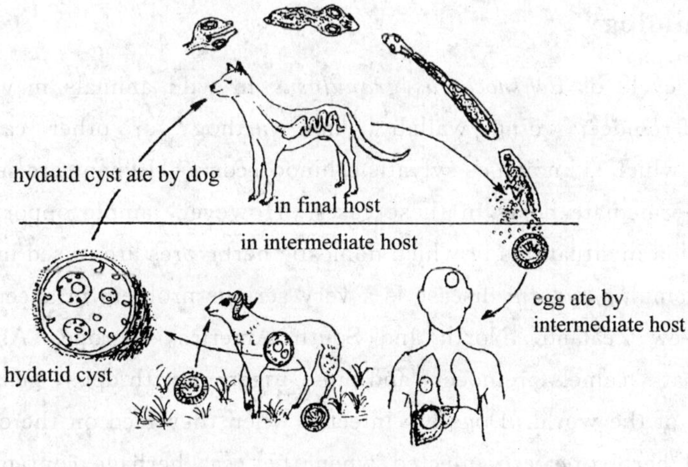

Figure 6-4-2 Life cycle of *Echinococcus granulosus*

Pathogenesis and Clinical Manifestation

The effects of a hydatid may not become apparent for many years after infection because of its usual slow growth. Up to 20 years may elapse between infection and overt pathogenesis. If infection occurs early in life, the parasite may be almost as old as its host.

The type and extent of pathological conditions depend on the location of the cyst in the host. As the size of the hydatid increases, it crowds adjacent host tissues and interferes with their normal functions. The results may be very serious. Hepatic involvement can result in abdominal pain, a mass in the hepatic area, and biliary duct obstruction. Pulmonary involvement can produce chest pain, cough, and hemoptysis. If the parasite is lodged in the nervous system, clinical effects may be manifested relatively early in the infection before much growth occurs. When bone marrow is affected, the growth of the hydatid is restricted by lack of space. Chronic internal pressure caused by the parasite usually causes necrosis of the bone, which becomes thin and fragile; characteristically, the first sign of such an infection is a spontaneous fracture of an arm or leg. When the hydatid grows in an unrestricted location, it may become enormous, containing more than 15 quarts of fluid and millions of protoscolices. Even if it does not occlude a vital organ, it can still cause sudden death if it ruptures. The host is sensitized to Echinococcus antigens during its long-standing infection, and sudden release of massive amounts in the hydatid fluid induces an adverse host reaction called anaphylactic shock, as well as cyst dissemination. Unconsciousness and death are nearly instantaneous in such instances.

Epidemiology

The life cycle of *Echinococcus granulosus* in wild animals may involve a wolf-moose, wolf-reindeer, dingo-wallaby, lion-warthog, or other carnivore-herbivore relationship, which is known as sylvatic echinococcosis. Humans are seldom involved as accidental intermediate hosts in these cases. However, ample opportunities exist for human infection in situations in which domestic herbivores are raised in association with dogs. For example, hydatid disease is a very serious problem in sheep-raising areas of Australia, New Zealand, North and South America, Europe, Asia, and Africa. Similarly, goats, camels, reindeer, and pigs, together with dogs, maintain the cycle in various parts of the world. Dogs are infected when they feed on the offal of butchered animals, and herbivores are infected when they eat herbage contaminated with dog dung. Humans are infected with hydatids when they accidentally ingest *Echinococcus* spp. eggs, usually as a result of fondling dogs.

The species *E. granulosus* is composed of a number of genetically differing strains. Strain differences include morphology, development, metabolism, DNA hybridization and restriction site analysis, and intermediate host specificity. Worms of one strain are adapted to one species of intermediate host, for example, cattle, horses, sheep, or pigs and they do not develop well in other species. The strains have considerable epidemiological significance for humans: Horse and pig strains in Europe probably do not infect humans, but sheep and cattle strains do.

Diagnosis

Symptoms of a tumor-like, slowly growing mass with eosinophilia are strongly suggestive, especially in an endemic sheep-raising area. Isolated hooks in the sputum suggest rupture of a lung cyst. Hepatic cysts require differentiation from liver abscess and hepatic carcinoma. The serologic tests that are currently most useful are indirect hemagglutination, latex agglutination, and ELISA. Ultrasound imaging (US), magnetic resonance (MR), and computed axial tomography (CT) have greatly improved the diagnosis of deep-seated lesions and also can demonstrate avascular fluid-filled cysts. Radiographs are less precise or useful, although they demonstrate the hollow cyst areas. The exploratory puncture for the purpose of obtaining fluid is contraindicated as a dangerous diagnostic procedure.

Prevention and Control

Treatment is chiefly by surgical resection. The typical surgical procedure involves incising the surrounding adventitia until the capsule is encountered and aspirating the hydatid fluid with a large syringe. Considerable delicacy is required at this point, since fluid spilled into a body cavity can quickly cause fatal anaphylactic shock. After aspiration of the cyst contents, 10% formalin is injected into the hydatid to kill the germinal layer. This fluid is withdrawn after five minutes, and the entire cyst is then excised. Recent work suggests that a long course of albendazole may kill the scoleces within the cyst and even reduce the size of the cyst. Long, continued use of mebendazole has also proved effective, although the results are variable. A recent approach involves percutaneous puncture under sonographic guidance, aspiration of cyst fluid, instillation of a protoscolecidal agent such as 95% methanol or cetrimide, and respiration (PAIR), along with albendazole treatment to reduce the danger of subsequently renewed disease from spillage. Some reports have suggested the use of albendazole or mebendazole for *Echinococcus multilocularis* infections.

Human infection of hydatid disease can be prevented if people are made aware of the risks and the proper safety precautions are taken. It is crucial to intercept the continuation of life cycle on farms and slaughterhouses by abstaining from feeding raw offal to dogs and enforcing thorough meat inspection procedures. In addition, exercising good hygiene is essential, which includes hand washing before meals, thoroughly cooking food, and wearing protective clothing and gloves when necessary to avoid contact with infected fecal material.

Current control strategies are aimed at improving primary health care of the population, which includes increasing access to diagnostic treatment and drug therapy, education, access to safe water, and improving sanitation and meat inspection.

More specific programs are aimed at eliminating *E. granulosus* directly by deworming dogs to kill tapeworms and controlling the stray dog population to prevent infection. Vaccines for sheep are being developed in Australia and could provide a breakthrough intervention strategy for the future.

Section 5 *Echinococcus multilocularis*

Echinococcus multilocularis is primarily boreal in its distribution. It is known from Europe, Asia, New Zealand, and South and North America. It has been reported from the United States as far south as Nebraska and Iowa and as far east as Ohio. Human cases in the United States occur most commonly from Alaska, but a human infection has also been reported from Minnesota. The adult is mainly a parasite of foxes, but dogs, cats, and coyotes may also serve as definitive hosts. The hydatid develops in several species of small rodents such as voles, lemmings, and mice.

The adult is very similar to *E. granulosus*, differing from it in the following characteristics: (1) *E. granulosus* is 3mm to 6mm long, whereas *E. multilocularis* is only 1.2mm to 3.7mm long; (2) the genital pore of *E. granulosus* is about equatorial, but it is preequatorial in *E. multilocularis*; and (3) *E. granulosus* has 45 to 65 testes with a few located anterior to the cirrus pouch, but *E. multilocularis* has 15 to 30 testes, all located posterior to the cirrus pouch.

The juvenile form differs in several respects from that of *E. granulosus.* Instead of developing a thick, laminated layer and growing into large, single cysts, this parasite has a thin outer wall that grows and infiltrates into the surrounding host tissues like a cancer. Each process may have several small, fluid-filled pockets containing several protoscolices. In humans and other unnatural hosts the pockets typically lack protoscolices. In natural intermediate hosts the cyst is more regular. In humans, pieces of the cyst sometimes break off and metastasize to other parts of the body. Because of its type of construction, this metacestode form is called an alveolar or multilocular hydatid(see Figure 6-5-1).

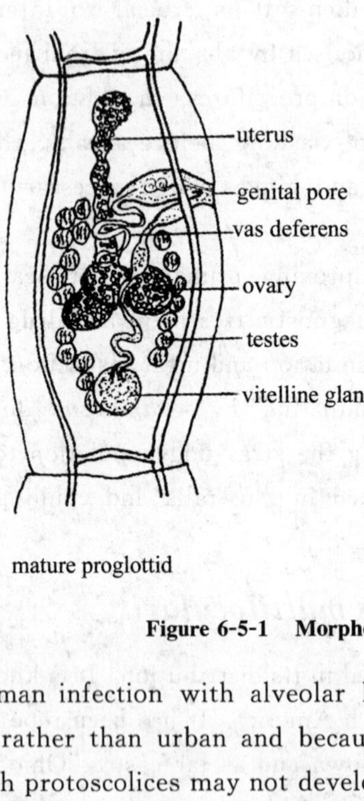

mature proglottid

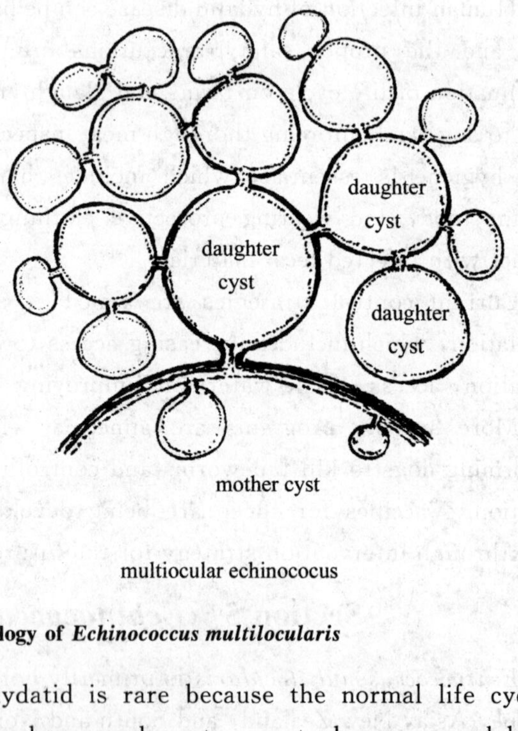

multiocular echinococus

Figure 6-5-1 Morphology of *Echinococcus multilocularis*

Human infection with alveolar hydatid is rare because the normal life cycle is sylvatic rather than urban and because humans do not seem to be very good hosts. Although protoscolices may not develop in human hosts, the germinal membrane is still viable. Anyone handling wild foxes may be exposed to infection. Thus, this disease is most common among professional trappers and among handlers of sled dogs that catch and eat wild mice as a regular part of their diet. There is some evidence that there are strains that differ in virulence. Some human infections seem to disappear spontaneously, while others seem to march inexorably toward death. Such differences may be explained by differing immune responses(see Figure 6-5-2).

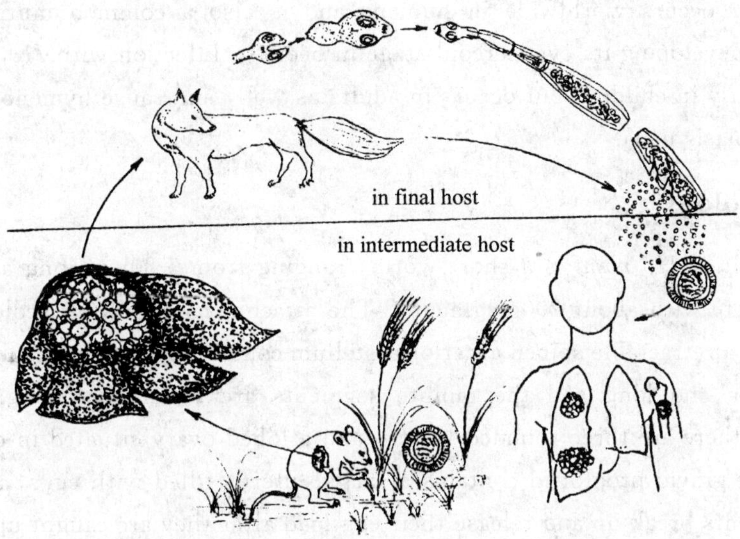

Figure 6-5-2 Life cycle of *Echinococcus multilocularis*

Diagnosis of an alveolar hydatid is difficult, particularly because the protoscolices may not be found. Even at necropsy cysts may be mistaken for malignant tumors. As a result of the difficulties of liver surgery, excision is usually practical only when the hydatid is localized near the tip of a lobe of the liver; infections of the hilar area are inoperable. The infiltrative nature of the cyst and its slow rate of growth may advance the disease to an inoperable state before its presence is detected. Praziquantel, the drug that is so effective for most flatworm parasites, may actually enhance growth of alveolar hydatids. Albendazole may be effective in some patients; encouraging results have been obtained in mice treated with albendazole-loaded nanoparticles.

Alveolar hydatidosis can be prevented only by avoiding dogs and their feces in endemic regions, by carefully washing all strawberries, cranberries, and the like that may be contaminated by dung, and by regularly worming dogs that may be liable to infection. Because this disease is a sylvatic disease and it is much more difficult to eradicate than *E. granulosus*.

(Guo Shuling)

Section 6 *Hymenolepis nana*

Hymenolepis nana, the dwarf tapeworm, was first found by Bilharz in 1851 in a child from Egypt. In 1852, V. Siebold named it *Taenia nana*, and renamed it *Hymenolepis nana* later. Grassi and Rovelli, in 1892, confirmed that the life cycle does not need intermediate hosts. About 40 years later, Bacigalupo approved that some insects may serve as the intermediate hosts and transmit the disease.

H. nana occurs worldwide in humans and is also a common murine parasite, occasionally developing its cysticercoid stage in beetles. Infection with *H. nana* is seen most frequently in children but occurs in adults as well, and cause hymenolepiasis nana or rodentolepiasis nana.

Morphology

The adult of *H. nana* is a short worm, ranging from 5-80mm long and 0. 5-1mm wide, complete with about 200 segments. The attachment organ, or scolex, has four suckers with a retractable spined anterior rostellum containing a row of hooks. The neck region is thin and long and the minute segments are wider than long. In mature proglottids, there are three rounded testes, and a lobed ovary situated in centre of the segment, the gravid proglottid contains a saclike uterus filled with eggs, and terminal gravid segments break up and release their egg load after they are caught up in the fecal bolus (see Figure 6-6-1).

Eggs are oval or subspherical and smaller, ranging 40-60μm by 30-50μm. On the inner membrane are two poles, from which 4 to 8 polar filaments spread out between the two membranes. The egg contains an oncosphere with six hooks, and the two polar thickenings on the membrane of which is with filaments extending into the space around the hexacanth embryo (see Figure 6-6-1).

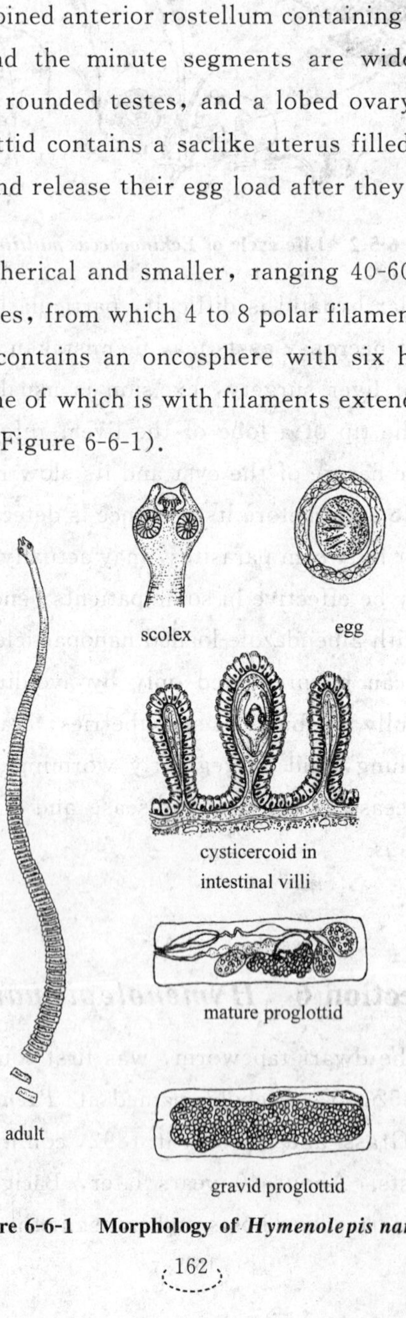

Figure 6-6-1 Morphology of *Hymenolepis nana*

Life Cycle

The life cycle of *H. nana* is shown in Figure 6-6-2.

Eggs are passed in the stool when released from segments through its genital atrium or when segments disintegrate in the small intestine.

The infection is acquired most commonly from eggs in the feces of another infected individual, which are transferred by contaminated food and drinking water. The ingested eggs hatch in the small intestine, and the six-hooked oncosphere burrows into the villi, where within a few days, it develops into a cysticercoid larva that emerges, 4 to 5 days later, into the gut lumen, and contains a scolex and neck. In 5 to 10 days, the scolex attaches to the mucosa, and the neck proceeds to strobilate. The larva grows into an adult worm that lives only a short time, perhaps 4 to 6 weeks. Rodents, such as mouse and squirrel, may also harbor these worms and serve as reservoir hosts, infecting humans via their pellets.

An alternate mode of infection consists of internal autoinfection, where the eggs release their hexacanth embryo, which penetrates the villus continuing the infective cycle without passage through the external environment. Since many eggs can be involved, this pathway can lead to massive infection with several thousand worms.

Remarkably, an indirect, two-host cycle may also occur, involving fleas, grain beetles, or other insect that feeds on infected rodent droppings, such as *Xenopsylla cheopis*, *Pulex irritans*, *Tenebrio* spp., and *Tribolium* spp. When eggs are ingested by an arthropod, intermediate host, they develop into cysticercoids, which can infect humans or rodents upon ingestion, and digestive enzymes then act on the cysticercoid to release the scolex, which attaches and develops into an adult worm in intestinal lumen of the final host.

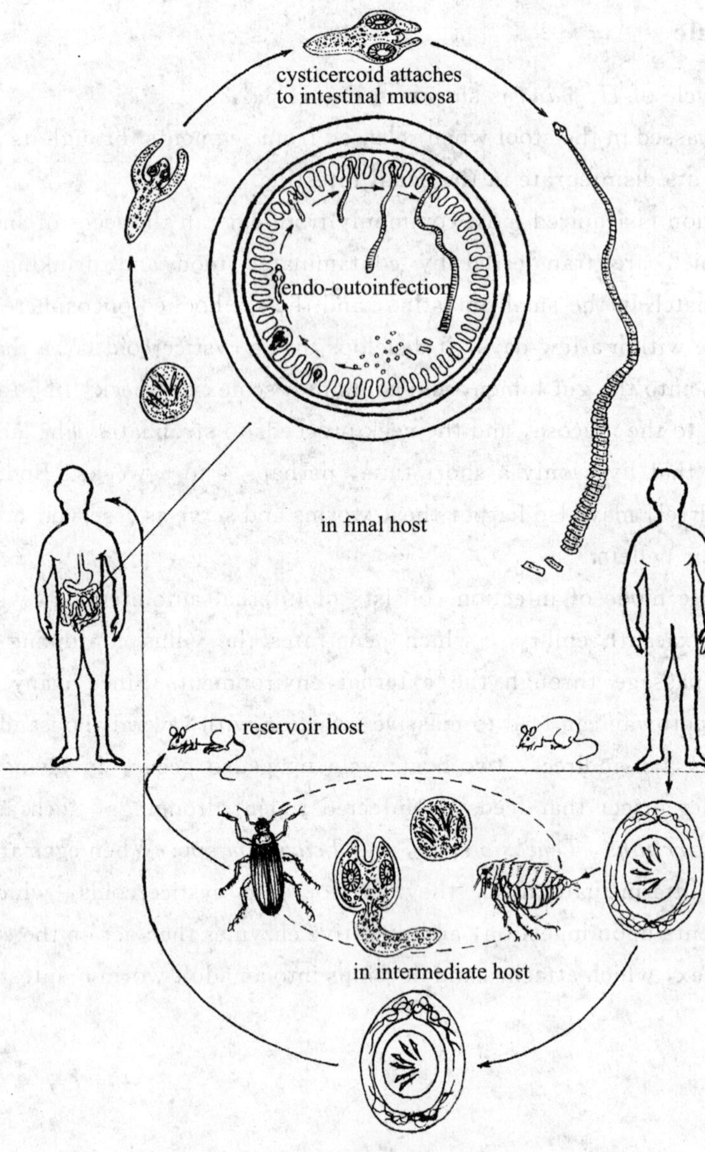

Figure 6-6-2 Life cycle of *Hymenolepis nana*

Pathogenesis and Clinical Manifestation

Attachment of adult worms to the intestinal mucosa and their secretion produce localized congestion, edema, hemorrhage and ulceration.

In cases with low intestinal parasite burden, there are no symptoms. However, in heavy infections, especially if autoinfection and hyperinfection occur, patients, especially children can experience nausea, vomiting, appetite loss, abdominal pain, diarrhea, headache, dizziness, fidget, insomnia, nervous disturbances, and anemia.

In experiment of rodents, the tissue phase of the direct cycle of *H. nana* initiates a profound cellular and humoral response, rendering most hosts immune to subsequent infection. In contrast, the indirect cycle through infected insects does not involve mucosal embryogenesis in humans and induces little or no immunity, even permitting occasional massive internal reinfection to occur. The immune response is seldom effective against the initial infection because tissues have already been invaded and a protective cyst formed when the response develops.

Laboratory Diagnosis

The diagnosis is usually suggested by the presence of characteristic *H. nana* eggs and gravid segments upon stool examination. Concentration techniques and repeated examinations will increase the likelihood of detecting light infection.

Epidemiology

In humans, infections with *H. nana* are encountered worldwide, that parasitization rate ranges between 0.3% and 50%. A relatively high prevalence has been reported in surveys conducted in Europe, Latin America, India, China and North America.

Humans and other animals become infected when they intentionally or unintentionally eat grain products contaminated by infected insects, intermediate hosts. On the other hand, *H. nana* is the only cestode that parasitizes humans without requiring an intermediate host. It is possible for the worm's entire life cycle to be completed in the bowel, so infection can persist for years. Congested areas, day-care centers, and crowded institutions such as nurseries, schools frequently have high levels of infection with *H. nana*.

Prevention and Control

Preventing fecal contamination of food and water in institutions and crowded areas is of primary importance. Eliminating rats, storing grains and flour properly in kitchens are also essential for prevention of *H. nana* infection.

Both praziquantel and niclosamide have been very effective and have minimal side effects. Cure rate of praziquantel is reported over 90 percent, in a single oral dose of 15-25mg/kg.

Section 7 *Hymenolepis diminuta*

Hymenolepis diminuta [(Rudolphi, 1819) Blanchard, 1891] is a tapeworm normally found in the mouse. It rarely infects humans, but may do so if a human eats a insect carrying cysticercoids of this worm, and causes hymenolepiasis diminuta.

Morphology

The adult of *H. diminuta* is similar to that of *H. nana*, but it is larger than the latter (see Figure 6-7-1). Several differences between two cestodes in detail are listed in Table 6-7-1.

Table 6-7-1 Morphological differences between *H. nana* and *H. diminuta*

		H. nana	*H. diminuta*
Adult	Size(mm)	(5-80)×(0.5-1.0)	(200-600)×(0.3-0.4)
	Proglottids	100-200	800-1000
	Scolex	Retractable, a row of hooks	not retractable, without hooks
	Gravid	Saclike uterus Proglottid	Saclike uterus, but the edge is irregular
Egg	Shape	Oval or subspherical	Elliptical
	Size(μm)	(40-60) ×(30-50)	(60-79) ×(72-86)
	Color	Colorless	Yellowish brown
	Morphological characteristics	Thin shell, two polar thickenings with filaments	Thick shell, without polar thickenings and filaments

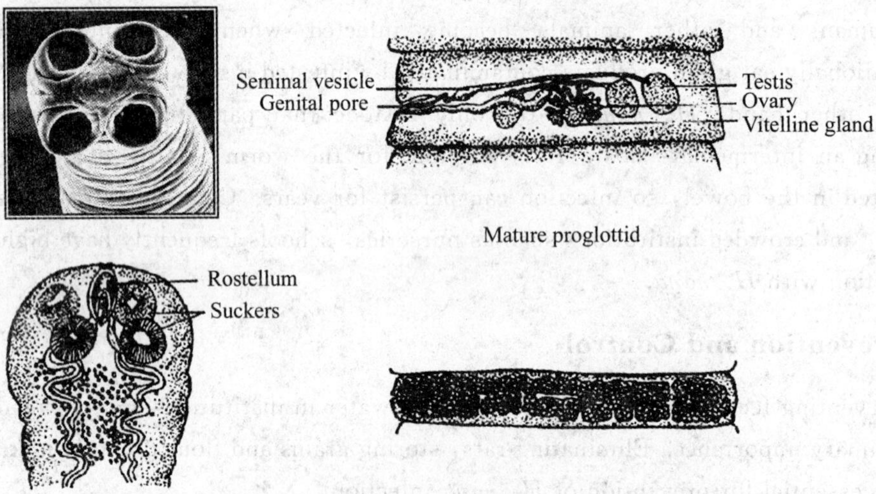

Figure 6-7-1 Morphology of *Hymenolepis diminuta*

Life Cycle

The life cycle of *H. diminuta* is similar to that of *H. nana*, but it is necessary that beetles (flour and grain beetles, *Tribolium* spp. and *Tenebrio* spp., respectively) serve as the intermediate host. The adult worms live in the intestine of the final hosts, normally rats but also sometimes dogs and humans. The beetles are infected when they eat the eggs passed from the definitive hosts. Once the egg is digested by the intermediate host, the oncosphere, a fully developed larva contained in the egg, is released. The oncosphere migrates to the haemocoel of the beetle where it will develope into a cysticercoid. The rat and human are infected when they eat an infected beetle. Within the definitive host's intestine, the cysticercoid evaginates its scolex, attaches to the intestinal mucosa and develops into an adult.

Pathogenesis and Clinical Manifestation

The infection with this tapeworm usually produces no pathology, but occasional patients may present mild complains such as headache, insomnia, nausea, abdominal pain, and diarrhea.

Laboratory Diagnosis

Diagnosis is made on finding characteristic eggs in the stool. Modified Kato's thick smear will increase the likelihood of detecting light infection.

Epidemiology

H. diminuta lives in all temperate zones throughout the world. In China, the parasitization rate is 0.13%.

The adult produces over 250,000 eggs per day. Humans can be accidentally infected through the ingestion of beetles in precooked cereals, or other food items; and directly from the environment (e.g., oral exploration of the environment by children), so the infection is most common in children.

Prevention and Control

It is important to propagandize hygienic knowledge for controlling the worm prevalence. Humans should be told to keep a favorable behavior including cleaning house, washing hands before taking food, not eating undercooked cereals. Eliminating rats is also effective for prevention of *H. diminuta*.

Treatment of hymenolepiasis diminuta is similar to that of hymenolepiasis nana.

Section 8 *Diphyllobothrium latum*

Diphyllobothrium latum (Linna, 1758) belongs to a group of tapeworms known as the pseudophyllideans. Its plerocercoid parasitizes in various fish and adult inhabits in the small intestine of a fish-eating final host, such as human, cat, and dog.

Morphology

The adult is the longest tapeworm found in man, ranging from 3-10m with

3,000-4,000 proglottids, each up to 2cm wide. The scolex is small, with a ventral and a dorsal bothrium. The mature and gravid proglottids are broader than long. There are 750-800 testes in each proglottid and the bilobed ovary lies in the posterior portion of the proglottid. A genital atrium in which the male and female genital pores open is located at the anterior part of ventral surface of proglottid. In the center of each segment is a rosette-shaped uterus connected to the outside by a uterine pore through which the eggs are passed (see Figure 6-8-1).

The egg with a thick shell is oval or ellipsoidal, light yellowish-brown in color, measuring 58-75μm by 40-50μm in size and contain an embryo with 3 pairs of hooklets, it is with an operculum at one end and with a small knob at the opposite end (see Figure 6-8-1).

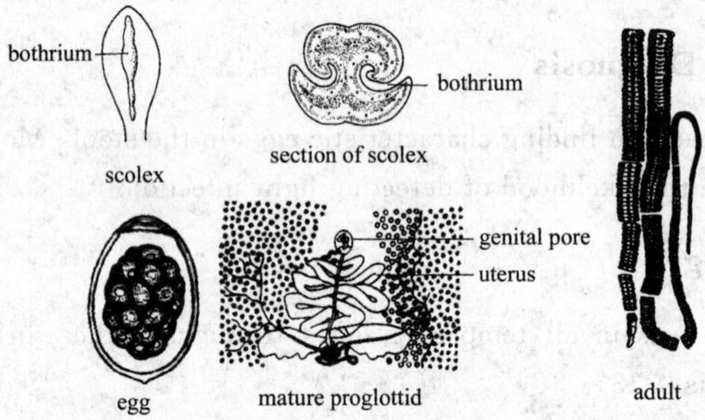

Figure 6-8-1 Morphology of *Diphyllobothrium latum*

Life Cycle

The definitive hosts of *D. latum* include human. Some freshwater fish-eating mammals are reservoir hosts, such as bear, dog, pig, cat, wolf, etc. Cyclops are first intermediate host. Freshwater fish are second intermediate host (see Figure 6-8-2).

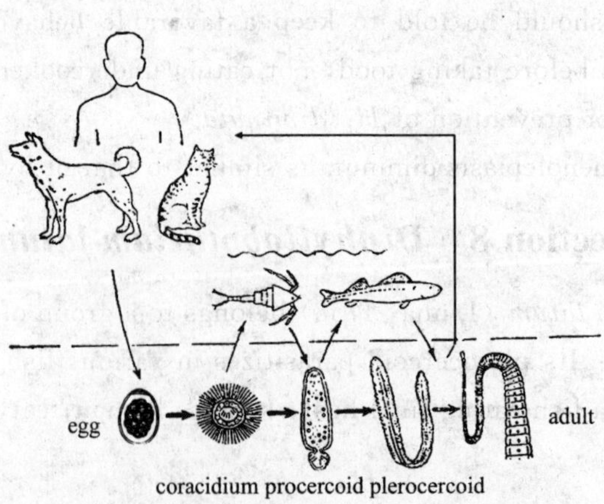

Figure 6-8-2 Life cycle of *Diphyllobothrium latum*

A human or other suitable mammalian host is infected by eating uncooked fish that contains plerocercoid larvae. The larvae attach to the small intestinal wall and mature into adulthood in 3 to 5 weeks. The life-span of adult worm in definitive host is about 5-13 years. The gravid proglottids and mature eggs are discharged in the feces of the definitive host. The eggs hatch ciliated coracidia in fresh water. The coracidia are ingested by Cyclops where they develop into procercoids. When freshwater fish consume the infected Cyclops, the procercoid penetrates the intestinal wall and develops into a plerocercoid (sparganum).

Pathogenesis and Clinical Manifestation

The presence of adult worms in the intestinal tract is usually asymptomatic in most infected persons. Some clinical symptoms may be mild, depending on the number of worms, that include abdominal discomfort, loss of appetite, vomiting, fatigue, loss of weight and some malnutrition. Massive infection may cause diarrhea and intestinal obstruction. Anemia and neurological problems associated with vitamin B12 deficiency are seen in heavily infected individuals because the adult worm can split the vitamin B12-intrinsic factor complex and prevent absorption of B12 by the human host.

Laboratory Diagnosis

Diagnosis is based on finding many characteristic operculated eggs and empty segments with the characteristic rosette-shaped uterus in the human stool.

Epidemiology

Fish tapeworm infection is distributed worldwide, in the subarctic and temperate regions. It is commonly found in Scandinavia, Russia, Japan, Australia, the Great Lakes of Canada, and Alaska, wherever undercooked, salted, or pickled freshwater fish is eaten by humans, but it is reported only several patients found in Heilongjiang, Guangdong and Taiwan in China. Human feces release eggs into the freshwater thereby infecting the fish.

Prevention and Control

In most areas, humans are the primary hosts of *D. latum*, and proper disposal of human feces will do much to break the infection chain. Plerocercoids in fish are quickly killed by thorough cooking, freezing at −10℃ for 15 minutes, or thorough pickling. Treatment of sewage before it enters lakes greatly reduces the prevalence of infection, as has been demonstrated in some countries such as Finland.

Treatment with praziquantel or niclosamide is effective. Cure rate of praziquantel is reported over 95%, in a single oral dose of 10mg/kg, but may cause headache, dizziness, nausea and abdominal pain in about 5% of treated patients. Vitamin B12 may be administrated for patients with its deficiency.

Section 9　Other Human Tapeworms

Dipylidium caninum

Dipylidium caninum [(Linnaeus, 1758) Railliet, 1892] is a tapeworm that commonly infects dogs and cats all over the world, but occasionally it is found in humans, especially children and causes dipylidiasis caninum. In 1758, Linnaeus described the morphological characteristics of adult. Later, that flea serves as the intermediate host was confirmed through experiments by Grassi and Rovelli in 1892, Joyeux in 1916, Chen Xintao in 1934, respectively.

Morphology

The adult of *D. caninum* measures 10-15cm in length and 0.3-0.4cm in width, with 200 proglottids (see Figure 6-9-1). The scolex bears four suckers and a retractable

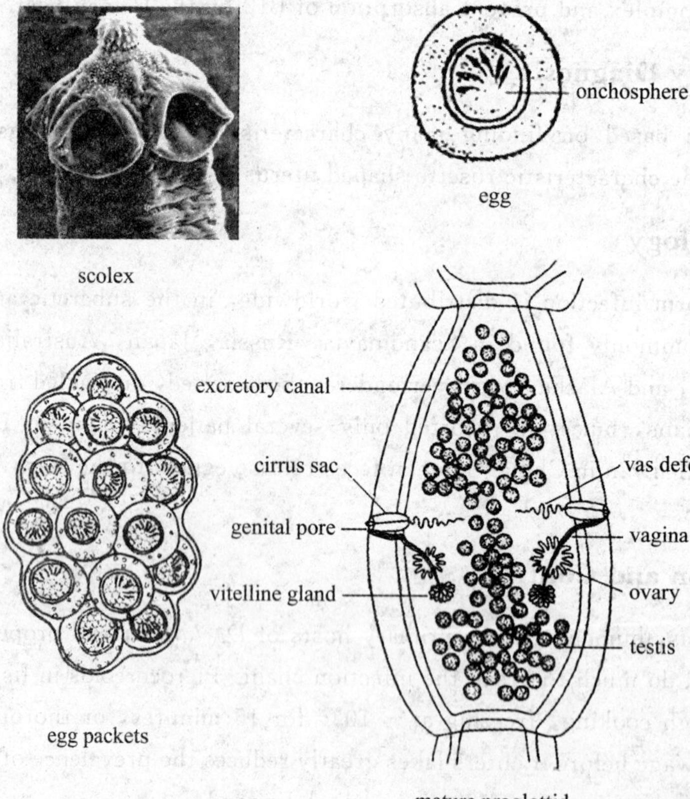

Figure 6-9-1　Morphology of *Dipylidium caninum*

rostellum with 1-7 circles of small hooks. Mature proglottids are longer than wide, and a characteristic feature of which is that they contain two sets of male and female reproductive organs. They therefore demonstrate two genital pores laterally sided that lead to their name as the "double-pored" tapeworm. The gravid proglottids measure 0.8-2.3cm, are elongated and resemble rice grains or cucumber seed, contain hyaline capsules with egg packets inside. Each packet contains 2-40 embryonated eggs which is spherical, measuring 35-50μm in diameter, with two layer of thin shell, and an oncosphere inside.

Life Cycle

The adult worms reside in the small intestine of the definitive hosts such as dogs, cats, foxes, where they attach to the intestinal mucosa by their scolex. The gravid proglottids detach from the tapeworm, and are passed in the stool. The segments contain egg packets. The eggs are released into the environment and then ingested by the larval stage of the intermediate host, a flea such as *Ctenocephalides canis*, *C. fells*, *Pulex irritans*. In the flea the oncosphere hatches, penetrates the intestinal wall, invades the hemocoel, and develops into a cysticercoid in about one month. When the infected flea bites, the dog or cat may eat flea with the cysticercoids. In the small intestine of the definitive hosts, the cysticercoids attach to the intestinal mucosa by its scolex and finally develop to the adult worm in three weeks. Humans occasionally get infection by ingesting the infected fleas. Children in close and continuous contact with pets are particularly prone to infection with *D. caninum*.

Clinical Manifestation

Light infections are often asymptomatic, but some patients may present with loss of appetite, malabsorption, abdominal pain, diarrhea, and anal pruritus.

Laboratory Diagnosis

Dipylidiasis caninum is diagnosed by examination of stool for characteristic gravid proglottids or, more rarely, egg packets. Special caution should be taken in identifying free eggs without shells.

Epidemiology

Distribution is worldwide. Several hundred human infections have been reported in Europe, Philipines, China, Japan, Argentina, and the United States.

In China, the parasitization rate of dogs is respectively 25.6% (Heilongjiang), 16% (Shanxi), 15.38% (Guizhou), and that of cats is 58.77% in Wuhan.

Prevention and Control

Health education is important for prevention. Ways to prevent infection include controlling the fleas and de-worming of pet dogs and cats. Praziquantel and Niclosamide are available for pet infection .

Praziquantel is very effective for human infection, given in a single oral dose of 10-25mg/kg, and Niclosamide may be an alternative.

Pseudanoplocephala crawfordi

Pseudanoplocephala crawfordi (Baylis, 1927) was first found by Baylis in small intestine of boar in Sri Lanka. The pig, boar and rattus norvegicus are definitive hosts. *Tribolium castaneum* may serve as the intermediate hosts. The human is infected by ingesting insects infected with cysticercoids of *P. crawfordi*.

Morphology

The adult is larger than that of *H. diminuta*, ranging from 97-167cm long and 0. 31-1. 01cm wide, with about 2, 000 segments. The scolex is spherical, has four suckers with a rostellum, without hooks. The proglottids are wider than long. In mature proglottids, there are 21-43 elliptic testes, and a cauliflower-shaped ovary situated in the centre of the segment. The gravid proglottid contains a saclike uterus filled with 2,000-5,000 eggs.

Eggs are spherical and brown, ranging 84μm × 108μm. The shell with granule protuberance is thick and friable, which encloses an oncosphere surrounded by an embryophore. The space between shell and embryophore is filled with colloid (see Figure 6-9-2).

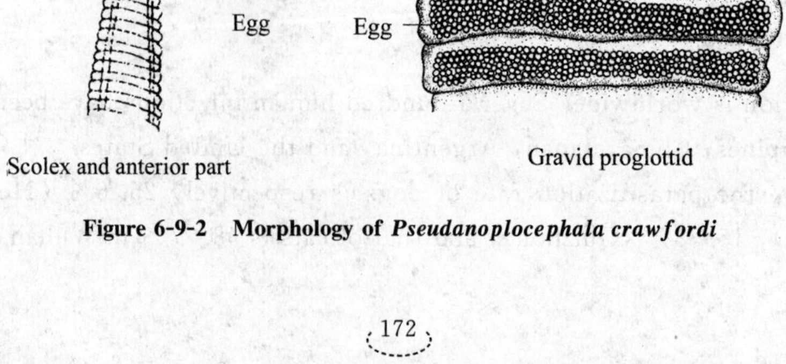

Figure 6-9-2 Morphology of *Pseudanoplocephala crawfordi*

Life Cycle

The adult worms parasitize in the small intestine of definitive hosts. The eggs and gravid segments are passed in faeces, and then ingested by intermediate hosts, in which they develop into cysticercoid within 29-35 days. The pig can be infected by ingesting *Tribolium castaneum* with cysticercoid which will develop into adult in the small intestine. The gravid proglottids detach from the adult and are passed with feces. Occasionally, human being is infected by ingesting intermediate host with cysticercoid.

Clinical Manifestation

Light infections are usually asymptomatic, but severe infections may present with loss of appetite, fatigue, loss of weight, abdominal pain, abdominal distention, nausea, vomiting. Dizziness and insomnia may occur.

Laboratory Diagnosis

Pseudanoplocephala crawfordi is diagnosed by detecting characteristic gravid proglottids or eggs in stool, and both of them should be distinguished from those of *H. diminuta*.

Epidemiology

P. crawfordi is found in Japan, India, Sri Lanka and China. In our country, the infections of pigs and boars are found in Shanghai, Shanxi, Gansu, Fujian, Guangdong. More than 20 cases are reported in China.

Prevention and Control

It is important to propagandize hygienic knowledge for controlling the worm prevalence. Humans should be told to keep a favorable behavior, including cleaning granary, eliminating grain beetle. Eliminating rats is also helpful for prevention of *P. crawfordi*.

Paromomycin and mebendazole are effective for human infection.

Spirometra mansoni

Spirometra mansoni (Cobbole, 1883) is a species of pseudophyllid tapeworms of wild and feral cats, the larval form of which may survive in human tissues and cause sparganosis mansoni.

Morphology

The adult is white in color, ranging from 60-100cm long and 0.5-0.6cm wide. The scolex is small and likes finger, measuring 1.0-1.5mm in length, 0.4-0.8mm in width, with a pair of linear sucking grooves called bothrium. A worm contains 1,000 segments, which are broader than long. In both mature proglottids and gravid segments are a set of male reproductive organs and a set of female reproductive organs. There are 320-540 testes in each proglottid and the bilobed ovary lies in the posterior portion of the segment. At the centre of proglottid, the uterus is conspicuous, spiral and there are three openings in total, including male-genital pore, female-genital pore, and uterine pore through which the eggs are passed (see Figure 6-9-3).

The egg with a thin shell is ellipsoidal, light brown in color, measuring 52-76μm × 31-44μm in size, containing one ovum and many yolk cells which are helpful in differentiating it from the eggs of Diphyllobothrium spp. The egg is tapered at two ends, one of which has a operculum (see Figure 6-9-3).

The plerocercoid or sparganum is a whitish, wrinkled, ribbon-shaped organism, about 0.7mm wide, 300mm long, and the anterior end is capable of invagination (see Figure 6-9-3).

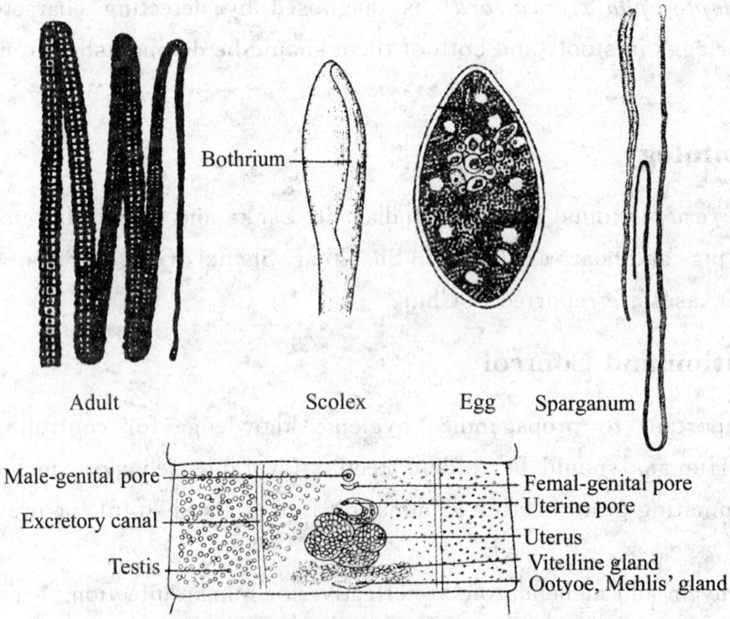

Figure 6-9-3 Morphology of *Spirometra mansoni*

Life Cycle

The development cycle requires three hosts. Main definitive host: dog, cat, tiger, fox, raccoon and human who can rarely be the final host. First intermediate host: a few species of copepods. Main second intermediate host or paratenic host: frog, snake, bird and pig (see Figure 6-9-4).

As shown in Figure 6-9-4, the adult parasitizes in the intestine of definitive host. Cyclops, the first intermediate host, ingests coracidia which are free, ciliated embryo and develop from the eggs when they reach the water with the feces of final hosts. In the hemocoel of the Cyclops, the coracidium turns into procercoid which develops into sparganum (plerocercoid) when a second intermediate host ingests an infected Cyclops. The sparganum can be harbored by many vertebrates, including amphibians, reptiles, birds, swine, rodents, insectivores, and humans. Numerous species of vertebrates are infected with plerocercoid by feeding on amphibians, but they may develop into sparganum after ingesting water containing cyclops infected by procercoids. Several animals are paratenic hosts.

When a definitive host ingests a second intermediate host, the plerocercoid reaches the intestine of the definitive host, it attaches to the mucosa and develops into an adult worm in 10 to 30 days. The lifespan of the adult cestode is three and half years in the cat.

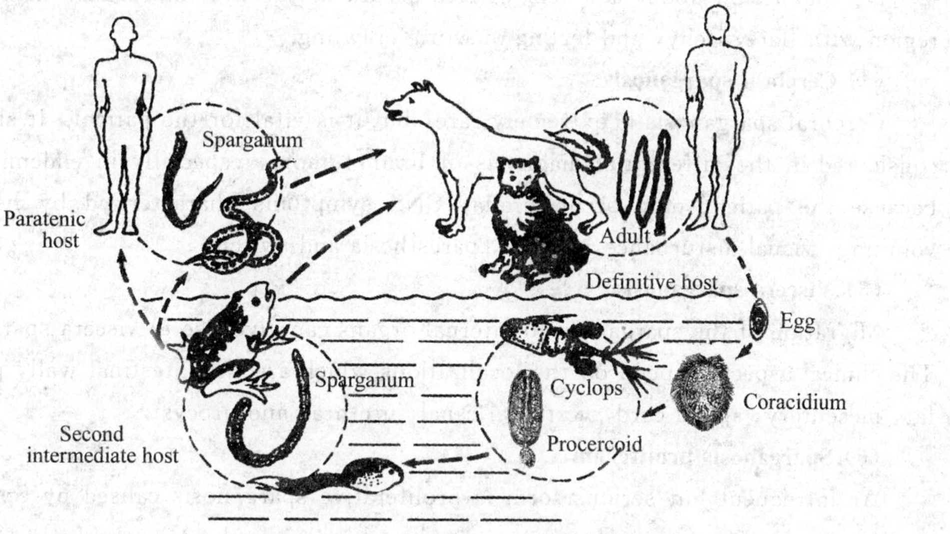

Figure 6-9-4 Life cycle of *Spirometra mansoni*

Pathogenesis and Clinical Manifestation

The adult of *S. mansoni* rarely parasitizes in the small intestine of human and hardly causes clinical aspects which are abdominal pain, vomiting, anorexia, and intermittent diarrhea.

The plerocercoid in the early migratory stage is asymptomatic, but when it has reached its final site and begin to grow, the sparganum may elicit an inflammatory reaction in the surrounding tissues and cause sparganosis mansoni which is as follows:

(1) **Ocular sparganosis**

Ocular sparganosis occurs mainly in Vietnam, Thailand, and a part of China. Its main symptoms consist of a painful edema of the eyelids with lacrimation and pruritus, since a nodule measuring 1 to 3cm forms on the upper eyelid. If the larvae inhabit retrobulbarly in position, the orbit may be forced out so that the lids are unable to close, and corneal ulcers occur.

(2) **Subcutaneous sparganosis**

The lesion is nodular, develops slowly, and can be found on any part of the body. The subcutaneous lesion resembles a lipoma, fibroma, or sebaceous cyst. The larva may be covered by a thin capsule of connective tissue if it stays at a site for a long period, but it may pass through the capsule and migrate from one location to another. The main symptom is pruritus, sometimes accompanied by urticaria. The patient may feel painful when there is inflammation.

(3) **Oral and maxillofacial sparganosis**

Nodular lesion about 0.5-3cm in size occurs in the oral mucosa or maxillofacial region with flare, itchy, and feeling of worm crawling.

(4) **Cerebral sparganosis**

Cerebral sparganosis is extremely rare, but it is vital for the patient. It should be considered in the differential diagnosis of brain tumors, especially in endemic areas, because the patient may occur similar CNS symptoms characterized by headache, vomiting, visual disturbance, seizure, paresthesia and twitch.

(5) **Viscera sparganosis**

Migration of the sparganum to internal organs can give rise to viscera sparganosis. The clinical aspects depend on the localizations which are the intestinal wall, perirenal fat, mesentery, spinal cord, vertebral canal, urethra, and urocyst.

(6) **Sparganosis proliferum**

An infrequent but serious form is proliferative sparganosis caused by Spirometra proliferum. Proliferating spargana may occur almost anywhere in the body, which is pleomorphic, with irregular branches and proliferative buds that detach from the larva and migrate to different tissues in the host, where they repeat the process and invade other organs.

Most patients have a single larva which is about 1mm wide, 10mm long, but multiple parasitism may sometimes be reported. The duration of parasitism is variable and may be more than 30 years.

Laboratory Diagnosis

The diagnosis of adult infection is based on microscopic observation of the eggs or proglottids eliminated in the feces. In the case of infection with a larva, it is useful to inquire history such as placing fresh frog meat on wounds or other lesions, drinking raw water with procercoids, or eating raw meat of second intermediate or paratenic hosts. Specific diagnosis can be made only by removing the nodular lesion and confirming the presence of the sparganum, which on section is seen to possess a rather homogeneous parenchyma in which are scattered the laminated, intensely basophilic calcareous corpuscles which is the characteristic of cestode tissue. Attempts have been made to identify the species of Spirometra larvae by infecting dogs or cats via the digestive route.

A presumptive preoperative diagnosis might be made on demonstration of a painful migratory subcutaneous nodule. If a tumor does not migrate, extensive clinical examinations and immunological studies are mandatory to differentiate it from cysticercosis, hydatidosis, and other diseases.

CT or MR may play a role in diagnosis.

Epidemiology

S. mansoni is found throughout the world, but human infection is not common and distributes in Japan and Russia. Several thousands of cases have been reported in China.

Sparganosis cases are mostly from Japan, China, Korea, and Southeast Asia. It has been reported in 21 provinces, cities and autonomous regions of our country, especially in Guangdong, Jilin, Fujian, Sichuan, Guangxi, and Hunan. Human is infected with the plerocercoid in several ways. (1) The infection of humans with the sparganum occurs from active migration of the larva from freshly split infected frogs used as a poultice for wounds, sore eyes, bruises, or ulcerations, because frogs are popularly believed to have an antiphlogistic effect. (2) Man acquires sparganosis by ingesting larvae contained in raw or undercooked meat of animals infected with spargana, such as amphibians, reptiles, birds, and wild mammals. (3) It is also probable that man can acquire sparganosis through drinking inadequately treated water with copepods infected by procercoids.

Prevention and Control

Human sparganosis can be prevented by avoiding drinking contaminated water, and by making sure that meat is sufficiently cooked. Public health education should emphasize the danger of using the tissue of frogs or other animals for medicinal purposes.

The use of praziquantel or albendazole is recommended for infection of adult.

Surgical removal of the sparganum larva is the effective treatment. Praziquantel, as a supplementary drug, has shown promising results in hastening recovery.

(Wang Yajing)

Raillietina celebensis

The tapeworm *Raillietina celebensis* mainly parasitize domestic rats as final host, but has also been found in humans, mostly children. The intermediate hosts are various species of ants. The adult is approximately 32cm in length, by 0. 2cm in width. It contains about 185 segments which are divided into scolex, neck and proglottids. There are 4 suckers and a large rostellum with about 72 tiny, hammer-shaped hooks in scolex. The mature proglottids are hermaphroditic. The gravid proglottids contains about 300-400 egg packets, each egg packet contains one to four large eggs measuring 45 by 27μm. The morphology of *Raillietina celebensis* shows in (see Figure 6-9-5).

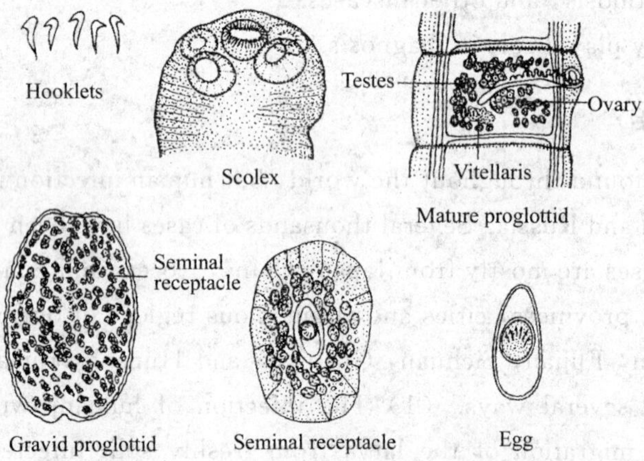

Figure 6-9-5 Adult and egg of *Raillietina celebensis*

The life cycle of *R. celebensis* is very simple. The adult parasitize the lumens of intestine of rats. The gravid proglottids depart from the adult and pass out with feces, and liberate the eggs. The egg enters the body of ants and develops as cysticercoids. When the ants were eaten by the rats, the cysticercoids will develop into an adult. This passage which happens in the human body is similar to that in the rat's body.

Most of the patients usually are asymptomatic in clinic, but some people shows nocturnal grinding teeth, dyspepsia, weight loss, abdominal pain, diarrhea and pruritus ani. The *raillietiniasis celebensis* may be confirmed if the eggs or gravid proglottids are found in feces.

Raillietina celebensis is widely distributed throughout the tropics and subtropics. It is prevalent in Thailand, Burma, Vietnam, the Philippines, Japan, and Australia *et al*. About 70 cases were reported in China, mainly in Taiwan, Fujian, Guangdong, Jiangsu, Zhejiang and Guangxi province. Most of the patients are 1-7 years old children because the children often play in ground and easily eat the ant.

(Si Kaiwei)

Mesocestoides lineatus

The adult of *Mesocestoides lineatus* mainly parasitize in various birds and mammals, especially in carnivores animal, as definitive host, and have occasionally been reported from humans in Denmark, Africa, the United States, Japan, and Korea.

The adult is 30-250cm in length. The scolex has four simple suckers, and no rostellum. Each proglottid has a single set of male and female reproductive systems. The genital pores are median and ventral. Otherwise, the morphology is typically cyclophyllidean, with a paruterine organ replacing the uterus.

The complete life cycle is not known, but it has a rodent or reptile intermediate host, in which a cysticercoid type of larva known as a tetrathyridium develops. Neither mammals nor reptiles can be infected directly by eggs, so a first host must be involved. As yet, such a host has not been identified.

Mesocestoides lineatus are widespread in carnivores such as dog, cat, fox, raccoon, leopard, throughout most of the world. About 20 cases of human Mesocestoidiasis lineatus were reported in the world, mainly distribute in Europe, Northern America, Korea and Japan. Only 4 cases of these diseases were reported in China, which were caused by taking the raw or undercooked flesh or blood of frog, snake or other animals. So the key of prevention is to avoid eating the raw or undercooked flesh, viscera or blood of frog, snake, bird, poultry or other wild animals. Praziquantel is used to treat this disease.

(Si Kaiwei)

Bertiella studeri

Bertiella studeri [(Blanchard, 1891) Stiles and Hassall, 1902] belongs to *Anoplocephalidae*, many species of which exist as parasites of nonhuman primates. Two species of the genus, *Bertiella studeri* and *B. mucronata*, can infect humans. More than 60 cases of human infection have been recorded, and the geographic distribution of cases shows that the tapeworm exists in countries in Asia, Africa, and the Americas.

Morphology

Adult: 150-450mm in length, proglottids average length is 0.1cm, each segment is 0.68-1.10cm in width. The scolex with 4 suckers measures approximately 800μm by 580μm, is globular in shape, and is devoid of hooks and a rostellum. The neck is short (2.65mm in length) and slender.

Egg: The eggs are spherical with a ranging in size from 50.0-65μm by 30.0-45μm and cover with a thin transparent shell 6-8μm thick. The oncospheres vary in size between 15μm and 19μm and had 6-8 slender hooklets each 7-9μm long. The pyriform apparatus range in size between 23μm, and 25μm and terminated into two clear arms (3. 88μm thick). Two filaments were also present, each consisting of a series of horn-like structures 11. 6μm in length, with two rounded or knob-like structures (each 8μm ×6. 5μm) at the extremities.

Life Cycle

The lifecycle of the cestode requires 2 hosts; nonhuman primates are generally the final host, while oribatid mites are the intermediate host, in which the infective cysticercoid of the cestode develops. Oribatid mites may exist in soil to maintain natural infection, and the definitive host is infected by eating or otherwise coming into contact with contaminated soil or food.

Clinical Manifestation

The infected children and the man had common signs and symptoms. All of these cases had intermittent epigastric pain after meals accompanied by nausea, diarrhea, and anorexia, with no fever and loss of weight. Except in one child, the abdomen was soft and tender.

Diagnosis

Diagnosis depends on detecting egg or gravid segment in stool.

Prevention and Control

It is a cestode from monkey and orangutan. Animal infection has been recorded in some provinces in China, and human bertiellosis has been recorded in Sri Lanka, Saudi Arabia, Vietnam, Japan, India, Thailand, Malaysia, and other Asian countries. Humans are infected by unconsciously swallowing infected mites, and in Mauritius, children were infected by eating guavas that had fallen on the soil.

Praziquantel and albendazole can be used for treatment.

(Li Wei)

Taenia asiatica

Asian *Taenia* is a human tapeworm which was first recognized in Taiwan aborigines and subsequently from Asian countries: Korea, Indonesia, Vietnam. It was originally described as *T. asiatica* (Eom and Rim, 1993) based on the morphology in its adult and larval stage. A taxonomic disagreement on whether it is species or subspecies level is mainly due to the morphological similarity of this tapeworm with *T. saginata*, but a sympatric distribution of these two tapeworms is also known in China.

Morphology

T. asiatica is morphologically different from *Taenia saginata* (Goeze, 1782) in having the unarmed rostellum on the scolex of adult, the large number of "uterine twigs" and the existence of "posterior protuberance". These structures in the gravid proglottids were used as taxonomic keys in taeniid tapeworms for the first time. *T. asiatica* metacestode (Cysticercus viscerotropica) was morphologically different from *T. saginata* metacestode (Cysticercus bovis) in having wart-like formations on the external surface of the bladder wall(see Table 6-9-1).

Table 6-9-1 Differential characteristics of *T. asiatica* and *T. saginata*

	T. asiatica	*T. saginata*
Numbers of segment	260-1016	1000-2000
Scolex diameter	1430-1197μm	935-1430μm
Numbers of testicle	354-1197	800-1200
Branch of uterus in gravid segment	11-32	14-32
Intermediate host	pig, boar	cattle
Cysticercus distribution	liver	muscle
Development time	4 weeks	10-12 weeks
Cysticercus length	450-2000μm	1650-5720μm
Width	580-1850μm	1160-3580μm
Scolex size of cysticercus	580-1850μm	1160-3580μm
Hooklet on scolex	2 circles	without

Moreover, the intermediate host involved is not cattle, but swine. The larval state of the Asian taeniid exhibits a liver tropism, though other organs may also be affected. In the intermediate host, the parasite has a cysticercus more similar to that of *T. solium* because the scolex possesses hooks; however, the cysticerci of the Asian *Taenia* are clearly smaller than those of *T. solium*. Cysticerci that have already lost their hooks may also be detected in swine.

Pathogenesis

To date, no clear evidence exists to substantiate the fact that the Asian *Taenia* causes human cysticercosis. This is the main remaining point to be clarified, in view of its importance to human health.

Diagnosis

Taeniasis can be diagnosed by demonstrating *Taenia* proglottids or eggs in the feces. Eggs may also be found in adhesive tape preparations taken near the anus. Repeated sampling may be necessary. *Taenia* spp. eggs cannot be distinguished from other tapeworms such as *Echinococcus* by their morphology; however, enzyme-linked immunosorbent assays (ELISAs) and PCR can differentiate the eggs of *T. solium* from *T. saginata*, and morphology can be used to distinguish these proglottids.

Epidemiology

The main epidemiological feature of this third form of human taeniid is that porcine cysticercosis is linked to the presence of *T. saginata* type adults rather than *T. solium* type adults. This epidemiological characteristic, peculiar to Taiwan (porcine cysticercosis *T. saginata* type adults in humans), stimulated the research that led to the discovery of this third taeniid.

In practical terms, the important point is that humans constitute the definitive host of three taeniids (*T. solium*, *T. saginata* and the Asian *Taenia*) instead of only two as believed until recently. In addition to serving as the definitive host, humans may also function as the intermediate host for *T. solium* with development of cysticercosis and especially neurocysticercosis, a serious and sometimes fatal disease. This is not the case with *T. saginata*, and it remains to be established whether humans are included in the range of possible intermediate hosts of the Asian taeniid.

This transcendental hypothesis is posed in view of the fact that it is precisely at the intermediate host level where both the Asian *Taenia* and the *T. solium* behave similarly and distinct to *T. saginata*. In this context, pigs serve as the intermediate host for both *T. solium* and Asian *Taenia*. Thus, if these parasites effectively share one intermediate host, the question may be posed of whether they are also able to share another, in this case, humans.

Prevention and Control

Prevention of taeniasis depends on avoiding raw or undercooked pork (*T. solium*), pork liver (*T. asiatica*) and beef (*T. saginata*). Potentially contaminated meat should be cooked to at least 56℃ throughout the meat. Freezing can also be beneficial.

Meat inspection reduces the risk of infection. Prevention of cysticercosis or coenurosis depends on good hygiene, including hand washing. In endemic areas, people should avoid eating raw fruits and vegetables that cannot be peeled. Only bottled water, filtered water, or water that has been boiled for at least one minute should be drunk. Human sewage can contain *Taenia* eggs and should not be used to irrigate crops.

The treatment is as outlined for taeniasis solium. Adult tapeworms in the intestines can be killed with anthelmintics such as praziquantel, niclosamide, buclosamide or mebendazole. Rare complications such as obstructed bile ducts or appendicitis may require surgery.

(Li Wei)

Chapter 7 *Acanthocephala*

Macracanthorhynchus hirudinaceus

Acanthocephalan or spiny-headed worm is a kind of parasitic worm in Phylum Acanthocephala. Acanthocephalan has many species, in general, adult worm parasitize in the intestinal tract of vertebrate living in fresh water, seawater and on land. Still, representatives inhabit the intestine of fishes, amphibians, reptiles (rarely), birds, and mammals, in which they occasionally cause serious disease. Some time acanthocephalan can infect human and cause acanthocephaliasis. Few zoologists and still fewer veterinarians and physicians ever encounter a thorny-headed worm. Compared with parasitic platyhelminths or nematodes, they are fairly rare.

The first recognizable description of an acanthocephalan in the literature is that of Redi, who, in 1684, reported white hooked worms in retractable proboscides in the intestines of eels. From the time of Linnaeus to the end of the 19th century, all acanthocephalan species were placed in the collective genus *Echinorhynchus* Zoega in Mueller. Hamam divided *Echinorhynchus*, which by then had become large and unwieldy, into *Gigantorhynchus*. *Neorhynchus*, and *Echinorhynchus*, thereby beginning the modern classification of the Acanthocephala.

Lankester proposed elevating the order Acanthocephala, proposed by Rudolphi in 1808, to the level of phylum. This suggestion was not widely accepted until Van Cleave convincingly argued in its favor. Today the Acanthocephala is widely accepted as a separate phylum.

Macracanthorhynchus hirudinaceus (thorny-headed worm) has a worldwide distribution and is most often associated with domestic swine. They are found in both temperate and tropical climates.

The giant thorny-headed worm of the pig, approximately the size of the giant roundworm (Ascaris); it inhabits the intestinal tract where nodules develop at the site of penetration of the spiny proboscis of each worm; it has occasionally been reported in humans; transmission is by ingestion of infected insects, frequently dung beetles or cockroaches that have fed on the feces of infected pigs containing viable eggs and have then developed the cystacanth stage infective to the vertebrate host, including humans.

Morphology

M. hirudinaceus is known as the giant thorny-headed worm of the hog. Generally they range from creamy white to yellow orange. The body is flat and gradually becomes smaller from the anterior to the posterior. Females are larger than males. Females can reach 650mm long by 7 to 8mm wide. Males range in size from 50 to 90mm long by 6 to 8mm wide. Each has a retractile proboscis that is cylindrical in shape and 0. 6 to 1. 0mm long and 0. 50 to 0. 92mm wide. The proboscis has six backward-curved hooks in each of six spiral rows. The hooks range in size from 0. 260 to 0. 432mm. The proboscis in connected to the trunk by the neck. There is a cerebral ganglion, i. e. , brain. There are flat lemnisci (extensions) that resemble a ribbon and range in size from 20 to 35mm long. Each lemniscus has approximately 6 giant nuclei. They extend from the base of the neck into the pseudocoelom. The function of the lemnisci is unknown. The testes of the male reside in the front half of the body along with the eight cement glands that are oval in shape. Females have embryos that range in size from 0. 092 to 0. 100mm long by 0. 051 to 0. 056mm wide.

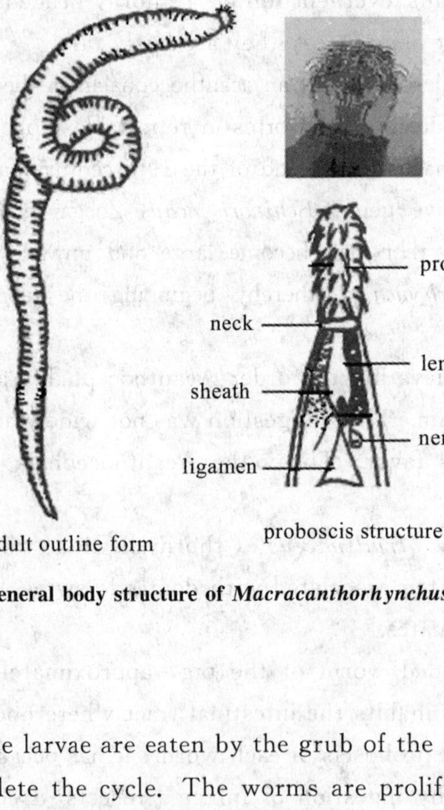

Figure 7-1-1 General body structure of *Macracanthorhynchus hirudinaceus* adult

Life Cycle

This is indirect, the larvae are eaten by the grub of the May beetle. The pig must then eat these to complete the cycle. The worms are prolific egg layers but they are uncommon parasites.

M. hirudinaceus uses an intermediate and definitive host. Intermediate hosts are usually white grubs. Definitive hosts are usually domestic swine but several vertebrates, including humans, are also known to be definitive hosts. Adult females produce a very large number of eggs. The female reproductive system has ovarian balls instead of discrete ovaries. The ovarian balls are within the ligament sac and float freely around. The eggs of *M. hirudinaceus* are deposited in soil when the feces of the definitive host come in contact with it. The beetle larvae eat the eggs in the soil. The larva that hatches from the egg is called the acanthor, a resting stage that doesn't develop until an intermediate host is found. Within an hour of being inside the beetle larva, the acanthor hatches from the egg and uses its bladelike hooks to cut through the gut of the beetle larva. It stops in the hemocoel, attaches to the serosa, and begins to feed. The acanthor begins development in approximately 5-20 days. Feeding triggers the developmental stage, the acanthella. At this stage it is a parasite of the beetle larva, feeding and growing. Once the organ system of the acanthocephalan larva is fully developed the acanthella stage terminates and the acanthocephalan is termed a juvenile. A juvenile infective to a definitive host is termed a cystacanth. When the definitive host eats the beetle larva the cystacanth uses its backward-curved hooks to attach to the intestinal wall of the host where it completes development into the adult, becoming infective in 60-90 days.

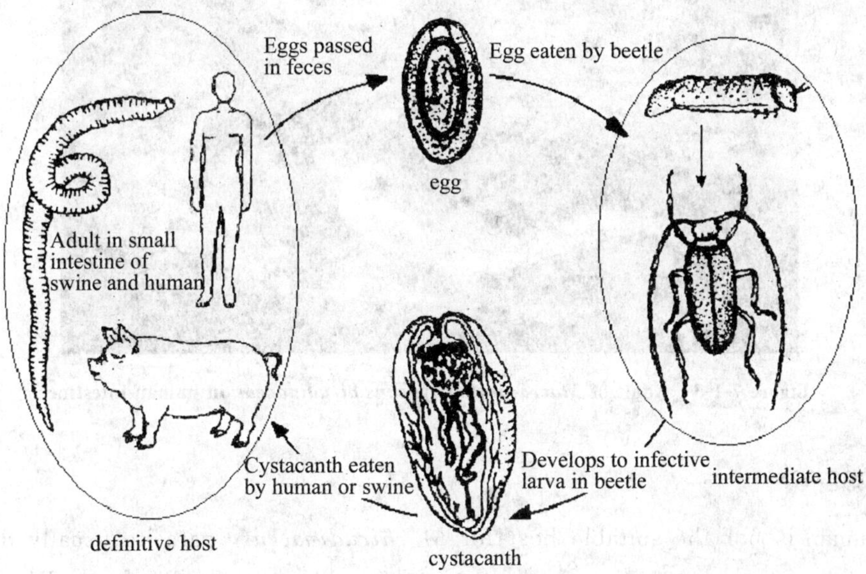

Figure 7-1-2 Life cycle of *Macracanthorhynchus hirudinaceus*

Pathogenesis

In definitive hosts the nature of damage to intestinal mucosa is primarily traumatic, by penetration of the proboscis, and is compounded by the tendency of the worm to release its hold occasionally and reattach at another place. Complete perforation of the gut sometimes occurs, and in mammals, at least, the results are often rapidly fatal (see Figure 7-1-3). Great pain accompanies this phase: Infected monkeys show evident distress, and Grassi and Calandruccio recorded the symptoms of pain and delirium experienced by Calandruccio after he voluntarily infected himself with cystacanths of

Moniliformis moniliformis. It is suspected that secondary bacterial infection is responsible for localized and generalized peritionitis, hemorrhage, pericarditis, myocarditis, arteritis, cholangiolitis, and other complications.

M. hirudinaceus infection show evidence that antigens are released from the proboscis, followed by an intense inflammatory response. It is clear that the pathogenesis caused by acanthocephalans can be severe, but little consideration usually is given to the role this group of parasites could play as a controlling factor of wildlife populations.

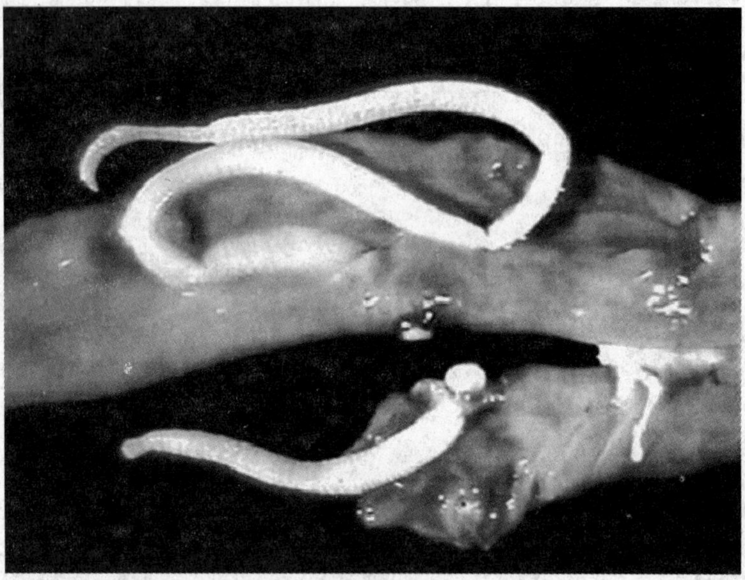

Figure 7-1-3 Adult of *Macracanthorhynchus hirudinaceus* in human intestine

Diagnosis

Human is not the suitable host for *M. hirudinaceus*, parasite usually does not develop into sexual maturation, and worm egg is seldom detected in feces. Diagnosis of the disease is based on the patient whether or not has eaten beetles by mistake and the clinical symptoms. To make a definite diagnosis should depend on the identification of parasite obtaining from natural released in feces, after taking orally diagnostic anthelminthin agent or operation. Use of the egg antigen intradermal test has some diagnostic value.

Epidemiology

Records of Acanthocephala in humans are few, no doubt because of the nature of the intermediate and paratenic hosts involved in the life cycle of the parasites. Few people of the world eat such animals as insects, microcrustaceans, toads, or lizards, at least without cooking them first. However, human infections with seven different species have been reported. *M. hirudinaceus* occasionally has been recognized as a parasite of humans from 1859 to the present.

Thus, it seems that the Acanthocephala do not pose much of a threat to human health. They are much more important as parasites of wild and captive animals, in which sudden epizootics have been known to kill a great number of individuals in a short time.

Epizootics are infrequent but are always possible among domestic swine. The chances of an epizootic wiping out an entire farm of domestic swine and negatively affecting revenue for the farmers are very small. If the acanthocephalan completely perforated the gut of the domestic swine, the pig could die from secondary infections. There are cases of humans being infected with *M. hirudinaceus* but they do not pose any major threat. This is mostly due to the nature of the intermediate host.

Prevention and Control

Little chemotherapy has been developed for acanthocephalans. Various authors have proposed chenopodium and castor oil, calomel and santonin, carbon tetrachloride, and tetrachloroethylene for primates and pigs, with varying results. Oleoresin of aspidium has been used successfully in human cases but is not recommended for children. Mebendazole was used successfully in a 12-month-old child. Control of intermediate hosts is helpful in preventing infection of domestic or captive animals.

(Yin Guorong)

Part III Medical Protozoology

Chapter 8 Introduction to Protozoa

The protozoa are one-celled eukaryotic organisms and are considered to be a subkingdom of the kingdom Protista. The Protozoa are named after the Greek term for first (proto) and animal (zoon). Their size varies greatly, ranging from a few micrometers (e. g., *Cryptosporidium*) up to several millimeters (e. g., opalinids). More than 65,000 species have been described, most of which are free-living organisms; and of which a fifth are parasitic. They are all organized according to the basic pattern of the eukaryotic cell. They are heterotrophic, lacking the ability to use light and inorganic materials to obtain energy and to synthesize structural components. Therefore, they must obtain preformed organic compounds. Apart from a few sedentary species, most Protozoa are motile. Because they have difficulty in retaining water, due in part to their small size, most live in aquatic (or at least moist) environments. Although the majority of Protozoa are free-living, many species are mutualists, commensals, or true parasites. Some are highly pathogenic to their plant or vertebrate hosts and hence are relevant to veterinary and human medicine and agriculture.

Protozoa are found in almost every possible habitat. Anton van Leeuwenhoek was the first person to see protozoa. Between 1674 and 1716, he described several free-living and parasitic protozoa. Virtually all humans have protozoa living in or on their body at some time, and many persons are infected with one or more species throughout their life. Protozoan diseases range from very mild to life-threatening. Parasitic protozoa still kill, mutilate, and debilitate more people in the world than any other group of disease organisms.

Morphology

Protozoa exhibit an enormous range of body form, even though they are largely microscopic, mainly ranging in size from 10-200μm. Most parasitic protozoa in humans are less than 50μm in size. The smallest (mainly intracellular forms) are 1 to 10μm long, but *Balantidium coli* may measure 150μm. a protozoan cell is composed of plasma membrane, cytoplasm and nucleus.

Nucleus

Protozoa are unicellular eukaryotes. As in all eukaryotes, the nucleus is enclosed in a membrane. In protozoa other than ciliates, the nucleus is vesicular, with scattered chromatin giving a diffuse appearance to the nucleus, all nuclei in the individual organism appear alike. One type of vesicular nucleus contains a more or less central body, called an endosome or karyosome. In the phylum Apicomplexa, on the other hand, the vesicular nucleus has one or more nucleoli that contain DNA. The ciliates have both a micronucleus and macronucleus, which appear quite homogeneous in composition.

Cytoplasm

The organelles of protozoa have functions similar to the organs of higher animals. The plasma membrane enclosing the cytoplasm also covers the projecting locomotory structures such as pseudopodia, cilia, and flagella. The outer surface layer of some protozoa, termed a pellicle, is sufficiently rigid to maintain a distinctive shape. In most protozoa the cytoplasm is differentiated into ectoplasm (the outer, transparent layer) and endoplasm (the inner layer containing organelles); the structure of the cytoplasm is most easily seen in species with projecting pseudopodia, such as the amebas. Some protozoa have a cytosome or cell "mouth" for ingesting fluids or solid particles. The trichomonads and trypanosomes have a distinctive undulating membrane between the body wall and a flagellum. Many other structures occur in parasitic protozoa, including the Golgi apparatus, mitochondria, lysosomes, food vacuoles, conoids in the Apicomplexa, and other specialized structures. A protozoan is more like an animal than like a single cell.

Classification of Protozoa

The protozoa are classified into six Phyla by a Committee on Systematica and Evolution of the Society of protozoologists (1985). This classification is based on the morphology of the protozoa as demonstrated by light and electron scanning microscopy. The Sarcomastigophora, the Apicomplexa and Ciliophora, are three important phyla which contain species of medical importance causing diseases in man (see Table 8-1-1). According to their locomotion organelles, protozoa can be divided into four groups: Amoebae, flagellates, ciliates and sporozoan. Protozoa in the category known as Sarcodina (amebae) move by means of pseudopodia ("false feet"). Protozoa classified as Mastigophora (flagellates) move by means of flagella. Protozoa in the category Ciliata or Ciliophora (ciliates) move by means of cilia. Protozoa classified as Sporozoa have no pseudopodia, flagella, or cilia, and therefore do not move. The common parasitic protozoa are list in Table 8-1-1.

Table 8-1-1 Common parasitic protozoa

Parasitic location	Scientific Species Name	Family	Order	Class
Mononuclear phagocyte system	*Leishmania donovani*	Trypanosomatidae	Kinetoplastida	Zoomastigophora
	Leishmania tropica			
	Leishmania braziliensis			
Blood	*Trypanosoma* sp.			
Urogenital canal	*Trichomonas vaginalis*	Trichomonadidae	Trichomonadida	
Oral cavity	*Trichomonas tenax*			
Intestine	*Trichomonas hominis*			
	Dientamoeba fragilis			
	Giardia lamblia	Hexamitidae	Diplomonadida	Lobosea
	Entamoeba histolytica	Entamoebidae	Amoebida	
	Entamoeba dispar			
	Entamoeba hartmanni			
	Entamoeba coli			
	Iodamoeba butschlii			
	Endolimax nana			
Oral cavity	*Entamoeba gingivalis*			
Brain	*Acanthamoebidae* sp.	Acanthamoebidae		
	Naegleria fowleri	Dimastiamoebidiae		
Erythrocyte	*Plasmodium vivax*	Plasmodidae	Eucoccidiida	Sporozoea
	Plasmodium malariae			
	Plasmodium falciparum			
	Plasmodium ovale			
Alveolus	*Pneumocystis* sp.	Undefined		
Karyocyte	*Toxoplasma gondii*	Toxoplasmatidae	Eucoccidiida	
Tissue	*Sarcocystis* sp.	Sarcocystidae		
Epithelium of small intestine mucosa	*Isospora* sp.	Eimeriidae		
	Cryptosporidium sp.	Cryptosporidae		
Colon	*Balantidium coli*	Balantidiidae	Trichostomatida	Kinetofragminophorea

Life Cycle

The life cycle of protozoa may be simple or complex. According to the mode of transmission, they can be divided into three types.

Transmission among humans

In this type, no intermediate host is needed. There is only one host in the life cycle. Transmission is from person to person. For example, the life cycle of intestinal amoebae, flagellates and ciliates is simple and completes in a single host. The parasites replicate only by asexual method of reproduction mostly in the trophozoite stage.

Under unfavorable circumstance, the actively growing trophozoites secrete a resistant cyst wall and are transformed into cysts. This process is called encystation. When the condition becomes favorable the cyst walls are lysed to liberate trophozoites. This process is called excystation. Both the processes of encystation and excystation take place in a single host. The parasites are transformed from one host to another host after encystation only.

Transmission between humans and animals

Some species of the parasitic Protozoa, like *Toxoplasma gondii*, needs more than one vertebrate to finish its life cycle, in which cat is the definitive host, man and others are the intermediate host, with sexual and asexual reproduction. The intermediate host and the definitive host can infect each other.

Transmission by vectors

Some protozoa need an arthropod vector in their life cycle. The transfer manner of these protozoa is person to insect and insect to person. In *Plasmodium* species, sexual reproduction occurs in one host (*Anopheles* mosquito) and asexual replication in another host (man). This process is known as alternation of generation accompanied by alternation of host.

Reproduction

Reproduction in the protozoa may be asexual, as in the amoebas and flagellates that infect humans, or both asexual and sexual, as in the Apicomplexa of medical importance.

Asexual reproduction

(1) **Binary fission**: The most common type of asexual multiplication is binary fission, in which the organelles are duplicated and the protozoan then divides into two complete organisms. Division is longitudinal in the flagellates and transverse in the ciliates; amoebas have no apparent anterior-posterior axis.

(2) **Multiple fission**: Multiple fission occurs in some amoebas and in the Apicomplexa. In this type of division the nucleus and other essential organelles divide

repeatedly before cytokinesis; thus a large number of daughter cells are produced almost simultaneously. During schizogony the cell is called a schizont, meront, or segmenter. The daughter nuclei in the schizont arrange themselves peripherally, and the membranes of the daughter cells form beneath the cell surface of the mother cell. The daughter cells are merozoites, and they finally break away from a small residual mass of protoplasm remaining from the mother cell to initiate another phase of merogony or begin gametogony. Schizogony to produce merozoites may be referred to as merogony. Another type of multiple fission is sporogony, which is multiple fission after the union of gametes.

Several forms of budding can be distinguished. Plasmotomy, sometimes regarded as budding, is a phenomenon in which a multinucleate individual divides into two or smaller, but still multinucleate, daughter cells. Plasmotomy itself is not accompanied by mitosis. External budding is found among some complex ciliates, such as the Suctorians. Here nuclear division is followed by unequal cytokinesis, resulting in a smaller daughter cell, which then grows to its adult size. Internal budding, or endopolygeny, differs from schizogony only in the location of the formation of daughter cells. In this process the daughter cells begin forming within their cell membranes, distributed throughout the cytoplasm of the mother cell rather than at the periphery. The process occurs in the schizonts of some coccidians. Endodyogeny is endopolygeny in which only two daughter cells are formed. It is a form of asexual division seen in *Toxoplasma* and some related organisms. Two daughter cells form within the parent cell, which then ruptures, releasing the smaller progeny which grow to full size before repeating the process.

Sexual reproduction

It occurs by conjugation of gametogeny. Sexual reproduction involves reduction division in meiosis, resulting in a change from diploidy to haploidy with a subsequent union of two cells to restore diploidy. The cells that join to restore diploidy are the gametes, and the process of producing the gametes is gametogony. Cells responsible for the production of gametes are gamonts. Reproduction may be amphimictic, involving the union of gametes from two parents, or automictic, in which case one parent gives rise to both gametes. The uniting gametes may be entire cells or only nuclei. When they are whole cells, the union is called syngamy. In syngamy the gametes may be similar (isogametes) or dissimilar (anisogametes). Although isogametes look similar, they will fuse only with isogametes of another "mating type". Anisogametes often differ in cytoplasmic contents, and in size (sometimes markedly). The larger, more quiescent of the pair is the macrogamete; the smaller, more active gamete is the microgamete. It is tempting to call these forms female and male, respectively, but it is debatable whether gender, in the commonly used sense, can or even should be distinguished in protozoa.

Fusion of the microgamete and macrogamete produces the zygote, which may be a resting stage that overwinters or forms spores that enable survival between hosts.

When only nuclei unite, the Process is termed conjugation. Conjugation is found only among the ciliates, whereas syngamy occurs in all other groups in which sexual reproduction is found.

Nutrition

The nutrition of all protozoa is holozoic; that is, they require organic materials, which may be particulate or in solution. Amoebas engulf particulate food or droplets through a sort of temporary mouth, perform digestion and absorption in a food vacuole, and eject the waste substances. Many protozoa have a permanent mouth, the cytosome or micropore, through which ingested food passes to become enclosed in food vacuoles. Pinocytosis is a method of ingesting nutrient materials whereby fluid is drawn through small, temporary openings in the body wall. The ingested material becomes enclosed within a membrane to form a food vacuole.

Pathogenesis and Defenses

Protozoal infection results in tissue damage leading to disease. In chronic infections the tissue damage is often due to an immune response to the parasite and/or to host antigens as well as to changes in cytokine profiles. Alternatively, it may be due to toxic protozoal products and/or to mechanical damage. Protozoa reproduce in their host, when the number is enough, they may destroy the infected cells, or invade other tissues and produce pathological changes.

Some symbiotic protozoa are nonpathogenic or cause only limited clinical symptoms in immunocompetent host, but give rise to serious damage in immunodeficient persons.

Resistance is the ability of a host to defend itself against a pathogen. Resistance to protozoan parasites involves three interrelated mechanisms: nonspecific factors, cellular immunity, and humoral immunity.

(**He Shenyi**)

Chapter 9 Amoebae

At least six to seven of amoebas are common inhabitants of the human intestinal tract, and belonging to four genera which have been definitely established as parasites of human being. Six belong to the genus *Entamoeba*: (1) *Entamoeba histolytica*, (2) *E. dispar* (3) *E. moshkovskii*, (4) *E. coli*, (5) *E. hartmanni*, (6) *E. gingivalis*. The other three species represent separate genus: *Anticlimax nana*, *Iodamoeba buetschlii* and *Dientamoeba fragilis*. The only parasitic amoeba of medical importance is *E. histolytica*, an important pathogenic parasite of humans, and cause severe disease in human. For this reason it is by far the most widely studies of intestinal parasitic protozoa with a literature spanning over 125 years.

Section 1 *Entamoeba histolytica*

In 1875 Löch discovered an amoeba in the feces of a Russian with dysentery; and reproduced the disease in dog, and he proposed the name of *Amoeba coli* for the new species. However, the association of the parasite with dysentery was not demonstrably established until 1887. In 1891 Councilman and Lafleur conduced an important study of the pathology at a patient with dysentery and hepatic abscess. They confirmed the pathogenic role of the amoebas and yielded the term "amebic dysentery" and "amebic liver abscess". In 1903 Schaudinn created the species name *Entamoeba histolytica* for Lösch's amoeba. In 1925, Emile Brumpt proposed that there were two species within what was being called *Entamoeba histolytica* in fact. One of these resulted in disease in human and the other did not, and the latter was named as *Entamoeba dispar*. As early as 1982, Sargeaunt and his colleagues were already suggesting that the 'non-pathogenic *E. histolytica* was synonymous with Brumpt's *E. dispar*. More recently, *E. histolytica* was formally redescribed to separate it from *E. dispar*, finally validating Brumpt's hypothesis after sixty-eight years.

E. histolytica is the causative agent of amoebic dysentery and extraintestinal abscess. It is prevalent in developing countries that cannot prevent its fecal-oral spread; the true prevalence of *E. histolytica* is perhaps closer to 1 to 5% worldwide, and leading to 50 million cases of invasive amebiasis and with an annual mortality of 40,000 to 110,000 deaths. Invasive amebiasis is a major health problem in worldwide, and on a global scale, it comes second to malaria among protozoan causes of death. All organisms considered in this chapter are grouped according to classification of protozoa as follows:

Phylum: Sarcomastigophora
  Subphylum: Sarcodina
    Superclass: Rhizopoda
      Class: Lobosea
        Order: Amoebida
          Family: Endamoebidae

Morphology

The development stages of *E. histolytica* in the feces include trophozoite, cyst, and precyst, a transitional form (see Figure 9-1-1).

Trophozoite: The trophozoite is distinguished from the other intestinal amoebas by morphologic characteristics of diagnostic importance. The living trophozoites of *E. histolytica* range in size from 10 to 60μm in diameter, but the average are from 15 to 30μm. Furthermore, the diameter of living trophozoites tends to be larger than that of fixed amoebas stain with Heidenhain's hematoxylin due to shrinkage induce by fixation. The trophozoite was with wide, clear, refractile, hyaline ectoplasm, sharply separated from endoplasm. Locomotion of trophozoite is depended on a single well-defined pseudopodium, extended rapidly, without clear differentiation between ectoplasm and endoplasm. The finely granular endoplasm often has ingested red blood cells when the trophozoites are isolated from dysenteric individuals, leukocytes, bacteria or foreign particles are visible sometimes. There is a fine single nucleus, it is spherical, and measuring 4 to 7μm in diameter, consisting of a clearly defined nuclear membrane lined with uniform in size and closely packed small granules of chromatin. The nucleus has a small spherical karyosome, often centrally located, and measuring 0.5μm in diameter, surrounded by an achromatic halo-like capsule.

When the trophozoites were observed by scanning electron microscopy, the surface of trophozoites appears rough with numerous circular openings 0.2 to 0.4μm in diameter that correspond to the mouths of micropinocytic vesicles. These openings are absent from the large protruding stomata of micropinocytic channels (2 to 6μm in diameter) and from pseudopodia. Transmission electron micrographs of trophozoites were shown that the cytoplasm is rich in glycogen and has ribosomes arranged in helices which aggregate. Transmission electron analysis has confirmed the absence of classical mitochondria in both the cytoplasm and nuclei of non-dividing amoebae. There is no classical rough endoplasmic reticulum, or visible Golgi apparatus. There is a heterogeneous population of vacuoles uniformly distributed throughout the cytoplasm.

Precyst: The trophozoites extrude all ingested material and present a spherical form, when it prepares for forming resistant cyst stage. The precystic amoebas are colorless, devoid of food inclusions and lack of a cyst wall. They are smaller than the trophozoite but larger than the cyst. The precyst is characterized by the presence of a larger vacuole and a thin rim of cytoplasm that contains a condensed nucleus. Pseudopodial action is sluggish, and there is no progressive movement.

Cyst: The cyst usually is the infective stage. Cysts are round or oval in shape, slightly asymmetrical hyaline bodies, ranging in diameter from 12 to 15μm. Cysts appear as hyaline bodies with a smooth, highly refractile, nonstaining wall about 125 to 150nm thick. The cytoplasm is colorless, and chromatoid bodies and nuclei are visible sometimes. Cyst nuclei are morphologically similar to those of trophozoites, but are smaller in the mature cyst. As the cyst matures, the number of nuclei changes from one to four. The cytoplasm of immature cysts contains glycogenic vacuoles and the chromatoid body with sausage-shaped, elongate bars with blunt or rounded ends. These chromatoid bodies, which contain ribonucleic, deoxyribonucleic acid, tend to disappear as the cyst matures.

Differentiation of *E. histolytica* from the commensal *E. dispar* is not possible by morphology but requires the use of species-specific monoclonal antibodies or species-specific primers using PCR techniques.

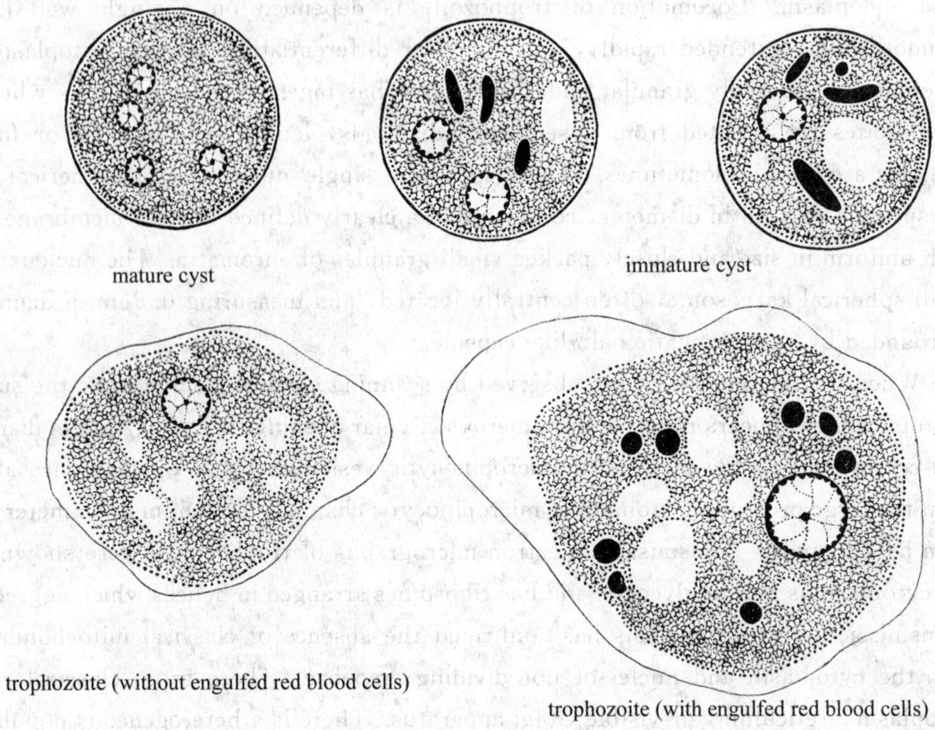

Figure 9-1-1 Trophozoites and cysts of *Entamoeba histolytica*

Life Cycle

The life cycle of *E. histolytica* is comparatively simple, which consists of an infective cyst stage and multiplying trophozoite stage. The mature cyst contains four nuclei, and it is the infective form for human. The cyst is ingested in fecal contaminated food or water and passes through the stomach and intestine. The trophozoite emerges in the terminal ileum or as the cyst forms in the lumen of the large intestine, pass out in the feces, and is immediately infective when the cyst is grown to mature. Few if any cyst is voided in acute dysentery, but it is predominant in chronic infections and carriers. The mature cyst, which is resistant to the acidic digestive juices of the stomach, passes to lower part of the small intestine, in the alkaline medium of caecum or low part of the small intestine, the cyst wall is damaged by the neutral or alkaline digestive juices or trypsin, liberating a four-nucleated trophozoite that undergoes three rounds of cytokinesis and one round of nuclear division into eight metacystic trophozoites. Each of the metacystic trophozoites is capable of developing from immature trophozoite into mature trophozoite. The trophozoite ingests bacteria and multiplies by binary fission during move downward to the colon where, response to unknown stimuli, they develop into precystic form and re-encyst. Cysts are evacuated periodically in the stool and completing their development cycle, and discharged into environment. Cysts remain viable and infective for several days in feces and water, but easily killed by desiccation (see Figure 9-1-2).

Trophozoites divide every 8 hours by binary fission. They are more easily destroyed than those are cysts; they survive up to 5 hours at 37℃ and 96 hours at 5℃. They are rapidly destroyed by heat, drying and chemical disinfectants. In contrast, the resistant cysts can survive for 2 days at 37℃ and up to 60 days at 0℃. Cysts can withstand freezing, but survival decreases rapidly at very low and elevated-temperature, for example, 7 hours at −28℃ or only 5 minutes at 50℃. Diamond's medium allows the growth of *E. histolytica* without living other organisms. Optimal cultivation occurs at 36℃±0.5℃, about pH 7.0 and under reduced oxygen tension.

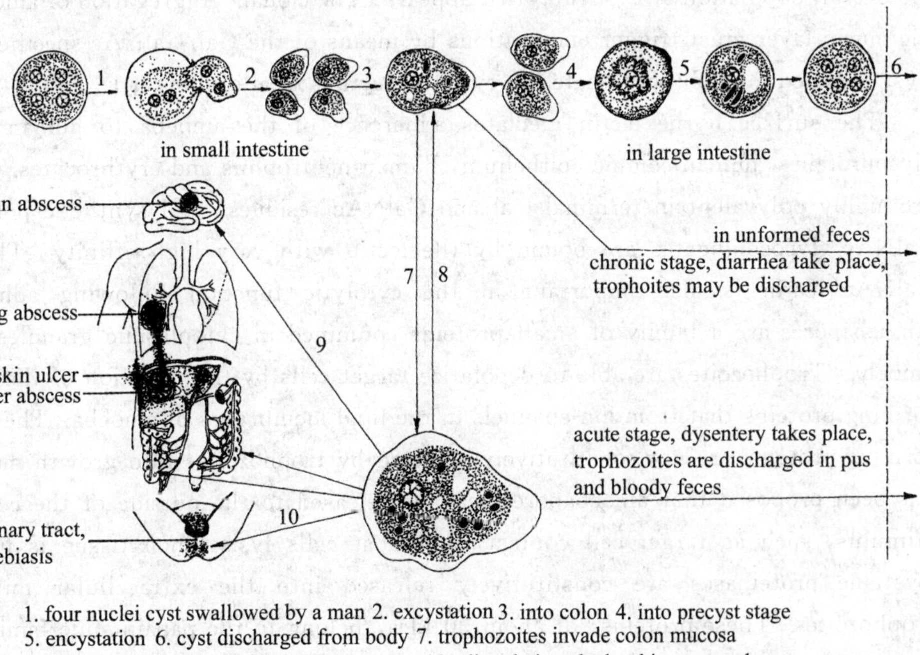

1. four nuclei cyst swallowed by a man 2. excystation 3. into colon 4. into precyst stage 5. encystation 6. cyst discharged from body 7. trophozoites invade colon mucosa 8. return to colon luman 9. via blood stream 10. directly invade the skin surround anus

Figure 9-1-2 Life cycle of *Entamoeba histolytica*

Pathogenesis and Clinical Manifestation

Pathogenicity

Ingestion of the quadrinucleate cyst of *E. histolytica* from focally contaminated food or water initiates infection. The cyst wall is resistant to the action of gastric juice. In the caecum or lower ileum, the cyst wall is damaged by the trypsin leading to excystation. Excystation in the intestinal lumen produces trophozoites. In invasive amebiasis, trophozoites are responsible for clinical syndromes, ranging from classical dysentery to extraintestinal disease with emphasis on hepatic amoebaisis, and they have the capacity to destroy almost all the tissues of human body. The intestinal mucosa, liver, brain or skin are affected most commonly. Several virulence factors contribute to pathogenesis of this parasite, and some might not be identified. However, three pathogenic factors have been studied and characterized at the molecular level extensively: the Gal/GalNAc lectin, mediating adherence to host target cells, the amebapores that form pores in host cell membranes, and the cysteine proteinases that are cytopathic for host tissue. The reproduction of trophozoites has no sexual cycle, and the overall population of *E. histolytica* appears to be clonal. Aggregation of amoebae in the mucin layer must trigger encystations by means of the Gal/GalNAc-specific lectin. Cyst excreted in stool perpetuate life cycle by further fecal-oral spread.

The surface borne lectin mediates adherence of the amoeba to human colonic glycoproteins, human colonic epithelium, human neutrophils and erythrocytes. Mucins are highly polyvalent in terminal Gal and GalNAc residues, and synthetic polyvalent GalNAc glycoconjugates are bound by the lectin with very high affinity. The Gal/GalNAc lectin is also important in the cytolytic function following adherence. Amoebapores are a family of small proteins contained in cytoplasmic granules in the amoeba. Trophozoites are able to depolarize target cells by the insertion of these pore-forming proteins that from ion-channels in the lipid membranes of amoeba. These pore-forming proteins are not constitutively secreted by trophozoites into growth media. It has been proposed that amoebapores may be released to the outside of the cell upon stimulus, such as target cell contact, and host cells lysis when tissue is invaded. Cysteine proteinases are constitutively released into the extracellular milieu by trophozoites. These proteins, of about 30 kDa, belong to the papain superfamily, and have been implicated in the cytopathic effect of *E. histolytica* upon target cells, resulting in the release of adherent cells from monolayers. Cysteine proteinases can cleave the extracellular structural matrix and can degrade fibronectin and laminin. Cysteine proteinases have also been confirmed to activate the alternate complement pathway by cleavage of C3.

Host factors that influence the course of infection include stress, malnutrition, alcoholism, corticosteroid therapy and immunodeficiency. Certain glycoproteins in the colonic mucus may bind avidly to the surface receptor of amoeba and thereby blocking their attachment to epithelial cells. Virulence of *E. histolytica* may also be influenced by the bacterial flora in the colon.

The attachment of *E. histolytica* tropozoites to the colonic mucosa is mediated by the Gal/GalNAc lectin. After attachment the parasite kills the host cell in an extracellular process that involves activation of host cell Caspase-3, leading to apoptotic death and engulfment of the host cell. Invasion of the colonic and cecal mucosa by *E. histolytica* begins in the interglandular epithelium. This is a site of low resistance where the intestinal cells are normally shed as the final stage in the renewal of the epithelium. Cellular infiltration occurs around the invading amoeba. There is lysis of the inflammatory cells and there is tissue necrosis. Intestinal amebiasis most commonly involves the cecum or appendix. Because the inflammatory cells are lysed, they are rarely found in biopsy samples or in materials from scraping rectal mucosal lesions. Ulceration may deepen and progress under the mucosa to form "flask ulcers." The typical flask-like primary ulcer has a crateriform appearance with a wide base and narrow opening with irregular, slightly elevated, and overhanging edges. These extend into the submucosa and produce microhemorrhage spots. The erythrocytes were found in trophozoites in stool specimens or in rectal scrapings, the finding of amoeba full of red cells is still the best indication of the amoebic nature of a case of dysentery or bloody diarrhea. The ulcers are initially superficial, with hyperemic borders and a necrotic base. There is normal mucosa between the sites of invasion. The complications of intestinal amebiasis include appendicitis, intestinal perforation, hemorrhage and stricture. The so-called ameboma or amebic pseudotumor of the colon is a proliferative reaction of *E. histolytica* and is composed of granulation tissue with chronic inflammation and fibrosis.

All lesions of extraintestinal amebiasis are bacteriologically sterile. In systemic amebiasis the liver is invaded chiefly and other organs less frequently. The primary intestinal focus is majorly disseminate to these organs by blood stream, but occurs by direct extension occasionally. The trophozoites reach the liver through the portal venous system causing periportal inflammation. There are authentic records of amebiasis of lung, pericardium, brain, spleen, genitalia, kidneys, urinary bladder, and testes. Cutaneous amebiasis is by direct spread, from the rectum perianally and from colostomy openings and sinuses draining liver abscess. Microscopy demonstrates liquefaction necrosis with few or no neutrophils, which is significantly marked contrast to the situation with bacterial abscesses. The trophozoites are searched at the periphery of an abscess, but not at the necrotic center.

The hepatic lesion is usually solitary, and most frequently is located in the right lobe, situated contiguously with the liver capsule. Variable in size, in some cases it may occupy more than 80% of the whole liver surface. The most serious complications of amebic liver abscess are rupture, particularly into the pericardium, and superinfection. Rupture into the pleura is most common and bacterial superinfection will present after repeated aspiration. Pleuropulmonary amebiasis is another most common complication of an amebic liver abscess, occurring in up to 35% of patients. Rupture of an abscess into the pleural space with empyema formation can cause respiratory compromise suddenly. The second most common complication of amebic liver abscess is intraperitoneal rupture, and result in peritoneal amebiasis. Pericardial amebiasis almost will be succeeding to rupture into pericardium of amebic liver abscess with high mortality rate (see Figure 9-1-3).

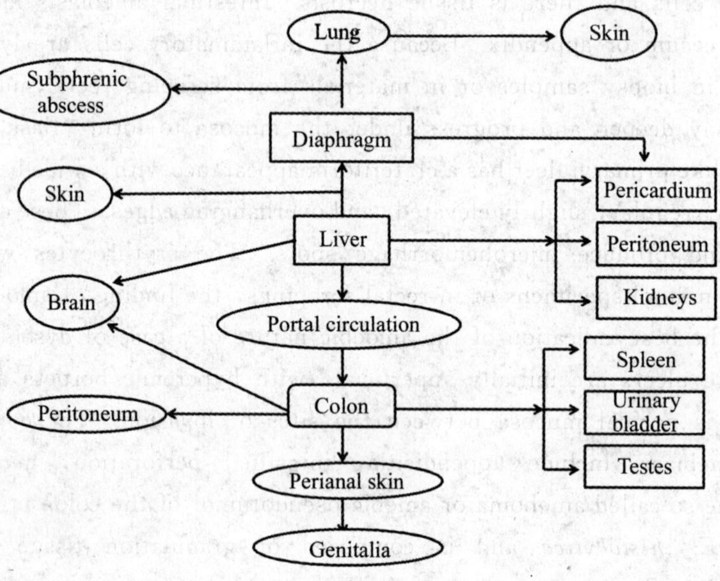

Figure 9-1-3 Summary of location affected by *Entamoeba histolytica*

Clinical Manifestation

The incubation period is highly variable, from 4 days to a year or longer. On an average it will be from 1 to 4 months. The clinical course is characterized by prolonged latency, intermissions and relapses.

In 1969, World Health Organization (WHO) adapted from the following clinical classification about amebiasis.

Ⅰ. Asymptomatic infection

Ⅱ. Symptomatic infection

A. Intestinal amebiasis

1. Dysenteric

2. Nondysenteric colitis

B. Extraintestinal amebiasis

1. Hepatic

a. Acute nonsuppurative

b. Liver abscess

2. Pulmonary

3. Other extraintestinal foci

Infection with *E. histolytica* may depend in large measure on the extent of tissue invasion and on whether the infection is confined to the intestinal tract or has affected other organs. Intestinal amebiasis may be asymptomatic. Patients with amebic colitis typically present with a several cramping abdominal pain, flatulence, anorexia, weight loss, chronic fatigue, and watery or bloody diarrhea. The amebic colitis does not always result in dysentery. Compared to bacillary dysentery, the amebic colitis is usually insidious in onset and the abdominal tenderness less and localized (see Table 9-1-1). The unusual manifestations of amebic colitis include acute necrotizing colitis, toxic megacolon, ameboma, and perianal ulceration. An ameboma, a chronic granulomatous lesion, develops most frequently in the cecal or rectosigmoid region. It may produce indistinguishable on X-ray examination from an annular carcinoma. Though acute necrotizing colitis is rare, the patients appear very ill, with high fever, bloody mucoid diarrhea, an aching abdominal pain with signs of peritoneal irritation. The acute necrotizing colitis is associated with a mortality rate of more than 40 percent.

Table 9-1-1 Differential features of amebic and bacillary dysentery

Features	Amebic dysentery	Bacillary dysentery
Clinical		
Onset	slow	acute
Fever	absent or low	present and high
Abdominal pain	localized	generalized
Diarrhea	6-8/day	over 10/day
Stool		
Color	deep red or dark red	bright red
Character	mixed with blood and mucus	blood and mucus only
Microscopy		
Cellular exudate	scanty	abundant
Red blood cell	clumped	discrete or in rouleaux
Charcot-Leyden crystals	present	absent
Trophozoite	motile trophozoite with RBC	absent

Hepatic involvement is overwhelmingly the most common extraintestinal manifestation of amebiasis. This complication is 10 times as common in adult men as in adult women and is a rare disease in children. Approximately 80 percent of patients with amebic liver abscess are 20 to 40-year-old males with typically two to four weeks fever, cough, and a constant dull abdominal pain in the right upper quadrant or epigastrium. Besides these prevailing symptoms, patients may also complain of malaise, nausea, vomiting, anorexia and weight loss. Hepatomegaly is the most important physical sign in amoebic liver abscess. The enlargement of the liver varies with the size and the site of the lesion. In the larger abscesses, a mass or a lump may be seen in the right hypochondria or epigastria. The tenderness may be diffuse or localized.

Complications of amebic liver abscess may arise from rupture of the abscess with extension into the peritoneum, pleural cavity, or pericardium. The amoebic abscess in lung, brain, and skin were described to result hematogenous spread from amebic lesion in the colon or other sites. The amebic abscess causes severe destruction of brain tissue and is fatal.

Immunity

E. histolytica infection will stimulate cell-mediated and humoral immune responses. Immunity to the infection is associated with a mucosal IgA response against the Gal/GalNAc lectin. As with other enteric organisms, antigen-specific secretory immunoglobulin A (IgA) antibodies have been found to mediate protection against intestinal infection by *Entamoeba* species. This mucosal secretory IgA against the Gal/GalNAc inhibitable lectin is associated with immunity to reinfection. In general, intestinal IgA antibodies prevent microbial binding to epithelial surfaces and promote clearance of pathogenic enteric organisms by agglutination and blocking of surface receptors essential for microbial pathogenesis and invasion. Local and systemic antibodies can be demonstrated within several days to one week of invasive infection, and in general are elicited after tissue invasion. The cell-mediated responses have been indicated in patients with amebic liver abscess, characterized by lymphocytes proliferation and cytokine secretion, such as interferon-γ, tumor necrosis factor-α or interleukin-2. Development of antibody responses may not correlate with protection against *E. histolytica*, because the trophozoites cap and degrade antibodies are attached to the surface. However, infection confers some degree of protection as evidenced by the very low frequency of recurrence of invasive colitis and liver abscesses in endemic areas. The activated macrophages could kill the trophozoites of a virulent strain of *E. histolytica* through a contact-dependent antibody-independent mechanism. A role of $CD4^+$ T cell in the outcome of the disease is also suggested. The good vaccine candidate should contain both B and T cells epitopes, and contribute to macrophage activation. The development of a vaccine against *E. histolytica* should be a priority. There are studies indicated that the course and severity of amebiasis do not seem to be affected by

HIV infection. Recently, some epidemiologic study in HIV-positive patients demonstrated that HIV infection is a risk factor for infection with *E. histolytica*.

Diagnosis

Traditionally, definitive diagnosis of amebiasis is made by detection of *E . histolytica* in tissues or discharge from the lesions by microscopy-cytological diagnosis. Cultures are not employed for routine diagnosis. Immunological test for antigen or antibody detection and DNA amplification of the parasite have been shown to be very helpful in diagnosis of amebiasis.

Microscopy-cytological diagnosis: The cytological diagnosis of amebiasis is neither specific nor sensitive. Since *E. histolytica* and *E. dispar* are morphologically identical, and fecal leukocytes or macrophages frequently have been misidentified as *E. histolytica* trophozoites, these make cytologic diagnosis extremely nonspecific. The identification of hematophagous trophozoites is the character of *E. histolytica* infection.

Trophozoites are sensitive to temperature or desiccation, and readily killed by water, urine, disinfector or antibiotics. The patient's feces with amebiasis are blood and mucous mixed, copious, semiliquid, dark red or brownish block in color. Frequently, a saline wet mount is used for the examination of trophozoites and iodine preparation shows the details of cysts. A sample of fresh feces consists of a few pus cells, epithelial cells and macrophages, except motile trophozoites throwing pseudopodia or containing erythrocytes. Charcot-Leyden crystals which are diamond shape and refractile are demonstrated in some cases. Iodine stained film shows that the cyst is a smooth and hyaline appearance; with clear and no more than four nuclei. The glycogen vacuoles and the sausage-shaped chromatoid bodies are stained sometimes. It is important to distinguish the differential characters of intestinal *Entamoeba* species, this is particularly true for *E. coli*, that is frequently detected in stool specimens isolated from individual exposed to contaminated food or water (see Table 9-1-2). A recent WHO special committee recommended that quadrinucleate cysts now are identified as *E. histolytica*/*E. dispar*. Stool culture is not used routinely but may prove positive in cases found negative by microscopy on occasion, however, stool culture is usually not available in clinical practice. In case of amebic liver abscess, trophozoites are usually only present in the capsule or the margins of abscess, so that the fluid obtained from the center of the abscess may not contain trophozoites. Since the trophozoites are rarely detected by aspiration, amebic liver abscess is difficult to diagnose by microscopic examination of the abscess fluid. Cysts are never seen in extraintestinal lesions. Because of the negative microscopy-cytological diagnosis, antigen detection or serology diagnosis and gene amplification can be an essential adjunct method.

Table 9-1-2 **Morphological identification of *E. histolytica* and *E. coli***

	E. histolytica	*E. coli*
Trophozoite(m)	10-60	15-50
Cyst(m)	12-15	15-30
Pattern of granules	fine, uniform	coarse
chromatin	ring	granules
Karyosome	central, sharp	moderately large, coarse
Ingested RBC	present	absent
Cyst with nuclei	1-4	1-8
Chromatoidal bars	smooth, round edges	splintered, irregular

Antigen detection and serology: Several kits marketed for antigenic diagnosis of *E. histolytica* in stool are currently available. Highly specific and sensitive ELISA reagents can differentiate between *E. histolytica* and *E. dispar* antigens, especially in early infection. Polyvalent immunochromatographic strip tests can detect *E. histolytica*/*E. dispar*, *Giardia* and *Cryptosporidium* antigens in stool samples. Detection of Gal-GalNAc lectin antigen in serum can be used to identify *E. histolytica* infection. Salivary antigen has also been tested as a predictor for invasive amebiasis, which assay shows moderate sensitivity and high specificity in early amebic colitis.

Serologic testing is still a major test for the diagnosis of invasive amebiasis. A number of different serological tests have been developed, including ELISA, indirect hemagglutination (IHA) test, latex agglutination (LA) test, cellulose acetate membrane precipitation (CAP) test, agar gel diffusion (AGD), counterimmunoelectrophoresis (CIE) and indirect fluorescent-antibody test (IFA). However, some serologic assays are less sensitive than antigen detection in early infection. Because serology remains positive for months to several years after exposure to *E. histolytica*, even after successful treatment, serology is not a specific marker for acute infection in all cases. Diagnosis of acute amebiasis based on a positive IFA titer of *E. histolytica* antibody is ≥1 : 256 may be valuable. More than 10% of patients acutely with an amebic liver abscess symptom may be shown to be seronegative, but the titer of IgG antibody detectable within a few days to two weeks. Detection of serum IgA antibodies might prove to be useful for diagnosis, since these antibodies were found in 83.8% of amebic colitis patients. The serologic assay could be very useful in determining if an asymptomatic cyst carrier in possessing *E. histolytica* if stool antigens detection is not available.

DNA amplification: A number of DNA amplification based test have been demonstrated for the detection of *E. histolytica* in stool. Detection of small rRNA genes or the repetitive regions in extrachromosomal DNA or other *E.* histolytica-specific DNA sequences by polymerase chain reaction (PCR) demonstrates extremely improved sensitivity over other methods. PCR is a powerful tool for amplification of *E. histolytica*-specific DNA in even in formalin-ether-sedimented stool sample. The *E.*

histolytica DNA from the abscess fluids of extraintestinal lesions also could be detected by using PCR. PCR-based tests are powerful tools for differentiating *E. histolytica* from *E. dispar* and other amoeba species.

Other diagnosis: Ultrasonography, noninvasive radiography, magnetic resonance imaging (MRI), and computed tomography (CT) scan are important in the early diagnosis of extraintestinal lesions, especially in amebic liver abscess. In the imaging study, an elevation of the right hemidiaphragm in chest radiography is a common find when there are abscess of the live right lobe. At sonography the amebic liver abscess tends to be oval or round. In some cases, the abdominal CT scan is valuable imaging procedure, with greater resolution and sensitivity for detection of hepatic lesions, especially the smaller ones, all excellent for early diagnosis. In the CT scan, an amebic liver abscess appears as a oval, well-defined, low-density lesion, with an homogeneous septated cavity, and with fluid. The colonoscopy examination may demonstrate intestinal amebiasis.

Epidemiology

The enteric protozoan *E. histolytica* is the intestinal protozoal parasite, it is responsible for an estimated 50 million cases of invasive amebiasis annually, including amebic colitis and liver abscess in human, and resulting in 40,000 to 100,000 deaths annually. Amebiasis is worldwide prevalent in persons residing in or travelling to endemic areas though it is more common in the tropical areas. The realizations that *E. histolytica* and *E. dispar* are morphologically identical species with markedly different pathological characteristics have demonstrated in aspects of amebiasis, which is notable on the epidemiology. Prevalence rates of amebiasis vary from as low as 0. 1 percent in affluent areas, to more than 20 percent in some poor sanitation areas. Usually the onset of the rainy season is associated with a sharp peak in prevalence. In addition, temperature, rainfall, and humidity also seem to be stimulative factors in this protozoa transmission. Recent studies from Japan, Republic of Korea, China (including Taiwan), and Australia, areas where *E. histolytica* endemicity is generally low, suggested that amebiasis is emerging parasitic infection that occurs exclusively in men who have sex with men (MSM). It could confirm that *E. histolytica* is one of major pathogens in the Gay bowel syndrome. It was suggested that the invasive amebiasis is emerging as an increasingly common infection, specifically in MSM population. It is also well known that the sexual transmission of *E. histolytica* has been widely documented; especially the clinical presentations of homosexual community often differ from those seen in the heterosexual population. Direct oral-anal sex contact is a common practice among homosexual men, leading to both fecal exposure and oral contact with a variety of intestinal pathogens.

Asymptomatic cyst passers or carriers are of utmost importance in the transmission of the disease. The patient with acute dysentery is of no importance as the source of infection, because his stool contains trophozoites only. Sometimes, carriers may shed the infective cysts for years. The human being is the reservoir host for *E. histolytica* and could transmit the infection to other humans, primates and so on. Amebiasis in animals may be important as a source of human infection. Intestinal infection occurs at all ages and there are no significant differences between males and females, though intestinal amebiasis is more common in less 14-year-old children or more than 40-year-old adults. Amebiasis is essentially an endemic disease though it could occasionally occur in epidemic form due to contamination of water. Contaminated food and water constitute the most important vehicles of infection.

The cyst stage is very resistant to environmental conditions and can remain for 2 months in water at 0℃ and 40 days at 2 to 6℃, viable in the soil for 8 days at 28 to 34℃, 30 minutes at 40℃ and 5 minutes at 50℃. In grossly contaminated water and sewage, the cysts may survive longer. They remain viable in moist soil up to 10 days, and resist 1/2,500 mercury bichloride. Cysts are removed by filtration or killed by 200 ppm of iodine, 5 to 10% acetic acid in 15 minutes, drying, boiling even by temperatures over 55℃. The asymptomatic cyst carrier who is a food handler may play one of the most important roles in transmission. Using night soil for fertilizer may play other important roles in some areas. Flies and cockroaches may act of epidemiologic importance as mechanical vectors.

Prevention and Control

Treatment

An ideal treatment is yet to be devised; therapy for invasive infection differs from that for asymptomatic intestinal amebiasis. For such noninvasive infections, treatment may not be strictly necessary, or may be treated with paromomycin. In case of invasive amoebiasis, which includes severe colitis with ulcerations and dysentery, hepatic abscess, and other extraintestinal sites, the patients should receive metronidazole, tinidazole, ornidazole as first-line agents. Tinidazole or ornidazole with longer half-lives, is a better tolerated and shorter periods of treatment. Although metronidazole is very effective in the treatment of amoebic systemic infection, it may be unable to eradicate amoebas from colon. This has suggested that these patients must receive sequentially, paromomycin or the second-line agent diloxanide furoate or iodoquinol to cure luminal infection and prevent relapse. The side effects of metronidazole consist of nausea, headache, diarrhea, and so on.

Therapeutic aspiration of an amebic liver abscess was a routine procedure, as an adjunct to metronidazole therapy. Drainage of the abscess may be necessary in the patient who has no clinical response to drug therapy within 7 days, in exceptional circumstance, for example, a high risk of abscess rupture, with the diameter of the cavity more than 5cm or by the presence of lesions in the left lobe of liver. The dangers that one can spread the amebic infection have to be considered, although the number of amebae within the aspirate is exceedingly small, and trophozoites incline to the edge of abscess. It has suggested that the aspiration is quite safe. Patients gradually respond to metronidazole therapy alone within a few days to a week, in the amoebic systemic infection, absence of complications, rapid clinical improvement is seen. The healing of abscess cavity of extraintestinal sites may occur within from 3 to 12 months and must be monitored by ultrasonography or CT scans.

There is some controversy on the approach to management of clinical amebiasis. In endemic areas, only patients with symptomatic amoebiasis should be treated, because of the frequency of reinfection. In nonendemic areas, every patient with amebiasis should be treated.

Prevention

It was known that most amebiasis is acquired through the contamination of foodstuffs and water, and the key point of general prophylaxis of infection will be breaking the chain of transmission. Consequently, improving basic personal hygiene and sanitation practices for all fecal-oral infection is one of the most effective methods. In addition, purification of water or elimination of the source of fecal contamination is also a required method to control the spread of amebic infection. It will be important that a thorough screening of food handlers by routine stool examinations, detection and treatment of carriers to limit the spread of infection. The spread of amebiasis among MSM presents a new problem for public health subject. There is no vaccine available against amebiasis. Several antigens of *E. histolytica* have been developed as possible immunogens, and yet these have been tried only in animal models. The control of invasive amebiasis could be achieved through improvement of living standards and the establishment of adequate sanitary conditions in countries where the amebiasis is endemic.

Section 2 Nonpathogenic Commensal Intestinal Amoeba

Entamoeba coli

E. coli is a one of nonpathogenic commensal intestinal amoeba that closely resembles *E. histolytica*. It was first described by Lewis (1870) and Cunningham (1871) in India, and it is present in healthy persons. It is worldwide in distribution. The trophozoites are about 15 to 50μm in diameter with sluggish motility with short, blunt pseudopodia and the cytoplasm contains bacteria. The nucleus is usually visible and has a characteristic karyosome surrounded by a coarse granules of chromatin and thick nuclear membrane. The cysts of *E. coli* are 10 to 30μm in diameter, and definitely greater than that of *E. histolytica*. The cytoplasm of cysts is with a prominent glycogen mass in immature stage, and the numbers of nuclei vary from one to eight in number, the mature cyst has eight nuclei (see Figure 9-2-1).

Entamoeba hartmanni

E. hartmanni is usually confused with *E. histolytica*, and formerly designated to be a "small race" *E. histolytica*. It is clearly distinguishable between this two species in size. It is considered a nonpathogenic commensal amoeba and accordingly treatment is not required to this infection. The size of rounded trophozoites of *E. hartmanni* measures from 4 to 12μm in diameter, and the cyst's size ranges from 5 to 10μm. Trophozoites do not ingest erythrocytes and show slow motility (see Figure 9-2-1). The cyst resembles that of *E. nana*.

Iodamoeba butschlii

I. butschlii is widely distributed, and less common than *E. coli* and *E. nana*. It is the most common amoeba of swine, and pig may be its original host. It is also frequently found in human. Trophozoites vary greatly in size, ranging 4 to 20μm in diameter, with conspicuous nucleus. The cytoplasm contains glycogen mass and bacteria. Yeasts and debris of erythrocytes are never ingested. The prominent karyosome is larger and in half size of the nucleus and surrounded by refractile granules. The cyst is oval, uninucleate, about 8-15μm in diameter, and the glycogen vacuole is prominent. *I. butschlii* is nonpathogenic, exceptionally has the presence of this protozoa been linked to symptomatic infection by human.

Entamoeba gingivalis

E. gingivalis was discovered in 1849, and the first parasitic amoeba of human to be described. It is often found from the pyorrheal pockets between teeth, tonsillar crypts, bronchial mucus, thus appearing in sputum, every discharge of pleural cavity. It is very similar to *E. histolytica* in morphology, and it is important to make identification between both. The trophozoite is about 10 to 20μm in diameter, and the cytoplasm contains food vacuoles with ingested bacteria, leukocytes and epithelial cells. The nucleus is round with a delicate central karyosome. *E. gingivalis* is the only species that could ingest these, and the cystic stage is apparently absent. It has been found in bronchial washings or aspiration of pleural cavity from cases of pulmonary suppuration and in sputum. It was reported that *E. gingivalis* has been found in vaginal and cervical smears from women using intrauterine devices, and they disappear spontaneously after removing these. No treatment is recommended. Although *E. gingivalis* is often discovered from individual with pyorrhea alveolaris, and even has been found in oral cavities of HIV infected patients with periodontal disease, it is still considered to be a nonpathogenic amoeba.

Entamoeba dispar

In 1925, Brumpt formulated the theory that there were in fact two species within what was being called *E. histolytica*. One of these was isolated from the individuals with amebic disease, and the other was not. The latter he named *E. dispar*, which could be correlated with the existence of two distinct but morphologically identical species. This hypothesis was dismissed at that time, but subsequent evidence which gave support to Brumpt's findings occured. In 1993, 68 years after the original discovery of *E. dispar*, *E. histolytica* and *E. dispar* were formally accepted as different closely related species on the basis of genetic, immunological, and biochemical analyses. The life cycle of *E. dispar* is essentially similar to that of the nonpathogenic intestinal amoeba, for example *E. coli*. *E. dispar* seems to be capable of causing focal intestinal lesion in experimental animal, but it does not seem to actually be able to invade the tissues. *E. dispar* is approximately nine times more prevalent than *E. histolytica*, and together they infect about 10% of the world's population. *E. dispar* does not cause symptomatic disease and does not require treatment, nor does it elicit the level of serum antibodies when *E. dispar* infection approach those seen with *E. histolytica*.

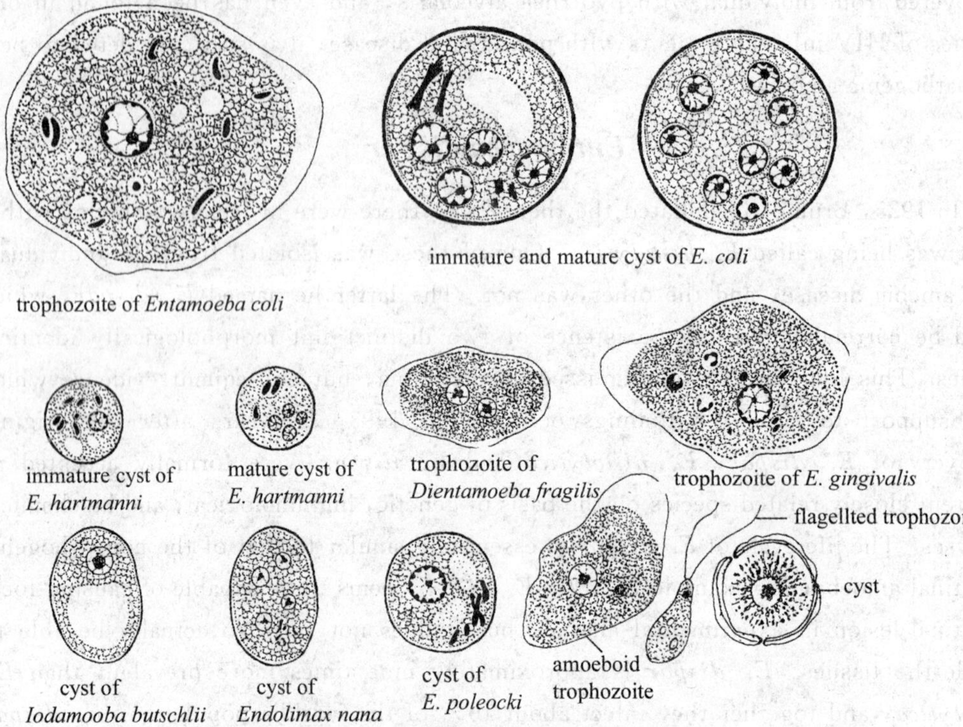

Figure 9-2-1 Morphologic characteristics of nonpathogenic intestinal amoeba

(Hiroshi Tachibana and Cheng Xunjia)

Section 3 Pathogenic free-living amoebae

In recent years, there has been a great deal of interest in a Group of small, free-living amoebae belonging to the genera *Naegleria* and *Acanthamoeba*. These amoebae are normally free-living in fresh, brackish, and salt water, moist soil, and decaying vegetation. They are capable of facultative parasitism in humans and are pathogenic. Their pathogenicity in humans was first noted in 1965, when fatal cases of primary amoebic meningoencephalitis (PAM) were diagnosed simultaneously in Australia and Florida. Since then, several hundred cases have been reported worldwide. Most victims have a history of recent exposure to stagnant, warm, fresh, or brackish water, such as that found in swimming pools, ponds, and lakes. Most cases with PAM can be ascribed to *Naegleria*; less commonly *Acanthamoeba* organisms are involved. Naegleria are characterized as ameboflagellates, able temporarily to assume a flagellate form while being completely devoid of flagella in the ameboid stage. *Acanthamoeba* never produce flagella.

Naegleria fowleri

Naegleria fowleri is the principal causative agent for PAM. Its life cycle includes flagellated and amoeboid trophozoites and cysts, with rapid transformation from one form to the other. The flagellated trophozoite possesses two flagella, while the amoeboid trophozoite displays a single, blunt pseudopodium with minutely pointed extensions on its end. In the free-living state, the organisms have contractile vacuoles (see Figure 9-3-1). Binary fission occurs only in the amoeboid trophozoite stage. The flagellated trophozoites are capable of rapid movement through the water, and transmission to humans most likely occurs when these forms invade the nasopharyngeal mucosa. The amoeboid trophozoite migrates through the nervous system via the cribriform plate to the brain, where inflammation occurs and death usually ensues. No cyst stage occurs in the human host, and flagellated trophozoites are observed only during the invasive stage. Diagnostic confirmation requires identification of the motile amoeboid trophozoite in cerebrospinal fluid under the microscope, but since death may occur in 5-7 days, most cases are diagnosed at autopsy.

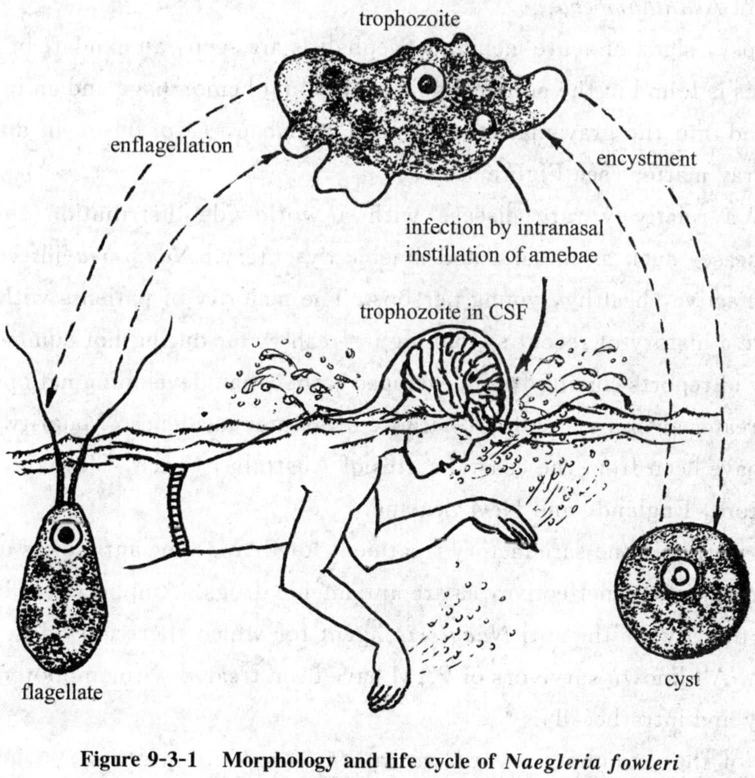

Figure 9-3-1 Morphology and life cycle of *Naegleria fowleri*

The clinical course of PAM is dramatic. A day or so of prodromal symptoms of headache and fever is followed by the rapid onset of nausea and vomiting accompanied by the signs and symptoms of meningitis with involvement of the olfactory, frontal, temporal, and cerebella area. Meningeal irritation may be accompanied by stiff neck, generalized seizures, and Kernig's sign. Olfactory lobe involvement is perhaps the most characteristic; disturbances in the sense of smell or taste may be noted early in the course of the disease but are not always seen. Patients often become irrational before lapsing into coma. Death occurs early; the entire clinical course seldom extends beyond 3 to 6 days.

Spinal puncture reveals a cloudy to frankly purulent or sanguinopurulent fluid, usually under increased pressure. The cell count ranges from a few hundred to more than 20,000 white blood cells per microliter, predominantly neutrophils, and the failure to find bacteria in such a purulent spinal fluid should alert physicians and laboratory technologists to the possibility of PAM. Spinal fluid protein is generally, though not invariably, increased, and glucose levels are low. Red blood cells are frequently present, and motile amoebae may be found in unstained preparation of spinal fluid. Their activity is characterized by the explosive formation of blunt pseudopodia, like those of *Entamoeba histolytica*, rather than the tapering, spiky projections seen on the pseudopodia of *Acanthamoeba*.

On autopsy, signs of acute meningoencephalitis are seen: an exudate of neutrophils and monocytes is found in the subarachnoid space, and hemorrhage and an inflammatory exudate extend into the gray matter. Rounded amoebae, 10 or 11μm in diameter, are seen in the gray matter (see Figure 9-3-1).

PAM is a relatively rare disease with a worldwide distribution comparing to protozoan diseases such as malaria and amebic dysentery. *Naegleria* infection is seen most often in active, healthy, young persons. The majority of patients with *Naegleria* infection have a history of recent swimming in fresh water during hot summer weather. The majority of reports coming from developed rather than developing nations, probably because of greater awareness and not because of greater incidence. Majority of reported PAM cases have been from the coastal states of Australia, Czech, Slovakia, the United States, Belgium, England, and New Zealand.

At present there is no satisfactory treatment for PAM. The antibiotics used to treat bacterial meningitis are ineffective, as are antiamebic drugs. Amphotericin B, a drug of considerable toxicity, is the anti-*Naegleria* agent for which there is evidence of clinical effectiveness. All known survivors of PAM have been treated with amphotericin B given intravenously and intrathecally.

Because of the swimming-related nature *of Naegleria* infection, swimming areas have been subjected to intensive investigation. People should avoid swimming and diving in the water in which *Naegleria* protozoa live. Given the present limited understanding of the ecology of *N. fowleri*, practical measures for the prevention and control of

Naegleria infection include public education, awareness in the medical community, and adequate chlorination of public water supplies, including swimming facilities.

Acanthamoeba

Four species of *Acanthamoeba* (*A. culbertsoni*, *A. polyphaga*, *A. castellanii*, and *A. rhysodes*) cause chronic PAM and have been positively implicated in human cases. It is possible that some of these may represent strains of a single species, *A. castellanii*, rather than separate species. Except for the absence of a flagellated trophozoite stage, the life cycle of *Acanthamoeba* is very similar to that of *Naegleria*. The amoeboid trophozoites of the two genera can be distinguished by their pseudopodia; the trophozoites of *Naegleria* form a single, lobose pseudopodium and move rapidly, while those of *Acanthamoeba* form small, pointed pseudopodia (acanthopodia) and move sluggishly. *Acanthamoeba* infections can be distinguished from those of *Naegleria* by the characteristic cysts of *Acanthamoeba* found in affected tissues. The cysts of *Naegleria* are round, while those of *Acanthamoeba* are square. Less common than *Naegleria*, *Acanthamoeba* is a facultative parasite of humans responsible for symptoms similar to but less severe than those of *Naegleria* infections. Central nervous system involvement, granulomatous amoebic meningoencephalitis (GAM), is relatively rare but usually fatal, especially in immunologically compromised patients. While there is no uniformly effective treatment for *Naegleria* infections, in a few cases there has been favorable response to intravenous administration of amphotericin B. New infections of *Acanthamoeba* respond favorably to sulfonamides, and established infections appear to respond to amphotericin B. Ocular keratitis, attributed to *Acanthamoeba* infecting wearers of soft contact lenses, is refractory to these drugs. Patients with ocular keratitis have been treated successfully with intensive topical chemotherapy consisting of miconazole nitrate, gramicidin B, and propamidine isethionate (see Figure 9-3-2).

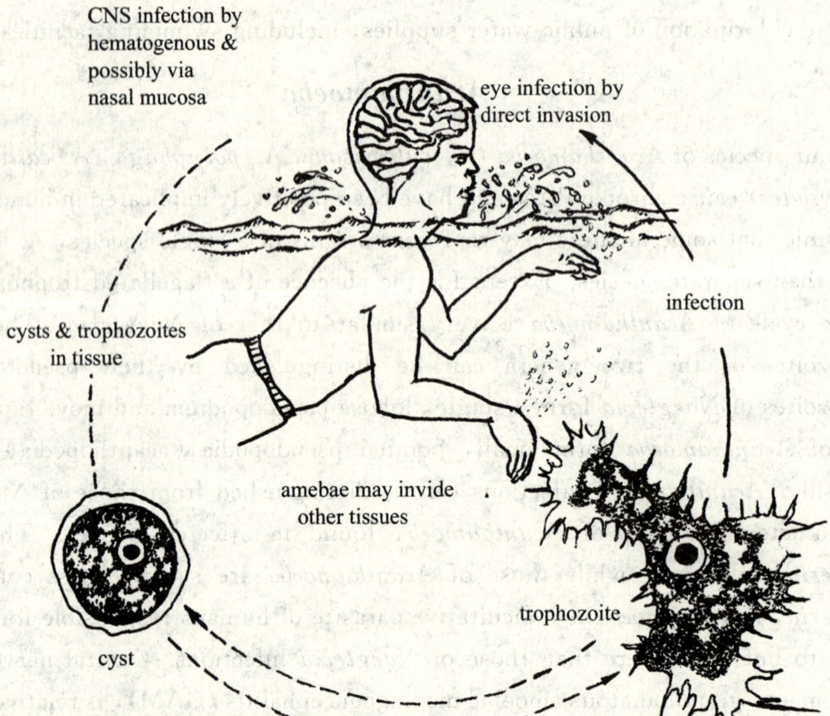

Figure 9-3-2 Morphology and life cycle of *Acanthamoeba*

(Yuan Fangshu)

Chapter 10 Flagellates

Section 1 *Leishmania donovani*

Leishmaniasis is a general term for diseases caused by species of the genus *Leishmania*, which are transmitted by the bite of infected sand flies. Several species of Leishmania are pathogenic for man: *L. donovani* causes visceral leishmaniasis (Kala-azar, black disease, dumdum fever); *L. tropica* (*L. t. major*, *L. t. minor* and *L. ethiopica*) cause cutaneous leishmaniasis (oriental sore, Delhi ulcer, Aleppo, Delhi or Baghdad boil); and *L. braziliensis* (also, *L. mexicana* and *L. peruviana*) are etiologic agents of mucocutaneous leishmaniasis (espundia, Uta, chiclero ulcer). The lesions of cutaneous and mucocutaneous leishmaniasis are limited to the skin and mucous membranes. The much more severe disease, visceral leishmaniasis, involves the entire reticuloendothelial system. The criteria used to differentiate *Leishmania* species are clinical, morphologic, behavioral (vector specificity, laboratory animal patterns, *in vitro* culture), immunologic (monoclonal antibodies), and biochemical (restriction enzymes, DNA probes, isoenzymes). The main species are *Leishmania tropica*, *L. major*, *L. aethiopica*, *L. mexicana*, *L. amazonensis*, *L. peruviana*, *L. braziliensis*, *L. panamensis*, and *L. guyanensis*.

Leishmania donovani (Laveran et Mesnil, 1903), one of the most important etiologic agents which cause visceral leishmaniasis, will be described in details in the following chapter.

Morphology

All species of *Leishmania* parasitic in man are morphologically similar and appear as intracellular amastigotes. Promastigotes develop in the intestine of the sand fly (see Figure 10-1-1). The organisms of different *Leishmania* species may be differentiated based on their geographic distribution, pathogenesis, kinetoplast DNA (kDNA) analysis, DNA hybridization and serologic testing.

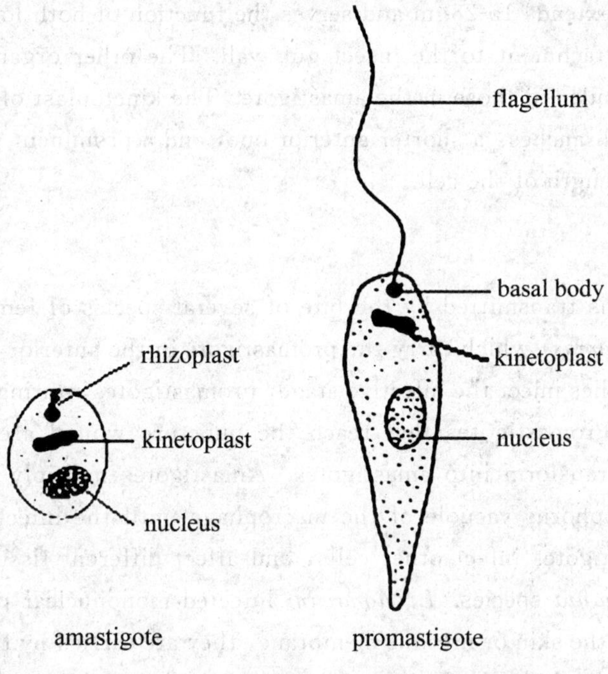

Figure 10-1-1 Amastigote and promastigote of *Leishmania* spp.

Amastigote (leishmanial form) is round or oval, and measures 2-5μm by 1-3μm (see Figure 10-1-1). Besides the eccentrically located nucleus and the rudimentary flagellum, the amastigote has a rod-shaped, unique organelle called the kinetoplast. When Giemsa stained, the kinetoplast is reddish purple and darker than the nucleus, contrasting with the pale blue cytoplasm. The kinetoplast appears to be a special part of mitochondrion and is rich in DNA. Two types of DNA molecules, *maxicircles* which encode mainly certain important mitochondrial enzymes, and *minicircles* which serve a function in the process of RNA editing, have been found in the kinetoplast.

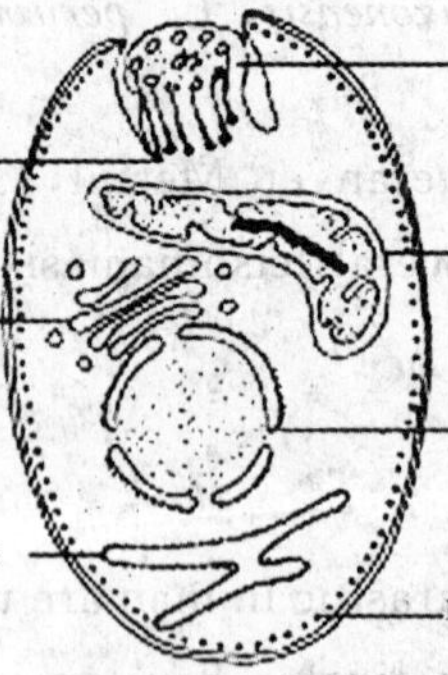

Figure 10-1-2 The ultrastructure of amastigote of *Leishmania* spp.

The promastigote (leptomonad) is more elongated, and measures 14-20μm by 1.5-4μm (see Figure 10-1-1). A single flagellum, which emerges from a basal body within the promastigote, extends 15-28μm and serves the function of both locomotion through the medium and attachment to the insect gut wall. The other organelles, except the kinetoplast, are similar to those in the amastigote. The kinetoplast of promastigote has two mitochondrial branches: a shorter anterior one, and a prominent posterior one that often extends the length of the cell.

Life Cycle

The organism is transmitted by the bite of several species of female phlebotomine sand flies (*Phlebotomus*) which carry the promastigote in the anterior gut and pharynx. The infected sand flies inject the infective stage, promastigotes, during blood meals on a mammalian host. Promastigotes that reach the puncture wound are phagocytized by macrophages and transform into amastigotes. Amastigotes multiply by binary fission within the parasitophorus vacuole of the macrophage until the infected cell ruptures. The released amastigotes infect other cells, and affect different tissues, depending in part on the *Leishmania* species. *L. donovani* infected mononuclear phagocytes do not remain confined to the skin or mucous membrane, they are carried by the bloodstream to lymphoid tissue throughout the body, especially to the spleen, liver and bone marrow. Amastigotes multiply in great numbers in these tissues, which originates the clinical manifestations of leishmaniasis. The sand fly acquires the organisms during the blood meal on an infected host when they ingest macrophages infected with amastigotes; the amastigotes differentiate into promastigotes, which multiply in the gut and migrate to the proboscis. Dogs and rodents are common reservoirs (see Figure 10-1-3).

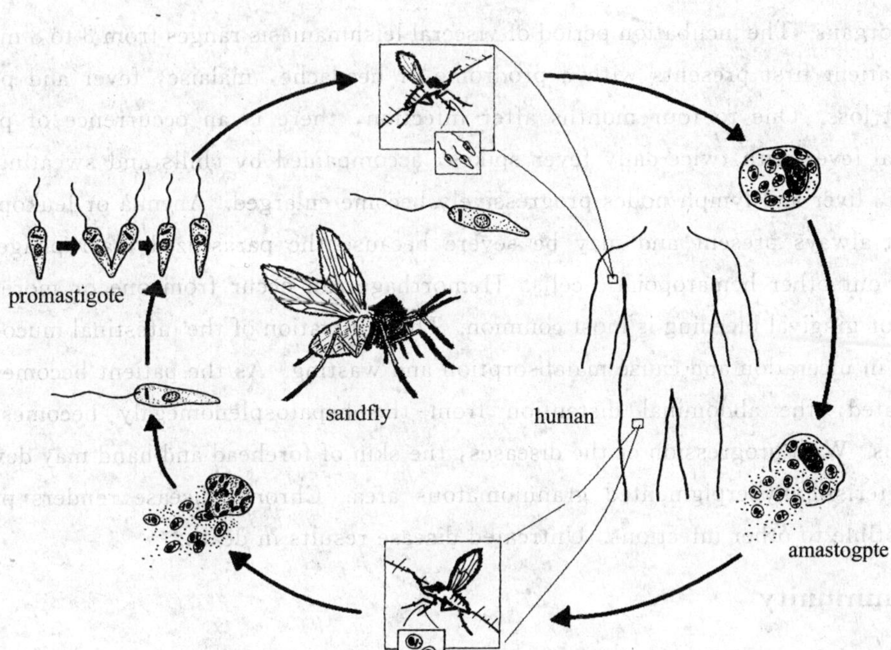

Figure 10-1-3 Life cycle of *Leishmania donovani*

Pathogensis and Clinical Manifestation

The amastigotes of *L. donovani* multiply in reticuloendothelial cells, especially macrophages in the spleen, liver, lymph nodes, and bone marrow. Hyperplasia of the amastigote-infected mononuclear phagocytes in the liver and spleen results in progressive hypertrophy. The spleen may enlarge massively as splenic lymphoid follicles are replaced by parasitized mononuclear cells. In the liver, a marked increase in the number and size of Kupffer cells, many of which contain amastigotes. Parasitized macrophages replace hematopoietic tissue in the bone marrow.

Pathogenesis of leishmaniasis is due to an immune reaction to the organism, particularly cell mediated immunity. Laboratory examination reveals a marked leukopenia with relative monocytosis and lymphocytosis, ancmia and thrombocytopenia. IgM and IgG levels are extremely elevated due to both specific antibodies and polyclonal activation. Patients with advanced disease are prone to superinfection with other organisms.

Symptom of visceral leishmaniasis

L. donovani organisms in visceral leishmaniasis are rapidly eliminated from the biting sites of sand flies, hence there is rarely a local lesion, although minute papules have been described in children. They are localized and multiply in the mononuclear phagocytic cells of spleen, liver, lymph nodes, bone marrow, intestinal mucosa and other organs. The incubation period of visceral leishmaniasis ranges from 3 to 8 months. The patient first presents with a prodrome of headache, malaise, fever and possible weight loss. One to four months after infection, there is an occurrence of periodic interval fever with twice-daily fever spikes, accompanied by chills and sweating. The spleen, liver and lymph nodes progressively become enlarged. Anemia or leukopenia is almost always present and may be severe because the parasitized macrophages may crowd out other hematopoietic cells. Hemorrhage can occur from one or more sites, nasal or gingival bleeding is most common. The infiltration of the intestinal mucosa may result in ulceration and cause malabsorption and wasting. As the patient becomes more emaciated, the abdominal distention from the hepatosplenomegaly becomes more obvious. With progression of the diseases, the skin of forehead and hand may develop a characteristic hyperpigmented granulomatous area. Chronic disease renders patients susceptible to other infections. Untreated disease results in death.

Immunity

Various *Leishmania* cell surface glycoproteins and lipopolysaccharides are being studied for possible use in species differentiation and with other purposes.

The glycoprotein gp63 on the surface membrane of promastigote, which is a ligand of CR3 complement receptors of macrophages, and a lipophosphoglycan play a prominent roles in the phagocytosis of promastigote. Intracellular survival of amstigotes is mediated by a surface lipophosphoglycan and an abundance of membrane-bound acid phosphatase, which inhibit the oxidative burst and / or inactivate lysosomal enzymes of macrophages.

The course of leishmaniasis is related to the response of T cell of the host. $CD4^+$ T cells of the Th1 type secrete interferon-γ in response to leishmanial antigens. Interferon-γ, in turn, activates macrophages to kill intracellular amastigotes by producing toxin nitric oxide. There is, however, a dramatic inhibition of the Th1 response in the infection with *L. donovani*. In individuals with progressive visceral leishmaniasis, the evidence of leishmania-specific Th1 responses is absent. Individuals with self-resolving infection of *L. donovani* and those have undergone successful chemotherapy usually manifest protective Th1 responses.

Infection of *L. donovani* results in suppression of cell-mediated immunity, leading to uncontrolled reproduction of the parasite and dissemination. There is increased production of globulins, with high levels of IgG and IgM. The major target for the humoral immune complexes is heat shock proteins. Circulating immune complexes involving IgA, IgG, and IgM can be found in the serum. Delayed-hypersensitivity responses to skin test antigens are suppressed or absent. With resolution of infection, the delayed-hypersensitivity reaction returns, and individuals recovering from infection are immune to re-infection of the parasite.

Visceral leishmaniasis is one of the important opportunistic infections among the immunocompromised individuals such as patients with HIV infection. Actually, the parasite may be a cofactor in the pathogenesis of HIV infection.

Diagnosis

Diagnosis of visceral leishmaniasis is based on a history of exposure to sand flies, symptoms and isolation of the organisms from the lesion aspirate or biopsy, by direct examination or culture. The typical symptoms, particularly hepatosplenomegaly and the pancytopenia, strongly suggest visceral leishmaniasis. The parasite usually can be demonstrated in stained or cultured bone marrow or spleen material. Giemsa stained slides of tissues biopsies from the spleen and liver are often used to demonstrate the diagnostic amastigote stage. The bone marrow and lymph node aspirations are often advised to obtain the specimen. Direct examination of stained smears and culture procedures are recommended. Culture samples on NNN medium will yield promastigotes.

Serologic tests (ELISA, immunofluorescent antibody) are useful, particularly in surveys. A skin test (Montenegro test, or leishimania test) and detection of anti-leishmanial antibodies by immuno-fluorescence are indicative of exposure. Montenegro test is a delayed hypersensitivity reaction provoked by a suspension of killed leishmanial promastigoes injected intradermally. A local inflammatory reaction appears at site of injection usually within 48-72 hours in a positive patient. Montenegro skin test is often used for screening of large population at risk for infection, but it is not reactive in patients with active disease, as the cell mediated immune responses are suppressed by the organisms, the delayed hypersensitivity response become reactive following successful treatment. Indirect fluorescence and molecular diagnostic technique are available in more advanced diagnostic laboratories.

Epidemiology

Leishmaniasis is prevalent worldwide: ranging from south-east Asia, Indo-Pakistan, Mediterranean, north and central Africa, south and Central America. The geographic distribution of *Leishmania* species that infect humans is listed in Table 10-1-1. *L. donovani* is found widely distributed throughout India, Pakistan, Thailand, northwestern areas of China, and parts of Africa. It is transmitted by Phlebotomus sand flies and is generally a disease of children and young adults. In China, the main vector for the disease involves *Phlebotomus chinensis*, *P. longiductus*, *P. wui*, and *P. alexandri*. Rodents and dogs serve as natural reservoirs in most endemic areas, but man appears to be only mammalian reservoir in India.

Visceral leishmaniasis can also be transmitted by the transfusion of blood contaminated with parasitized macrophages, or by an accidental contaminated needle stick injure in a laboratory. On rare occasions, it causes congential infection.

Leishmaniasis is an important public health problem. World Health Organization statistics suggest that 12 million people are currently infected with leishmaniasis in 88 countries. Another 350 million people in those countries are at risk of becoming infected. It is estimated that the new cases grow by 2 million per year and only about 600,000 of those cases are reported. The increased cases of leishmaniasis are related to man's encroachment into the sand fly habitat. Economic development, such as mining, harvesting lumber, and expanding cultivation in the primary forests, as well as rapid urbanization worldwide, have elevated the number of reported incidences.

Table 10-1-1 Geographic distribution of *Leishmania* species

Leishmania species	Clinical manifestation & Geographic distribution
Leishmania donovani complex	Visceral Leishmaniasis
L. donovani	India, Pakistan, Thailand, China, parts of Africa
L. infantum	Mediterranean area, Europe, Africa, the Near East, parts of former Soviet Union
L. chagasi	Central and South America
Leishmania tropica complex	Old World Cutaneous Leishmaniasis
L. tropica	Mediterranean area, Middle East, India, Kenya
L. aethiopica	Ethiopia, Kenya, Southern Yemen
L. major	Turkmenistan, Uzbekistan, Kazakhstan, Norther Africa and the Sahara, Iran, Syria, Israel, Jordan
Leishmania mexicana complex	New World Cutaneous Leishmaniasis
L. mexicana	Belize, Guatemala, the Yucatan peninsula
L. pifanoi	Amazon river basin, Brazil, Venezuela
L. amazonensis	Amazon basin of Brazil
L. venezuelensis	Venezuela
L. garnhami	Venezuelan Andes
Leishmania braziliensis complex	Mucocutaneous Leishmaniasis
L. braziliensis	Mexico to Argentina
L. panamensis	Panama, Columbia
L. peruviana	Peruvian Andes
L. guyanensis	Guiana, Brazil, Venezuela

Prevention and Control

Control of *L. donovani* infection involves the prompt diagnosis and treatment of infected individuals, vector control and avoidance.

Sodium stibogluconate (Pentostam) is the drug of choice for the infection of *L. donovani*. Pentamidine isethionate is used as an alternative. Patients with Indian Kala azar tend to respond rapidly to the treatment and have a good prognosis. If the disease does not respond to either therapeutic agent, amphotericin B is advised. If the treatment with these regimens fails, combination drug regimens exist using either allopurinol or gamma interferon along with pentostam.

The spraying of residential insecticide in homes and sand fly breeding areas effectively interrupts the spread of the disease. Avoidance of outdoor activities when the sand flies are most active (dusk to dawn), the use of mechanical barriers such as protective clothing, screens and bed netting, and the use of insect repellents are effective measures.

Immunization has not been effective.

Section 2 Trypanosomes

Trypanosoma brucei gambiense and *Trypanosoma brucei rhodesiense*

Trypanosomes are hemoflagellates of the family *Trypanosomatidae* that live in the blood and tissues of their human hosts. The organisms of two subspecies of *Trypanosoma brucei* cause African trypanosomiasis (African sleeping sickness).

African trypanosomiasis includes two clinical forms, a slowly developing disease caused by *Trypanosoma brucei gambiense* (Dutton, 1902), and a rapidly progressing disease caused by *T. brucei rhodesiense* (Stephens & Fanthan, 1901). It is not possible to differentiate the two species of trypanosomes on their morphology and reservoir hosts. Differentiation is based on clinical signs and geographic area, and isoenzyme characteristics and DNA and RNA methods.

Morphology

T. b. gambiense and *T. b. rhodesiense* are two subspecies, which are morphologically indistinguishable. In their life cycles, two trypanosomal forms can be observed (see Figure 10-2-1). Amastigote stage in human in African trypanosomiasis is only suspected and not confirmed, although amastigote has been seen in the choroid plexus in mice.

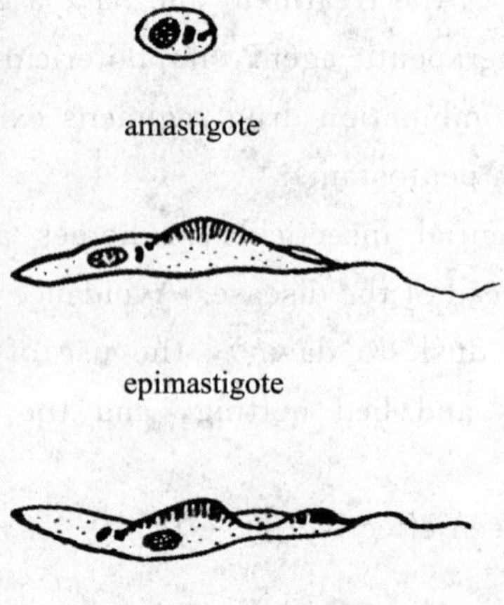

Figure 10-2-1 Morphology of trypanosomes

The epimastigote lives in the gut of the vector tsetse fly, and trypomastigote lives in the blood, cerebrospinal fluid, lymph nodes of human or animal hosts. In epimastigote form, the nucleus is posterior to the kinetoplast, in contrast to the trypomastigote, in which the nucleus is anterior to the kinetoplast. With Giemsa or Wright's stain, the granular cytoplasma of trypomastigote is pale blue and contains dark blue granules and possibly vacuoles. The reddish nucleus is centrally located. The reddish kinetoplast is at the posterior end. The flagellum arises from the kinetoplast, and runs along the edge of the undulating membrane until the undulating membrane merges with the trypanosome body at the anterior end of the organism. At this point, the flagellum becomes free to extend beyond the body. The trypomastigote varies in different forms in same blood smear, and measures 14 to 33μm in length and 1. 5 to 3. 5μm in width. The forms range from long, slender-bodied organisms with a long flagellum to short, fat, stumpy without a free flagellum. The short stumpy forms do not divide in the bloodstream but are the infective stage for the tsetse fly. The trypomastigotes multiply by longitudinal binary fission.

The outer surface of the trypomastigote is densely coated with a layer of glycoprotein, the variable surface glycoprotein (VSG), which can changes about every 5 to 7 days (antigenic variation) and is helpful to evade the host immune response.

Life Cycle

The life cycles of both *T. b. gambiense* and *T. b. rhodesiense* are similar (see Figure 10-2-2). African trypanosomiasis is transmitted by the tsetse fly (*Glossina* spp.) The infective metacyclic trypomastigotes is injected into the primary host (human or animals) during a bite by the tsetse fly. The organism transforms into a trypomastigote (dividing form) as it enters the draining lymphatic and blood stream. Trypomastigotes can traverse the walls of blood and lymph capillaries into the connective tissues and, at a later stage, traverse cross the choroid plexus into the brain and cerebrospinal fluid. The trypomastigote enters the vector during the blood meal and moves through the alimentary tract to the salivary gland where it proliferates as epimastigote and matures to infectious metacyclic trypomastigotes. The organisms can also be transmitted through blood transfusion.

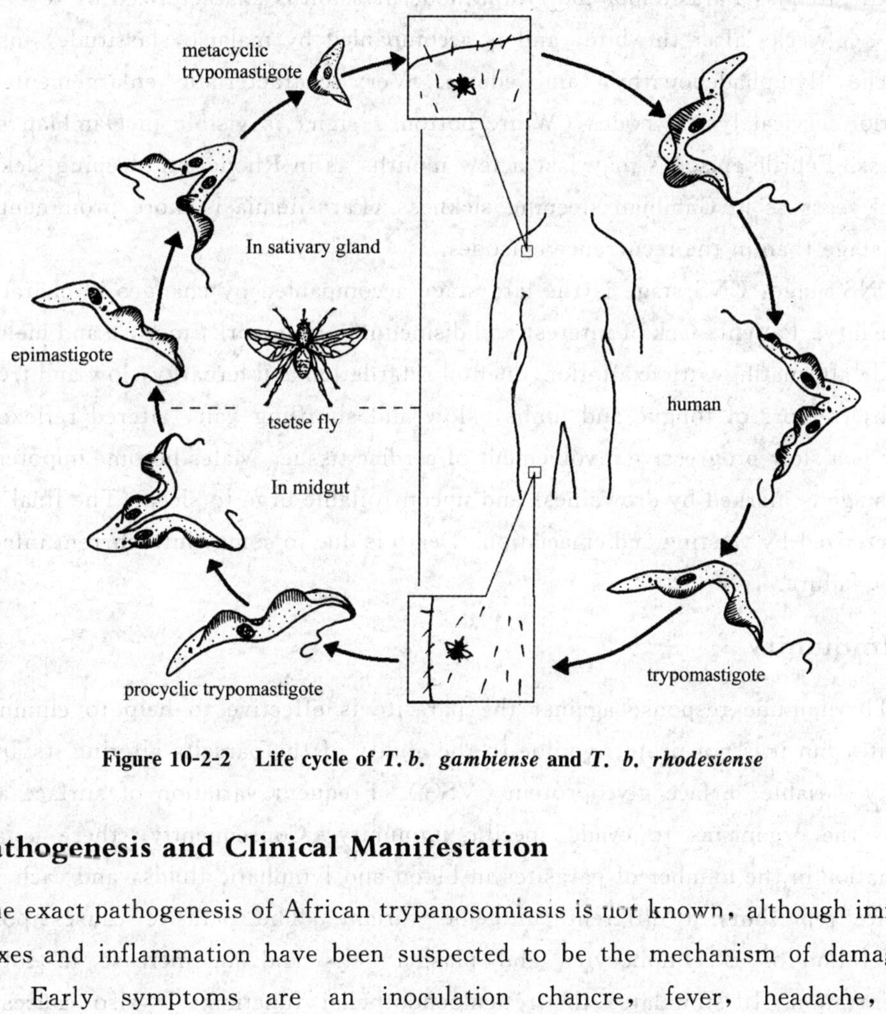

Figure 10-2-2 Life cycle of *T. b. gambiense* and *T. b. rhodesiense*

Pathogenesis and Clinical Manifestation

The exact pathogenesis of African trypanosomiasis is not known, although immune complexes and inflammation have been suspected to be the mechanism of damage to tissues. Early symptoms are an inoculation chancre, fever, headache, and lymphadenopathy. Victims later develop meningoencephalitis, become somnolent, and die unless treated. The clinical features of Gambian and Rhodesian trypanosomiasis are similar, although they vary in severity and duration. Rhodesian trypanosomiasis progresses more rapidly and the symptoms are often briefer and more acute. The acuteness and severity of disease do not allow typical sleeping sickness. Death results from cardiac failure within 6-9 months.

Symptoms

Classically, the progression of African trypanosomiasis can be classified into 3 stages: the bite reaction (chancre), parasitemia (blood and lymphoid tissues), and CNS stage.

Bite reaction: 1-3 weeks after a bite by the tsetse fly, a non-pustular, painful, itchy chancre forms, lasts 1-2 weeks, and leaves no scar.

Parasitemia: Parasitemia and lymph node invasion is characterized by fevers which starts 2-3 weeks after the bite, and is accompanied by malaise, lassitude, insomnia, headache, lymphadenopathy, and edema. Very characteristic enlargement of the posterior cervical lymph nodes (Winterbottom's sign) is visible in Gambian sleeping sickness. Febrile episodes may last a few months as in Rhodesian sleeping sickness or several years as in Gambian sleeping sickness. Parasitemia is more prominent in the acute stage than in the recurrence episodes.

CNS Stage: CNS stage is the late stage accompanied by changes in character and personality. Patients lack of interest and disinclination to work, morose and melancholic attitude alternating with exaltation, mental retardation and lethargy, low and tremulous speech, tremors of tongue and limbs, slow and shuffling gait, altered reflexes, etc. There is a slow progressive involvement of cardiac tissue. Males become impotent. The later stage is marked by drowsiness and uncontrollable urge to sleep. The final stage is characterized by wasting and emaciation. Death is due to coma, intercurrent infection or cardiac failure.

Immunity

The immune response against the parasite is effective to help to eliminate the parasite, but it is not protective due to the ability of the parasite altering its antigens, namely variable surface glycoprotein (VSG). Frequent variation of surface antigens allows the organisms to evade specific immunity. Consequently, there is a cyclic fluctuation in the number of parasites in blood and lymphatic fluids, and each wave of parasite represents a different antigenic variant. The parasite causes polyclonal proliferation of B lymphocytes and plasma cells and an increase in total IgM concentration. It stimulates the reticuloendothelial function. It also causes severe depression of cell mediated and humoral immunity to other antigens.

Diagnosis

The parasites appear first in the blood and lymph nodes and later in the cerebrospinal fluid. Therefore, detection of parasite in the bloodstream, lymph secretions and enlarged lymph node aspirate provides a definitive diagnosis in acute stages. The parasite in blood can be concentrated by centrifugation or by the use of anionic support media. Cerebrospinal fluid must always be examined for organisms. Immuno-serology (enzyme-linked immune sorbent assay, enzyme-linked immune assay, immunofluorescence) may provide presumptive diagnosis. The diagnosis is also made by inoculating susceptible laboratory animals.

Epidemiology

T. b. gambiense is predominant in the west and central Africa, whereas *T. b. rhodesiense* is restricted to the east Africa. 6,000 to 10,000 human cases are documented annually. 35 million people and 25 million cattle are at risk. *T. b. gambiense* is maintained mainly in domestic animals; *T. b. rhodesiense* is maintained in various mammals of open savannahs.

Prevention and Control

The blood stage of African trypanosomiasis can be treated with Pentamidine isethionate or Suramin. These drugs are also effective in prophylaxis although they may mask early infection and thus increase the risk of CNS stage of trypanosomiasis. Cases with CNS involvement should be treated with the organic arsenic compound, Melarsoprol.

The most effective prevention is to avoid biting by tsetse flies. Immunization has not been effective due to antigenic variation of the parasites. Vector eradication is impractical due to the vast area involved.

Trypanosoma cruzi

American trypanosomiasis, also known as Chagas' disease, is caused by the protozoan trypanosome, *Trypanosoma cruzi* (Chagas, 1909).

Morphology

The organism of *T. cruzi* occurs in three different forms depending on its host environment(see Figure 10-2-1).

The trypanosomal (trypomastigote) form, found in mammalian blood, is 15-20μm long and morphologically similar to African trypanosomes. When the trypomastigote is stained with Giemsa stain, the cytoplasm is blue and the nucleus, kinetoplast, and flagellum are red or violet. The nucleus is in the center of the body, with a large oval kinetoplast located at the posterior end. A flagellum arises from the basal body and extends along the outer edge of the undulating membrane until it reaches the anterior end of the body, where it projects as a free flagellum.

The epimastigote form is found in the insect intestine, its morphological structures are similar to those of trypomastigote except the location of kinetoplast, which is anterior to the nucleus.

The amastigote form, found intracellularly or in pseudocysts in mammalian viscera (particularly in myocardium and brain), is round or oval in shape, measures 2-6μm in diameter, and lacks a prominent flagellum. The amastigote contains a large nucleus and rod-shaped kinetoplast that stains red or violet with Giemsa stain, and its cytoplasma is blue.

Life Cycle

More than one hundred mammalian species of wild and domestic animals including cattle, pigs, cats, dogs, rats, armadillo, raccoon and opossum are naturally infected by *T. cruzi* and serve as a reservoir host. The organism of *T. cruzi* is transmitted to mammalian host by many species of kissing bug (riduviid), which normally bites in the facial area of a person, most prominently by *Triatoma infestans*, *T. sordida*, *Panstrongylus megistus* and *Rhodnius prolixus*. Transmission occurs during the bug's feeding and defecating. The metacyclic trypamastigotes in the feces of the insect gain access to the mammalian tissue through the wound which is often rubbed by the individual that is bitten. Subsequently, the trypomastigotes enter various cells, including macrophages, where they differentiate into amastigotes and multiply by binary fission. The amastigotes differentiate into nondividing trypomastigotes and the cells rupture to release them into the blood. A variety of host cells can become infected, and the trypomastigotes once again form amastigotes inside these cells. Uninfected riduviid bugs acquire the organism when they feed on infected animals or people containing trypomastigotes in their blood. Inside the bug's alimentary tract, the trypomastigotes differentiate into epimastigotes and divide longitudinally in the mid and hindgut of the insect where they develop into infective metacyclic trypomastigotes (see Figure 10-2-3). Transmission from man to man may also occur by blood transfusion, by the transplacental route (congential infection), or by organ transplantation.

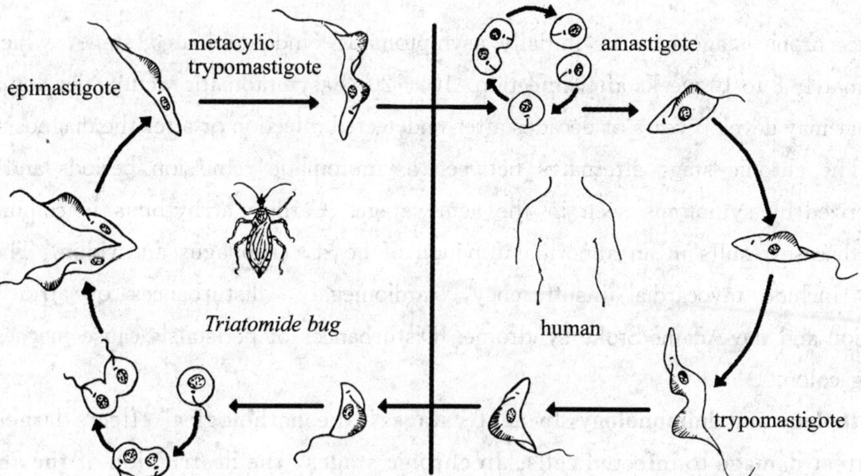

Figure 10-2-3 Life cycle of *Trypanosoma cruzi*

Pathogenesis

The clinical syndromes associated with Chagas' disease include three stages: the primary lesion, the acute stage, and the chronic stage. The incubation period in human is about 7 to 14 days but is somewhat longer in some patients.

Primary lesion, also known as chagoma, appears at the site of infection, within a few hours of a bite. It is usually found on the face, eyelids, cheek, lips or the conjunctiva, but may occur on the abdomen or limbs. The chagoma consists of a slightly raised, flat non-purulent erythematous plaque surrounded by a variable area of hard edema. When the primary lesion is on the face, there is an enlargement of the pre- and post- auricular and the submaxillary glands on the side of the bite. Infection in the eyelid often results in a unilateral conjunctivitis and orbital edema. The chagoma is painful and may take 2 to 3 months to subside.

Acute stage symptoms appear 7-14 days after infection, and are characterized by restlessness, sleeplessness, malaise, increasing exhaustion, chills, fever and bone and muscle pains. Other manifestations of the acute stage include cervical, axillary and iliac adenitis, hepatomegaly, erythematous rash and acute myocarditis. There is a general edematous reaction due to the lymphadenopathy. Diffuse myocarditis, sometimes accompanied by serious pericarditis and endocarditis, is very frequent during the initial acute stage. In children, Chagas' disease may cause meningoencephalitis and coma. Death occurs in 5%-10% infants. Hematologic examination reveals lymphocytosis and parasitemia. The symptoms of acute stage last for 4 to 8 weeks and then may subside, even without therapy, therefore, the acute stage is often not recognized and usually resolves with little or no immediate damage, the victim remains an asymptomatic carrier.

The chronic stage may be initially asymptomatic (indeterminate) stage, which begins approximately 8 to 10 weeks after infection. 10%-20% asymptomatic victims develop a chronic stage that may develop years or decades after undetected infection or after the diagnosis of acute stage. The chronic stage alternates between asymptomatic remission periods and relapses characterized by symptoms seen in the acute stage. Cardiac arrhythmia is common. The chronic disease results in an abnormal function of heart, esophagus and colon. The cardiac changes include myocardial insufficiency, cardiomegaly, disturbances of atrioventricular conduction and the Adams-Stoke syndrome. Disturbances of peristalsis cause megaesophagus and megacolon.

Pathology and immunology: In acute stages, the pathological effects largely result from direct damage to infected cells. In chronic stages, the destruction of the autonomic nerve ganglions may be of significance. *T. cruzi* stimulates both humoral and cell mediated immune responses. Both cell mediated and humoral immune mechanisms involving reaction to the organism and to autologous tissues have been implicated in pathogenesis.

Immunity: *T. cruzi* does not alter its antigenic coat. Antibody can lyse the organism, but rarely causes eradication of the organism, perhaps due to its intracellular localization. Cell mediated immunity may be of significant value. The activated macrophages can kill the organism. Antibodies directed against heart and muscle cells have been detected in infected patients suggesting that there is an element of autoimmune reaction in the pathogenesis of Chagas' disease. The infection of *T. cruzi* causes severe depression of both cell mediated and humoral immune responses. Immunosuppression may be due to induction of suppressor T-cells and/or overstimulation of macrophages.

Diagnosis

The diagnosis of Chagas' disease should be considered if there is a history of consistent exposure to reduviid bug bites, residence in or travel to the endemic areas of the disease, recent blood transfusion in the endemic area, or laboratory accident.

Acute Chagas' disease should be suspected in any individual from the endemic areas of the disease who has an acute febrile illness with lymphadenopathy and myocarditis. Cardiac dilation, megacolon and megaesophagus in individuals from endemic areas indicate present or former infection. Clinical diagnosis is usually easy among children in endemic areas. Definitive diagnosis requires the demonstration of trypomastigotes in the blood, amastigotes in tissues, or positive serologic tests. Methods used for examination of blood are similar to those used for the diagnosis of African trypanosomiasis. Trypomastigotes may be detected in blood by using thin and thick blood films or by buffy coat concentration techniques. The most sensitive methods for detection of trypomastigotes are concentration techniques. Aspirates from chagomas lymph nodes can be examined for amastigotes and trypomastigotes. Aspirates, blood, and tissues can be cultured for examination of epimastigotes.

In the chronic stage of Chagas' disease, trypomastigotes are very rare or absent in the peripheral blood except during febrile exacerbation. Diagnosis depends primarily on culture, serologic tests, or xenodiagnosis. Serologic tests include complement fixation, indirect fluorescent-antibody, indirect hemagglutination tests and ELISA. In xenodiagnosis, trypanosome-free bugs are allowed to feed on the suspected individuals of Chagas' disease, and examined monthly for flagellated forms over a period of 3 months. Alternative diagnostic techniques include PCR and immunoblotting methods for confirming of Chagas' disease.

Epidemiology

Chagas disease occurs throughout Mexico, and central and southern America, where it continues to pose a serious threat to health. The overall prevalence of human *T. cruzi* infection is estimated at 16 to 18 million cases. Approximately 120 million people, i. e., 25% of the inhabitants of Latin America, are at risk of contracting infection; 25% to 30% of those infected with the parasite will progress to irreversible cardiac, and esophageal and colonic pathology, causing considerable morbidity and mortality.

The disease is vectored by triatomine bugs and may also be transmitted congenitally and by transfusion. Outbreaks are associated with mud, thatched, or dirt-floored dwellings that harbor the vector bugs. Chagas' disease is a zoonosis. Animal reservoirs include opossums, armadillos, rodents, dogs, and cats.

Prevention and Control

There is no effective therapy available. Most drugs are either ineffective or highly toxic. The experimental drugs, benznidazole and nifurtimox, are effective in the acute stage of Chagas' disease, however their side effects limit their prolonged use in chronic cases. Drug therapy has little effect on reducing the progression of chronic Chagas' disease. Symptoms associated with megaesophagus and megacolon may be treated with dietary measures or may require surgery.

Attempts to develop a vaccine have not been very successful.

Control relies on interrupting transmission by killing vector insects in houses, improving housing to render them unsuitable for colonization by vector insects, and comprehensive health education initiatives, systematic screening of blood donors in all endemic countries, detection and treatment of congenital transmission, and treatment of acute cases and children. Travelers can avoid the disease by not sleeping in infested housing and ensuring that any transfusions are with blood that have been screened.

Laboratory personnel working with *T. cruzi* must be aware of the hazard in handling the highly infectious trypomastigote form. Precautions include the use of gloves and eye protection. All clinical specimens must be handled by using universal precaution.

(**Ye Bin**)

Section 3 *Giardia lamblia*

Giardia lamblia, also known as *G. duodenalis* and *G. intestinalis*, is a protozoan parasite that colonizes the upper portions of the small intestine. It has a worldwide distribution and is one of the most common intestinal protozoans throughout the world. The incidence is estimated at 200 million cases per year. Typically *Giardia* is non-invasive and quite often results in asymptomatic infections. Humans infected with *Giardia* may have acute diarrhea or chronic diarrhea with malabsorption, weight loss and failure to thrive.

Giardia was first described in 1681 by Antony van Leeuwenhoek. It was reported in more details in 1859 by Lambl, after whom the human species was named (*Cercomonas intestinalis* Lambl, 1859). It was renamed *Giardia lamblia* by Stiles in 1915. However, it has only been in the last 50 years that its real role in diarrheal syndromes has been described.

Morphology

The *Giardia* belongs to the class Zoomastigophorea, the order Diplomonadida and the family Hexamitidae. Its life cycle involves two stages: the trophozoite and the cyst. It is one of the oldest eukaryotic organisms, and lacks many of the organelles typical of higher eukaryotes, such as mitochondria, peroxisomes and a typical Golgi apparatus.

Trophozoite: The *Giardia* trophozoite exhibits a characteristic pear, or tear-drop, shape with bilateral symmetry when viewed from the top (see Figure 10-3-1). It is typically 9-21μm long, 5-15μm wide, and 2-4μm thick, contains four sets of posteriorly directed flagella. Three pairs of flagella emerge from the dorsal surface (anterior, posterior-lateral, caudal) and one pair emerges from the ventral surface. Trophozoites exhibit a distinctive erratic twisting motion, sometimes compared to that of a falling leaf. Characteristic features of the stained trophozoite include: two nuclei with central karyosomes, fibrils running the length of the parasite, and median bodies. The large karyosome and lack of peripheral chromatin gives the nuclei a halo appearance. The fibrils are called axonemes and are formed from the proximal regions of the flagella within the body of the trophozoite. The median bodies are a pair of curved rod-shaped structures which lie posterior to the nuclei. The function of the median bodies is not known, they may involve with the adhesive disk and its formation. An adhesive disk occupies the ventral side of the anterior end.

Cyst: the oval cyst measurs 8-14μm in length and 7-10μm in breath, and can often be seen to contain two to four nuclei at one end and prominent diagonal fibrils (see Figure 10-3-1). A thick wall surrounds it. The cyst consists of cytoplasm, which is finely granular and is separated from the cyst wall by a clear space. The mature cyst contains four nuclei, which is the infective stage of *G. lamblia*.

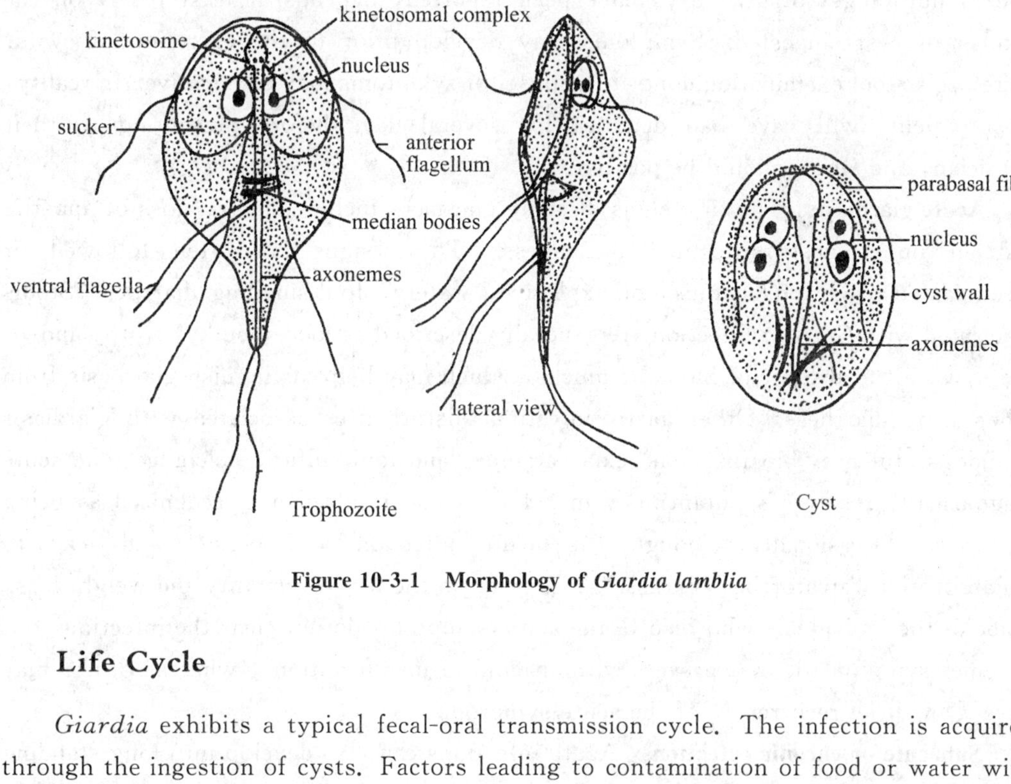

Figure 10-3-1 Morphology of *Giardia lamblia*

Life Cycle

Giardia exhibits a typical fecal-oral transmission cycle. The infection is acquired through the ingestion of cysts. Factors leading to contamination of food or water with fecal material are correlated with transmission. The exposure of cysts to host stomach acidity and body temperature triggers excystation, which is completed in the small intestine with the emergence of trophozoites that promptly attach to host intestinal epithelium.

The trophozoite, lives in the upper two-thirds of the small intestine (duodenum and jejunum) and multiplies by binary fission. Trophozoites that are swept into the fecal stream lose their motility, round up, and are excreted as dormant, resistant cysts.

Excreted trophozoites disintegrate. The cyst is sufficiently hardy to survive host-to-host transfer. For example, some *Giardia* cysts excyst successfully after more than 2 months' storage in water at refrigerator temperatures.

Clinical Manifestations

Giardia infection may be asymptomatic or it may cause disease ranging from a self-limiting diarrhea to a severe chronic syndrome and malabsorption. Children exhibit clinical symptoms more frequently than adults and subsequent infections tend to be less severe than initial infections. It can be estimated that 5%-15% of infected persons will become asymptomatic cyst passers, 25%-50% will have a diarrheal syndrome, and 35%-70% will have no trace of infection. The incubation period for acute giardiasis is 1-3 weeks, but ranges of 1-75 days have been reported, depends at least partly on the number of cysts ingested. Symptoms may develop prior to the excretion of cysts; therefore a stool examination done at the onset of symptoms may be negative. In reality, most patients will have had diarrhea for several days before presenting to their physician, and stools should be positive.

Acute giardiasis: The first signs of acute giardiasis include nausea, loss of appetite and an upper gastro-intestinal uneasiness. These signs are often followed or accompanied by a sudden onset of explosive, watery, foul-smelling diarrhea. Stools associated with *Giardia* infection are generally described as loose, bulky, frothy and/or greasy with the absence of blood or mucus, which may help distinguish giardiasis from other acute diarrheas. Other gastro-intestinal disturbances associated with giardiasis include: flatulence, bloating, anorexia, cramps, and foul sulfuric belching. The acute stage usually resolves spontaneously in 3-4 days and is often not recognized as being giardiasis. Occasionally, though, an acute infection will persist and lead to malabsorption, steatorrhea (excessive loss of fat in the feces), debility and weight loss. Some of the individuals who resolve the acute symptoms do not clear the infection, but become asymptomatic cyst passers without clinical manifestations, whereas others may have a few brief recurrences of the acute symptoms.

Subacute or chronic infections: Acute infections can also develop into long-standing subacute or chronic infections which in rare cases last for years. The typical chronic stage patient presents with recurrent brief episodes of loose foul stools which may be yellowish, frothy and float, accompanied by intestinal gurgling, abdominal distention and flatulence. Between episodes the stools are usually mushy, but normal stools or constipation can also occur. Cramps are uncommon during chronic infections, but sulfuric belching is frequent. Anorexia, nausea, and epigastric uneasiness are additional frequent complaints during chronic infections. In the majority of chronic cases the parasites and symptoms spontaneously disappear.

Most *Giardia* infections are asymptomatic. For this reason, and because these organisms are so widespread, it was earlier believed that *Giardia* was a nonpathogenic commensal. Enough evidence has accumulated, however, to show that *G. lamblia* can cause disease.

Some patients with giardiasis develop a severe disease that is not self-limited. Signs and symptoms may include interference with the absorption of fat and fat-soluble vitamins, retarded growth, weight loss, or a celiac-disease-like syndrome. Although most cases are seen in hosts with some concurrent condition, such as an immune deficiency, protein-calorie malnutrition, or bacterial overgrowth of the small intestine, some cases of severe giardiasis occur in apparently normal hosts. Another feature of giardiasis is the duration of symptoms by the time a patient presents. Most persons will have been sick for 7-10 days. This feature, combined with weight loss, help distinguish giardiasis from most viral and bacterial etiologies of diarrhea, which usually have shorter durations of illness.

Different strains of *G. lamblia* possibly vary in virulence.

Pathogenesis

The precise pathogenic mechanisms are not known but appear to be multifactorial. Attachment of trophozoites to the brush border could produce a mechanical irritation or mucosal injury. In addition, normal villus structure is affected in some patients. *Giardia* infection can also lead to lactase deficiency as well as other enzyme deficiencies in the microvilli. The reduced digestion and absorption of solutes may lead to an osmotic diarrhea and could also explain the malabsorption syndromes. Additional mechanisms of pathogenesis may well exist. For example, mechanical blockage of the intestinal mucosa, competition for nutrients, inflammation of the intestinal mucosa, bacterial induced deconjugation of bile salts, and altered jejunal motility with or without overgrowth of intestinal bacteria and yeast. Thus far, no single virulence factor or unifying mechanism explains the pathogenesis of giardiasis.

Host Defenses

The fact that many *Giardia* infections in humans and experimental animals resolve spontaneously implies that an effective host immune response develops. There is evidence that both humoral and cellular immune mechanisms are involved. Hosts with gamma globulin deficiencies are prone to severe disease, suggesting that humoral immunity plays a role. Although the fact that milk from immune mothers can prevent infection in suckling mice seems to indicate a role for IgA, the nature of this protection is not clear. Furthermore, experiments with nude mice (congenitally athymic) suggest that the thymus-dependent (T-cell mediated) immune system also plays a role. In these mice, wasting and premature death may result from *Giardia* infection, whereas nude mice "reconstituted" with thymus transplants are able to reduce the numbers of infecting *Giardia*.

In vitro studies have found that normal human milk (but not cow's milk or goat's milk) kills trophozoites of both *G. lamblia* and *Entamoeba histolytica*, and that this killing does not depend on secreted IgA. This finding raises the possibility that even mother's milk that does not have antiprotozoal antibody may protect infants exposed to these parasites.

Diagnosis

The symptoms of giardiasis are not pathognomonic. Diagnosis is confirmed by finding cysts or trophozoites in feces or in duodenojejunal aspirates or biopsies. In the case of giardiasis, cysts are found in formed stool. Diarrheal specimens may also contain trophozoites. If still motile, the trophozoites exhibit a typical "falling leaf" movement. Because cysts are often shed intermittently, three stool specimens should be obtained at approximately 48-hour intervals. Examination of these specimens permits detection of the organism in most cases. The chance of finding cysts in a light infection increases if the stool specimen is subjected to a concentration method, such as the zinc sulfate centrifugal flotation technique. Watery or loose stools may contain motile trophozoites which are detectable by the immediate examination of wet smears. Otherwise the specimen should be preserved and stained due to trophozoite lability. The harder cysts are relatively easy to recognize in either direct or stained smears.

Diagnosis can also be made by examining duodenal fluid for trophozoites. Duodenal fluid is obtained by either intubation or the Enterotest (also called "string test"). The Enterotest consists of a gelatin capsule containing a nylon string of the appropriate length. The free end of the string is taped to the patient's face and the capsule is swallowed. After four hours to overnight the string is retrieved and the bile-stained mucus on the distal portion of the string is scraped off and examined by both wet mount and permanent staining. A small intestinal biopsy, preferably from multiple duodenal and jejunal sites, may also reveal trophozoites attached to the intestinal epithelium.

In addition, diagnostic kits based on immunological methods for detection of antigens are also available.

Epidemiology

Giardia infection occurs worldwide, with an incidence of world surveys ranging from 2.4 to 67.5 percent. *G. lamblia* infection also widely distributes in China, with an incidence varying from 0.48 to 10 percent.

Higher incidences are likely where sanitary standards are low. Although people of all ages may harbor these organisms, infants and children are more often infected than adults. Carriers are probably more important in the spread of these organisms than symptomatic patients because cysts are less likely to be present in diarrheal stool.

Like other diseases spread by the fecal-oral route, giardiasis can be a problem in institutions, nurseries, and day-care centers.

Giardia is one of the most common agents identified in water-borne outbreaks of diarrhea. Recent outbreaks, some of epidemic proportions, have occurred. These outbreaks have been caused by drinking contaminated water from community water supplies or directly from rivers and streams. Several factors contribute to the frequency of water-transmitted disease. First, *Giardia* is widely distributed in both humans and other mammalian species, allowing for frequent contamination of surface water supplies. Second, the cyst form of *Giardia* can survive for weeks in cold fresh water. Third, *Giardia* cysts are relatively resistant to chlorination alone. Therefore, when water supplies are only treated by chlorination, there is the possibility that *Giardia* will escape inactivation. And fourth, only a few parasites are necessary to establish infection.

Evidence for animal-to-human transmission is limited, despite the wide distribution of *Giardia* organisms in non-human mammalian hosts. On the other hand, evidence suggests some of the *Giardia* strains that parasitize animals may also infect humans and vice versa. Infected beavers are believed to be one source of water-borne giardiasis. Beaver *Giardia* isolates were found capable of infecting dogs and humans. Canines thus may be another source of human giardiasis.

It has been recognized that *Giardia* infection may be transmitted by sexual activity, particularly among homosexual men, but also heterosexually.

Prevention and Control

Giardiasis can be prevented and controlled by improved water supply, proper disposal of human feces, maintenance of food and health education. Attention to personal hygiene is the key to preventing the spread of giardiasis. Controlling the spread of *Giardia* in drinking water should be possible where community water treatment methods (e. g. , disinfection and filtration) are available. For example, iodine and chlorine kill *Giardia* cysts under appropriate conditions. Destruction of *Giardia* cysts is more difficult if the water is near freezing or contains considerable organic matter, because under such conditions so much iodine or chlorine must be added that the water is not palatable. Boiling promptly inactivates *Giardia* cysts and it is the best solution.

The drug of choice for treating *Giardia* infections is metronidazole, it is highly effective. One drawback is that it frequently causes headache and nausea; another is that it is believed to be carcinogenic in rodents and mutagenic in bacteria. Its use in pregnant women is generally contraindicated, particularly in the first trimester. Other effective drugs include: quinacrine, tinidazole, furazolidone, and paromomycin. Paromomycin is not absorbed and may be useful during pregnancy.

Section 4 *Trichomonas vaginalis*

Trichomonas vaginalis was first described from purulent vaginal discharges in 1836 by a French scientist Alfred Donné, and is the etiological agent of trichomoniasis. Trichomoniasis is a common sexually transmitted disease with a worldwide distribution. *T. vaginalis* infects both men and women. In females the organism inhabits the vagina, and in males it is usually found in the prostate or epididymis and the urethra in both sexes.

Morphology

Trichomonas vaginalis occurs only as a trophozoite. The trophozoites of *Trichomonas*, are pear-shaped, measuring 7-30μm by 5-15μm, have a single nucleus, four anterior flagella and a single lateral flagellum attached to pellicle to form an undulating membrane (see Figure 10-4-1). The inner margin of this membrane is supported by a filament. They are actively motile; with characteristic twitching or "bobbling"motility. A hyaline rod-like structure, the axostyle, runs through the length of the body and exits at the posterior end. The cytoplasm contains a large number of hydrogenosomes which functions in anerobic metabolism. Trophozoite is the infective form of the parasite.

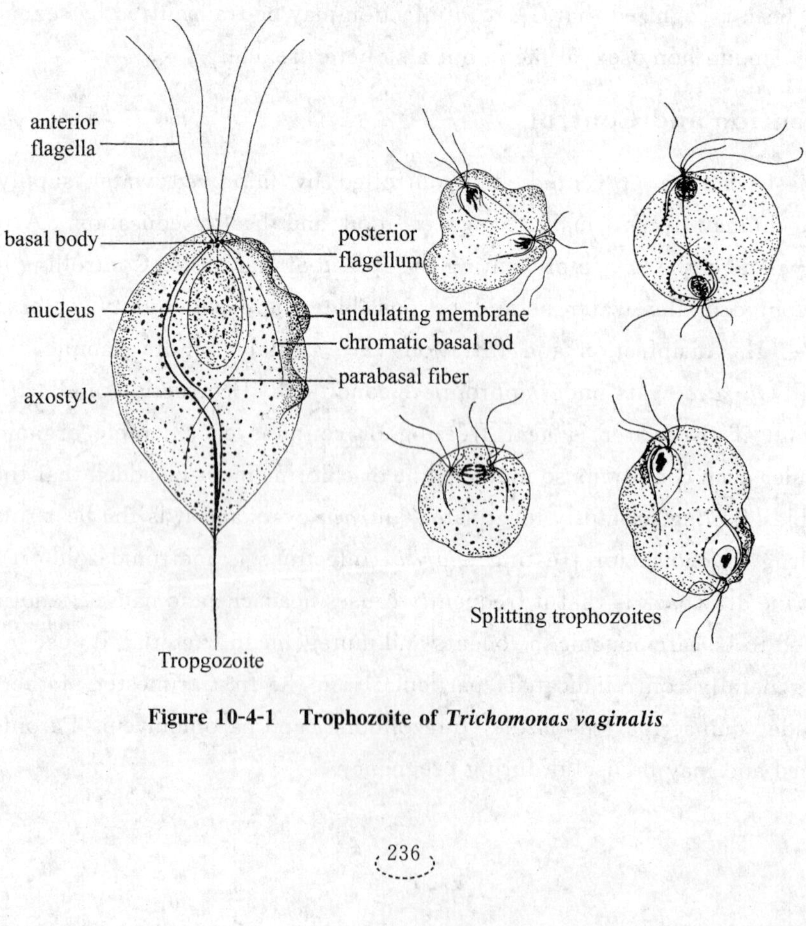

Figure 10-4-1 Trophozoite of *Trichomonas vaginalis*

Life Cycle

The life cycle consists only of a trophozoite stage which is transmitted by direct contact during sexual intercourse. Because there is no resistant cyst, the parasite does not survive well in the external environment, transmission from host to host must be relatively direct. The trophozoites live closely associated or attached to the epithelium of the urogenital tract, where they replicate by longitudinal binary fission. Non-venereal transmission is rare, but possible since the trophozoites can survive 1-2 days in urine and 2-3 hours on wet sponge. In addition, neonatals have been infected during the birth process.

Clinical Manifestations

The incidence of *T. vaginalis* infections varies widely. Trichomoniasis is one of the commonest sexually transmitted diseases. More women than men are infected with *T. vaginalis*. In both sexes, most infections are asymptomatic or mild. Symptomatic infection is common in women, rare in men.

The incubation period ranges from 5-28 days. In females the infection can present as an asymptomatic vaginitis, an acute or chronic vulvovaginitis, or urethritis. The onset or exacerbation of symptoms commonly occurs during or immediately after menstruation. The most common complaint is a persistent mild vaginitis associated with a copious, foul-smelling discharge that is often accompanied by burning or itching. The discharge is most often gray, but can be yellow or green and is sometimes frothy or blood tinged. The discharge diminishes as the infection becomes more chronic. Many women also experience painful or difficult coitus. Urethral involvement occurs in a large number of cases and is characterized by painful and frequent urination.

Males are likely to be asymptomatic and the infection tends to be self-limiting. Occasionally, urethritis, epididymitis, and prostatitis can occur. Common symptoms include: urethral discharge (ranging from scant to purulent), dysuria, and urethral pruritus.

Pathogenesis

Little is known about the pathogenesis associated with *T. vaginalis* infection, but is presumably due to interactions between the parasite and host epithelial cells. In vitro studies indicate that *T. vaginalis* can destroy cells in a contact dependent manner. It may be the mechanical irritation resulting from contact between the parasite and vaginal epithelium. *Trichomonas vaginalis* is an obligate parasite which cannot live without close association of the vaginal, urethral or prostatic tissues. The vaginal walls are usually erythematous and may show petechial hemorrhages. Punctate hemorrhages of the cervix (strawberry cervix) are a distinctive pathological observation associated with trichomoniasis.

However, inflammation can occur in areas where parasites are not found, suggesting that the full explanation may be more complicated.

A number of putative virulence factors have been tentatively identified but the relationship between them and the observed signs and symptoms is far from clear.

In women the nature of the vaginal epithelium and the resident bacterial flora are both profoundly affected by hormonal status. After puberty the vaginal stratified squamous epithelial cells are rich in glycogen and the microbial flora is dominated by lactobacilli; the pH is low (about 4.5, partly but not exclusively because of bacterial lactic acid production). These conditions discourage colonization by anaerobic bacteria. They are also far from ideal for *T. vaginalis* to grow. Nevertheless, it is in this milieu that the organism grows most luxuriantly under natural conditions. Interestingly, in infected women lactobacilli tend to disappear, the pH rises and anaerobic bacteria join the vaginal flora. *T. vaginalis* may bring about this change.

Host Defenses

Relatively little is known about the human immune response to *T. vaginalis* infection. Studies employing experimental animals suggest that antibody may play a protective role.

Whatever protective antibodies are elicited are short-lived, however, and disappear completely in 6 to 16 months.

Diagnosis

Diagnosis is still frequently carried out by the demonstration of trophozoites in vaginal, urethral, prostatic secretions, or urine sediment (following prostate massage). Microscopic examination of wet mounts of fresh vaginal discharge, preferably collected with a speculum on a cotton-tipped applicator, is the most practical method of diagnosis; Specimens should be mixed with a drop of saline and examined as soon as possible, as the size and jerky motility of a living trophozoite are all but diagnostic. Specimens can also be fixed and stained with Giemsa or fluorescent dyes. In vitro culture will sometimes reveal organisms when direct examination is negative.

A number of immunological methods have been marketed. Both DNA probe- and PCR-based tests have been developed. PCR-based methods offer exciting new possibilities for making an accurate diagnosis on specimens obtained in less invasive ways.

Epidemiology

Trichomoniasis probably is the commonest sexually transmitted diseases worldwide with at least 170 million new infections acquired per annum (WHO, 1995). Although sexual intercourse is believed to be the usual means of transfer, some infections probably are acquired occasionally through fomites such as towels, toilet seats, and sauna benches; the organisms may spread through mud and water baths as well. Survival studies of *T. vaginalis* in vaginal discharges have shown that these trophozoites can be cultured from toilet seats for 30 minutes or more.

Women with trichomoniasis may occasionally infect their female babies while giving birth. Infected women and men harboring trophozoites of *T. vaginalis* in the genital tract are the chief reservoir of infection and the source of transmission.

Prevention and Control

The drug of choice for treatment is metronidazole. Treatment of both sexual partners at the same time is recommended to prevent reinfection. Some drug resistance has been reported. Tinidazole is an alternate drug. Measures used in the control of other sexually transmitted diseases, such as avoidance of sexual contact with infected partners and use of condoms, are also effective in preventing trichomoniasis.

(He Shenyi)

Section 5 Other trichomonads

Trichomonas hominis

Trichomonas hominis (Davaine, 1860), found in the cecum where it forms a harmless infection, is of cosmopolitan distribution.

T. hominis has no cystic stage. Its trophozoite measures from 5 to 15μm in length and from 7 to 10μm in width. The trophozoite is pyriform and has an axostyle which runs from the nucleus down the centre of the body and extends from the end of the body. The undulating membrane extends the entire length of the body. *T. hominis* has a variable number of anterior flagella (three to five) but typically five. It is characterized by the presence of four free flagella and an undulating membrane bordered by a flagellum that is free posterior, and a vesicle-like nucleus located in the anterior end (see Figure 10-5-1).

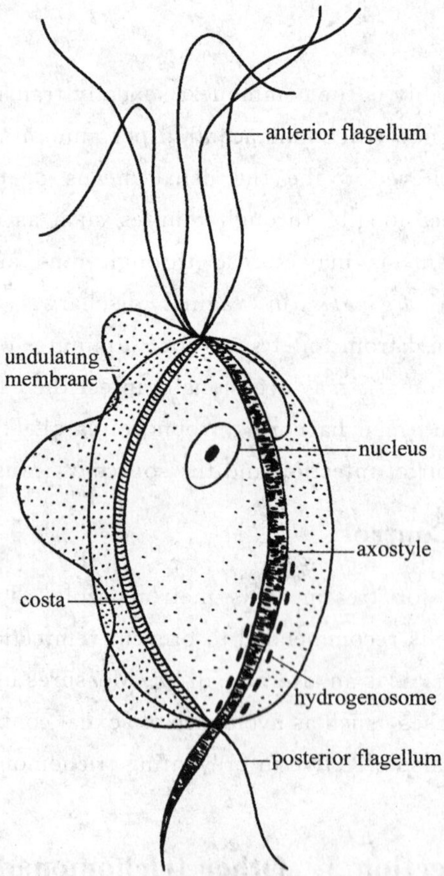

Figure 10-5-1 Trophozoite of *Trichomonas hominis*

The flagellate is thought to be non-pathogenic although it has been associated with diarrhoeic stools. The transmission may occur through contaminated food and drinking water. Infection of the host is by the oral route. The flagellate is often identified in human diarrheic stools. The diagnosis depends upon finding of the trophozoites in unformed stool that contains considerable mucus. In a fresh stool, the flagellates move very rapidly in a jerky, non-directional manner. A stained preparation (usually stained with trichrome or iron hematoxylin) provides an accurate identification of the organisms.

Because of the fecal-oral transmission rout, infection with *T. hominis* is more frequently reported in children than in adults. Although infections with the trichomonads in some world regions are as often as with Giardia, no prevention and optimal treatment are defined, chlorhexidine and metronidazole were used.

Trichomonas tenax

There is only trophozoite stage in the life cycle of *Trichomonas tenax* (O. F.

Müller, 1773; Dobell, 1939). The trophozoite is pyriform in shape and small, measuring 5 to 16μm in length by 2 to 15μm in width. There is a typical axostyle and a single nucleus, and four anterior free flagella. The fifth flagellum recurved and merged with an undulating membrane that extends almost the length of the body (see Figure 10-5-2).

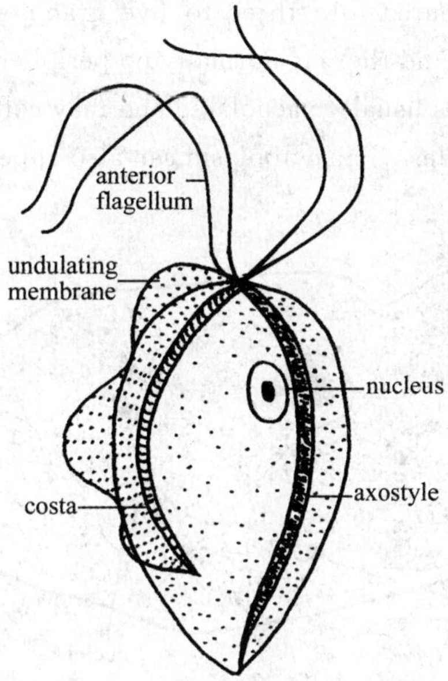

Figure 10-5-2 Trophozoite of *Trichomonas tenax*

T. tenax is a protozoa in the mouth of man, inhabits in the tartar around the teeth, and carious teeth. Although the organism is not considered to be pathogenic, its infection indicates a poor oral hygiene. The flagellate will not survive passage through the stomach and cannot establish infection in vagina, but there are reports of respiratory infection and thoracic abscesses.

It is worldwide in distribution. Prevalence rates reach to 25%. The exact transmission mode is not known, it is assumed to be by direct contact, usually kissing, or use of contaminated dishes and glasses.

Diagnosis is based on the recovery of the protozoa from the teeth, gums, or tonsillar crypts. Therapy is not necessary. Better oral hygiene will eliminate its infection.

Dientamoeba fragilis

Dientamoeba fragilis (Jepps & Dobell, 1918) is an amoeba-flagellate with a cosmopolitan distribution. The parasite was originally thought to be an amoeba but recent ultrastructural and immunological studies indicate it is more closely related to *Trichomonas*.

D. fragilis live in the lumen of the caecum and upper colon. The organisms have only a trophozoite stage (see Figure 10-5-3). Trophozoite is relatively small, round in shape, varying from 3 to 22μm in diameter and there can be considerable variation in size among organisms in the same fecal sample. In a permanently stained preparation, one, two or rarely three nuclei can be seen, two being the most common. The nuclear chromatin is usually fragmented into three to five granules but these have not been visualized by Giemsa Stain, and there is normally no peripheral chromatin on the nuclear membrane. The cytoplasm is usually vacuolated and may contain ingested debris as well as some large uniform granules. The cytoplasm can also appear uniform and clean with a few inclusions.

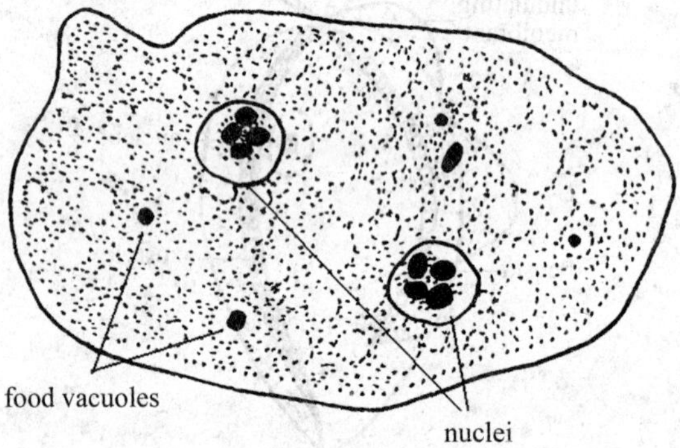

Figure 10-5-3 Trophozoite of *Dientamoeba fragilis*

The life cycle of the organism is not known. Because the parasite does not form cysts and trophozoites cannot survive passage through the small intestine, the details of transmission is unknown, although eggs of the intestinal nematode *Enterobius* spp. and *Ascaris* have been suggested as possible carriers. The pathogenesis of the flagellate is a controversial area. The organism has been reported in association with mucous diarrhea, abdominal pain and tenderness. Nausea, vomiting and low-grade fever have also been reported in a number of cases. But most parasitologists now believe that other parasites were the cause of diarrhea, as *D. fragilis* is usually never found alone. The precise role of this organism as a cause of disease remains to be determined.

The organism of *D. fragilis* has been associated with a wide range of symptoms, although its pathogenic status is still not well defined. Case reports of children infected with the protozoa reveal a number of symptoms, such as intermittent diarrhea, abdominal pain, nausea, anorexia, malaise, fatigue, poor weight gain. The most common symptoms appear to be intermittent diarrhea and fatigue. In some patients, both the parasite and the symptoms persist or reappear until the appropriate treatment is initiated.

Diagnosis depends upon proper collection of stool (at least three fecal specimens) and examination of the fresh direct wet preparation or permanently stained smears prepared from unformed or formed stools with mucus. It is important that permanently stained smears of stool preparations should be examined, because survival times of the organism in terms of morphology, is very limited and specimens must be examined immediately or preserved in a suitable fixative as soon as possible after defaecation. The recommended stains are Fields' and Giemsa stain (trophozoites are destroyed in a formol-ether concentrate).

Symptomatic relief or clinical improvement has been observed in the infected individuals to follow appropriate therapy with tetracycline, diiodohydroxyquin, or metronidazole. Current recommendations are iodoquinol, paromomycin, or tetracycline.

D. fragilis is worldwide in distribution. The parasite may be infrequently recovered and identified; low incidence or absence from survey studies may be due to poor laboratory techniques and a general lack of knowledge concerning the protozoa.

Because fecal-oral transmission is possible, the appropriate hygienic and sanitary measures to prevent contamination with decal material would be an effective prevent mode.

(Ye Bin)

Chapter 11 Sporozoa

Section 1 *Plasmodium*

The causal agents of malaria are blood parasites of the genus *Plasmodium*, family Plasmodiidae in the suborder Haemosporina. There are approximately 156 named species of *Plasmodium*, which infect various species of vertebrates. Four are known to infect humans, *P. falciparum*, *P. vivax*, *P. ovale* and *P. malariae*. In China, *P. falciparum* and *P. vivax* are common; *P. ovale* and *P. malariae* infection are rarely seen.

Morphology

As it is important to recognize the forms of human plasmodium in blood, the morphology of the diagnostic differences among the two species of human infecting plasmodium is described. Malarial Blood Stage Parasites include trophozoite and gametocyte. In the Blood Smears, trophozoites are generally ring shaped, 1-2 microns in size, although other forms (ameboid and band) may also exist. The sexual forms of the parasite (gametocytes) are much larger and 7-14 microns in size. *P. falciparum* is the largest and is banana shaped while others are smaller and round. *P. vivax* causes stippling of infected red cells (see Plate III).

Table 11-1-1 **Comparisons of erythrocyte changes in *Plasmodium* species infection**

Plasmodium species	Stages found in blood	Appearance of Erythrocyte (ABC)
P. vivax	Ring form	Normal to 11/4 ×, round; occasionally fine Schüffner's dots; multiple infection of RBC not uncommon
	Trophozoite	Enlarged 11/2 to 2 ×; may be distorted; fine Schüffner's dots
	Schizont	Enlarged 11/2 to 2 ×; may be distorted; fine Schüffner's dots
	Gametocyte	Enlarged 11/2 to 2 ×; may be distorted; fine Schüffner's dots
P. falciparum	Ring form	Normal; multiple infection of RBC more common than in other species
	Trophozoite	Normal; rarely, Maurer's clefts (under certain staining conditions)
	Schizont	Normal; rarely, Maurer's clefts (under certain staining conditions)
	Gametocyte	Distorted by parasite

Life Cycle

There are two phases in the life cycle: the sexual cycle, which occurs primarily in mosquitoes, and the asexual cycle, which occurs in humans, the intermediate hosts. The vector and definitive host is the female *Anopheles* mosquito (only the female take blood meal). During a blood meal, a malaria-infected female *Anopheles* mosquito inoculates sporozoites into the human host.

Exo-erythrocytic stage (EE stage)

Sporozoites infect liver cells and mature into schizonts, which rupture and release merozoites. (Of note, in *P. vivax* and *P. ovale* a dormant stage (hypnozoites) can persist in the liver and cause relapses by invading the bloodstream weeks, or even years later.) After this initial replication in the liver (exo-erythrocytic schizogony), the parasites undergo asexual multiplication in the erythrocytes (erythrocytic schizogony).

In *P. vivax*, hypnozoites are found inside the liver parenchyma. These are single-nucleated parasites measuring 4-6μm in diameter and are the dormant stages of the parasite. Relapse in vivax malaria is caused by these hypnozoites, which after a period of time become active and develop into pre-erythrocytic schizonts, thereby causing malaria. In *P. falciparum*, only a single generation of exo-erythrocytic stage takes place, and secondary EE stage is absent. Recent evidences indicate that hypnozoites are found in the liver phase of *P. malariae*. The single nucleated intra-hepatocellular hypnozoites of

P. ovale resemble those of *P. vivax*.

Erythrocytic stages

Merozoites are released from the liver cells and infect red blood cells. During the erythrocytic phase, the organism differentiates into a ring-shaped trophozoite. The ring stage trophozoites mature into schizonts, which rupture releasing merozoites. After release, the merozoites infect other erythrocytes. Some parasites differentiate into sexual erythrocytic stages (gametocytes). Blood stage parasites are responsible for the clinical manifestations of the disease.

In mosquito

The sexual cycle begins in the human red blood cells when some merozoites develop into male and others into female gametocytes. The gametocyte-containing red blood cells are ingested by the female *Anopheles* mosquito and, within her gut, a female macrogamete and eight spermlike male microgametes are produced. After fertization, the diploid zygote differentiates into a motile ookinete that burrows into gut wall, where it grows into an oocyst within which many haploid sporozoites are produced. The sporozoites are released and migrate to the salivary glands, ready to complete the cycle when the mosquito takes her next blood meal.

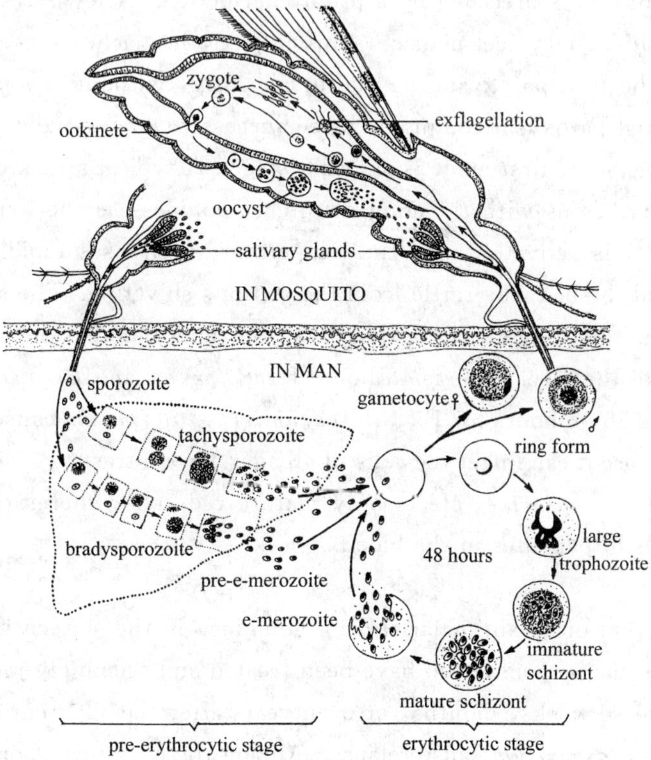

Figure 11-1-1 Life cycle of *Plasmodium*

Pathogenesis and Clinical Manifestation

Most of pathologic findings of malaria result from the destruction of red blood cells. Red cells are destroyed both by the release of the merozoites and by the action of spleen to first sequester the infected red cells and then to lyse them. The enlarged spleen is due to congestion of sinusoids with erythrocytes, coupled with hyperplasia of lymphocytes and macrophages.

Incubation period

Usually after humans get infection, the symptoms will not appear immediately, and there is an incubation period. It is the time interval between the infective bite of *Anopheline* mosquito and the onset of the clinical symptoms. It includes the period of the time for the sporozoite to reach the liver, the duration of the development in the liver, and the time of development in the RBC to produce sufficient erythrocytic merozoites to cause clinical symptoms. The incubation period in *P. vivax* varies from 8 to 31 days; 7 to 27 days in *P. falciparum*. In *P. malariae*, the incubation period is relatively longer and varies from 18 to 35 days; In *P. ovale*, it is 16 to 18 days.

Malarial paroxysm

Malarial paroxysm is preceded by a prodromal period. A few days before the first paroxysm, the patient may feel malaise, muscle pain, headache, loss of appetite, and slight fever; or the first paroxysm may occur abruptly, without any prior symptoms. The classic malarial paroxysm comprises three successive stages: cold stage, hot stage and sweating stage. The first stage is the cold-stage. A typical attack of benign tertian or quartan malaria begins with a feeling of intense coldness as the hypothalamus, the body's thermostat, is activated, and the temperature then rises rapidly to 41℃. The teeth chatter, and the bed may rattle from the victim's shivering. The skin is warm and dry. Nausea, vomiting, severe headache, backache, and hypotension are usual.

The timing of the fever cycle is 48 hours for *P. vivax* and *P. ovale*, 72 hours for *P. malariae*, and 36-48 hours for *P. falciparum*. *P. falciparum* causes a high level of parasitemia, because it can infect red cells of all ages. In contrast, *P. vivax* infects only reticulocytes and *P. malariae* infects only mature red cells; therefore, they produce much lower levels of parasites in the blood.

Relapse

Since the advent of an antimalarial drug (quinine) in the sixteenth century, it has been noted that some persons, who have been treated and seemingly recovered, relapse back into the disease weeks, months, or even years after the apparent cure. However, not all species of *Plasmodium* cause relapse. Among the parasites of primates, only *P. vivax* and *P. ovale* of humans cause true relapse.

Two populations of exoerythrocytic forms have now been shown. One develops rapidly into schizonts, as previously described, but the other remains dormant as hypnozoites ("sleeping animalcules"). These have been demonstrated for *P. vivax*, *P. ovale*, and *P. cynomolgi*, but they have not been found in any species that does not cause relapse. How long the hypnozoite can remain capable of initiating schizogony and what triggers it to do so are unknown. Primaquine has been shown to be an effective hypnozoiticide.

Recrudescence

Recrudescence is not relapses; it is a feature of *P. malariae* and *P. falciparum*. It also occurs in *P. vivax* and *P. ovale*. This occurs over many years, due to persistence of small numbers of viable erythrocytic forms of the parasite in the internal organs. This is believed to be due to change of the surface antigens of the parasites, thus evading themselves from the immune responses of the host. Attacks have also been reported even up to 40 years after the initial infection, notably after splenectomy.

Complications of malaria

Malaria caused by *P. falciparum* is more severe than that caused by other plasmodia. It is characterized by infection of far more red cells than the other malarial species and by occlusion of the capillaries with aggregates of parasitized red cells. This leads to life-threatening hemorrhage and necrosis, particularly in the brain (cerebral malaria). Furthermore, extensive hemolysis and kidney damage occur, with resulting hemoglobinuria. The dark color of the patient's urine has given rise to the term, "blackwater fever". The hemoglobinuria can lead to acute renal failure. Malaria caused by the other three plasmodia is usually self-limited, with a low mortality rate. However, relapses of *P. vivax* and *P. ovale* malaria can occur up to several years after the initial illness as a result of hypnozoites latent in the liver. Splenomegaly is seen in most patients, and hepatomegaly occurs in roughly one-third. Anemia is prominent.

Congenital malaria

It is a recognized entity in malaria. It is caused by transmission of erythrocytic asexual forms of the parasite through the placenta, when the latter is injured. Neither EE forms nor sporozoites lead to infection. Congenital malaria is usually acquired during parturition. The conditions are known to occur more frequently in non-immune infected mothers than in highly immune mothers, with intense parasitisation of the placenta. It is a relatively rare condition seen only in highly endemic areas.

Transfusion malaria

Transfusion of infected blood and the use of contaminated needle of the intravenous drug addicts can cause transfusion malaria. Pre-erythrocytic development is absent, and incubation period is short. Clinically, it behaves like a naturally acquired infection. Relapse does not occur.

Immunity

Host immunity in malaria broadly has two types: natural or innate immunity and acquired immunity.

Natural (innate) immunity

Natural immunity in malaria refers to the inherent but non-immune mechanisms of the host defense against malaria. It is mainly based on the nature of the red cells. The nature of the red blood cells that determine the susceptibility of the cells to invasion by malaria parasites and development in the cells include (1) Age of red blood cell, (2) Nature of haemoglobin, (3) Enzyme content of erythrocyte, and (4) Presence or absence of certain factors.

Individuals with sickle cell trait (heterozygotes) are protected against malaria because their red cells have too little ATPase activity and cannot produce sufficient energy to support the growth of the parasite. People with homozypgous sickle cell anemia are also protected but rarely live long to obtain much benefit. The receptor for *P. vivax* is the Duffy blood group antigen. People who are homozygous receive for the genes that encode this protein are resistant to infection by *P. vivax*. More than 90% of black West Africans and many of their American descendants do not produce the Duffy antigen and are thereby resistant to vivax malaria. People with glucose-6-phosphate dehyfrogenase(G6PD) deficiency also protected against the severe effects of falciparum malaria. G6PD deficiency is an X-linked hemoglobinopathy found in high frequency in tropical areas where malaria is endemic. Both male and female carriers of the mutated gene are protected against malaria.

Acquired immunity

People residing in malaria-endemic regions acquire immunity to malaria through natural exposure to malaria parasites. This naturally acquired malarial immunity that is protective against parasites and clinical disease results only after continued exposure from multiple infections with malaria parasites over time. Clinical immunity generally provides protection against severe effects of malaria but fails to provide strong protection against infection with malaria parasites, and generally develops first. After several years of continued exposure people develop immunity that limits high-density parasitemia; however, it does not lead to sterile protection.

Specific acquired immunity in malaria involves both humoral and cellular immunities. The specific immunity restricts the level of parasitemia and eventually confers protection from the disease but not from infection. The development of protection immunity in malaria is the result of a complicated interaction between the malaria parasites and immune system of the host, which involve both humoral and cellular immunities. These immune responses include antibodies, lymphocytes, monocytes, macrophages, natural killer (NK) cells, and neutrophils. Experimental studies have shown that antibodies, cells and cellular factors can mediate protection in malaria as well as disease.

Humoral immunity

Circulating antibodies against sporozoites, asexual blood stages and sexual blood stages develop in persons repeatedly exposed to malaria. Antibody response is strongly against the asexual blood forms of the parasite, which have consequently evolved various methods of immune evasion.

Humoral antibodies against asexual blood forms may protect against the malaria parasites by inhibiting red cell invasion or by inhibiting growth inside the red blood cells and sequestration of parasitised red blood cells. These antibodies are responsible for the decreased susceptibility of the host to malarial infection and disease. Antibodies against sexual stages are suggested to reduce malaria transmission. Acquired antibody-mediated immunity is transferred from mother to foetus across the placenta. This passively transferred immunity protects the baby from severe malaria in the first few months of life. It disappears within 6 to 9 months.

Cell-mediated immunity

Recent work suggests that a variety of cellular mechanisms may play a role in conferring protection against malaria. The cellular mechanism is mainly of non-specific type. In acute *P. falciparum* infection, a positive correlation has been found between natural killer (NK) and resistance to malaria. Activated macrophages may phagocytose and induce extra-cellular killing of target cells. These reactions may be specifically amplified or induced by antibodies bound to target cell surfaces. These may also be induced non-specific by endotoxin-like substances derived from malaria parasites. The mediators released from activated macrophages are responsible for various pathogical changes found in the infected hosts during acute malarial infections.

Immunological factors have been implicated in the pathogenesis of several complications of malaria such as glomerulonephritis, cerebral malaria, tropical splenomegaly syndrome (TSS) and anemia.

Diagnosis

The diagnosis of malaria can be based on clinical criteria and/or techniques for parasites. The condition is considered in any person who has a febrile illness and who has come from the area endemic for malaria, received blood transfusion or used intra venous drugs.

Laboratory diagnosis of malaria is established by parasitological methods by demonstration of malaria in blood. Serological methods are useful only in the epidemiology studies. Molecular diagnosis techniques can complement microscopy, especially in species identification.

Microscopy detection

Microscopic identification is the method most frequently used to demonstrate an active infection. A blood specimen collected from the patient is spread as a thick or thin blood smear, stained with a Romanovsky stain (most often Giemsa), and examined with a 100X oil immersion objective. Visual criteria are used to detect malaria parasites and to differentiate (when possible) the various species.

Thin smear is used for detecting parasites and for determining the species of the infecting parasite. The thin smears are air-dried rapidly, fixed in methanol and stained. The red blood cells in the tail end of the smear are examined under oil-immersion for the parasite. This technique remains the gold standard for laboratory confirmation of malaria. However, it depends on the quality of the reagents, of the microscope, and on the experience of the laboratorian.

Immunodiagnosis

In addition to microscopy and molecular methods, there are methods for detecting malaria parasites on the basis of antigens and antibodies.

(1) Detection of an antigen (histidine rich protein-2, HRP-2)

Detection of an antigen is associated with malaria parasites (especially *P. falciparum* and *P. vivax*). The detection of HRP-2 and of pLDH forms the basis for diagnostic kits that have been evaluated. Various test kits are available to detect antigens derived from malaria parasites. Such immunologic ("immunochromatographic") tests most often use a dipstick or cassette format, and provide results in 2-15 minutes. These "Rapid Diagnostic Tests" (RDTs) offer a useful alternative to microscopy in situations where reliable microscopic diagnosis is not available.

(2) Detection of antibodies

Malaria antibody detection can be performed using various techniques. For the clinical laboratory, the most practical approach is the indirect fluorescent antibody (IFA) test and ELISA.

Molecular diagnosis

Parasite nucleic acids are detected using polymerase chain reaction (PCR). This technique is more accurate than microscopy. However, it is expensive, and requires a specialized laboratory (even though technical advances will likely result in field-operated PCR machines).

Epidemiology

Epidemic situation

Today approximately 40% of the world's population mostly living in the world's poorest countries are at risk of malaria. The disease was once more widespread but it was successfully eliminated from many countries with temperate climates during the mid 20th century. Today malaria is found throughout the tropical and sub-tropical regions of the world and causes more than 300 million acute illnesses and at least one million deaths annually.

Ninety percent of deaths due to malaria occur in Africa south of the Sahara mostly among young children. Malaria kills an African child every 30 seconds. Many children who survive an episode of severe malaria may suffer from learning impairments or brain damage. Pregnant women and their unborn children are also particularly vulnerable to malaria, which is a major cause of perinatal mortality, low birth weight and maternal anemia.

Malaria is still an important problem of public health in China, especially in the southern and central parts. Yunnan and Hainan still faced a severe situation of malaria endemic with the spread of *Plasmodium falciparum*, particularly the imported malaria cases in 25 border counties in Yunnan. In the central parts of the country, especially in Anhui Province the malaria prevalence increased considerably with the highest incidence and over half of the total malaria cases in 2006, rank of P/M/A were basically in concordance in the two systems, which revealed new challenges to the National Malaria Control Program in China.

Epidemic factors

A variety of interrelated factors contribute to the level of natural transmission of the disease in a given area.

(1) Reservoir

The prevalence of the infection in humans, and in some cases other primates, with high enough levels of parasitemia to infect mosquitoes; this would include persons with symptomatic diseases and tolerant individuals.

(2) Vector

Suitability of the local anophelines as hosts; their breeding, flight, and resting behavior; feeding preferences; and abundance. Of the approximately 390 species of *Anopheles*, some are more suitable hosts for *Plasmodium* than are others. Of those, which are good hosts, some prefer animal blood to human; therefore, transmission may be influenced by the proximity with which humans live to other animals. The preferred breeding and resting places are very important. Some species breed only in fresh water, others in brackish; some like standing water around human habitations, such as puddles, or trash that collects water, such as bottles and broken coconut shells. Water, vegetation, and amount of shade are important, as are whether the species enters dwellings and rests there after feeding and whether the species flies some distance from breeding areas. *Anopheles* spp. exhibits an astonishing variety of such preferences. *Anopheles sinensis*, *A. anthropophagus*, *A. dirus* and *A. minimus* are important vectors in China.

(3) Susceptible population

That means new hosts—availability of nonimmune hosts.

(4) Local climatic conditions

(5) Local geographical and hydrographical conditions and human activities that determine availability of mosquito breeding areas.

One must thoroughly study and understand all these factors before understanding a malaria control program with any hope of success. Sometimes deliberate government policy exacerbates transmission of malaria.

Prevention and Control

Treatment of infected individuals

Acute attacks by any of malaria parasites should be treated with chloroquine. *P. vivax* and *P. ovale* infections acquired through mosquito bites may have persistent hepatic forms (hypnozoites). These must be eliminated with primaquine to prevent relapse. For *P. falciparum*: as a response to increasing levels of antimalarial resistance, WHO recommends the following therapeutic options: artemether/lumefantrine, artesunate plus amodiaquine, artesunate plus sulfadoxine/pyrimethamine (in areas where SP efficacy remains high), artesunate plus mefloquine (in areas with low to moderate transmission), and amodiaquine plus sulfadoxine pyrimethamine.

Mosquito control

Valuable actions in mosquito control include destruction of breeding places when possible or practical, introduction of mosquito predators such as the mosquito-eating fish *Gambusia affinis*, and judicious use of insecticides. The efficacy and economy of DDT have been a boon to such efforts in underdeveloped countries. Although we now seem to be aware of the supposed environmental dangers of DDT, we consider these dangers preferable and minor compared with the miseries of malaria. Unfortunately, reports of DDT-resistant strains of Anopheles are increasing, and this phase of the battle will become more difficult in coming years. For exterminating susceptible *Anopheles* spp. that enter dwellings and rest there after feeding, spraying the insides of houses with residual insecticides can be effective and cheap, without incurring any environmental penalty. Unfortunately, some *Anopheles* rest in houses only for a short time before or after feeding, and sufficient quantities of DDT are becoming difficult to obtain on the world market.

Prevention from mosquito bite

These include: (1) personal protection by proper use of mosquito nets while sleeping, (2) Wearing protective clothings that minimize contact with mosquitoes, and (3)Use of mosquito repellants.

(Wu Zhongdao)

Section 2 *Toxoplasma gondii*

Toxoplasma gondii belongs to the phylum Apicomplexa and is a coccidian parasite with the cat as the definitive host but any warm-blooded animal, including humans, act as intermediate hosts. It was discovered by Nicolle and Manceaux in 1908 in Tunisia in a small rodent, *Ctenodactylus gundi*. It has cosmopolitan distribution and causes infection in over 200 species of birds and mammals, including man. *T. gondii* is an obligate intracellular parasite, which is found inside the reticuloendothelial cells and many other nucleated cells. Infections by *T. gondii* are widely prevalent in humans and animals worldwide and have emerged as one of the most common opportunistic infections in patients with AIDS.

Morphology

There are three infectious stages of *T. gondii*: the tachyzoites (intracellular trophozoites or proliferative forms), the bradyzoites (in tissue cysts) and the sporozoites (in oocysts). These are important stages seen during the life cycle of the parasite (see Figure 11-2-1). All these stages are infectious to man.

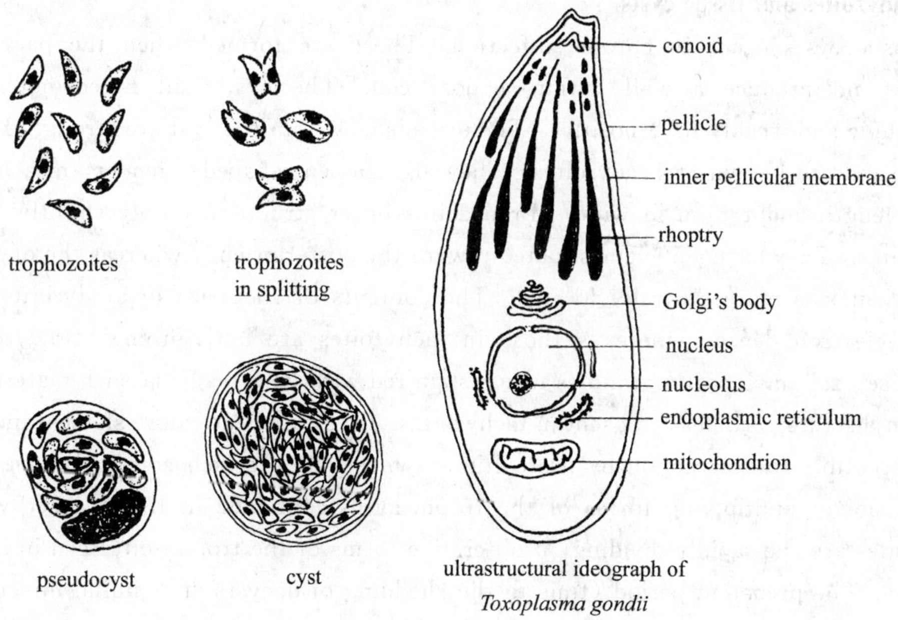

Figure 11-2-1 Morphology of *Toxoplasma gondii*

Tachyzoite

The term "tachyzoite" (tachos=speed in Greek) was coined by Frenkel to describe the stage that rapidly multiplies in any cell of the intermediate host and in non-intestinal epithelial cells of the definitive host. Tachyzoites have also been termed endodyozoites or endozoites. It is crescent-shaped with a pointed anterior and a rounded posterior end. It measures 6μm in length and 2μm in breadth. Ultrastructurally, the tachyzoite consists of various organelles and inclusion bodies including a pellicle (outer covering), apical rings, polar rings, conoid, rhoptries, micronemes, micropore, mitochondrion, subpellicular microtubules, endoplasmic reticulum, Golgi complex, ribosomes, nucleus and a multiple membrane bound plastid like organelle which has also been called a Golgi adjunct or apicoplast. The nucleus is spherical or rounded and is usually situated towards the posterior end or in the central area of the cell.

Tachyzoite is the active multiplying form seen during the acute stage of infection. It enters the host cell by active penetration of the host cell membrane. After entering the host cell the tachyzoite assumes an oval shape and becomes surrounded by a parasitophorous vacuole, which appears to be derived from both the parasite and the host cell. It multiplies asexually within the host cell by repeated endodyogeny or internal budding, a specialized form of reproduction in which two daughter tachyzoites being formed within the parent cell. When the host cell becomes distended with the parasites it disintegrates releasing the trophozoites which infect other cells. Groups of proliferating tachyzoites within a host cell are known as pseudocyst.

Bradyzoites and tissue cysts

Tissue cysts occur in chronic infection. These are formed when the parasites multiply and produce a wall within a host cell. The cyst wall is eosinophilic, argyrophilic and weakly PAS-positive. The organisms within the cyst are strongly PAS-positive and are known as bradyzoites. They are crescent shaped, slender, measuring 7μm in length and 1.5μm in width. Bradyzoites differ structurally only slightly from tachyzoites. They have a nucleus situated toward the posterior end, whereas the nucleus in tachyzoites is more centrally located. The contents of rhoptries in bradyzoites are usually electron dense, where as those in tachyzoites are labyrinthine. Bradyzoites contain several amylopectin granules which stain red with PAS reagent; such material is either in discrete particles or absent in tachyzoites. Bradyzoites are more slender and are less susceptible to destruction by proteoltic enzymes than are tachyzoites. Bradyzoites are the slowly multiplying forms of the trophozoites contained in tissue cyst, while tachyzoites are the rapidly dividing, proliferative forms of the trophozoite seen in acute infection. The prepatent period (time to the shedding of oocysts after initial infection) in cats following feeding of bradyzoites is shorter than that following feeding of tachyzoites.

Young tissue cysts may be as small as 5μm in diameter and contain only two bradyzoites, while the older ones may contain hundreds of bradyzoites. In histological sections of brain, tissue cysts rarely reach a diameter of 60μm, whereas intramuscular cysts may reach a diameter of 100μm. Although tissue cysts may develop in visceral organs, including the lungs, liver and kidneys, they are more prevalent in the neural and muscular tissues, including the brain, eyes, and skeletal and cardiac muscles. Intact tissue cysts probably do not cause any harm and can persist for the life of the host without causing a host inflammatory response.

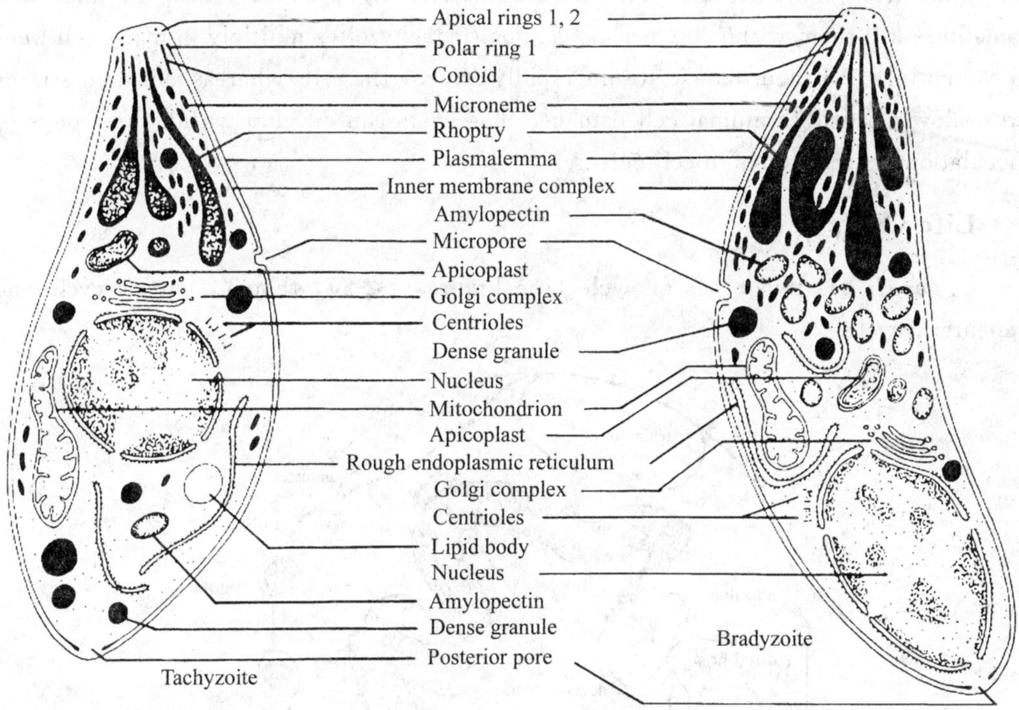

Figure 11-2-2　Morphological difference between Tachyzoite and Bradyzoite

Oocyst

This stage is present in cat and other felines and not in humans. It is oval or spherical, 10-12μm in diameter and contains a sporoblast. The oocyst wall contains two colourless layers. Sporulation of oocysts occurs outside the cats within 1 to 5 days of excretion depending upon aeration and temperature. Sporulated oocysts are subspherical to ellipsoidal and are 11 by 13μm in diameter. Sporoblast divides and forms two sporocysts and four sporozoites develop inside each sporocyst.

Tachyzoites and tissue cysts represent stages of asexual multiplication (schizogony), while the oocyst is formed by sexual reproduction (gametogony). All three forms occur in domestic cat and other felines which are the definitive hosts and which support both schizogony and gametogony. Only the asexual forms, tachyzoites and tissue cysts are present in other mammals, including man and birds, which are the intermediate hosts.

Cultivation

T. gondii can be cultured in laboratory animals, chick embryos and cell cultures.

Mice, hamsters, guinea pigs and rabbits are all susceptible but mice are generally used as hosts because they are more susceptible. After intraperitoneal inoculation of any of the three infectious stages, i. e. tachyzoites, bradyzoites and oocysts of *T. gondii*, some strains grow in the peritoneal cavity producing ascites, and tissue cysts are prominent in the brain after eight weeks. Virulent strains usually produce illness in mice and sometimes kill them within 1-2 weeks. *T. gondii* tachyzoites multiply in many cell lines in cell culture. Virulent mouse strains rapidly destroy the cells whereas avirulent strains grow slowly causing minimal cell damage. The cysts can develop within three days of inoculation of tachyzoites in cell culture.

Life Cycle

T. gondii has two types of cycle (see Figure 11-2-3), that is, enteric cycle and exoenteric cycle.

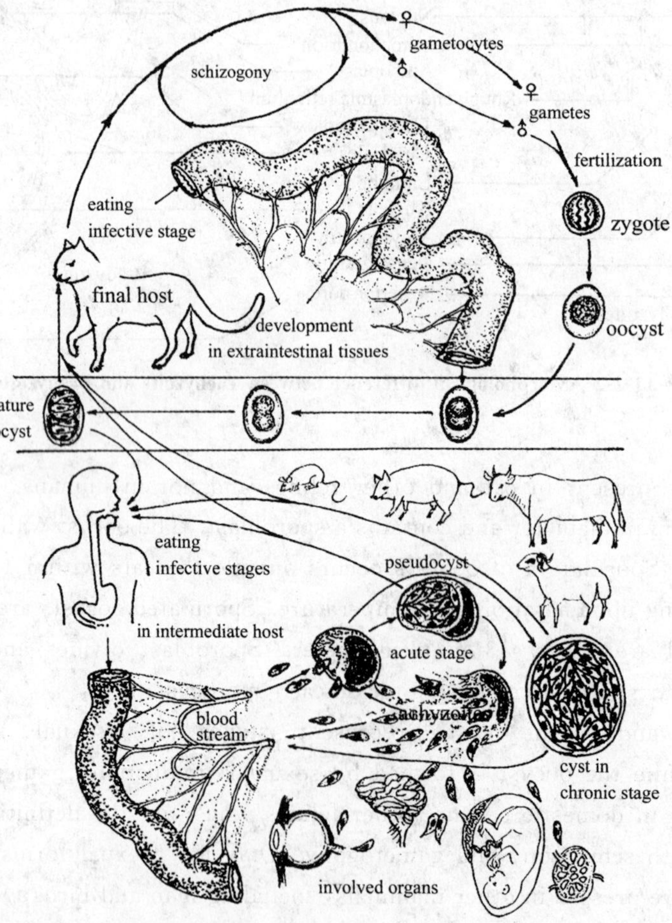

Figure 11-2-3 Life cycle of *Toxoplasma gondii*

Enteric cycle

Enteric cycle occurs in domestic cat and other felines which are definitive hosts. It includes both asexual multiplication (schizogony) and sexual reproduction (gametogony) within the mucosal epithelial cells of the small intestine. Cat acquires infection by ingestion of any of the three infectious stages of *T. gondii*, i. e. tachyzoites, bradyzoites from tissue cysts and sporozoites from oocysts. These invade mucosal cells of cat's small intestine in which they undergo several cycles of asexual generation before the sexual cycle begins with the formation of male and female gametocytes which give rise to male and female gametes respectively. After sexual fusion (fertilization) of male and female gametes, oocysts develop, exit from host cell into the gut lumen, and pass out in the faeces. Freshly passed oocyst contains a sporoblast and is not infectious. It becomes infectious only after development in soil for a few days. During this time, the sporoblast divides into two. These then become sporocysts by acquiring a cyst wall. Four sporozoites develop inside each sporocyst. The mature cyst containing eight sporozoites is the infective form of the parasite. It can remain infective in the soil for about one year. When ingested, it can either repeat its cycle in a cat or if ingested by rodent or other mammal, including humans or certain birds, can establish an infection in which it reproduces asexually.

Exoenteric cycle

Humans, mice and other mammals and certain birds, which are the intermediate hosts acquire infection by ingestion of food and water contaminated with cat's faeces containing sporulated oocysts, and also by ingestion of undercooked meat (mutton, pork and rarely beef) containing tissue cysts. In duodenum, the oocysts release sporozoites and tissue cysts release bradyzoites. These pass through the gut wall, circulate in the body, and invade various cells, especially macrophages, where they form tachyzoites, multiply, break out and spread the infection to other organs. Subsequently they enter into the neural and muscular tissues, such as the brain, eye and skeletal and cardiac muscle where they multiply slowly (as bradyzoites) to form tissue cysts, initiating chronic stage of the disease. Tissue cysts may also develop in other organs such as lungs, liver and kidneys. Tissue cysts, when ingested by both definitive and intermediate hosts, are infective.

Transmission

Human toxoplasmosis may occur in two ways:

Congenital

Foetus is infected in utero through transplacental route. Infection occurring in early months of pregnancy results either in abortion or still birth of foetus. If infection occurs in later months, the foetus is free from any sign of disease which however develops 2 to

3 months after birth. If mother is infected during the puerperium, a breast-fed infant may acquire the infection through mother's milk.

Acquired

Infection may occur in children as well as in adults. The infective forms may enter by the following routes:

(1) By ingestion of undercooked meat (containing pseudocyst), cow's milk and eggs. Major route of infection is by ingestion of oocysts discharged in the faeces of infected cats.

(2) By inhalation (droplet infection): The infective forms are found in the bronchial secretions and sputum. Pneumonitis is a common feature of toxoplasmosis in animals. Infection can also occur when oocysts are inhaled in air or dust contaminated with cat's faeces.

(3) By inoculation (through skin): Contact with infected tissues of animals. Toxoplasma can penetrate through cracks and small abrasions in the skin.

Laboratory contamination, blood transfusion and organ transplantation are other modes of infection in humans. Persons handling the parasite in the laboratory may be infected accidentally.

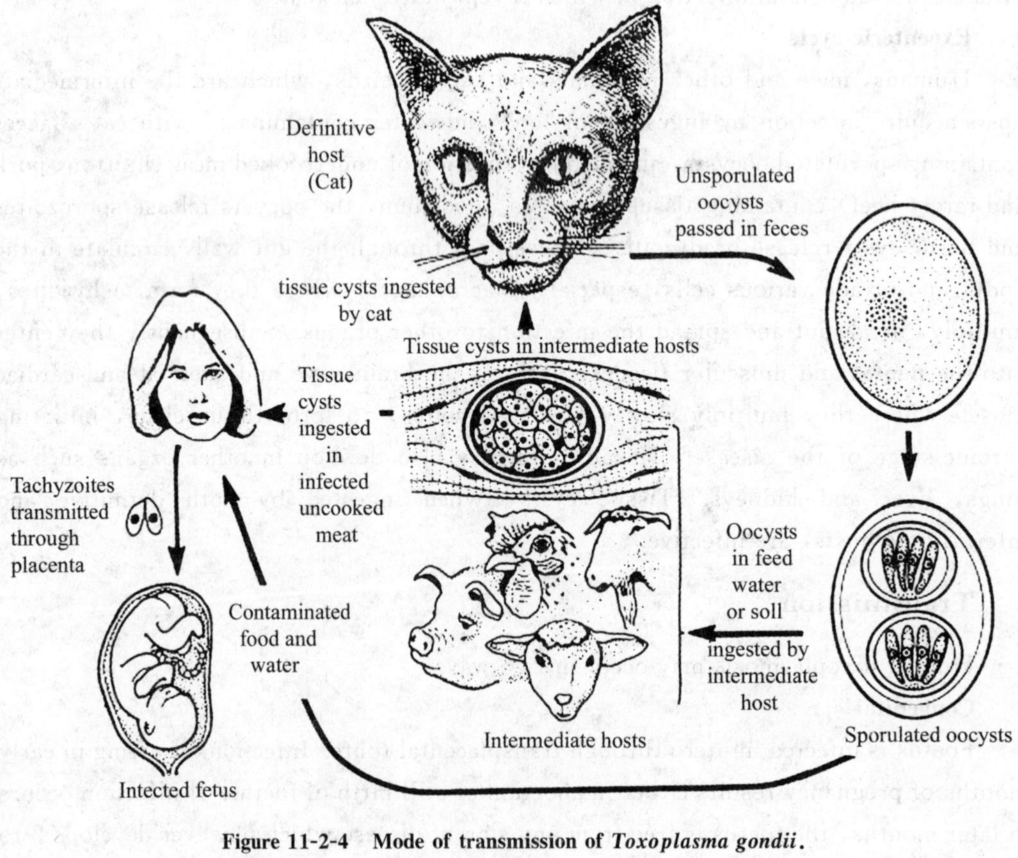

Figure 11-2-4 Mode of transmission of *Toxoplasma gondii*.

Pathogenesis

T. gondii infection is widespread among humans and its prevalence varies from 16% to 80%. Most infections in humans are asymptomatic. However, fulminating fatal infections may develop in patients with AIDS. Infection may be congenital or postnatally acquired.

The pathological lesion is characterized by an area of focal necrosis, surrounded by inflammatory cells (monocytes, plasma cells and lymphocytes). A large number of parasites may be found inside the cell which is enlarged, forming the pseudocysts. Toxoplasmosis has been recognized both as a neonatal infection and as an acquired infection in children and adults. Congenital toxoplasmosis is generally fatal and lesions are widespread, having a special predilection for the developing nervous system of the foetus. Congenital infections are always symptomatic but acquired infections on the other hand are usually asymptomatic, occurring in adults as latent infections.

Congenital infection

Congenital infection develops when mothers are infected during pregnancy. Although the mother rarely has symptoms of infection, she does have a temporary parasitaemia. Focal lesions develop in the placenta and the foetus may become infected. Congenital infection leads to stillbirths, chorioretinitis, intracerebral calcification, psychomotor disturbances, and hydrocephaly or microcephaly. Prenatal toxoplasmosis is a major cause of blindness and other congenital defects. Infection during the first trimester generally results in stillbirth or major central nervous system anomalies. Second and third trimester infections induce less severe neurologic damage, though they are far more common. Clinical manifestations of these infections may be delayed long after birth.

Postnatally acquired infection

Postnatally acquired toxoplasmosis is much less severe than congenitally acquired disease. The commonest manifestation is lymphadenopathy. Although any lymph node may be involved, the most frequently involved are the deep cervical lymph nodes. Lymphadenopathy may be associated with fever, malaise, headache, muscle pain, fatigue and sore throat. The illness is self-limited, though the lymphadenopathy may persist. Rarely there may be pneumonitis, myocarditis and meningoencephalitis, which may be fatal in some cases. Encephalitis is the most important manifestation of toxoplasmosis in immunosuppressed patients. Approximately 10% of AIDS patients in the USA and up to 30% in Europe are estimated to die from toxoplasmosis.

Diagnosis

Laboratory diagnosis

Specimens: Blood (buffy coat of heparinized sample), sputum, bone marrow, cerebrospinal fluid and exudates, lymph node, spleen and brain biopsy material, and ventricular fluid.

Microscopic examination

Smears and sections stained with Giemsa or other special stains, such as periodic acid-Schiff may show the organisms. Tachyzoites of *T. gondii* in the smear are crescent-shaped and in sections round to oval. Tissue cysts are usually spherical and lack septa, and the cyst wall stains with silver stains. The bradyzoites are strongly PAS-positive. The densely packed cysts, chiefly in the brain or other parts of the central nervous system, suggest chronic infection. The immunohistochemical staining of parasites with fluorescent or other types of labelled *T. gondii* antiserum can aid in the diagnosis.

Animal inoculation

T. gondii can be isolated by intraperitoneal inoculation of body fluids or ground tissues into young laboratory mice that are free from infection. If no death occurs, the mice are observed for about six weeks, and tailor heart blood is then tested for specific antibody. The diagnosis is confirmed by demonstration of tissue cysts in the brain of inoculated mice.

Inoculation of tissue culture

T. gondii can also be isolated by inoculation of tissue culture.

Polymerase chain reaction

Toxoplasmal DNA can be detected in the specimens by PCR.

Serology

Numerous serological tests are available for the detection of humoral antibodies. The Sabin-Feldman dye test depends upon the appearance in 2-3 weeks of antibodies that will render the membrane of laboratory-cultured living *T. gondii* impermeable to alkaline methylene blue, so that organisms are unstained in the presence of positive serum. Other tests include indirect haemagglutination assays, indirect fluorescent antibody assays, direct agglutination tests, latex agglutination tests and enzyme-linked immunosorbent assays. Two samples should be collected from the same patient, the second 2-4 weeks after the first. A 16-fold increase in antibody titre indicates an acute infection.

Prevention and Control

Treatment

A combination of pyrimethamine and sulphadiazine is widely used for the treatment of toxoplasmosis. These drugs act synergistically by blocking the metabolic pathway involving P-aminobenzoic acid and the folic-folinic acid cycle respectively. Alternative drugs include spiramycin, clindamycin and trimethoprim-sulphamethoxazole. Prednisolone is given in ocular toxoplasmosis.

Prevention

The measures recommended for prevention of toxoplasmosis include:

- Avoidance of human contact, particularly of pregnant women with negative serologic tests with cat faeces and uncooked meat.
- Proper cooking of meat.
- Hands of the people handing meat, all cutting boards, sink tops, knives and other materials coming in contact with uncooked meat should be washed thoroughly with soap and water.

At present there is no effective subunit or killed vaccine for immunization against *T. gondii*.

(Chen Xiaoguang)

Section 3 *Cryptosporidium*

Cryptosporidium spp. belongs to the family Cryptosporidiidae, which is a member of the phylum Apicomplexa. The exact placement of Crptosporidiidae in Apicomplexa is uncertain. It was long considered a member of the class Coccidea, in the order of Eimeriida or Eucoccidiorida. Recent phylogenetic studies, however, indicate that *Cryptosporidium* spp. is more related to gregarines than to coccidia. Extracellular gregarine-like reproductive stages in *C. andersoni* and *C. parvum* have been described. Thus, *Cryptosporidium* spp. is no longer considered coccidian parasites.

Recently, the taxonomy of Cryptosporidium has gone through revisions as the result of extensive molecular genetic studies and biologic characterizations of parasites from various animals. There are at least 16 established *Cryptosporidium* species in fish, reptiles, birds, and mammals. There are also many host-adapted Cryptosporidium genotypes that do not yet have designated species names, such as Cryptosporidium horse, rabbit, mouse, ferret, deer mouse, skunk, squirrel, bear; deer, deer-like, cervine, fox, mongoose, wildebeest, duck, woodcock, snake, tortoise, goose I and II, muskrat I and II, opossum I and II, marsupial I and II, and pig II genotypes.

To date, eight *Cryptosporidium* spp. have been reported to exist in humans: *C. hominis*, *C. pmrvum*, *C. meleagridis*, *C. felts*, *C. canis*, *C. muris*, *C. suis*, and *Cryptosporidium cawine genotype*. Humans are most frequently infected with *C. hominis* and *C. parvum*. The former almost exclusively infects humans and thus is considered an anthroponotic parasite, whereas the latter infects mostly humans and domestic and wild ruminants and thus is considered a zoonotic pathogen.

Morphology and Life Cycle

The only extracellular stages in *Cryptosporidium* life cycle are oocysts, which are the environmental stage of the parasite, *Cryptospogdium* oocysts in humans generally measure 4 to 6μm (see Figure 11-3-1). Occasionally, *C. muris* oocysts are also found, which are more elongated and measure 6 to 9μm. Oocysts released sporozoites, merozoites, and microgametes, which are briefly in the lumen of the digestive tract. However, recently, a gregarine-like extracellular stage has been described for *C. andersoni* and *C. parvum*, which undergoes multiplication through syzygy, a sexual reproduction process involving the end-to-end fusion of two or more parasites.

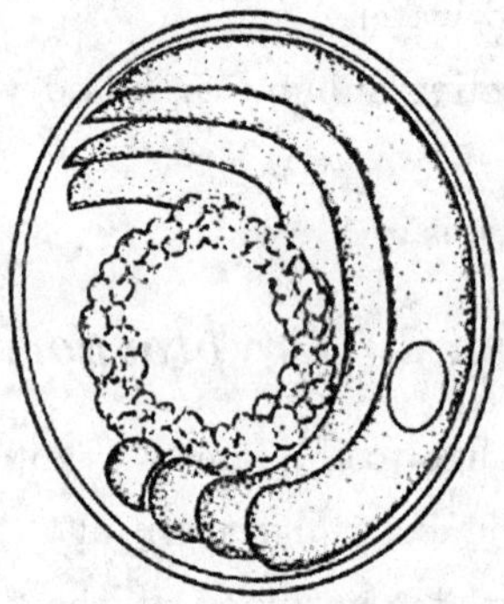

Figure 11-3-1 Oocyst of *Cryptosporidium* spp.

Cryptosporidium infections in humans or other susceptible hosts start with the ingestion of viable oocysts. Upon contact with gastric and duodenal fluid, four sporozoites are liberated from each excysted oocyst, invade the epithelial cells, and develop to trophozoites surrounded by a parasitophorous vacuole. Within the epithelial cells, trophozoites undergo several generations of asexual amplification called merogony, leading to the formation of different types of meronts containing 4 to 8 merozoites. The latter differentiate into sexually distinct stages called macrogamonts and microgamonts (containing microgametes) in a process called gametogony. New oocysts are formed in the epithelial cells from the fusion of macrogamonts and microgametes, sporulate in situ in a process called sporogony, and contain four sporozoites. It is believed by some that about 20% are "thin walled" and may excyst within the digestive tract of the host, leading to the infection of new cells (autoinfection). The remaining 80% of oocysts are excreted into the environment; are resistant to low temperature, high salinity, and most disinfectants; and can initiate infection in a new host without further development upon ingestion. The time from ingestion of infective oocysts to the completion of endogenous development and excretion of new oocysts varies with species, hosts, and infection doses; it is usually between 4 and 14 days (see Figure 11-3-2).

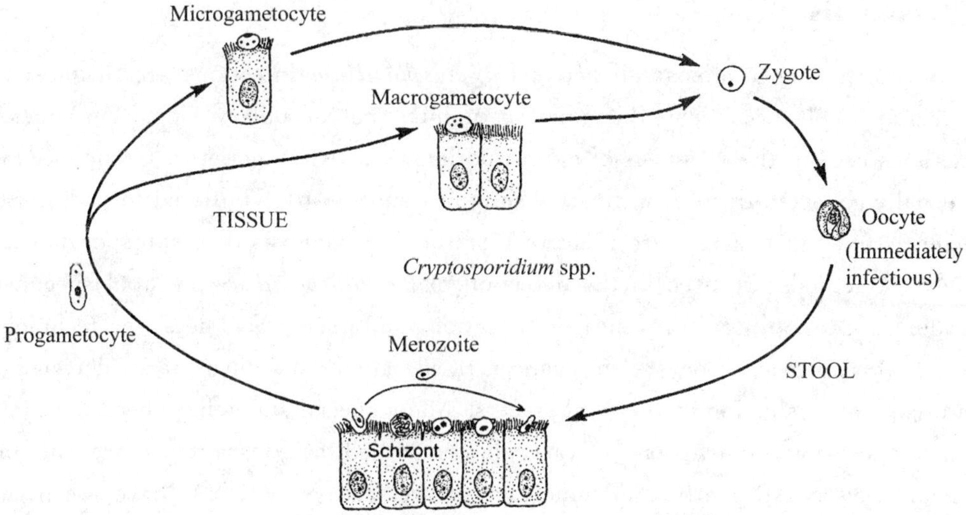

Figure 11-3-2 Life cycle of *Cryptosporidium* spp. (Illustration by Sharon Belkin)

Pathogenesis, Clinical Manifestation and Immunity

Cryptosporidium spp. inhabit the brush borders of the gastrointestinal and respiratory epithelium of various vertebrates, causing enterocolitis and cholangiopathy in humans. The infection site varies according to species, but almost the entire development of *Cyptosporidium* spp. occurs between the two lipoprotein layers of the apical membrane of the epithelial cells, with the exception of *C. molnari* and *C. scophthalmi*, for which oogonial and sporogonial stages are located deeply within the epithelial cells.

Cryptosporidiosis is common in immunocompromised persons, including AIDS patients, persons with primary immunodeficiency, and cancer and transplant patients under going immunosuppressive therapy. In HIV-positive persons, the occurrence of cryptosporidiosis increases as the $CD4^+$ lymphocyte cell counts fall, especially below 200 cells/L. Cryptosporidiosis is considered an AIDS-defining illness and is associated with increased mortality and shortened survival among AIDS patients.

Frequent symptoms include diarrhea, abdominal cramps, vomiting, headache, fatigue, and low grade fever. Immunocompetent children and adults with crptosporidiosis usually have a short-term illness accompanied by watery diarrhea, malabsorption, and weight loss. The diarrhea can be voluminous and watery but usually resolves within 1 to 2 weeks without treatment. In immunosuppressed persons, however, the infection can be protracted and life-threatening.

Children can have multiple episodes of cryptosporidiosis, implying that the anti-Cryptosporidium immunity in children is short-lived or incomplete.

Diagnosis

At the moment, almost all active *Cryptosporidium* infections are diagnosed by analysis of stool specimens. Examination of intestinal or biliary biopsy specimens is sometimes used in the diagnosis of cryptosporidiosis in AIDS patients. Stool specimens are usually collected fresh or in fixative solutions such as 10% buffered formalin. Stool specimens fixed in formalin are preferred for routine diagnosis of cryptosporidiosis. A variety of methods are used in the detection of *Cryptosporidium* in stool specimens, including microscopy, culture, antigen detection, and nucleic acid detection techniques.

Cryptosporidium oocysts in concentrated stool specimens are detected by microscopy after staining of the fecal smears. Many special stains have been used in the detection of *Cryptosporidium* oocysts, but modified acid-fast stains are the most commonly used. Recently, immunofluorescence assays (IFA) have been used increasingly in *Cryptosporidium* oocyst detection by microscopy. Compared to acid-fast staining, IFA has higher sensitivity and specificity.

The in vitro cultivation of *Cryptosporidium* spp. remains inefficient despite recent advances. Thus, the low parasite yields and oocyst production have limited the usefulness of parasite culture in the diagnosis of *Cryptosporidium* infection. The recent development of procedures for long-term maintenance of *C. parvum* and *C. hominis* in cell and cell-free culture could promote the use of in vitro cultivation methods in routine diagnosis of *Cryptosporidium* infection.

Cryptosporidium infection can also be diagnosed by the detection of *Cryptosporidium* antigens in stool specimens by immunoassays. Antigen capture-based enzyme immunoassays (EIA) have gained popularity because they do not require experienced microscopists and can be used to screen a large number of samples.

Molecular techniques, especially PCR and PCR-related methods, have been developed and used in the detection and differentiation of *Cryptosporidium* spp. for many years. Several PCR-restriction fragment length polymorphism based genotyping tools have been developed for the detection and differentiation of *Cryptosporidium* at the species level. Most of these techniques are based on the small subunit rRNA gene.

Epidemiology

Cryptosporidium spp. has a worldwide distribution, and their oocysts are ubiquitously present in the environment. Humans can acquire cryptosporidiosis through several transmission routes, such as direct contact with infected persons or animals and consumption of contaminated water (drinking or recreational) or food. However, the relative role of each in the transmission of *Cryptosporidium* infection in humans is unclear.

Studies have shown that cryptosporidiosis is more common in homosexual man than in persons in other human immunodeficiency virus (HIV) transmission categories, indicating that direct person-to-person or anthroponotic transmission of cryptosporidiosis is common. Contact with persons with diarrhea has been identified as a major risk factor for sporadic cryptosporidiosis in the United States, the United Kingdom, and Australia. This is exemplified by the high prevalence of cryptosporidiosis in day care facilities and nursing homes in developed countries.

In the United States, the United Kingdom, and Australia, contact with farm animals is a major risk factor in sporadic cases of human cryptosporidiosis. Contact with pigs, dogs, or cats is also a risk factor for cryptosporidiosis in children in Guinea-Bissau and Indonesia. Nevertheless, recent subtyping studies based on sequence analyses of the 60-kDa glycoprotein (GP60) gene have shown that not all *C. parvum* infections in humans are results of zoonotic transmission.

Cryptosporidium are well recognized water- and food-borne pathogens, having caused many outbreaks of human diarrheal disease. Epidemiologic studies have frequently identified water as a major route of *Cryptosporidium* transmission in areas where the disease is endemic. In most tropical countries, *Cryptosporidium* infections in children usually peak during the rainy season, and waterborne transmission is considered a major route of cryptosporidiosis in these areas. The role of food in the transmission of cryptosporidiosis is much less clear. Nevertheless, it is estimated that about 10% of *Cryptosporidium* infections in the United States are food-bone.

Prevention and Control

As for any pathogens that are transmitted by the fecal-oral route, good hygiene is the key in preventing tile acquisition of *Cryptosporidium* infection Immunosuppressed persons especially should take necessary precautions in preventing the occurrence of cryptosporidiosis. These include washing hands after going to bathrooms, changing diapers, and contacting pets or soil (including gardening); avoiding drinking water from lakes and rivers, swallowing water in recreational activities, and drinking nonpasteurized milk, milk products, and juices; and following safe-sex practices (avoiding oral- anal contact). During cryptosporidiosis outbreaks or when a community advisory to boil water is issued, individuals should boil water for 1 minute to kill the parasite or use a tap water filter capable of removing particles less than 1μm in diameter. Immnunosuppressed persons also should avoid eating raw shellfish and should not eat uncooked vegetable salads and unpeeled fruits when traveling to areas where cryptosporidiosis is endemic (such as tropical countries).

Numerous pharmaceutical compounds have been screened for anti-*Cryptosporidium* activities in vitro or in laboratory animals. Some of those showing promising results have been used in the experimental treatment of cryptosporidiosis in humans, but few have been shown to be effective in controlled clinical trials. Oral or intravenous rehydration is used whenever severe diarrhea is associated with *Cryptosporidium* infection. Nitazoxanide (NTZ) is the only FDA-approved drug for the treatment of pediatric cryptosporidiosis in USA. The most effective treatment and prophylaxis for cryptosporidiosis in AIDS patients is the use of highly active antiretroviral therapy (HAART). It is believed that the eradication and prevention of the infection are directly related to the replenishment of $CD4^+$ cells in treated persons, rather than anti-parasitic activities of these drugs.

Section 4 *Pneumocystis*

Pneumocystis organisms were first identified in 1909 by Carlos Chagas and named *Pneumocystis carinii* by Delanoë in 1912. The taxonomic problems have plagued the organisms since their original description. In the late 1980s, phylogeneric analyses based on the nuclear small subunit rRNA sequence alignments showed that *P. carinii* was a member of the fungal kingdom. Subsequently, additional gene sequence comparisons and cDNA and genomic sequence data emerging from the *Pneumocystis* Genome Project showed that the closest extant relative to *P. carinii* was the fission yeast *Schizosaccharmyces pombe*. Based on generic and morphologic criteria, *P. carinii* was placed with *S. pombe* in the Phylum Ascomycota within a newly described Class, Archiascomycetes, without designation of an order. In contrast, Erikkson proposed the creation of the Family *Pneumocystidaceae*, Order *Pneumocystidales*, based solely on gene sequence comparisons.

The morphological characteristics of *Pneumocystis* organisms are very similar regardless of the host origin. Until 1976, "*P. carinii*" was thought to represent a single zoonotic species. However, it is now clear that the organism first identified as "*P. carinii*" is actually a family of related organisms that exhibit mammalian host specificity. Almost every mammal examined to date appears to harbor at least one species of *Pneumocystis* that is not found in any other mammal. Four species have been formally described: *P carinii* and *P. wakefieldiae* infect rats; *P. murina* is found in the lungs of mice; and *P. jirovecii* is the name given to the organisms that cause infection in human beings. The name *P. jirovecii* has not been without controversy, and it remains to be seen if this epithet will be retained by the scientific community.

Morphology

Three developmental forms are generally recognized: the trophozoite (trophic stage) 1 to 5μm; the precyst (sporocyte), 5 to 8μm; and the cyst (spore case) about 8μm (see Figure 11-4-1). Pneurnocystis organisms reproduce extracellularly within the mammalian lung alveoli. The trophic forms appear ameboid in structure in electron micrographs, but in freshly prepared specimens, they are ellipsoidal and often occur in dusters with other trophic forms and developmental stages. The nucleus and (often) the mitochondrion are visible in rapid Wright-Giemsa-stained specimens by light microscopy. The trophic forms do not stain with fungal stains designed to complex with the cell wall, such as methenamine silver. The sporocyte is smaller than the mature cyst and frequently oval. This stage contains a rigid cell wall lacking in the trophic forms and is visualized with fungal cell wall stains. At the sporocyte stage, the nuclei are at varying levels of nuclear division (from 2 to 8 nuclei) but have not yet been compartmentalized into separate spore structures. Aggregates of mitochondria can also be seen in this stage. The mature cyst is spherical; contains eight spores, although these may not all be visible; has a thick cell wall that excludes stains such as the rapid Wright-Giemsa stain; and stains with cell wall complexing stains such as methenamine silver. It is considered the diagnostic morphological form.

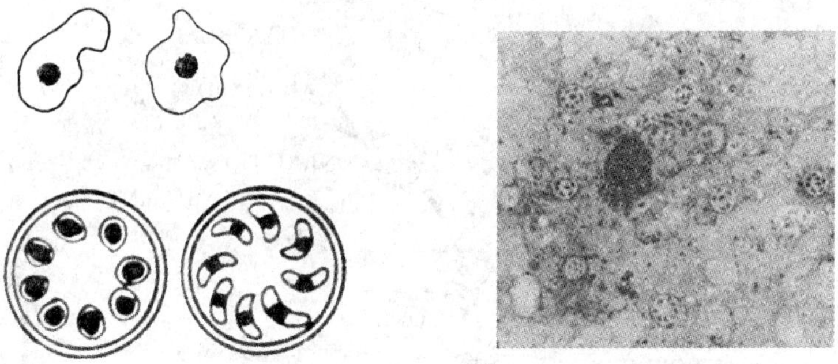

A B

Figure 11-4-1 ***Pneumocystis*** **cyst and trophozoites**

A. Diagram of the cysts and trophozoites. B. Giemsa stain of a smear specimen showing the rounded cysts contain 6-8 intracystic bodies, whose nuclei are stained by Giemsa; the walls of the cysts are not stained.

Putative Life Cycle

Histochemical and ultrastructural studies form the basis of the current understanding of the life cycle of *Pneumocystis*, due to a historic lack of a long-term cultivation method outside the lung. Thus, any life cycle should be considered presumptive until definitive kinetic analyses are able to be performed. There is no evidence for an intracellular phase although the organisms can be frequently observed within macrophages as a result of the host response to the infection.

The portal of entry for *Pneumocystis* organisms has not been firmly established; inhalation is a likely mode of transmission. Trophic forms are presumed to be the vegetative stages of the *Pneumocystis* life cycle and reproduce asexually by binary fission, not budding, as do most yeasts, it is likely that they also participate in the sexual mode of reproduction using a process similar to yeast mating type systems, although these processes are only now beginning to be defined. Several fungal meiosis-specific and mating type gene homologs have been identified in cDNA and genomic *P. carinii* databases, lending credence to the existence of these processes. Subsequent to the mating process and karogamy (nuclear fusion), the zygotic nucleus undergoes meiosis and sporogenesis is initiated, resulting in formation of the precyst, or sporocyte. Following meiosis, an additional mitotic replication occurs, with subsequent compartmentalization of the nuclei and organdies into eight ascospores. The end product of sporogenesis is the spherical cyst, or spore case. The process of spore release has not been described but may involve a localized thickening at one pole of the spore case (cyst). It should be noted that unlike other fungi, all the developmental stages of *Pneumocystis* contain a double membrane (see Figure 11-4-2).

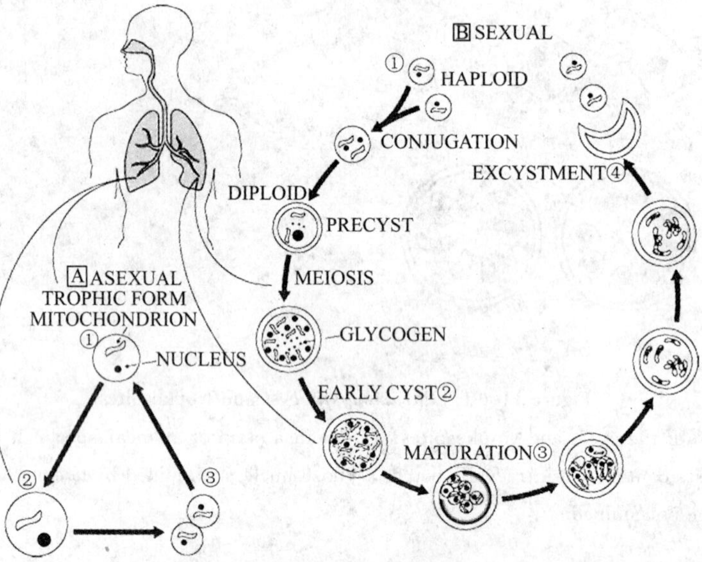

Figure 11-4-2 Life cycle of *Pneumocystis* in lung

A. Asexual phase: trophic forms ①replicate by mitosis ②to ③. B. Sexual phase: haploid trophic forms conjugate ① and produce a zygote or sporocyte (early cyst) ②. The zygote undergoes meiosis and subsequent mitosis to produce eight haploid nuclei (late phase cyst) ③. Spores exhibit different shapes (such as, spherical and elongated forms). It is postulated that elongation of the spores precedes release from the spore case. It is believed that the release occurs through a rent in the cell wall. After release, the empty spore case usually collapses, but retains some residual cytoplasm ④. A trophic stage, where the organisms probably multiply by binary fission is also recognized to exist. (This is a generalized life cycle proposed by John J. Ruffolo, Ph. D. (Cushion, MT, 1988) for the various species of *Pneumocystis*.

Pathogenesis and Clinical Manifestation

The organism is low virulence that seldom produces disease in a host with normal T-lymphocyte function. In susceptible (immunocompromised) hosts, the organism occurs in massive numbers and resulted in pneumocystis pneumonia (PCP). PCP remains the leading opportunistic infection associated with AIDS patients, even in the era of highly active antiretroviral therapy(HAART). Within the mammalian lung, the trophic forms of *Pneumocystis* adhere to the type I pneumocytes presumably through macromolecular bridges. Type I cells are responsible for the gas exchange between the alveolar capillaries and the alveolar lumen. Besides attachment to the type I cells, the various developmental stages of the parasite adhere to one another, producing large clusters that extend outwardly into the alveolar lumen. In severe, untreated infections, most of the alveoli are filled with organisms. Direct attachment to the cells responsible for gas exchange combined with the accumulation of organisms within the alveoli results in impaired gas exchange and altered lung compliance, as well as other physiologic changes associated with the pneumonia, such as hypoxia.

Histopathologic findings can be characterized by two traits: (1) alveolar interstitial thickening and (2) a frothy eosinophilic honeycomb-like exudate in the lumina of the lung. The interstitial thickening is a result of hyperplasia and hypertrophy of the type II pneumocyte, interstitial edema, mononuclear cell infiltration, and in some cases mild fibrosis.

PCP in children can be associated with cyanosis, flaring of the nasal alae, a mild cough without fever, and retractions of intercostals in severe disease. Of note, whereas adults with $CD4^+$ cell counts of less than 200 per microliter are at increased risk for PCP, children less than a year old who developed the pneumonia had $CD4^+$ counts greater than 1,000 per microliter. Adults with PCP frequently present with dyspnea, nonproductive cough, inability to breathe deeply, chest tightness, and night sweats. A low-grade fever (e. g. 38.5°C) and tachypnea are often present, while hemoptysis or sputum production is rare. Upon physical examination, few pronounced abnormalities are detected, but various degrees of respiratory distress, small respiratory volumes, and fine basilar rales can be observed. Patients with AIDS often have amore insidious progression to clinical disease than do those not infected with HIV but who are immunosuppressed.

The incidence of *Pneumocystis* organisms in sites other than the lung has been reported in 1% to 3% of postmortem examinations of patients with pulmonary *P. jirovecii* infections. This is likely an underestunate due to the limited number of autopsies performed and the lack of suspicion of extrapulmonary pneumocystosis. *P. jirovecii* has been detected in the adrenal glands, gastrointestinal tract, genitourinaty tract, thyroid, ear, liver, pancreas, eyes, skin, and other sites. The extrapulmonary clinical manifestations range from incidental autopsy findings to progressive multisystem disease. Infection of multiple extrapulmonary sites was associated with a rapidly fatal outcome. Pathological findings correlated with the organ where the infection was present.

Immunity

The nature of the immunodeficiencies in patients with pneumocystosis points to the primacy of cell-mediated immunity in resolution of infection with Pneumocystis. Alveolar macrophages are the first line of defense, with activated macrophages and $CD4^+$ lymphocytes playing essential roles in the resolution of the infection. Activated macrophages release several cytotoxic factors, including O_2-derived radicals, reactive nitrogen intermediates, and cytokines (tumor necrosis factor-α, interleukin-2). Specific antibody responses to the special antigens appear in the course of pneumocystosis. A significant role for humoral immunity is suggested by the ability of MSG antibody to protect against experimental PCP in animals.

Laboratory Diagnosis

The definite diagnosis of PCP relies on finding organisms of typical morphology in pulmonary tissue or lower airway fluids. The organism can be detected in a variety of respiratory specimens including induced sputum, bronchoalveolar lavage fluid (BALF), tracheal aspirate fluid, tissue obtained by transbronchial biopsy, cellular material obtained by bronchial brush, pleural fluid, and tissue obtained by open thorax lung biopsy. The diagnostic yield is dependent upon the underlying disease state of the patient and the expertise of the staff obtaining the sample. For infants and young children who are unable to produce sputum or for whom this method is not warranted, tracheal aspirate fluid, open-thorax lung biopsy, or respiratory specimens must be obtained by a special pediatric bronchoscopy service.

The diagnosis of extrapulmonary pneumocystosis relies on accurate sampling of the infected organ and subsequent staining of the histological sections.

A variety of slams have been used for the identificatkm of *P. jirovecii* organisms. One of the most common stains used by pathologists for tissue sections, hematoxylin and eosin, does not stain the organism but rather the foamy exudates within the lung alveoli, often described as "honeycombed" in appearance.

A common staining procedure used for the diagnosis of PCP is methenamine silver. Silver-stained cysts have a distinctive, black, cup-shaped morphology against green-colored host cell architecture. In some staining reactions, cyst wall thickenings appear as a "double comma" morphology. More often the folds in the wall stain a dark brown to black to produce a crinkled, raisin-like appearance. Intracystic daughter forms cannot be seen with this stain, and cysts that are empty (nonviable) appear the same as those with the full contingent of eight spores. Other stains that complex with components of the cyst wall include periodic acid-Schiff; toluidine blue, cresyl echt violet, and calcofluor white.

In contrast to the cyst wall stains, Giemsa and rapid Giemsa-like stains do not stare the cyst wall but instead stain the nuclei of all the various life cycle stages a reddish purple and stain the cytoplasm a light blue. The cyst wall excludes the dyes and appears with a circumscribed clear zone surrounding the reddish purple nuclei of the daughter forms within. Originally used for quantitation of rat *P. carinii* organisms, the rapid variants of the Giemsa stain are recommended for the diagnosis of PCP by using BALE induced sputum, or impression imprints because of the low cost, ease, and rapidity of the staining procedure.

Direct and indirect fiuorescein-conjugated monoclonal anti-*P. jirovecii* antibodies used for immunofiuorescent assay are targeted to a family of surface glycoproteins that contain both common and distinct epitopes, within and among Pneumocystis species.

Serologic studies for antibodies and antigen are not helpful in establishing a specific diagnosis.

Amplification of *P. jirovecii* DNA is not yet used routinely for the diagnosis of PCP in the clinical laboratory setting.

Epidemiology

Pneumocystis pneumonia (PCP) has historically been one of the leading causes of disease among persons with AIDS. The introduction of highly active antiretroviral therapy in industrialized nations has brought about dramatic declines in the incidence of AIDS-associated complications, including PCP. In the adult population, the incidence of PCP has significantly decreased, but it remains among the most common AIDS-defining infections. Similar declines have been documented in the pediatric population.

In much of the developing world, PCP remains a significant health problem, although its incidence among adults in sub-Saharan Africa has been debated. Although fewer cases of PCP occur in industrialized countries, increasing drugresistant HIV infections, possible drug-resistant PCP, and the tremendous number of AIDS cases in developing countries make this disease of continued public health importance.

Pneumocystis infection was likely transmitted by an airborne route. *Pneumocystis*-free rats could acquire the infection from infected rats housed in the same room or from infected cage mates. Transmission through water, food, or ingestion of infected lungs was not observed in the same experimental studies. Although Pneumocystis DNA could be detected in air samples from patient rooms and from an orchard after extensive sampling, no laboratory has been able to identify the agent of transmission.

Prevention and Control

Two drugs constitute the mainstay of therapy for acute PCP, trimethoprim-sulfamethoxazole (TMP-SMX) and pentamidine isethionate. TMP-SMX is preferred because of its low toxicity and greater efficacy, and is the treatment of choice for all forms of pneumocystosis. Unfortunately, AIDS patients have a high incidence of adverse effects to TMP-SMX, particularly the sulfonamide component. This requires the use of other antimicrobics (e. g. clindamycin, primaquine, dapsone) alone or in combination with TMP. Secondary treatments such as atovaquone and clindamycin-primaquine have been used for milder forms of the disease, and treatment with corticosteroids has been used to improve the clinical outcome for some patients. The disease can be prevented by prophylactic administration of trimethoprim-sulfamethoxazole, aerosolized pentamidine or dapsone.

Section 5 Other Sporozoa

Sarcocystis

There are numerous species of *Sarcocystis* in the literature with most of them being named with respect to the host in which they are found. Two well-described species are *Sarcocystis bovihominis* (cattle) and *S. suihominis* (pigs). Some publications refer to *S. bovihominis* as *S. hominis*. The organism first observed in man by Lindemann in 1868. It has been authentic that humans may become infected by 3 species: *S. lindemanni*, which cause muscular sarcosporidiosis; *S. suihominis* and *S. hominis*, which cause intestinal sarcosporidiosis.

Morphology and Life Cycle

Sarcocystis is found in many animals. The organism in man differs morphologically from the species in animals. The sporocysts 13-19 by 8-19μm, containing 4 sporozoites (see Figure 11-5-1). The tubes or sarcocysts are columniform or spindly, 1-5cm in length by 0. 1-1cm in wide.

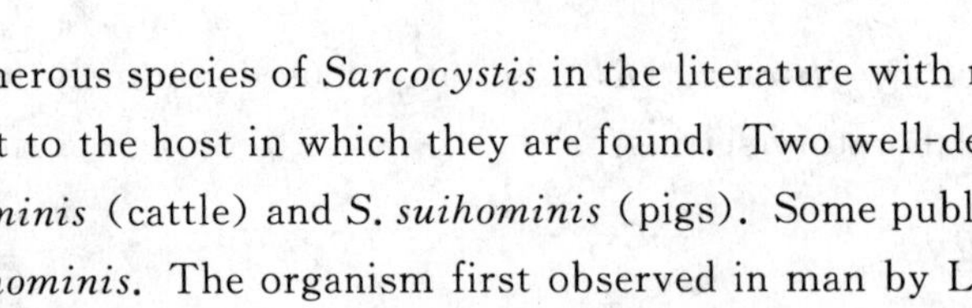

Figure 11-5-1 *Sarcocystis* spp. : A. Sporulated oocyst; B. sporacyst; C. Sarcocyst

The life cycle of *S. hommis* is heteroxenous (see Figure 11-5-2). Humans are definitive hosts for *S. hommis*, and *bovids* are the intermediate hosts, infection occurs when infected meat which is not cooked or is not thoroughly cooked is ingested. Known intermediate hosts include cattle, American bison, water buffalo, and European bison or Wisent. These intermediate hosts harbor sarcocysts (muscle cysts) that are infective when ingested by humans. Infective bradyzoites (dormant merozoite-like stages) are present in the sarcocysts. The bradyzoites penetrate the human intestinal epithelium and develop as sexual stages (macrogametocytes and microgametocytes) in cells in the lamina propria of the intestine. Fertilization occurs and the oocysts sporulate in the lamina propria. The oocysts are "Isospora" like and contain two sporocysts each with four sporozoites. The oocyst wall often ruptures as the oocyst makes its way to the intestinal lumen. This results in the shedding of individual sporocysts in the feces. Both oocysts with two sporocysts and individual sporocysts can be seen in the feces of humans with intestinal *Sarcocystis* infection.

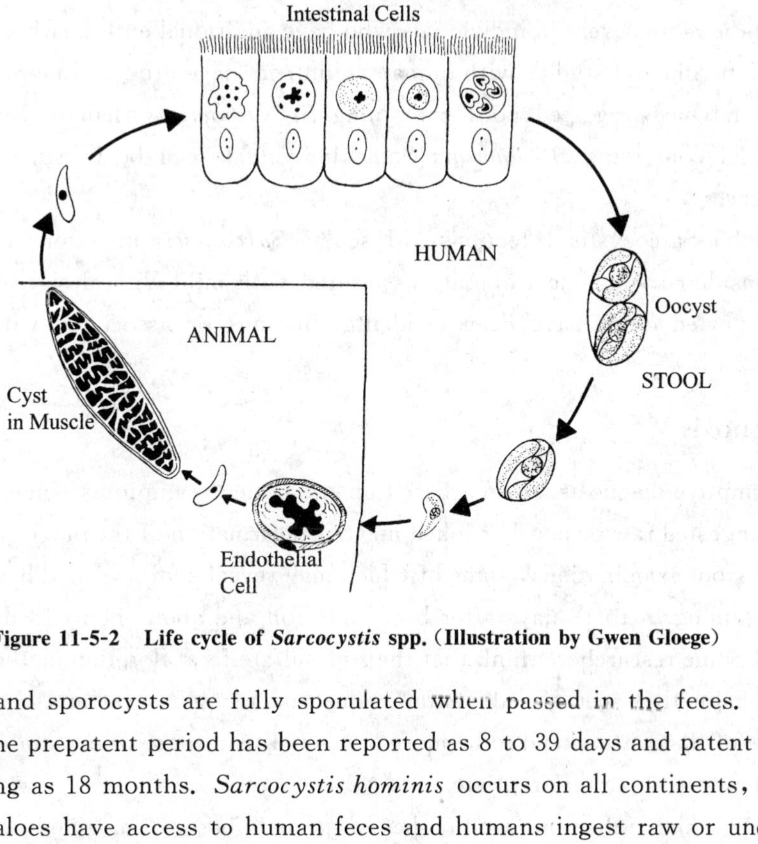

Figure 11-5-2 Life cycle of *Sarcocystis* spp. (Illustration by Gwen Gloege)

Oocysts and sporocysts are fully sporulated when passed in the feces. In human volunteers, the prepatent period has been reported as 8 to 39 days and patent infections can last as long as 18 months. *Sarcocystis hominis* occurs on all continents, anywhere cattle or buffaloes have access to human feces and humans ingest raw or undercooked beef.

The life cycle of *S. suihominis* is similar to that described above for *S. hominis* except that pigs are the intermediate hosts. The prepatent period is 9 to 10 days, and patency is in excess of 36 days. *S. suihominis* presumably occurs on all continents, anywhere swines have access to human feces and humans ingest raw or undercooked pork.

Human Muscular *Sarcocystis* Infection: Sarcocysts have been reported as incidental findings from both skeletal and cardiac muscle of nearly 60 humans worldwide. Where are at least seven distinct types of sarcocysts present in human muscles. Many of these sarcocysts appeared to be similar to sarcocysts found in nonhuman primates. Humans seem to be an occasional incidental intermediate host for some *Sarcocystis* spp. in wildlife.

Pathogenesis and Clinical Manifestation

Intestinal *Sarcocystis* Infections: Clinical *Sarcocystis* infections in humans can manifest primarily as intestinal disease if infected meat is ingested or as muscular disease if sporocysts are ingested. Intestinal disease occurs soon after consumption of infected meat (3 to 6h) and is characterized by nausea, abdominal pain, and diarrhea, Intestinal disease can be more severe in individuals who have additional enteropathogens present in the gut. Experimental studies with human volunteers have produced more severe disease in those who have ingested pork containing *S. suihominis* than in those who have ingested beef containing *S. hominis* Some individuals can be infected and show no clinical signs.

Muscular Sarcocystis Infections: Muscular *Sarcocystis* infections in humans are usually considered subclinical or only associated with mild clinical signs. Many of the over 50 reported cases have been incidental findings or associated with eosinophilic myostitis.

Diagnosis

Presumptive diagnosis is often based on the patient symptoms, including a history of having ingested raw or poorly cooked meat. Confirmation of the diagnosis may depend on several stool examinations, some of which may reveal sporocysts. They are generally passed beginning 14 to 18 days after beef ingestion and about 11 to 13 days after pork ingestion. Some researchers think that the zinc sulfate fecal flotation method is preferred to the formalinethyl acetate sedimentation method for sporocyst and oocyst recovery. Sporocysts of *S. hominis* tend to be more elongated than those of *S. suihominis*, but the two may be difficult to differentiate.

Intramuscular infection would be suspected based on symptoms, including persistent myalgia, episodic weakness, subcutaneous nodules, dermatomyositis, eosinophilia, and elevated muscle creatinine kinase levels. Often these symptoms, coupled with a history of travel to or living in tropical locations, suggest the next step, which would be a muscle biopsy. Sarcocysts in biopsy specimens can be identified by microscopy of routine histologic sections stained with hematoxylin and eosin. Stain variability is common, and PAS positivity of rile sarcocyst wall is not always seen.

Sarcocystis can be detected in meat by using routine histologic methods. Most sarcocysts in humans have been identified in skeletal and cardiac muscle; however, muscles in the larynx, pharynx, and upper esophagus have also been involved. Artificial digestion fluids can also be used on the meat source; after centrifugation, the sediment can be examined microscopically for the presence of bradyzoites.

Epidemiology

Human intestinal *Sarcocystis* species is potentially present in any region in the world where cattle, buffaloes, and swines have access to human feces and the life cycle can be maintained. Cultural habits that include ingestion of raw meat or undercooked meat products help maintain this life cycle in areas of endemicity. Cooking meat until an internal temperature above 67℃ is achieved kills *T. gondii* tissue cysts, and this temperature should also kill tissue cysts of human infective *Sarcocystis* species in meat products. Preventing cattle, buffaloes, and swine from consuming human feces will also break the cycle in areas of endemicity.

Most cases of human muscular *Sarcocystis* infection have been reported from the Far East. It is presumed that humans become infected by ingesting sporocysts in contaminated water or food.

Prevention and Control

There is no known treatment or prophylaxis for intestinal infection, myositis, vasculitis, or related lesions in humans due to sarcocystosis. Given the efficacy of trimethoprim-sulfamethoxazole against other coccidian infections and its activity in vitro against *Sacocystis neurona*, it is reasonable to assume that this drug may have some efficacy in *Sarcocystis* infection. There is a case report of albendazole having efficacy in an outbreak of eosinophilic myositis due to *Sarrocystis* spp.

Isospora belli

Isospora belli is a coccidian parasite of the intestinal epithelium. Both sexual and asexual reproduction can occur in the intestinal epithelium, resulting in tissue damage.

Morphology and Life Cycle

The life cycle stages, i. e., schizonts, merozoites, gametocytes, gametes, and oocysts, are structurally similar to those species in the other coccidia.

Size of oocyst: 20-23μm by 10-19μm. The oocyst contains two sporocysts, and this is typical of the genus *Isospora* (see Figure 11-5-3). Immature oocysts containing one sporocyst are released in the feces into the external environment. Under ideal environmental conditions, the oocyst matures and develops two sporozoites that serve as the infective form. On ingestion of infective oocysts in contaminated food or water by a human host, excystation takes place in the intestine. The released sporocysts invade the mucosal epithelial cells in which schizogony takes place. Mature sporozoites are released from the intestinal cells. In the process of gametogenesis male and female gametocytes are formed. After fertilization of the female gametocyte by sperm released from the sporozoite, an oocyst with a thick cell wall develops. Release of these immature oocysts into the external environment completes the life cycle (see Figure 11-5-4).

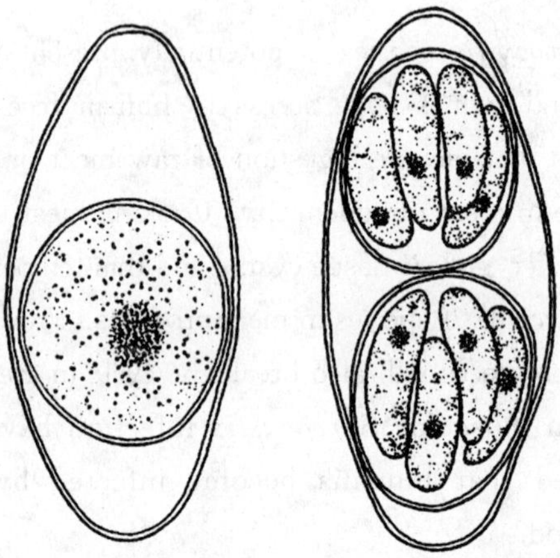

Figure 11-5-3 Unsporulated and spulated oocysts of *Isospora belli*

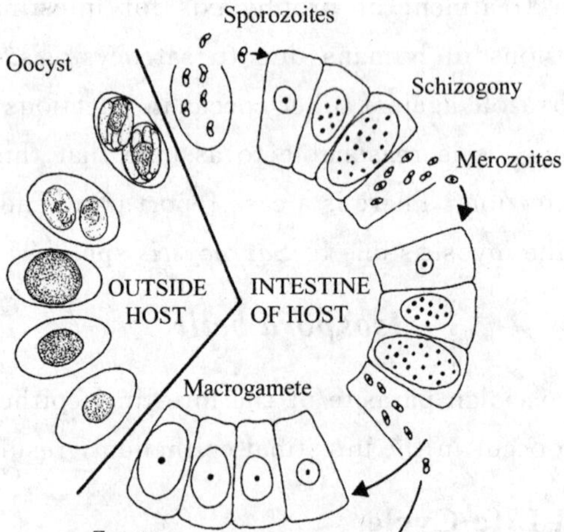

Figure 11-5-4 Life cycle of *Isospora belli* (Illustration by Gwen Gloege)

Pathogenesis and Clinical Manifestation

I. belli can cause serious and sometimes fatal disease in immunocompetent humans. Symptoms of *I. belli* refection include diarrhea, steatorrhea, headache, fever, malaise, abdominal pain, vomiting, dehydration, and weight loss. Blood is not usually present in the feces. Eosinophilia is observed in many patients. The disease is often chronic, with parasites present in the feces or biopsy specimens for several months to years. Recurrences are common. Disease is more severe in infants and young children. Clinical disease in *I. belli* infections is usually more severe in immunocompromised patients than in immunocompetent patients. Diarrhea produced by *I. belli* infection in AIDS patients is often very fluid and secretory-like and leads to dehydration requiring hospitalization. Fever and weight loss are also common findings. Other opportunistic pathogens are also common copathogens in these patients. *I. belli* induced intestinal lesions and responses to chemotherapy are usually similar to those observed in immunocompetent patients. *I. belli* has been observed in patients with concurrent Hodgkin's disease, non-Hodgkin's lymphoproliferative disease, human T. cell leukemia virus type I-associated adult T-cell leukemia, and acute lymphoblastic leukemia. These patients respond to specific anti-*I. belli* treatment. It was suggested in one report that treatment with prednisolone led to transient immunosuppression and severe *I. belli* infection in one patient. The patient recovered without specific treatment.

Infections with *I. belli* in the gallbladder epithelium and endometrial epithelium have been reported. Clinical signs in patients with parasites in these locations are not specific for coccidiosis, and parasites are located after tissue biopsy as part of a diagnostic workup.

Diagnosis

Examination of a fecal specimen for the oocysts is recommended. However, wet preparation examination of fresh material either as the direct smear or as concentrated material is recommended rather than the permanent stained smear. The oocysts are very pale and transparent and can easily be overlooked. They can also be very difficult to see if the concentration sediment is from polyvinyl alcohol-preserved stool. The light level should be reduced, and additional contrast should be obtained with the microscope for optimal examination conditions. It is also quite possible to have a positive biopsy specimen but not recover the oocysts in the stool because of the small numbers of organisms present. These organisms are acid fast and can also be demonstrated by using auramine-rhodamine stains. Organisms tentatively identified by using auramine-rhodamine stains should be confirmed by wet smear examination or acid-fast stains, particularly if the stool contains other cells or excess artifact material (more normal stool consistency).

Detection of *I. belli* by PCR using primers based on small-subunit ribosomal RNA sequences and Southern blot hybridization has been reported (61). This method was effective for detecting *I. belli* DNA in duodenal biopsies and in stool samples. A slight cross reactivity to *T. gondii* was observed in a nested-PCR version of this test.

Epidemiology

I. belli is primarily found in tropical, subtropical, and warm temperate regions, but reports of indigenous infections from temperate areas have also been published. Most cases of infection in temperate areas involve foreign travel or homosexual contact. Large outbreaks of isosporiasis have nor been reported. Recently, however, this parasite has been reported with increasing frequency in healthy and immunocompromised patients.

Transmission is via ingestion of sporulated oocysts and possibly the ingestion of raw or under-cooked tissues from unknown paratenic hosts.

Prevention and Control

Effective eradication of the parasites has been achieved with co-trimoxazole, TMP-SMX, pyrimethamine-sulfa-dlazine, primaquine phosphate-nitrofurantoin, and primaquine phosphate-chloroquine phosphate. Other drugs proven to be ineffective include dithiazanine, tetracycline, metronidazole, phanquone, and quinacrine hydrochloride. The drug of choice is TMP-SMX, which is classified as an investigational drug for treatment of this infection. TMP (160mg)-SMX (800mg) is given every 6h for 10 days and then twice a day for 3 weeks. Pyrimethamine alone (50 to 75mg daily) has cured infections in patients allergic to sulfonamides. In immunosuppressed patients with recurrent or persistent infection, therapy must be continued indefinitely.

Improved personal hygiene measures and sanitary conditions will eliminate possible fecal-oral transmission from contaminated food, water, and possibly environmental surfaces.

Microsporidia

Microsporidia are true eukaryotes because they have a membrane-bound nucleus, an intracytoplasmic membrane system, and chromosome separation on mitotic spindles, but they are unusual eukaryotes in that they have bacterium-like ribosomes, no recognizable mitochondria, no peroxisomes, and simple vesicular Golgi membranes. The small-subunit (SSU) rRNA genes of microsporidia, for example, are significantly shorter than those of other eukaryotes and even those of some prokaryotes. Also, structural features of the organisms such as the presence of chitin in the spore wall, diplokaryotic nuclei, and electron-dense spindle plaques associated with the nuclear envelope suggest a possible relationship between fungi and *Microsporidia*.

More than 150 microsporidial genera and 1,200 species that are parasitic in every major animal group have been identified. To date, seven genera (Enterocytozoon, Encephalitozoon, Nosema, Pleistophora, Vittaforma, Trachipleistopora, and Brachiola) and unclassified microsporidia, assigned to the collective group *Microsporidium*, have been implicated in human infections.

Interest in the microsporidia has grown tremendously with the recognition of new species that cause opportunistic infections in AIDS patients.

Morphology and Life Cycle

Microsporidia are small single-celled, obligate intracellular parasites. The mature and infectious spores of the microsporidia species that infect mammals are relatively small, measuring 1.0-3.0μm by 1.5-4.0μm, and usually round, oblong, ovate or rod-shaped (see Figure 11-5-5). The spores are surrounded by an outer electron-dense glycoprotein layer and an electron-lucent endospore layer composed primarily of chitin. A plasma membrane encloses the cytoplasm, which contains an anterior anchoring disc, Golgi-like apparatus, nucleus, posterior vacuole, and polar filament that originates at the anterior end and coils in the posterior region of the spore.

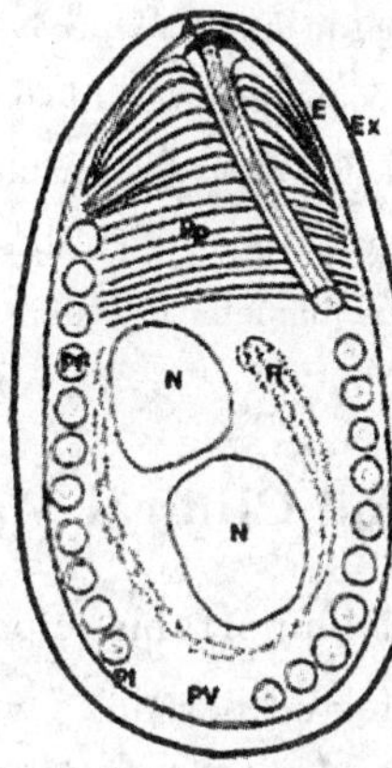

Figure 11-5-5 A diagram of a microsporidian spore in cross section

Microsporidia develop intracellularly exclusively, and have no metabolically active stages outside tile host cell. A life cycle (see Figure 11-5-6) involving a proliferative merogonic sequence followed by a sporogonic sequence results in environmentally resistant spores of unique structure. The polar filament distinguishes the *microsporidia* from other single-celled organisms and is used for infecting the host cell. A change in osmotic pressure or pH results in swelling of the posterior vacuole due to an influx of water, or possibly, the generation of water, and the ensuing pressure leads to the propulsion of the nucleus and cytoplasmic contents through the everting polar filament into the host cell. Organisms then undergo merogony, during which nuclear division occurs, followed by sporogony, during which differentiation and maturation occur. Cytokinesis occurs after either merogony (e. g. *Encephalitozoon* species) or sporogony (e. g. *Enterocytozoon bieneusi*).

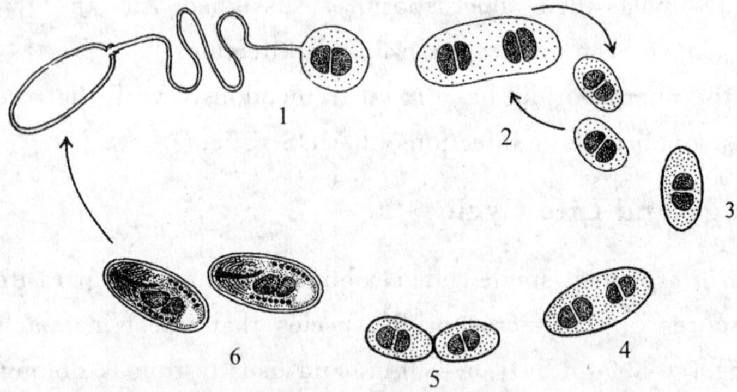

Figure 11-5-6 Basic life cycle illustrated by Nosema

1. Sporoplasm: the infective stage emergent from the spore, it may have unpaired nuclei (monokaryotic) or two nuclei in close apposition (diplokaoyotic), depending on the genus. 2. Merogony: proliferative stage. It may have a simple plasma membrane, but a surface coat is present in *Brachiola*, *Pleistophora*, and *Trachipleistophoya*. Division can be by binary or multiple fission into two or more individuals. 3. Sporont: the first stage of sporogony. If not already present, a surface coat is added (this step is delayed in *Enterocytozoon*). 4. Sporogony: divisions culminating in spore production. Binary or multiple fissions give rise to sporoblasts. 5. Sporoblasts: end products of sporogony, which mature into spores. 6. Spores: resistant stages for transmission. Spores are characterized by an extrusion apparatus (polar tube), which serves to conduct the sporoplasm into a host cell. The polar tube may be of uniform diameter (isofilar) or show a sharp decrease in diameter in the most posterior coils (anisofilar).

Pathogenesis, Immunity and Clinical Manifestation

Microsporidia are predominantly opportunistic pathogens capable of causing disease in severely immunodeficient HIV-infected persons (with CD4 cell counts below 200/μl) and otherwise immunocompromised patients including organ transplant recipients and patients with idiopathic or other CD4 T lymphocytopenia, as well as in immunocompetent individuals. Microsporidiosis has been associated with abnormalities in structures and functions of infected organs, but the mechanisms of pathogenicity of the different microsporidial species are not sufficiently understood. Patients with severe cellular immunodeficiency appear to be at the highest risk for developing microsporidial disease. Unfortunately, little is known about immunity to this infection, although the importance of T cells has been demonstrated in experiments with athymic mice. It is not understood whether microsporidiosis in immunocompromised patients is primarily a reactivation of latent infection acquired prior to the state of suppressed immunity or whether microsporidial disease is caused by recently acquired infection.

Clinical symptoms and disease associated with microsporidiosis vary with the species causing the infection and the status of the host's immune system. *E. bieneusi* infects the enterocytes of the small intestine and epithelial cells of the biliary tree and respiratory tract. Clinical disease is probably caused by the continuous excess loss of epithelial cells. Enterocytozoon infection may be accompanied by alterations in small bowel physiology such as decreased brush border sucrase, lactase, and maltase activities, as well as malabsorption. *E. bieneusi* is estimated to be one of the most important HIV-associated intestinal pathogens, present in 5% to 30% of patients with chronic diarrhea, weight loss, or cholangiopathy, particularly when CD4 lymphocyte counts are low. Upper or lower respiratory tract infections have been detected in a few patients, but systemic infection due to *E. bieneusi* has not been documented. Case reports have documented that the parasite is also a cause of diarrhea in organ transplant recipients.

In immunocompetent adults and in children, *E. bieneus* is associated with self-limited watery diarrhea (lasting up to 2 to 3 weeks), particularly among persons who reside or have traveled in tropical countries. Furthermore, the parasite has been identified among elderly persons with acute or chronic diarrhea.

Encephalitozoon spp. infect epithelial and endothelial cells, fibroblasts, macrophages, and possibly other cell types, as reported for humans and mammals. Encephalitozoon (identifled as *E. cuniculi* because this was the only species known at that time) was initially identified in two children with a seizure disorder. The spectrum of recognized *E. cuniculi*- and *E. hellem*-associated disease in patients with AIDS, organ transplant recipients, and otherwise immunocompromised patients includes keratoconjunctivitis, intraocular infection, sinusitis, bronchiolitis, pneumonitis, nephritis, ureteritis, cystitis, prostatitis, urethritis, hepatitis, sclerosing cholangitis, peritonitis, diarrhea, and encephaliti. Clinical manifestations may vary substantially, ranging from an asymptomatic carrier state to organ failure.

E. intestinalis infects primarily enterocytes, but the parasite is also found in intestinal lamina propria, and dissemination to the kidneys, airways, and biliary tract appears to occur via infected macrophages. Chronic diarrhea and disseminated disease due to *E. intestinalis* have been diagnosed mainly in immunodeficient patients. A case of nodular cutaneous *E. intestinalis* infection was observed in a patient with AIDS. Furthermore, *E. intestinalis* has been detected in stool specimens from otherwise healthy children and adults, with or without diarrhea, living in Mexico and among travelers with diarrhea returning from tropical countries.

Other *Microsporidia* infective: Different microsporidial species have been isolated from otherwise healthy persons who presented with keratoconjunctivitis, severe keratitis, or corneal ulcers. Also, kera-toconjunctivitis due to microsporidia has been diagnosed ill an immunocompetent contact lens wearer.

In immunocompromised patients, myositis has been linked to infections with different rnicrosporidia, including *Pleistophora* spp., *P. ronneafiei* spp. nov., *T. hominis*, *B. vesicularum*, and *B. algerae*. *B. algerae* has also been isolated from erythematous skin nodules from a boy with acute lymphocytic leukemia.

T. anthropophthera has been identified at autopsy in cerebral, cardiac, renal, pancreatic, thyroid, hepatic, splenic, lymphoid, and bone marrow tissue of patients with AIDS who initially presented with seizures. Disseminated infection due to *B. connori* was found at autopsy in a 4-month-old athymic male infant.

Diagnosis

Specimens

Spores of enteropathogenic microsporidia can be detected in stool specimens or duodenal aspirates that have been fixed in 10% formalin or ill sodium acetate; acetic acid-formalin, fresh stool samples, or biopsy specimens. The spores of microsporidia causing disseminated infection can usually be detected in fresh or fixed urine sediments, other body fluids (including sputum, bronchoalveolar lavage fluid, nasal secretions, cerebrospinal fluid, and conjunctival smears), corneal scrapings, or tissue. For histological examination, tissue specimens are fixed in formalin. For electron microscopy, fixation of tissue with glutaraldehyde is preferred. Collection of fresh material (without fixative) may be useful for cell culture and for molecular identification. Microsporidial spores are environmentally resistant and, if prevented from drying, can remain infectious for periods of up to several years.

Detection procedures

The most robust technique for the diagnosis of microsporidial infection is light microscopic detection of the parasites themselves. Spores, the stages at which microsporidia pathogenic in humans are usually identified, are small, ranging in size from 1 to 4μm. Evaluation of patients with suspected intestinal microsporidiosis should begin with light microscopic examination of stool specimens, and microsporidia which cause systemic refection are best detected in urine sediments or other body fluids. Definitive species identification of microsporidia is made by electron microscopy, antigenic analysis, or, preferably, molecular analysis.

For stool specimens, smears are prepared using 10 to 20μl of unconcentrated stool that is very thinly spread onto slides. The most commonly used stains are chromotrope-based stains and chemofluorescent optical brightening agents, including calcofiuor white M2R, the Fungi-Fluor kit, Fungiqual A, Cellufluor, Uvitex 2B, and other chemofluorescent stains. Regardless of which staining technique is used, the use of positive control material is essential.

Microsporidial spores are ovoid and have a specific appearance when stained with chromotrope stains. The spore wall stains bright pinkish red, some spores appear transparent, and other spores show a distinct pinkish red-stained belt-like stripe that girds the spores diagonally or equatorially. Most background debris in stool specimens counterstains a faint green (or blue, depending the staining technique). Some other fecal elements, such as yeasts and some bacteria, may also stain reddish, but they are distinguished from microsporidial spores by their sizes, shapes, and staining patterns.

Epidemiology

Human rnicrosporidial infections have been documented globally. The sources of *microsporidia* infecting humans and their modes of transmission are uncertain. Ingestion of the environmentally highly resistant spores is probably the normal mode of transmission. Possible transmission by the aerosol route has also been considered because *microsporidia* have been found in respiratory specimens. Studies with mammals suggest that *Encephalitozoon* spp. can be transmitted transplacentally from mother to offspring, but no congenitally acquired human infections have been reported. Direct zoonotic transmission of *microsporidia* infecting humans has not been verified but appears likely because many microsporidial species can infect both humans and animals.

Epidemiologic studies suggest water contact as a risk factor for microsporidiosis, and *E. bieneusi*, *E. intestinalis*, and *V. corneae* homologous DNA has been detected in sewage effluent, groundwater, and surface water. Nevertheless, the importance of possible waterborne transmission requires further investigation.

Prevention and control

Albendazole has been found to cause growth deformities of *Encephalitozoon* and *Vittaforma* and to reduce or eradicate the parasites propagated in cell cultures but does not destroy mature microsporidial spores, so these may sustain infection. Numerous antiprotozoal drugs and antibiotics have been tested in vitro, with negative findings. In vitro systems to investigate *E. bieneusi* are not available.

Observational studies showed that an improvement of immune functions by potent antiretroviral combination therapy results in complete clinical response and normalization of intestinal architecture which parallels the clearance of intestinal microsporidia.

Blastocystis hominis

Blastocystis hominis, initially described by Alexieff in 1911, is a common inhabitant of the human gastrointestinal tract. It was named in 1912 by Brumpt, who considered it to be a yeast. At present, *B. hominis* is an organism of uncertain taxonomic classification. Zierdt recently classified *B. hominis* as a protozoan and placed it in the suborder Blastocystina, order Amoebida, pending confirmation at a molecular level. The role of *B. hominis* as a human pathogen is controversial and at present unresolved.

Morphology and Life Cycle

B. hominis is a strict anaerobic protozoan of variable size (5 to 40μm). It lacks a cell wall and has three morphologic forms: vacuolated, ameba-like, and granular. The vacuolated form, characterized by a large membrane-bound central body, which may be involved with carbohydrate and lipid storage (visually like a large vacuole), is most commonly identified in human fecal samples (see Figure 11-5-7). The more amebic form is occasionally seen in diarrheal fluid but may be extremely difficult to recognize.

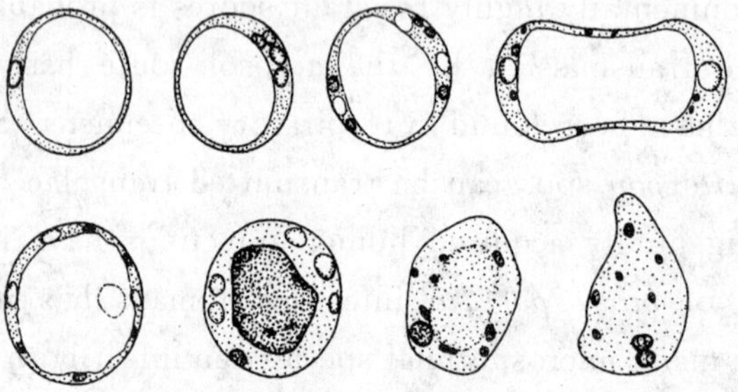

Figure 11-5-7 Vacuolated and anaerobic form of *Blastocystis hominis* (from Faust)

B. hominis resides primarily in the cecum and large bowel, divides by binary fission. The vacuole takes up 90% of tile cell and functions in sexual and asexual reproduction. Other structures with unknown function are not yet defined. The organism is strictly anaerobic, normally requires bacteria for growth, and is capable of ingesting bacteria and other debris. A new study reports the presence of thin- and thick-walled cysts. It is suggested that the thin-walled cysts are auto-infectious, leading to multiplication of the organism in the intestinal tract. The thick-walled cysts are responsible for externaltransmission via the fecal-oral route. This type of life cycle might explain the high percentage of positive carriers in many studies, showing that the percentage of patients with *B. hominis* is often much higher than those who are infected with other intestinal protozoa.

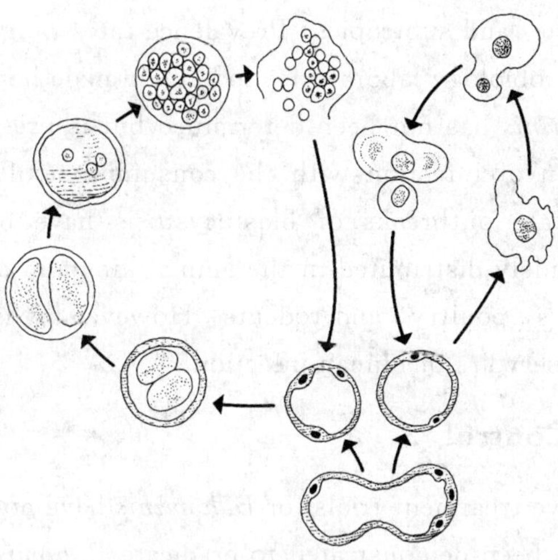

Figure 11-5-8 Life cycle of *Blastocystis hominis* (After Zierdt, 1973)

Pathogenesis and Clinical Manifestation

Pathogenic mechanisms for *B. hominis* have not been identified. Infections with *B. hominis* were increasingly reported in the 1980s and 1990s in both immunocompromised and immunologically intact hosts, in the absence of other identified microorganisms, several authors consider *B. hominis* to be a possible pathogen. Symptoms attributed to infection include diarrhea, abdominal pain, flatus, nausea, vomiting, anorexia, and malaise. However, virtually all the studies that have evaluated the clinical significance of blastocystosis have been retrospective case series from which a definitive answer is not forthcoming. Two prospective cas-control studies assessing the role of *B. hominis* as a possible intestinal pathogen in travelers gave opposite results.

Diagnosis

The diagnosis of blastocystosis is made by demonstrating the organism in unstained or permanently stained stool smears. The vacuolated form is most often identified and stains well with iron hematoxylin or trichrome. Concentration techniques may result in lysis of the organism. Heavy infections may obscure the identification of other intestinal protozoa in stool.

Both ELISA and fluorescent antibody tests have been developed for detection of serum antibody to *B. hominis* infections.

Epidemiology

B. hominis has a worldwide distribution, but some evidence suggests that it may be more common in the tropics and subtropics. Prevalence rates range from 3% to 20% in samples submitted to microbiology laboratories to 52% in male homosexuals. The mode of transmission of *B. hominis* has not been determined but is presumed to be fecal-oral because of the association of infection with the consumption of untreated water and travel to the tropics. Rare outbreaks of blastocystosis have been reported. Also, infection appears to be widely distributed in the animal kingdom and has been reported in pigs, monkeys, reptiles, poultry, and rodents. However, it is not known whether animals are significant reservoirs of human infection.

Prevention and Control

Controlled prospective treatment trials for *B. hominis* have not been performed. No antimicrobial agents have been demonstrated to eradicate *B. hominis* infection reliably, but metronidazole (Flagyl) is frequently prescribed. Diiodohydroxyquin (Floraquin) has also been effective. Limited *in vitro* susceptibility testing has shown activity against *B. hominis* by emetine, metronidazole, furazolidone, co-trimoxazole, quinacrine, and pentamidine (in order of efficacy).

Prevention would probably involve improved personal hygiene and sanitary conditions.

In summary, B. hominis is a frequently recognized colonic protozoan of uncertain pathogenic potential. Clarification of its role in human disease will require properly controlled prospective studies of pathogenicity and specific therapy. At present, little evidence is available.

(An Chunli)

Chapter 12 Ciliates

Balantidium coli

Ciliates are a large and diverse group of protozoa in the phylum Ciliophora. Most ciliates are free-living, but many are commensals of vertebrates and invertebrates, and a few are parasitic and are found in a variety of habitats. As the name implies, ciliates possess cilia at some point during their life cycles. The cilia are generally arranged in longitudinal rows and typically cover the surface of the organism. Ciliates are also characterized by nuclear dimorphism in that they have two distinct nuclei. The large kidney-shaped macronucleus is involved in the somatic functions of the cell, whereas the smaller spherical micronucleus contains the complete genome. Ciliates undergo both an asexual reproduction and a sexual reproduction involving conjugation, autogamy and cytogamy.

Balantidium coli is a protozoan parasite responsible for the disease Balantidiasis. It is the largest protozoan and the only ciliate known to parasitize humans. *B. coli* most commonly infects pigs, humans and other primates, with strains adapted to various other hosts. It is found world wide, but is more prevalent in the tropics. *B. coli* infection is most often asymptomatic, but the parasite can invade the large intestine leading to diarrhea, dysentery, colitis, and abdominal pain.

Morphology

B. coli has two developmental stages: a trophozoite stage and a cyst stage. Living trophozoites and cysts are yellowish or greenish (see Figure 12-1-1).

Trophozoites

Trophozoites are covered in cilia and have boring or rotary motility. *B. coli* is known for being the largest protozoan parasite of humans. They are ovoid, spheroid, or more slender, measuring between 30-150μm long by 25-120μm wide. In trophozoites, the two nuclei are clearly visible. The macronucleus is long and kidney-shaped, and the spherical micronucleus is nestled next to it. Trophozoites are characterized by a vestibulum, a cystostome-cytopharyngeal complex, at the pointed anterior end. There are two contractile vacuoles, which function in osmotic regulation, one near the middle of the body and the other near the posterior end. Food vacuoles contain erythrocytes, cell fragments, starch granules, and fecal and other debris.

Cysts

Cysts are smaller than trophozoites, measuring 40-60μm across. They are round and have a tough, heavy cyst wall made of one or two layers. Usually only the macronucleus and perhaps cilia and contractile vacuoles are visible in the cyst.

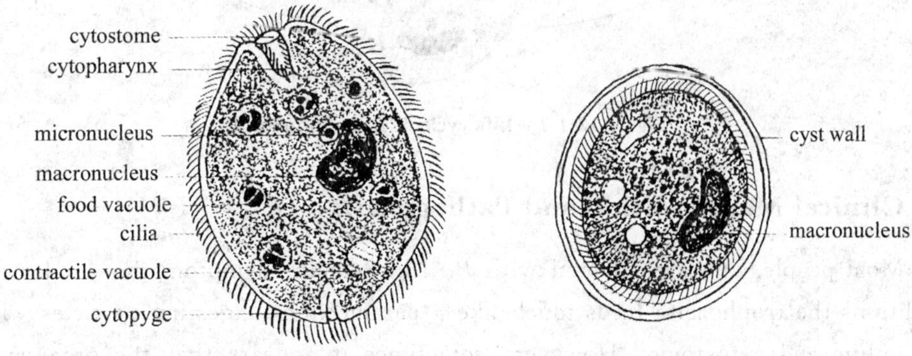

Figure 12-1-1 Morphology of *Balantidium coli*

Life Cycle

The ciliate *B. coli* lives in the cecum and colon of humans, pigs, and many other mammals and exhibits a typical fecal-oral life cycle consisting of trophozoite and cyst stages (see Figure 12-1-2). The infective stage is the cyst. Once the cyst is ingested via feces-contaminated food or water, it passes through the host digestive system. The cyst can resist degradation in the acidic environment of the stomach and the basic environment of the small intestine until it reaches the large intestine. There, excystation takes place.

The motile trophozoite then resides in the lumen of the large intestine, feeding on intestinal bacterial flora and intestinal nutrients. Trophozoites multiply by asexual transverse binary fission or rarely sexual conjugation. The trophozoite may become invasive and penetrate the mucosa of the large intestine. Encystation takes place in the rectum of the host as feces are dehydrated or soon after the feces have been excreted. Cysts in the environment are then ready to infect another host.

Although *B. coli* infection of humans is rare, it is most likely to occur in places where humans and pigs live in close contact.

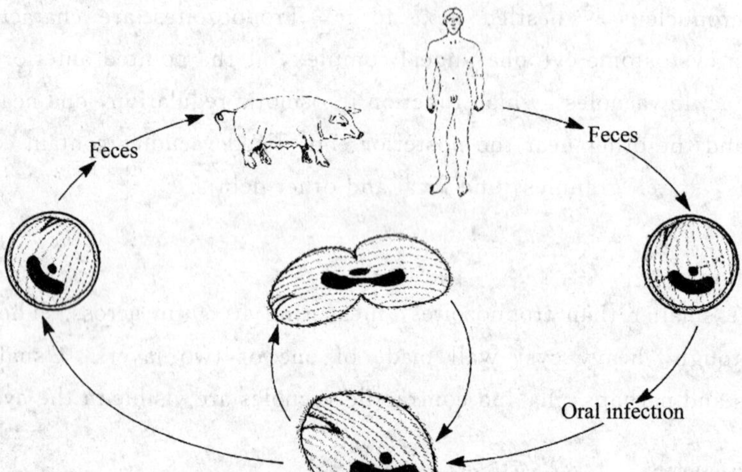

Figure 12-1-2 Life cycle of *Balantidium coli*

Clinical Manifestation and Pathogenesis

Most people who are infected with *B. coli* remain asymptomatic. Under normal conditions the trophozoite feeds much like a paramecium, ingesting particles with the vestibulum and cytostome. However, sometimes it appears that the organisms can produce proteolytic enzymes that digest away the intestinal epithelium of the host. The parasite secretes a substance called hyaluronidase enzyme, which helps degrade intestinal tissue and facilitates penetration of the mucosa. Other bacteria in the intestine may enter the ulcer along with *B. coli*, leading to secondary infections. The ulcer usually is flask-shaped, like an amebic ulcer, with a narrow neck leading into an undermining saclike cavity in the submucosa. The colonic ulceration produces lymphocytic infiltration with few polymorphonuclear leukocytes, and hemorrhage. Fulminating cases may produce necrosis and sloughing of the overlying mucosa and occasionally perforation of the large intestine or appendix, as in amebic dysentery. Death often follows at this stage. In contrast to *E. histolytica*, *B. coli* rarely invade extraintestinal tissues, but, secondary foci, such as the liver or lung, may become infected. Urogenital organs are sometimes attacked after contamination, and vaginal, uterine, and bladder infections have been reported.

After ingestion of an infective *B. coli* cyst, days to weeks may pass before infection occurs. Common symptoms of Balantidiasis include chronic diarrhea, occasional dysentery, nausea, foul breath, colitis, abdominal pain, weight loss, deep intestinal ulcerations, and possibly perforation of the intestine. Left untreated, it is reported to have a case fatality rate of 30%. Dysentery due to hemorrhaging can lead to shock and death.

Diagnosis

Although Balantidiasis is an uncommon infection, it should be considered if the patient has above-mentioned clinical manifestation and works closely with pigs or other livestock, lives in or has recently traveled to a region with poor water sanitation, or has had contact with infected persons.

Balantidiasis is diagnosed by microscopic examination of a patient's feces. A stool sample is collected and a wet mount is prepared. Cysts or trophozoites can be detected in the feces. *B. coli* is passed periodically, therefore stool samples should be collected frequently and examined immediately in order to make a definitive diagnosis.

Trophozoites can also be detected in tissue from the large intestine by a sigmoidoscopy procedure. A physician can look for bleeding, ulcers, and inflammation in order to diagnose the cause of diarrhea and other gastrointestinal complaints, and can take a tissue biopsy for inspection.

Since the symptoms of Balantidiasis are similar to those of amebiasis, it is important to identify the correct protozoan responsible for the disease.

Epidemiology

Balantidiasis in humans can be found almost anywhere in the world. It is reported to be more common in the tropics. Countries that are known to have had incidences of

B. coli infection include the Philippines, Bolivia, and Papua New Guinea, etc. Many cases of balantidiasis have been reported from China in 22 provinces/autonomous regions/municipalities.

Generally the disease is considered rare and occurs in less than 1% of the human population. Higher infection rates have been reported among institutionalized persons. Balantidiasis is common among those who are in close contact with swine. However, in pigs the infection rate may be quite high; Prevalence in pigs has been reported from 20% to 100%. Pigs typically do not show signs of infection; indeed, *B. coli* is believed to live commensally in the large intestines of swine.

Primates other than humans sometimes are infected and may represent a reservoir of infection to humans. Cysts can remain alive for weeks in pig feces, if the feces do not dry out. The pig is probably the usual source of infection for humans, but the relationship is not clear. There may be strains of *B. coli* that vary in their adaptability to humans. Infections often disappear spontaneously in healthy persons, or they can become symptomless, making infected persons carriers.

Prevention and Control

Several drugs are commonly used to combat infections of *B. coli*, including Tetracyclines 500mg four times daily for 10 days (contraindicated in pregnant women and children younger than 8 years of age), Metronidazole 750mg three times daily for 5 days, and Iodoquinol 640mg three times daily for 20 days.

Most cases of *Balantidium coli* infection are asymptomatic. If possible, asymptomatic individuals should still be treated in order to halt further transmission of the disease. Many people clear the infection spontaneously without treatment. Infected individuals usually respond well to treatment using one of the aforementioned drugs. If left untreated, Balantidiasis can become chronic. Persistent diarrhea can lead to high fluid loss and dehydration. Abdominal bleeding can lead to death.

Prevention and control measures are similar to those for *Entamoeba histolytica*, except that particular care should be taken by those who work with pigs. Like many diseases transmitted by a fecal-oral route, Balantidiasis can be prevented by improved hygiene practices, water sanitation, and proper disposal of fecal material.

(He Shenyi)

Part IV Medical Arthropodology

Chapter 13 Introduction

Arthropods are the largest group of animals, which belong to Phylum Arthropoda in Kingdom Animalia in zoological taxonomy. The Arthropoda makes up 75% of all animals on Earth with over a million modern species (about 1,200,000 species) described, usually including the insects, arachnids, crustaceans and other similar creatures. The Arthropods are common throughout marine, freshwater, terrestrial, and even aerial environments, as well as including various symbiotic and parasitic forms. They range in size from about 0. 1mm up to several meters long. Medical arthropods are extraordinarily important group of pests, which may directly injure human beings or transmit some diseases (especially some zoonoses) in many ways. The subject related to medical arthropods is called medical arthropodology or medical entomology.

The arthropods usually have some common features and scientists often identify them through their morphological features (see Figure 13-1-1). The most important features of arthropods include: (1) the segmented body with appendages on each segment; (2) bilaterally symmetric body; (3) covered by a hard exoskeleton that is made out of chitin, a polysaccharide; (4) a dorsal heart with hemocele and a nervous system on the ventral side of their bodies; (5) ecdysis (molting) and metamorphosis (an arthropod sheds this covering periodically when it molts and this covering prevents the arthropod from drying out, but also prevents arthropods from growing too big).

Section 1 Major Groups of Medical Arthropods

In the field of arthropods, medical arthropods only take account for a small proportion and most arthropods are of no medical significance. In Phylum Arthropoda, some species in five classes are closely related to medicine and these five classes are namely Insecta, Arachnida, Crustacea, Chilopoda and Diplopoda. Sometimes Chilopoda and Diplopoda are combined into one class, Myriapoda (or Multipoda). The Class Insecta is the most important class in the field of medical arthropodology (medical entomology) and Class Arachnida comes next (see Table 13-1-1, Figure 13-1-1, Figure

13-1-2, Figure 13-1-3 and Figure 13-1-4).

Table 13-1-1 Morphological features of major classes of medical arthropods

Major groups (Classes)	Morphological features
Insecta	The body is divided into three regions (head, thorax and abdomen) with one pair of antennae on the head. There are three pairs of legs on both sides of thorax. Some species have one or two pairs of wings.
Arachnida	The body has two regions (cephalothorax and abdomen) or is syncretized into one part (idiosoma) without antennae and wings. The adult has four pairs of legs. There are chelicerae and pedipalps in the front of gnathosoma.
Crustacea	The body is divided into two parts (cephalothorax and abdomen) without wings. There are two pairs of antennae and five pairs of walking legs. Most are aquatic and use gills for respiration.
Chilopoda	The body is divided into two parts (head and long segmented idiosoma or body segments) with one pair of antennae, but without wings. There is one pair of legs on both sides of every body segment.
Diplopoda	The body looks like a tube and has two parts (head and long idiosoma or body segments) with one pair of antennae, but without wings. There are two pairs of legs on both sides of every body segment.

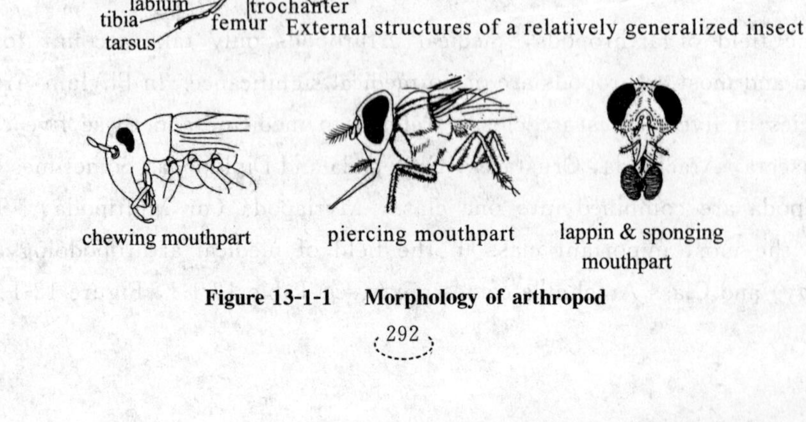

Figure 13-1-1 Morphology of arthropod

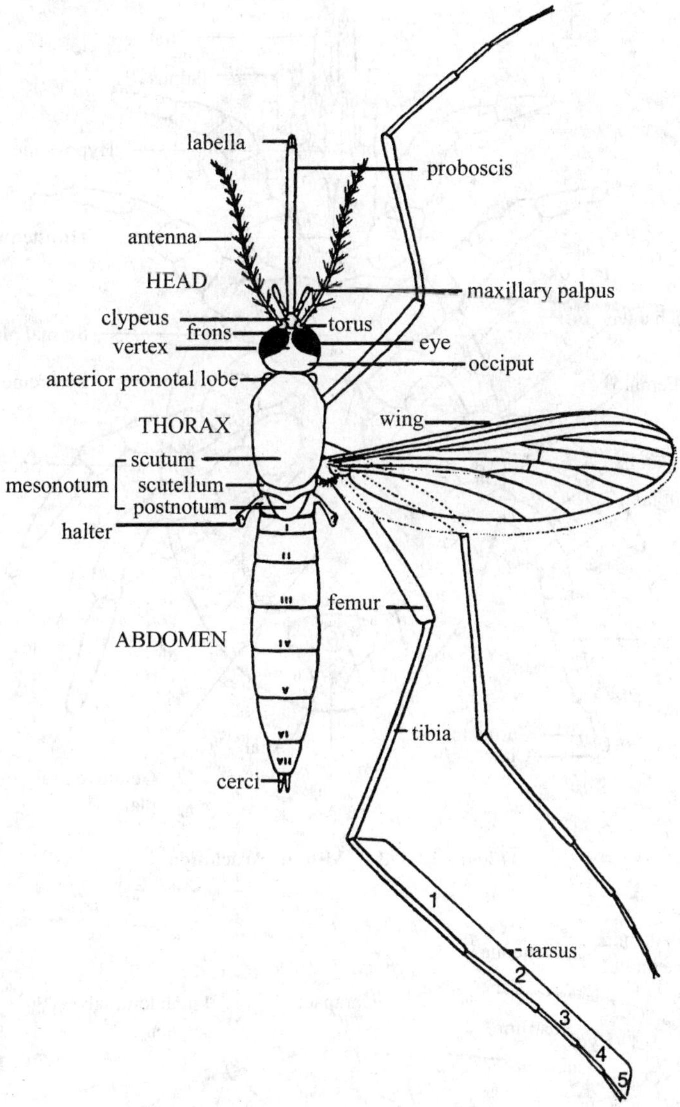

Figure 13-1-2 Mosquito in Insecta

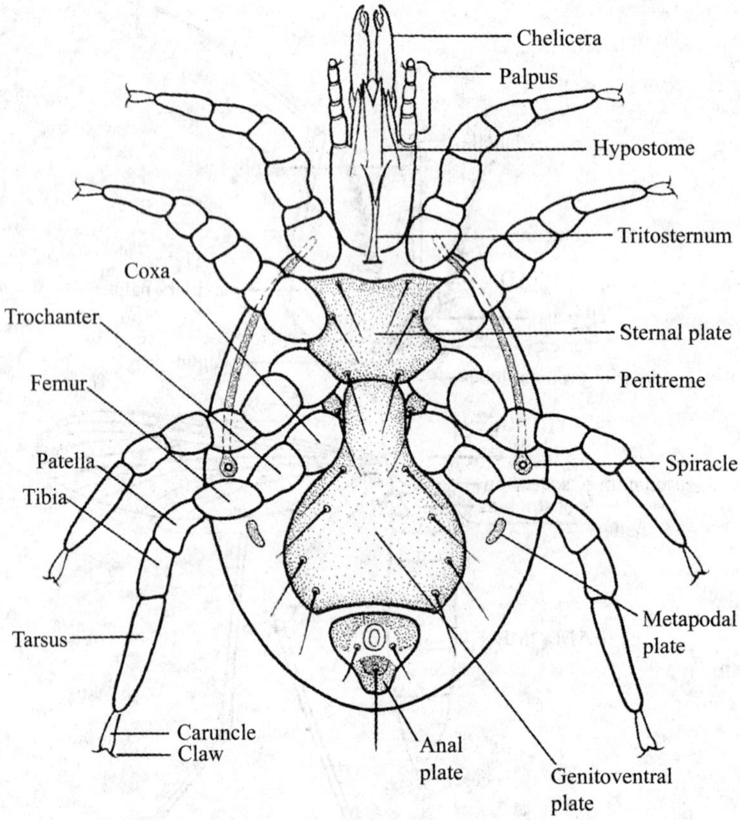

Figure 13-1-3 Mite in Arachnida

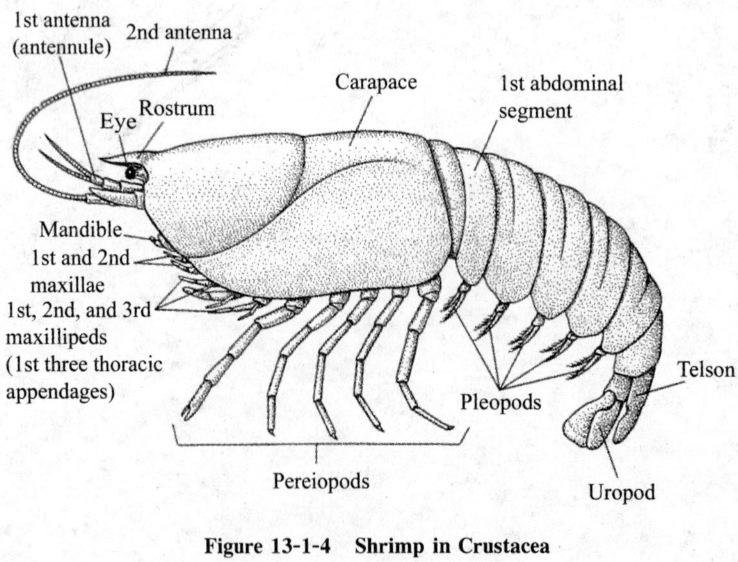

Figure 13-1-4 Shrimp in Crustacea

Of the above five classes of arthropods, Order Diptera in Insecta and subclass Acari in Arachnida are the most important groups in medical arthropodology (medical entomology). The major groups of medical arthropods are listed in Table 13-1-2.

Table 13-1-2 Representative groups of medical arthropods

Classes	Orders	Representative groups
Insecta	Diptera	Mosquitoes, flies, sandflies, biting midges, black flies and tabanid flies(horse and deer flics), etc.
	Siphonaptera	Fleas
	Anoplura	Sucking lice including body louse, head louse and crab louse (pubic louse), etc.
	Blattarria	Cockroaches
	Hemiptera	Bedbugs and conenose bugs.
	Others	Mulberry caterpillars and pine caterpillars in order Lepidoptera; Rove beetles in order Coleoptera; Ants, bees and hornets (wasps) in Hymenoptera.
Arachnida	Parasitiformes	Ticks and gamasid mites.
	Acariformes	Chigger mites, itch mites, follicle mites and dust mites, etc.
	Others	Black widow spider in subclass Aranea, scorpions in subclass Scorpiones.
Others	Crabs, shrimps and copepods (*Cyclops* and *Diaptomus*), etc. in Class Crustacea; Centipedes in Class Chilopoda; Diplopods and millipedes in Class Diplopoda.	

Section 2 Medical Arthropods and Diseases

Relationship Between Arthropods and Medicine

Medical arthropods can be harmful to human health directly or indirectly. Some arthropods can transmit some diseases as vectors. The diseases transmitted by arthropod vectors are called vector born diseases, which are the most important harm way of arthropods to human health. The disease transmission is done in two ways, mechanical transmission and biological transmission. Tick paralysis, myiasis, tungiasis, scabies, demodicidosis and dust mite asthma are the examples of direct impairment of arthropods while malaria, filariasis, epidemic encephalitis B, visceral leishmaniasis (kala-azar), plague, murine typhus and scrub typhus, etc. are vector born diseases.

Impairment of Arthropods to Human Beings

Direct impairment

Arthropods may directly injure an animal host in many ways. Some types of direct impairment may be caused by insect feeding such as blood sucking activity and other arthropod activities may also be damaging. There are usually four major categories of direct effects from arthropods.

(1)Biting, stinging, blood sucking and annoyance

Some medical arthropods directly injure humans and animals through their biting (or stinging) animals' skin or sucking blood from animal hosts. The common stinging or blood-sucking arthropods include mosquitoes, sandflies, biting midges, black flies and tabanid flies (horse and deer flies), fleas, sucking lice, bedbugs, conenose bugs, ticks, chiggers, centipedes and scorpions, etc. Annoyance may come from the disruptive activities of blood-sucking arthropods or non blood-sucking ones, such as flying around or landing on the head, and from feeding (blood-sucking activities). Arthropods usually do not remove sufficient blood to cause a medical problem, although anemia and significant blood loss caused by insects have been documented with livestock. Nevertheless, annoyance is not a trivial effect of arthropods. Human activities may be disrupted by arthropods (especially insects), and in some instances, such as when recreational facilities cannot be used because of insects. With livestock, annoyance is of even greater importance. Continuous irritation from insects may reduce weight gain in cattle, may disrupt milk production, and may contribute to increased susceptibility to other stresses.

(2) Envenomization

Envenomization is the introduction of a poison into the body of humans and animals. Tick paralysis caused by salivary venom of some hard ticks is a typical example of arthropod envenomization. Few arthropods have sufficiently toxic poisons to kill humans outright. However, humans and other animals do die from arthropod venoms and envenomization: ① biting, as occurs with spiders; stinging, as occurs with scorpions, ticks and some Hymenoptera (such as ants, bees, and wasps); ② contact, passively or inadvertently touching a poisonous feature, such as urticating hairs (hairs that produce wheals and itching) which are found on many Lepidoptera larvae and some spiders (such as tarantulas); ③ active projection, contacting poisons that are secreted or expelled such as vesicating fluids (acid or alkaline liquids causing skin irritation or blistering), that occur in some beetles; and ④ingestion, accidentally eating poisonous insects (e. g. , horses can be killed by ingesting hay containing some poisonous beetles).

(3) Allergic reaction (anaphylaxis)

Arthropods may give rise to allergic reaction (anaphylaxis) which is a hypersensitive response to arthropod proteins. Dust mites are the very common source of allergen, which usually lead to asthma and allergic rhinitis. Some people are even allergic to cockroach proteins. All mechanisms of envenomization also involve allergic reaction. Human deaths from bee and wasp stings usually are associated with hypersensitive reaction rather than direct effect of a toxin.

(4) Direct parasitism

Some arthropod species directly parasitize on the body surface of humans or other animals or inside the host body as ectoparasites or endoparasites. Dermatitis and dermatosis are common problems caused by arthropod activities. Dermatitis is an inflammation of the skin, dermatosis a disease of the skin. Many mite species, such as scabies mites and chiggers, produce acute skin irritations. Human scabies, a skin disease caused by infestations of the itch mite (*Sarcoptes scabiei*) is an important public health problem. In livestock, mange, any persistent skin inflammation caused by mites can seriously weaken animals. Follicle mites are common ectoparasites of human and livestock, and they may cause demodicidosis. Fleas in genus *Tunga* (*Tunga penetrans*, for example) may penetrate into animals' skin and cause tungiasis. Myiasis is the invasion and feeding on living tissues of humans or animals by dipterous larvae, especially fly larvae (maggots). Fortunately, myiasis is a rare condition in humans, but it commonly occurs in livestock. Acariasis is the invasion by the direct parasitism of some mites. A number of mite species in superfamily Acaroidea can be the pathogen of acariasis, which can enter the digestive, respiratory or urinary tracts and give rise to intestinal acariasis, pulmonary acariasis and urinary acariasis.

Indirect impairment

The indirect impairment of medical arthropods focuses on disease transmission. Disease transmission is more important than any other effect produced by medical arthropods. Organisms that produce disease are called pathogens, and arthropods capable of transmitting pathogens are called vectors. Some diseases may depend on only a single host and a vector; however, other diseases may include multiple host species, and even multiple vectors. In any of these instances, an organism that maintains the infective agent (the pathogen source) when active transmission does not occur is termed a reservoir. Arthropods can be as reservoirs in the transmission of diseases (especially some zoonoses). The diseases transmitted by the vectors of arthropods are usually called vector-borne diseases. The ability of a pathogen to survive and remain infective in or on a vector species is a critical factor in disease transmission. Two mechanisms of transmission are possible, mechanical transmission and biological transmission.

(1) Mechanical transmission

Mechanical transmission is the transfer of a pathogen from an infectious source to a susceptible host by a vector, without obvious reproduction and development of the pathogen in the vector. Flies and cockroaches are typical examples of mechanical transmission and they often mechanically carry some pathogens (the pathogenic bacteria of dysentery, typhoid fever or cholera, amebic cysts and eggs of some helminths, etc.) on their body parts or inside their body (alimentary tracts, for example). Generally, mechanical transmission is an inefficient mechanism for disease transmission and the transmission can be made with or without arthropod vectors.

(2) Biological transmission

In biological transmission, the pathogen either reproduces or develops (or both) in the vector, and arthropod vectors are a necessary link in the transmission (The transmission can not be finished without the vectors). Biological transmission is the most effective and significant mechanism for disease transmission by arthropods. It usually needs some time when the pathogen enters arthropods and then develops (or reproduces) into an infective stage, and this time period is called extrinsic incubation period. Biological transmission is further divided into the following four styles: ① developmental biological transmission with the pathogenic organisms having a period of development in the arthropod vectors (e. g. when mosquitoes transmit filariasis); ② propagative biological transmission with the pathogens multiplying in the vectors (e. g. when fleas transmit plague); ③ cyclopropagative biological transmission with the pathogens developing and multiplying in the vectors (e. g. when mosquitoes transmit malaria); ④ transovarial biological transmission with the pathogens being transferred to the next generation of vectors through their eggs (e. g. when ticks and mites transmit some viruses).

Arthropod-associated Diseases

Diseases by the direct impairment of arthropods

Apart from some non-specific direct impairment such as annoyance, envenomization, allergic reaction and dermatitis, some arthropods can also cause a series of special diseases as arthropod pathogens themselves, including asthma, acariasis, scabies, dermodicidosis, tick paralysis, tungiasis and myiasis, etc. Some diseases like asthma, scabies and dermodicidosis are quite common in clinical practice while others like tick paralysis, tungiasis and myiasis are very occasional in humans. Although there may be a variety of causes in the onset of asthma, dust mites are often regarded as an important element. Allergic asthma induced by dust mites is frequently found in humans, especially in children. Table 13-2-1 lists major diseases by the direct impairment of arthropods.

Table 13-2-1 Major diseases by the direct impairment of arthropods

Names of diseases	Arthropod pathogens	Lesion sites	Mechanisms
Allergic asthma and rhinitis	Dust mites	Respiratory system	Allergic reaction
Acariasis	Some mite species (especially mites in Acaroidea)	Digestive, respiratory and urinary tracts	Direct parasitism of the mites
Scabies	Itch mites	Skin	Direct parasitism of itch mites
Demodicidosis	Follicle mites	Skin or viscera	Direct parasitism of follicle mites
Tick paralysis	Some hard tick species	Nerve system	Nerve toxicity
Tungiasis	Some flea species	Skin	Direct parasitism of fleas
Myiasis	Dipterous larvae (especially fly maggots)	Skin, eyes and digestive tracts, etc.	Direct parasitism of the larvae.

Major diseases mechanically transmitted by arthropods

Flies and cockroaches often carry some pathogens on or in their body and mechanically transmit some diseases. The involved pathogens include viruses, bacteria and protozoa, etc. Table 13-2-2 summarizes major pathogens mechanically transmitted by arthropods.

Table 13-2-2 Major pathogens mechanically transmitted by arthropods

Pathogens	Arthropod vectors	Diseases	Victims
Virus			
Poliovirus	Flies and cockroaches	Poliomyelitis	Humans
Myxomatosis virus	Mosquitoes	Myxomatosis	Rabbits
Bacterium			
Bacillus anthracis	Tabanidae	Anthrax	Humans and various animals

Francisella tularensis	Tabanidae	Tularemia	Humans
Salmonella	Flies, cockroaches and eye gnats	Salmonellosis	Humans
Shigella	Flies	Shigellosis	Humans
Vibrio cholerae	Flies	Cholera	Humans
Spirochete			
Treponema pertenue	Flies and eye gnats	Yaws	Humans
Protozoa			
Entamoeba histolytica	Flies and cockroaches	Amebic dysentery	Humans
Toxoplasma gondii	Cockroaches	Toxoplasmosis	Humans and cats, etc.

Major diseases biologically transmitted by arthropods

The most important significance of medical arthropods focuses on biologically transmitting a series of diseases, especially some zoonoses. Table 13-2-3 presents some important biologically-transmitted diseases by arthropod vectors.

Table 13-2-3 Major pathogens biologically transmitted by arthropods

Pathogens	Arthropod vectors	Diseases	Victims	Distribution
Virus				
JEV	*Culex*, *Anopheles* & *Aedes*	Epidemic type B encephalitis	Humans & pigs, etc.	Eastern Asia
Dengue virus	*Aedes*	Dengue fever & dengue hemorrhagic fever	Humans & monkeys	Southeast Asia, North America
YF virus	*Aedes*	Yellow fever	Humans & monkeys	Africa, Central & South America
Sand fly fever virus	*Phlebotomus*	Sand fly fever	Humans	Africa, Asia, Europe

Bluetongue virus	*Culicoides*	Bluetongue	Sheep & horse	Africa, Asia, United States
Forest encephalitis virus	*Ixodes*	Forest encephalitis (Russian spring-summer encephalitis)	Humans, wild mammals & birds	Russia & China
CCHF virus (XHF virus)	*Ixodes*	Xinjiang haemorrhagic fever (XHF) or Crimean-Congo hemorrhagic fever	Humans, livestock & wild animals	Africa, Asia & Europe
Hantaan virus	Some gamasid mites and chigger mites	Hemorrhagic fever with renal syndrome (HFRS)	Humans & rodents	China, Korea & North America
Rickettsia				
Rickettsia prowazekii	*Pediculus humanus*	Epidemic typhus (louse-borne typhus)	Humans	Africa
Bartonella quintana	*Pediculus humanus*	Trench fever	Humans	Africa, Asia, Europe, Central & South America
Rickettsia typhi (R. mooseri)	Siphonaptera (fleas)	Endemic typhus (murine typhus)	Humans and rodents	Central & North America, Europe
Rickettsia tsutsugamushi (R. orientalis)	*Leptotrombidium*	Tsutsugamushi disease (scrub typhus)	Humans and rodents	Southeast Asia
Bacterium				
Yersinia pestis	Siphonaptera (fleas)	Plague	Humans & rats	World

Spirochete				
Borrelia recurrentis	*Pediculus humanus*	Epidemic relapsing fever (louse-borne relapsing fever)	Humans	Africa
Borrelia burgdorferi	*Ixodes*	Lyme disease	Humans & other mammals	United States
Borrelia persica, B. latyschevi & B. hermsii, etc.	*Ornithodoros* (soft tick)	Endemic relapsing fever (Tick-borne relapsing fever)	Humans & rodents	Africa, Asia, Europe, North America, South America
Protozoa				
Plasmodium (*P. vivax*, *P. falciparum*, *P. malariae* & *P. ovale*)	*Anopheles*	Malaria	Humans	World (tropics)
Trypanosoma	*Glossina*	Trypanosomiasis (sleeping sickness)	Humans, livestock & wild animals	Tropical Africa
Leishmania	*Phlebotomus*	Leishmaniais	Humans, dogs and rodents, etc.	World
Nematode				
Wuchereria brancrofti	*Culex*, *Anopheles* & *Aedes*	Bancroftian filariasis	Humans	World (tropics)
Brugia malayi	*Anopheles* & *Aedes*	Brugian filariasis	Humans & other mammals	Southeast Asia
Onchocerca volvulus	*Simulium*	Onchocerciasis	Humans	Africa, tropical South America
Loa loa	*Chrysops*	Loiasis	Humans	Africa

Dipetalonema perstans, *D. streptocerca* & *Mansonella ozzardi*	*Culicoides*	Three types of filariasis	Humans	Africa & South America
Thelazia callipaeda	House flies	Thelaziasis	Dogs and cats, etc.	World

Determination of Vector Arthropods

It is very important to determine the arthropod vectors in the surveillance and control of vector-born diseases. Generally, the determination of arthropod vectors often comes from the following evidences: (1) Biological evidence: The suspected arthropods are very close to humans and they usually bite (or sting) humans for bloodmeal or lap our food with a bigger population and longer life span. (2) Epidemiological evidence: The seasonal fluctuation of the arthropod population is consistent with the epidemic trend of the suspected diseases. (3) Laboratory evidences for natural infection and artificial infection: The corresponding pathogens can be successfully isolated from the suspected arthropods from the foci of the prevailing diseases. The suspected arthropods should be also artificially (manually) infected with the pathogens in laboratory.

Section 3 Ecology and Control of Medical Arthropods

Ecology of Medical Arthropods

Ecology is a big branch of life science, which is to study the interactions between organisms and their environments. An organism's environment usually includes abiotic component and biotic component. The abiotic component of an environment is all of the non-living components of an organism's environment. These include such things as temperature, light, water, wind, nutrients and substrate (e. g. rock and soil), etc. The abiotic component of an environment can and does have a dramatic impact on the ability of organisms to survive and reproduce. The biotic component of an environment is all of the other organisms found in an environment with which an organism makes contact, directly or indirectly. These organisms may be competing, preying upon, being preyed upon, providing shelter, or in some other way impact on the environment. Generally, organisms make a significant impact on other organisms within an environment.

Ecological studies are usually made on three levels of ecological organization, individual, population, community and ecosystem. An organism itself is an individual such as a bacterium, a plant and an animal, etc. A population contains many individuals of the same species in a certain space and time. For instance, all the individuals of *Anopheles sinensis* (a species of mosquitoes) in a specific area form a population of *Anophele sinensis*. A community is the assemblage of different species of organisms within a given environment. For example, different species of mosquitoes (mosquito larvae) in a given rice field are a mosquito community. The ecosystem is the highest level of ecological organization and it is actually the combination of the community and its abiotic environment.

Control of Medical Arthropods

The fundamental threat posed by medical pests is disease transmission and therefore the control for medical arthropods should focus on some important transmitting vectors, which is an effective way to prevent and control the related vector-born diseases. Chemical control by insecticides (or pesticides) has long been a major way of controlling medical arthropods and other pests. In temperate regions, some diseases have been eliminated or greatly diminished through reducing vector populations. Although attempts have been made to eradicate insect vectors, these efforts have not been very successful. In fact, by subjecting pest populations to heavy, continual insecticide (or pesticide) pressure, insecticide resistance has developed in a number of medically-important species. Some insecticides are two-side chemicals, which have killed some other non-targeted animals (especially some natural enemies of pests). In addition, insecticides have also become an important source of environment pollution.

Because of insecticide resistance, the control of medical arthropods is becoming more and more difficult and a single procedure of management usually does not work in the campaign of controlling pests. Since it is usually impossible to thoroughly eliminate the medical arthropod and other pests, the fundamental rule of controlling vector arthropods is to adopt an integrated management (integrated control). Integrated management is based on ecological, economic and social criteria and integrates multidisciplinary methodologies into pest management strategies that are practical and effective to protect public health and the environment and improve the quality of life. Integrated management strategies are usually employed in concert with insecticide. These include environment management, physical control, chemical control, biological control, genetic control and legislation management (some limiting methods by laws), etc.

Environment management

The environment management is to remove or control the arthropods' habitat where they live and breed. In mosquito control, for example, it may includes: (1) to eliminate standing water in rain gutters, old tires, buckets, plastic covers, toys, or any other container where mosquitoes can breed; (2) to empty and change the water in bird baths, fountains, wading pools, rain barrels, and potted plant trays to destroy potential mosquito habitats; (3) to drain or fill temporary pools of water with dirt; (4) to keep swimming pool water treated and circulating.

Physical control

The physical management is to use some mechanical ways (instrument, heat, light, sound and electricity, etc.) to kill the pests or to avoid their annoyance, biting or stinging. It is an easy way in physical management to use head nets, long sleeves and long pants if you venture into areas with high populations of blood-sucking arthropods. For the prevention of flying insects such as house fly and mosquito, window screen (and door screen) and mosquito-net are often recommended.

Chemical control

The chemical control has long been a predominant way in the campaign of pest control and it is to use a number of chemicals (insecticides and repellents) to eliminate the pests or avoid arthropods' disturbance. The excellence of insecticides is usually evaluated from: (1) highly efficient on the pests with low quantity; (2) wide spectrum of killing most pests; (3) low toxicity to human beings and non-targeted animals (especially natural enemies); (4) degradable in environment without severe environment pollution; (5) low potentiality to creat insecticide resistance; (6) cheap and convenient to be used. The common insecticides include organochlorides (DDT, benzene hexachloride or BHC, Lindane, etc.), organophosphates (malathion, phoxin, fenitrothion or sumithion, pirimiphos methyl, temephos or abates, fenithion or baytex, dichlorvos or DDVP, etc.), carbamates (landrin, sunside or propoxur, etc.) and pyrethroid (allethrin, tetramethrin, resmethrin, permethrin, deltamethrin or decamethrin, etc.), etc. In the control of mosquito adults, ultra-low volume (ULV) sprays are recommended. ULV sprayers dispense very fine aerosol droplets that stay aloft and kill flying mosquitoes on contact. ULV applications involve small quantities of pesticide active ingredient in relation to the size of the area treated, which minimizes exposure and risks to people and the environment.

Biological control

The biological control is a comparatively safe way to environment and non-targeted animals (human being, livestock and natural enemy, etc.). It is to use some predators, parasites, fungi, bacteria and even viruses to diminish the pest populations. Mosquitofish (*Gambusia affinis*) are usually used in a variety of mosquito breeding situations where chemical treatment may be ineffective and environment management (source reduction) infeasible.

Genetic control

It is to use genetic measures to reduce the genetic potentiality of pests and then to diminish their natural populations. Male sterilization is a typical genetic measure, in which male insects are treated by radio rays or chemicals to make them sterilized. The sterilized males without the ability of fertilization should maintain the potentiality to mate with natural females in the actual practice and field application. Scientists have made a series of scientific researches on the genetic control of medical arthropods, but lots of them are still under laboratory experiment and transgenic mosquito is an example.

Legislation management

Legislation management is to make some laws and regulations (some limiting methods by laws) to control the spread of pests. In some instances, legislation management can be carried out through customs quarantine and health supervision.

(Guo Xianguo)

Chapter 14 Insecta

Section 1 Introduction

Insecta (commonly called insects) is a class in zoological taxonomy, which is the largest and most widely distributed taxon in Phylum Arthropoda. Insects may be found in nearly all environments on the planet. They comprise the most diverse group of animals on the earth (with over 800, 000 species described—more than all other animal groups combined), but the species associated with medicine (medical insects) are only a small proportion and most species of insects have no medical significance.

Generally, insects can be easily identified morphologically from the following characteristics: (1) apparent three parts of body, head, thorax and abdomen; (2) one pair of antennae, pedipalps and compound eyes on the head with mouth parts in the front of head; (3) three pairs of legs on both sides of thorax with 1-2 pair(s) of wings in some species. The function of antennae is for olfactory and tactile sensation. Apart from compound eyes, some insects have ocelli or single eyes (see Figure 13-1-1).

The mouthparts of medical insects are usually divided into three types, chewing mouthparts as in cockroaches, lapping mouthparts as in house flies and piercing-sucking mouthparts as in mosquitoes. The thorax of an insect has three parts, prothorax, mesothorax and metathorax. Three pairs of legs have five segments, coax, trochanter, femur, tibia and tarsus with a claw. Wings have special veins and cells. The pattern of wing venation is constant within a species and therefore is often of value in taxonomy. In

Diptera, the metathoracic wings (hind wings) have modified into knobbed structures, called halteres (a balancing organ). The abdomen of adult insects consists basically of 11 somites plus a terminal telson, but all these segments usually can be discerned only in the embryo. Appendages of the genital segments are called external genitalia consisting of penis or aedeagus on the ninth segment of males and the ovipositor is formed of the eighth and ninth segment appendages of females. The eleventh segment may also have appendages, the cerci, which range from vestige in size to longer with sensory function (see Figure 13-1-1).

Metamorphosis is an apparent feature of medical insects, which includes a series of morphological, physiological, behavioral and ecological changes from egg to matured adults, and it is actually postembryonic development. During metamorphosis, insects (also including other arthropods) have to shed their cuticle (covering) periodically since the cuticle prevents them from growing. The shedding process is called molts or ecdyses, through which all arthropods go during their development. The stages of the animal between each molt are referred to as instars. There are a few types of metamorphosis and the most common ones associated with medical insects are complete metamorphosis (holometamorphosis) and incomplete metamorphosis (hemimetamorphosis). Insects with complete metamorphosis undergo four basic stages (eggs, larvae, pupae and adults) in their life cycle and their larvae bear little resemblance to the adults. After several larval instars, the insects enter a nonfeeding period calling the pupa stage, in which the animal is completely recognized and the wing buds grow internally. The typical life cycle for complete metamorphosis may be simply described as: eggs → larvae (one or several instars) → pupae → adults. Insects with incomplete metamorphosis, however, undergo three basic stages (eggs, nymphs and adults) and the nymphs are similar to adults morphologically. The life cycle of insects with incomplete metamorphosis may be summed up as: eggs→nymphs (one or several instars)→adults. Some insects have more than one stage of larvae or nymphs. The insects in Anoplura and Hemiptera exercise incomplete metamorphosis while diptera, siphonaptera, lepidoptera and Hymenoptera complete metamorphosis.

(Guo Xianguo)

Section 2 Mosquitoes

The family Culicidae contains more than 3,500 described species that are divided into three subfamilies: Anophelinae, Culicinae, and Toxorhvnchitinae. Some of their recognition features are as follows:

1. *Toxorhynchitinae*. Larvae predaceous with large jaws for capturing other mosquito larvae on which they feed. Adults are relatively large with a long, curved proboscis; not blood feeders, but rather are plant feeders. *Toxorhynchites*.

2. *Anophelinae*. Larvae lack a breathing tube on the eighth abdominal segment; the body of the larva lies parallel to the surface of the water. Pupae have short, broad trumpets or breathing tubes, which have large openings that continue as a split down the front. Adult males and females both have maxillary palps at least as long as the proboscis, and in the males they are clubbed at the distal ends; the scutellum is often trilobed. Eggs are laid singly and have floats on their sides. Adults have a characteristic resting and feeding posture with the head down and the hind legs raised. *Anopheles*, *Chagasia Bironella*.

3. *Culicinae*. Larvae have a long breathing tube on the eighth abdominal segment; the body of the larva hangs head down from the surface of the water. Pupae in Culex have long slender breathing tubes that are not split, but other genera may have short trumpets, some of which may be split. Adults have short maxillary palps in the females and long ones in the males. The scutellum is usually rounded. Eggs are laid in rafts and they lack floats. The resting and feeding positions of the adult females are with the body parallel to the surface and usually with all of the legs on the surface, further subdivided into the tribes Culicini and Aedini. *Culex*, *Aedes*, *Mansonia*, *Culiseta*, *Wyeomyia*, *Psorophora*, and so on.

Morphology

Mosquitoes are generally 3 to 6mm long, but a few exceed 9mm. They have large numbers of flat scales on both wings and to body; the scales on the wings are on the veins and the margins. The wings have an unforked vein between two forked veins on the distal margin. Mouthparts are a long proboscis or fascicle adapted for sucking blood and plant juices; the females have mandibles, but the males usually lack them and cannot take blood, only plant juices. The thorax is broader than the head, antennae are long and plumose in the males, but the females have only a few sparse hairs. Larvae are aquatic, and have a well defined head, thorax, and abdomen; an air tube arises on abdominal segment 8 (see Figure 14-2-1, Figure 14-2-2, Figure 14-2-3 and Figure 14-2-4).

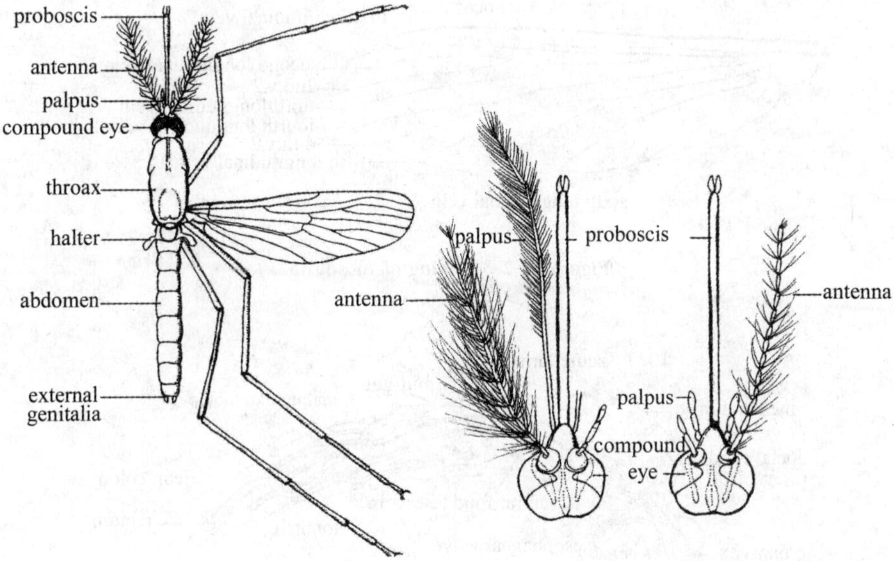

Figure 14-2-1 Morphology of mosquito

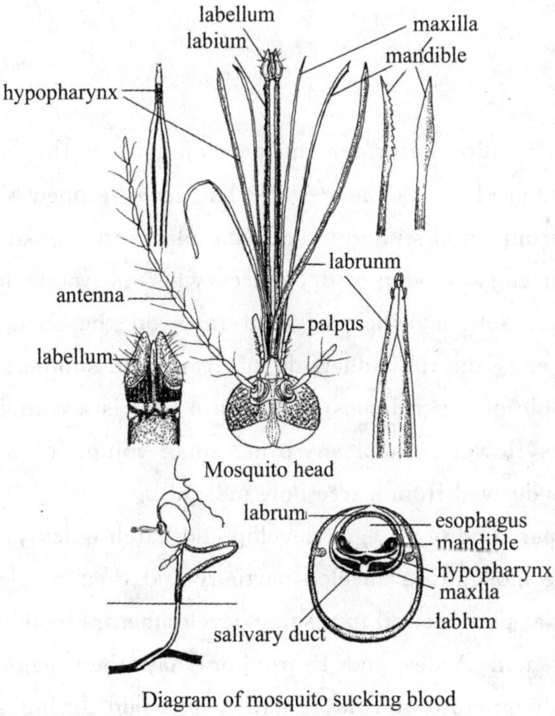

Figure 14-2-2 Mouthpart of female mosquito

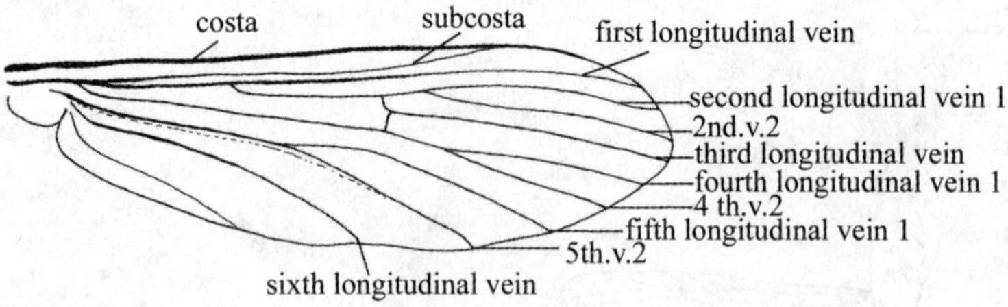

Figure 14-2-3 Wing of mosquito

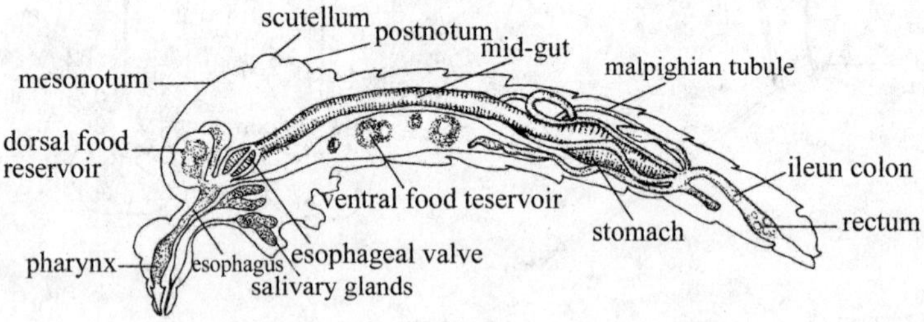

Figure 14-2-4 Internal structure of mosquito

Life Cycle

All mosquitoes require water for the development of the larvae and pupae (see Figure 14-2-5). Eggs are laid in or near water but never in open water. Females respond to a number of environmental stimuli in choosing places to deposit their eggs. Aedes and Psorophora lay their eggs in damp or dry places, whereas Anopheles lays its eggs in the water. Culex and Culiseta lay their eggs in rafts on the surface of the water, and Mansonia lays its eggs on the underside of leaves of submerged vegetation. *Aedes aegypti* is an example of a peridomestic mosquito that is a container breeder; eggs are laid in tin cans, tires, flower pots, or any other small volume of water near houses. *Ae. aegypti* is probably derived from a tree-hole mosquito.

Under the proper conditions, eggs develop and hatch quickly, often within 24 to 48 hours. Some aedine mosquitoes develop partially and then require a stimulus such as cooling or a particular photoperiod to resume development. Floodwater mosquitoes, some members of the genera Aedes and Psorophora, lay their eggs in areas that flood periodically, and in temperate or cold climates, eggs laid during summer do not hatch until the following spring when the area is flooded. They typically come out in hordes at that time.

Most mosquito larvae trap little bits of food in their mouth fans; they are sometimes said to be filter feeders, but it is more accurately referred to as trapping. Food consists of bits of organic debris and microorganisms such as protists and rotifers. A few mosquito larvae, notably the larvae of Toxorhynchites, are predaceous and typically feed on other mosquito larvae.

The four larval stages may last for as short a time as three days to more than a month depending upon temperature and species. For example, *Psorophora confinnis* goes from egg to adult in three days at 46℃ in the California desert. Culiseta inornata requircs 28 to 30 days to complete development at 14℃. The development of the yellow fever mosquito, *Ae. aegypti*, come almost to a standstill below about 26℃. Most culicine mosquitoes complete development in about seven days. Oxygen is required for larval development, and most larvae obtain it from the air by coming to the surface where they apply their breathing tubes; however, in Mansonia oxygen is obtained from plants by puncturing them with a posterior stylet.

The fourth larval stage is the last one before the pupa, and it typically does not feed but rather prepares itself to become a pupa. The head and thorax of the pupa are fused to form a cephalothorax. The pupa is free swimming but nonfeeding and usually lasts only two to three days. Pupae require oxygen and have breathing tubes, usually called trumpets, on the cephalothorax. In two genera, Mansonia and Coquillettidia, the trumpets are modified to penetrate plant tissue so as to obtain oxygen.

Adults emerge from the pupa at the surface of the water; 10 to 15 minutes are required for emergence, drying of the body, and extension of the wings. During this time, mosquitoes are quite susceptible to predation. Females are not ready to take a blood meal until one to three days after emergence. This is the beginning of the phase called the gonotrophic cycle. During this time the ovarian follicles develop.

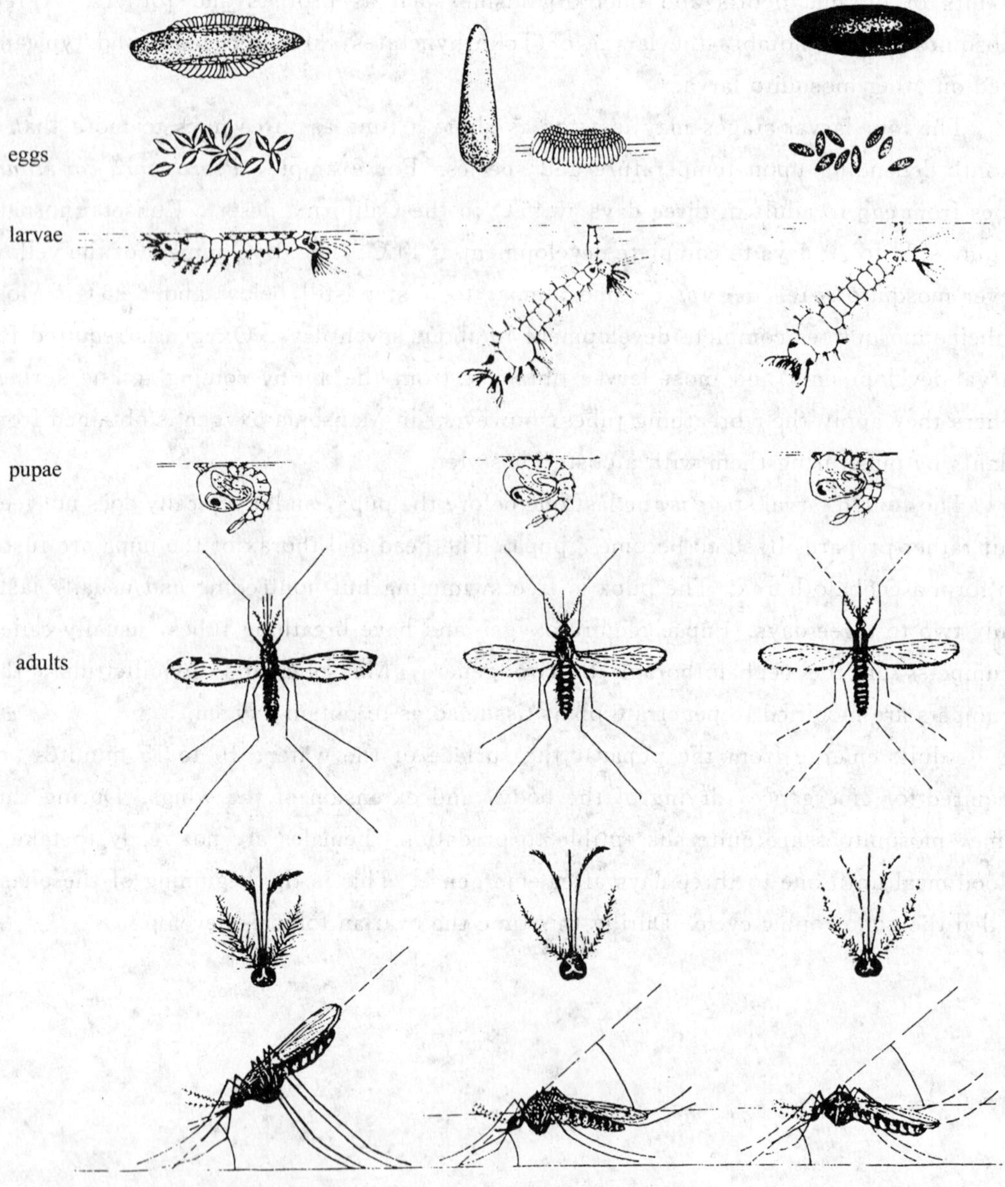

Figure 14-2-5 Life cycle of mosquito

The females are then ready to mate, and it takes place in swarms of males. Females enter the swarm, pair up with a male, and they then probably leave the swarm, although this is difficult to determine. Males may mate several times, but females mate only once.

The next phase, host seeking, lasts for 3 to 10 days during which time they seek hosts, take a blood meal, and then rest somewhere while the eggs develop. Egg laying takes place over about a three-day period. The gonotrophic cycle, except for copulation, is then repeated, and one female may have as many as five cycles of egg laying. It should be noted that in the biological transmission of disease agents of all sorts, the female is infected at one feeding, lays eggs, and then must take another blood meal for transmission to occur.

Old Tires and *Aedes*

An automobile tire is maniacally designed to hold water. There is no way that a tire can be oriented so that water will drain from it; trying to empty one is an exercise in frustration. In investigating the sporadic cases and outbreaks of LaCrosse encephalitis in Wisconsin, the vector was determined to be Aedes triseriatus, a tree-hole mosquito. A tree hole is a cavity likely to hold water for a period of time and in which the female mosquito oviposits. An old tire is as good as a tree-hole and females oviposit readily in them as well. In a number of instances, old tires were found to be the breeding sites of mosquitoes near houses.

Old tires were also determined to be the culprit in the importation of Ae. albopictus into the United States in 1985. Interestingly, in Asia used truck tires are not recapped but rather are sent in container ships to the United States where they are recapped and put back on the road. Old tires serve as oviposition sites for Ae. albopictus and the eggs withstand the sea voyage from eastern Asia to West Coast ports and to ports on the Gulf Coast. *Ae. albopictus* was first identified in the Houston, Texas, area, but it was later found to have been introduced into ports in California as well. This mosquito is an excellent vector of about 23 viruses. Of greatest interest to those living in the United States is that it is an efficient vector of the viruses causing St. Louis encephalitis, Dengue, and yellow fever. Fortunately Ae. albopictus has not been proven to have transmitted any disease agents in the United States yet.

We see in these examples that economics, rapid transport, and the adaptability of potential vectors intersect both in the distribution of vectors and their likelihood of transmitting a pathogen to humans. If it were economical to recap truck tires in Asia, *Ae. albopictus* might not have been imported into the United States. Since it is now a resident here, a whole industry has sprung up to decipher the biology of the mosquito as well as to determine its potential as a vector and means of controlling it.

Ecology

Certain biological and behavioral characteristics of mosquitoes are important in relation to their ability to serve as vectors of disease agents. The categories are used principally in relation to humans, but they apply equally well to domestic animals:

(1) Domiciliated species that have sites of larval development in or near houses readily enter dwellings and feed primarily on human blood; they usually rest in houses. They usually fly only a few hundred meters from the site of emergence. Aedes aegypti and Culex pipiens are examples of mosquitoes that transmit arboviruses. Several species of Anopheles that vector malaria fall into this group; *An. stephensi* is an example of a malaria vector that is a truly urban mosquito.

(2) Species that regularly come into contact with humans outdoors and may enter

houses but do not rest there. They breed in wet fields, irrigation ditches, swamps, and standing water that is either natural or made by humans such as tree holes, banana trees, tin cans, or old tires. *Culex tarsalis*, *Ae. albopictus*, and *Mansonia* are examples.

(3) Salt- or fresh-water marsh, temporary rain pool breeders, or floodwater breeders. Eggs are laid in dry or damp areas and adults emerge five days after rain or flooding or emerge the following season. Concentrations of preadults may be extraordinarily high: as many as 20 million larvae/hectare (50 million/acre). *Ae. sollicitans* and *An. taeniorhynchus* are examples; they may migrate 70km (40 miles) from the site of emergence. *Psorophora* spp. are also included since they are single brood per year mosquitoes in the Arctic and high mountain areas.

(4) Forest canopy mosquitoes breed in tree holes or water-holding portions of leaves such as the axils of bromeliads. These species come into contact with humans only under special circumstances such as lumbering where trees are cut and thereby carry mosquitoes down to the ground or when trees are planted for shade near dwellings. *Ae. africanus* is an example.

Another classification of mosquito habitat relies on the type of water rather than emphasizing the association with humans: flowing stream, ponded stream, lake edge, swamp and marsh, shallow permanent pond, intermittent ephemeral puddle, natural container, and artificial container.

The feeding preferences of mosquitoes are important in their abilities to serve as vectors as well as their being pests of humans and domesticated animals. Most mosquitoes have preferences for certain groups of vertebrates: birds, reptiles, amphibia, or mammals, but in some instances they switch hosts as the situation demands. Certain floodwater or marsh mosquitoes are bird feeders and do not feed on humans. *Culex tarsalis* is the principal vector of St. Louis encephalitis (SLE) in the western United States. SLE has its reservoir in birds, and in the spring, *Cx. tarsalis* feeds on nestling birds, which are the amplifying hosts; as the summer progresses, nestlings fledge and are no longer readily available. *Cx. tarsalis* then switches to mammals for blood and may come to feed on humans thereby transmitting the virus. The anopheline vectors of malaria must have humans as their preferred hosts for transmission to be optimized.

We tend to think that blood feeding is essential for mosquitoes, and this is true in some species. However, some species and some demes can lay eggs without a blood meal; this capability is called autogeny. Usually only a few eggs are laid, perhaps 10% of the normal complement, but it is sufficient to keep the genetic line intact.

(5) Both male and female mosquitoes take nectar as a source of energy, but only the females take blood. Nectar is an essential nutrient for the males both for the energy

it provides as well as the water that is needed for survival. Although autogeny is a heritable trait, larvae that do not have good nutrition and do not carry over food reserves to the adult stage cannot produce eggs autogenously. Parenthetically, it should be noted that autogeny is not parthenogenesis, males are needed to fertilize the eggs.

Blood provides a good source of protein for production of eggs, but it is not by any means a perfect food. It is lacking in carbohydrate and fat so these sources of energy are not available. Energy must be sought from blood components such as proline. Also, blood has antibodies and leukocytes that may be harmful to a hematophagous insect. Blood also is low in vitamin content, and this lack is often made up by symbiotic bacteria in the cells of the intestine.

The female mosquito finds a host through a series of stereotyped maneuvers. The female flies at a right angle to the wind so that aromas drifting downwind cross its flight path. Once having encountered a plume of CO_2 or body odor from a potential host, the female turns upwind. As the mosquito approaches a host, it uses visual clues, heat, and moisture to decide that there is something worthwhile nearby.

Having reached a potential host, the female probes the skin to determine whether it should attempt to feed. Both lactic acid and octenol are stimulants to feeding. The mosquito salivates and probes searching for a capillary. When a capillary is found, or the mouthparts enter a hematoma formed by probing, the cibarial pump is activated and the midgut is filled. Stretch receptors in the midgut respond in order to stop feeding.

Knowing When to Quit

If left undisturbed, a mosquito will feed to repletion. A female mosquito may take up to four times her body weight in blood during two or three minutes of feeding. Blood, unlike other nutrients such as nectar, goes directly to the midgut. A fully fed mosquito is laden with an enormous quantity of fluid, and the meal is reduced in volume by excretion of water via the Malpighian tubules. Thus concentrated, the blood meal is then more manageable.

It is essential that a mosquito not take too much blood. The signal to terminate blood feeding comes from stretch receptors in the wall of the abdomen. This can be clearly demonstrated in a mosquito that has had its ventral nerve cords severed at the point where they enter the abdomen. Such a mosquito can feed, but it doesn't know when or how to quit. It continues to ingest blood until it literally explodes, showering the area with blood. It is not a pretty sight.

Relationship with Diseases

Cosmopolitan. "Ubiquitous" might be a better term for mosquitoes since they are everywhere that has the tiniest amount of water in which the larvae can develop. It is difficult to overstate the importance of mosquitoes to human and animal welfare. Not only do they suck blood and make life intolerable at certain times and places, but they also transmit a huge number of disease agents of humans and other animals (see Table

14-2-1). In addition to the few organism listed in the tabulation, mosquitoes transmit hundreds of arboviruses (arthropod-borne viruses) such as Cache Valley virus, Crimean Hemorrhagic Fever virus, and Japanese Encephalitis B virus; there are so many that it is not possible to give anything other than a brief glimpse of the agents. All of these agents (except dengue virus) cycle silently in the wild and may be transmitted to humans or livestock under certain conditions.

Table 14-2-1 Some Disease Agents Transmitted by Mosquitoes

Disease agent and disease	**Hosts Natural**	**Hosts Tangential**	**Vectors**
Eastern equine Bird encephalitis	Bird	Human	*Coquilletidia perfurbans*
Venezuelan encephalitis	Small mammal	Human horse	*C. pipiens*, etc.
Western equine encephalitis	Bird	Human horse	*C. tarsalis*
Dengue	Human		*Ae. aegypti*, *Ae. albopictus*
Japanese encephalitis	Swine	Human	*C. tritaeniorhynchus*
St Lonis encephalitis	Bird	Human	*C. pipiens*, *C. nigripalpus*
Yellow fever	Primate	Human	*Ae. Aegypti* *Ae. afticanus*
LaCrosse encephalitis	Rodent	Human	*Ae. triseriatus*
Apicomplexa			
Malaria	Human		*Anopheles* spp.
Malaria	Bird		*Culex* spp.
Filarioid Nematode			
Wuchereria bancrofti	Human		*Culex*, *Mansonia*
Brugia malayi	Cat	Human	*Culex*, *Matlsorlia*
Dirofflaria Canid immitis	Canid	Human	*Culex*, *Aedes* spp.

The most important significance of mosquitoes focuses on the mosquito-borne diseases though they may give rise to annoyance through their biting. There are four main diseases transmitted by mosquitoes in China: malaria, filariasis, epidemic type B encephalitis (Japanese encephalitis) and dengue fever.

Malaria

Malaria is an infectious disease of humans, which is caused by 4 species of protozoa, that is, *Plasmodium vivax*, *P. falciparum*, *P. malariae* and *P. ovale*.

Only *Anopheles* mosquitoes are the transmitting vectors of malaria. The important vectors for malaria in China are *Anopheles sinensis*, *An. minimus*, *An. anthropophagus* and *An. dirus*, etc.

Filariasis

Eight species of filariae of human beings have been documented in the world, causing various types of filariasis, which involves different kinds of vectors. In China, two important types of filariasis (bancrofian filariasis and brugia filariasis) caused by *Wuchereria bancrofti* and *Brugia malayi* are transmitted by mosquito vectors. The most important vectors of Wuchereria bancrofti in China are *Culex pipiens pallens*, *C. pipiens quinquefastiatus* and *Anopheles sinensis* while the vectors of *Brugia malayi* are *Anopheles anthropophagus* and *An. sinensis*, etc.

Epidemic type B encephalitis

Epidemic type B encephalitis is also called Japanese B encephalitis and its pathogen is Japanese encephalitis virus (JEV). The disease mainly distributes in eastern Asia and it is transmitted through the biting of mosquitoes. *Culex tritaeniorhychus* is the most important vector of the disease.

Dengue fever and dengue hemorrhagic fever

Dengue fever and dengue hemorrhagic fever are the virus diseases, caused by dengue virus, distributing in Southeast Asia and North America. *Aedes albopictus* is important vector in China.

Others

In some other parts of the world, mosquitoes are also the vectors of Chikungunya disease, yellow fever, eastern equine encephalitis, western equine encephalitis, Venezuelan equine encephalitis and St. Louis encephalitis, etc. All these diseases are virus diseases. There probably exists Chikungunya disease in some regions of China (Yunnan Province, for example).

Epidemiology and Control

Control of mosquito populations requires an area-wide program except in instances where the rooms of a dwelling might be sprayed to clear them of adults. The definition on an area depends on the particular mosquito(s) of concern as well as drainages, water courses, and prevailing winds. Different species of mosquito have different flight ranges, and as indicated earlier, different types of breeding sites. In short, the type of control program is determined by the species of mosquito that is the pest or vector.

Because their habitats and foods are so different, the control of larval and adult mosquitoes is also radically different.

Larval Control

(1) Chemical

① No. 2 diesel oil may be applied to the surface of water. Larvae come to the surface of the water to obtain air (except for Mansonia and Co-quilletiddia) and are killed by becoming covered in oil. Diesel oil also has a component that is directly toxic to larvae.

② Insecticide is placed in the water. The materials most often used now are second- and third-generation insecticides. The organochlorine insecticides have been phased out in most countries, and organophosphates and carbamates are currently being used. Among third-generation insecticides, juvenile hormone (JH) mimetics can be used in waters where food products are not consumed by humans. JH mimetics have the advantage of not causing environmental contamination, and they are specific for insects; the second-generation insecticides may affect fish, birds, and mammals in addition to the target organisms.

(2) Biological

① Predators

a. Fish such as Gambusia

b. *Toxorhynchites* larvae

c. Nematodes such as *Romanomermis petersoni*

d. Planaria that prey on larvae

② Disease agents

a. Microspora such as *Nosema algerae*

b. Bacteria such as *Bacillus thuringiensis israeliensis* (Bti) and *B. sphaericus*. Bti is a toxi-cant rather than a disease agent since it kills mosquito larvae when they ingest the spores that have a crystal of toxin; no reproduction of the bacterium takes place; that said, it is usually included among biological control agents.

(3) Source reduction or habitat management

This method refers specifically to the techniques that do not use chemicals directly to kill insects and are not included under biological control; it can be thought of as physically altering the environment. For mosquitoes, the methods are as follows:

① Fill or drain swampy areas.

② Remove aquatic plants that impede water flow or provide oviposition sites.

③ Remove manufactured sources of standing water such as tin cans, tires, and flower pots.

④ Use irrigation water properly so that ditches can be flushed or waste water does not accumulate in ditches or at the low ends of fields.

Adult Control

(1) Insecticides

① Direct action

Insecticide is sprayed into the air and kills mosquitoes that fly into the spray. Compounds used are carbamates, organophosphates, and pyrethrins.

② Residual action

Insecticide is sprayed onto a surface or released from a carrier into a closed space. Organochlorine insecticides usually have a long residual action when sprayed onto surfaces in homes; because of environmental damage, organochlorines have been banned in many parts of the world. Organophosphates have only a short residual action but can be released slowly from a plastic carrier.

Personal Protection

(1) Repellents or barriers

① Deet repels insects and may be placed on the skin or impregnated into clothing as has been developed for military personnel. A combination of Deet and a synthetic pyrethroid has been successful both spread on the skin or impregnated into clothing.

② Screening of houses and use of mosquito netting at night. It is interesting to note that in areas of the United States where mosquitoes and mosquito-borne diseases have been historically important, they have become less so. Since the late 1940s both air conditioning and television have become common, and people spend less time in the cool evening air when mosquitoes are searching for a blood meal.

③ Use of barrier animals or zooprophylaxis. Since mosquitoes have feeding preferences, those which prefer animals other than humans may be kept away by providing an ox, say, as a diversion. Although possible to use, this method is not ordinarily purposefully employed.

(2) Traps

Various kinds of devices that emit ultra-violet light lure insects so that they are either electrocuted or drowned in a detergent solution. They may reduce mosquito populations as well as those of other harmless insects.

(3) Sound generators are sometimes marketed with the claim that certain frequencies drive away mosquitoes. These claims have not been substantiated.

(4) Birds

Purple martins are known to eat large numbers of insects, and some people provide houses to encourage their nesting near homes. Whether the birds actually reduce mosquito populations is unknown.

(Chen Xiaoguang)

Section 3 Fly

In zoological taxonomy, fly belongs to suborder Cyclorrhapha, order Diptera in class insecta. Over 10,000 known fly species have been recorded in the world and more than 1,500 species in China. Most species of flies associated with human diseases belong to four families, namely Muscidae, Calliphoridae, Sarcophagidae and Oestridae. The most important species mechanically transmitting human diseases are *Musca domestica vicina*, *Chrysomyia megacephala*, *Aldrichina grahami*, *Lucilia sericata*, *Boettcherisca peregrina* and *Stomoxys calcitrans*, etc.

Morphology

An adult fly has a pair of compound eyes, three ocelli and a pair of antennae on the head. The compound eyes are widely separated in females (wider spacing between two eyes) while narrowly separated in male (narrower spacing between two eyes) in most flies except Sarcophagidae. Each antenna has a special structure called arista. Most fly species have a lapping mouthpart which is composed of base proboscis with a pair of pedipalps, middle proboscis and labellum. There are many pseudotracheae on the ventral side of the labellum. Some bloodsucking flies have a piercing-sucking mouthpart like female mosquitoes while some others have a degenerated mouthpart. Of three parts of thorax, mesothorax is the most developed and obvious, with many bristles and stripes on its scutum. On the thorax, there are three pairs of legs, and each leg has a claw pad (pulvillus) with lots of tiny thin hairs at the end. The special venation on the two wings is composed of costa, subcosta and six longitudinal veins without branches. Of 10 segments of abdomen, five segments are visible while others evolved to external genitalia (see Figure 14-3-1 and Figure 14-3-2).

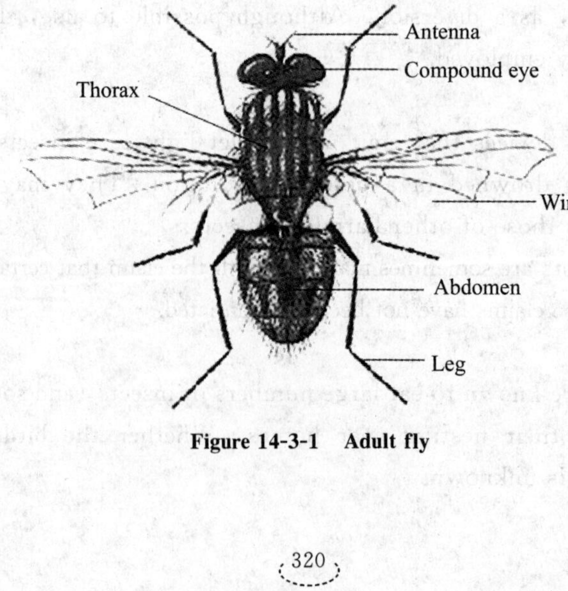

Figure 14-3-1 Adult fly

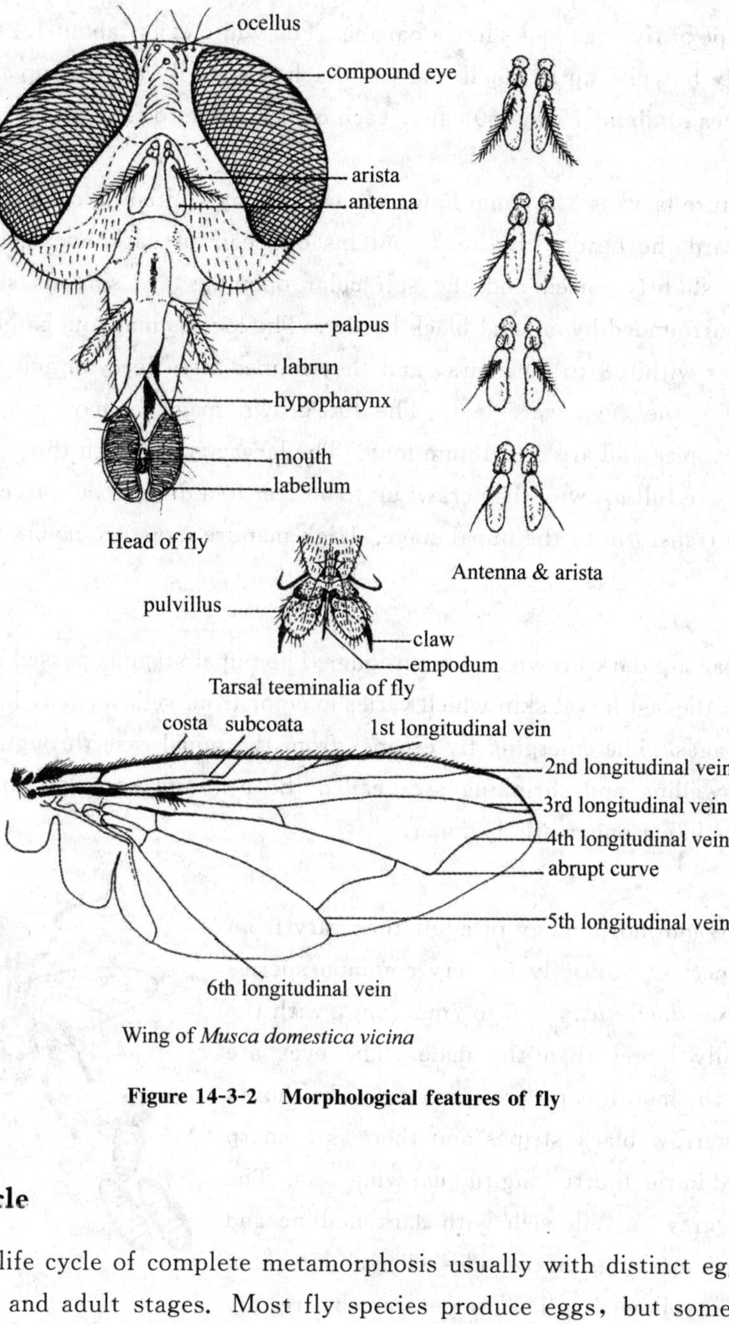

Figure 14-3-2 Morphological features of fly

Life Cycle

Fly has a life cycle of complete metamorphosis usually with distinct egg, larva or maggot, pupal and adult stages. Most fly species produce eggs, but some species in Sarcophagidae may directly produce larvae. Generally, fly overwinters in either larval or pupal stage under manure piles or in other protected locations. Warm summer conditions are optimum for the development of house fly, and it completes its life cycle in as little as seven to ten days, and as many as 10 to 12 generations may occur in one summer (see Figure 14-3-3).

Egg

The shape of fly eggs looks like a banana. The white eggs, about 1.2mm in length, are laid singly but pile up in small masses. Each female fly can lay up to 500 eggs in several batches of about 75 to 150 eggs, each over a three to four day period.

Larva

The mature larva is 3 to 9mm long, typical creamy whitish in color, cylindrical but tapering toward the head. The head contains one pair of dark hooks. The posterior spiracles are slightly raised and the spiracular openings are sinuous slits which are completely surrounded by an oval black border. The legless maggots hatch from eggs in warm weather within 8 to 20 hours, and they immediately feed on and develop in the material where the eggs were laid. The full-grown maggots have a greasy, cream-colored appearance and are 8 to 12mm long. The larvae go through three instars. When the maggots are full-grown, they crawl up to 50 feet to a dried, cool place near breeding material and transform to the pupal stage. High manure moisture favors the survival of fly larvae.

Pupa

Fly pupae are dark brown and 8mm long. The pupal stage is passed in a pupal case formed from the last larval skin which varies in color from yellow, red, brown, to black as the pupa ages. The emerging fly escapes from the pupal case through the use of an alternately swelling and shrinking sac, called the ptilinum, on the front of its head which it uses like a pneumatic hammer.

Adult

The size and morphology of adult flies vary from species to species. Housefly (a very common species of fly), *Musca domestica*, is 6 to 7mm long, with the female usually larger than the male. The eyes are reddish and the mouth parts are sponging. The thorax bears four narrow black stripes and there is a sharp upward bend in the fourth longitudinal wing vein. The abdomen is gray or yellowish with dark midline and irregular dark markings on the sides. The underside of the male is yellowish. The sexes can be readily separated by noting the space between the eyes, which in females is almost twice as broad as in males.

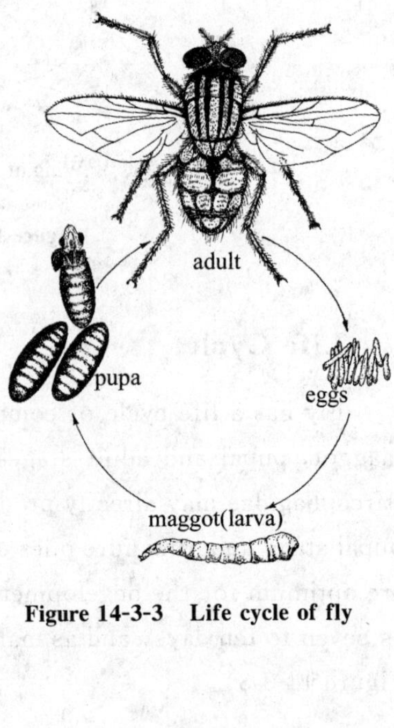

Figure 14-3-3 Life cycle of fly

Ecology

Female flies usually produce their eggs in feces, garbage, putrid plants or decaying flesh, etc. The larvae of most flies (houseflies for example) feed on organic substance, and their breeding places are usually the same as oviposition sites. Three feeding types of adult flies have been documented: (1) Most fly species are omnivorous, house fly or *Musca domestica*, for example. They have lapping mouthparts and do not piercing for bloodmeal, but instead feed on a variety of food, including feces, decaying animals or plants, excretory substance and humans' food, etc. Omnivorous flies are usually guttlers (engorging omnivores) with no-stopping eating habit. They often vomit and excrete while eating, which is very important in mechanically transmitting diseases. (2) Some adult flies with piercing-mouthparts have to suck blood from animals or humans for their development as seen in *Stomoxys calcitrans* and tsetsefly, and both their males and females feed on blood. (3) Some others with degenerated mouthparts do not eat at all at their adult stages. Flies are skillful at flying and they usually fly around at daytime. They have preference to light. Most flies hibernate at pupa stage while others hibernate at larvae or adult stages.

Relationship with Diseases

Direct injury

Main direct injury of most flies comes from their annoyance and direct parasitism. Myiasis is an infection caused by the direct parasitism of the larvae of some *Diptera* insects, especially the maggots of flies. The term, myiasis, is useful in describing the location of the larvae: gastrointestinal myiasis for invasion of the digestive system; nasopharyngeal myiasis for nose, sinuses and pharynx; auricular myiasis for the ears; ophthalmic myiasis for the eyes; cutaneous myiasis when the larvae burrow through the skin. Some flies bite painfully, sucking blood from humans and animals.

Indirect injury

Three kinds of indirect injury are associated with flies: (1) Tsetse flies are known to be the vector of African trypanosomiasis (sleeping sickness). An individual will get African trypanosomiasis if he is bitten by tsetse flies (*Glossina* infected with the *Trypanosoma* parasite. The tsetse fly is common only in Africa. (2) House flies may serve as intermediate hosts for *Thelazia callipaeda* (a species of parasitic nematodes) which is the pathogen of thelazia in dogs and cats, etc. (3) Most species of omnivorous flies can mechanically transmit more than 100 pathogens. For example, house flies may mechanically spread diseases such as conjunctivitis, dysentery (shigellosis), amebic dysentery, cholera, poliomyelitis, salmonellosis, typhoid fever, tuberculosis, anthrax, leprosy and yaws, etc.

Control

The more common measures in the control of flies are sanitation, use of traps, and insecticides, but in some instances the integrated control is also recommended.

Environment management

Sanitation or cultural control is the basic step in all fly management. Food and materials on which the flies can lay their eggs must be removed, destroyed as a breeding medium, or isolated from the egg-laying adult. Killing adult flies may reduce the infestation, but elimination of breeding areas is necessary for good management. Garbage cans and dumpsters should have tight-fitting lids and be cleaned regularly. Dry garbage and trash should be placed in plastic garbage bags and sealed up. All garbage receptacles should be located as far from building entrances as possible. For control at waste disposal sites, refuse should be deposited onto the same area as inorganic wastes to deteriorate the capacity of breeding resources, or the disposed refuse should be covered with soil or other inorganic wastes (about 15cm in thickness).

Physical control

Fly traps may be useful in some fly control programs if enough traps are used, if they are placed correctly, and if they are used both indoors and outdoors. House flies are attracted to white surfaces and to baits that give off odors. Indoors, ultraviolet light traps collect the flies inside an inverted cone or kill them with an electrocuting grid.

Chemical control

The application of adulticides or larvicides (similar to mosquito control) can directly or indirectly suppress adult densities. Residual wall sprays can be applied where the flies congregate. Resistance to some insecticide (permethrin, for example), however, develops more rapidly in fly populations, at this situation, the insecticide applied should be alternated.

Biological control

With the increasing incidence of insecticide resistance in fly populations and environmental pollution, some other alternative control strategies including biological control have been taken into account. The use of biological control, however, at present time, in fly management is still at a relatively early stage.

Section 4 Sand Fly

Morphology

Sand flies are small insects and the adults are about 1. 5mm to 4mm long with a pair of dark compound eyes on their head and many tiny hairs on their body. Female adults have a piercing-sucking mouthpart and they have a pair of thin-long antennae on the head and two membranous wings on the thorax. Female sand flies suck the blood of humans and other animals through their piercing-sucking mouthparts, but males' mouthparts are not suitable for piercing skin (see Figure 14-4-1 and Figure 14-4-2).

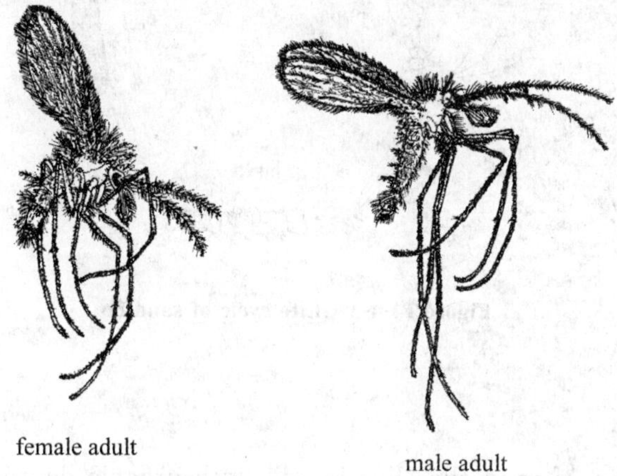

Figure 14-4-1 Adult of sand fly

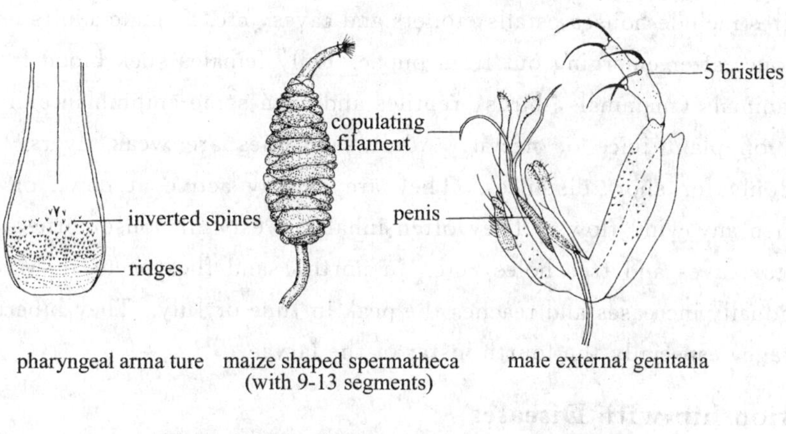

Figure 14-4-2 Important structures of sand fly

Life Cycle

Sand flies undergo a complete metamorphosis in their life cycle: eggs, larvae, pupae and adults. Each female lays oval eggs that hatch in 6 to 12 days into larvae. The larvae have 4 instars. Larvae grow and pupate in 25 to 30 days. The life cycle from egg to adult may be from 6 to 8 weeks in warm weather (see Figure 14-4-3).

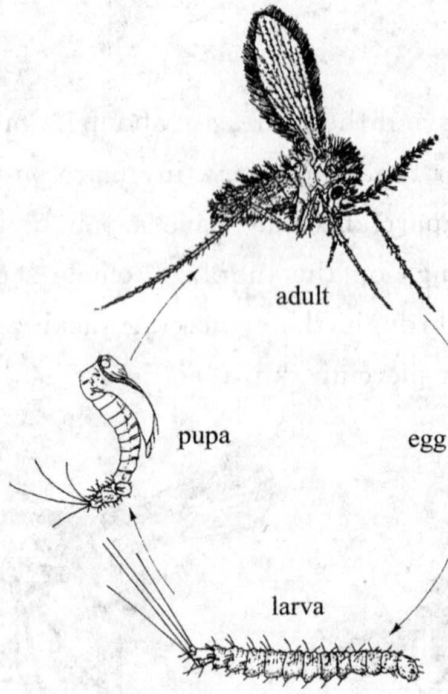

Figure 14-4-3 Life cycle of sand fly

Ecology

The early stages of sand flies live in soil with organic debris on which the larvae feed, and they are often found 10-12cm deep under the surface of the soil. The suitable breeding sites include houses, stalls, toilets and caves, etc. Female adults usually mate with male ones after emerging out from pupae. Only females suck blood from humans and other animals (mammals, birds, reptiles and even some amphibian animals) while males feed on plant juice or nectar. Adult sand flies are weak flyers, capable of navigation only for short distances. They are usually active at dawn or dusk, but inactive when any wind flows. They often inhabit (rest) in house corners, crevices, animal nests, caves and tree holes, etc. In north, sand flies occur in May, and the density gradually increases and reaches the peak in June or July. They hibernate in soil at larval stage, especially the fourth instar of the larvae.

Relationship with Diseases

Direct injury

Sand flies are blood-sucking insects and their blood sucking activities can give rise to some annoyance.

Indirect injury

The indirect impairment of sand flies focuses on their disease transmission, especially as the vectors of some zoonoses. The sand fly born diseases include leishmaniasis, sand fly fever (pappataci fever) and bartonellosis, etc.

Leishmaniasis widely distributes in the world, and the pathogen of leishmaniasis is *Leishmania* protozoa, including *L. donovani*, *L. tropica*, *L. mexicana* and *L. braziliensis*, etc. Visceral leishmaniasis (Kala-azar) is caused by *L. donovani*, cutaneous leishmaniasis by both *L. tropica* and *L. mexicana* while mucocutaneous leishmaniasis by *L. braziliensis*. All types of leishmaniasis are transmitted by sand flies, and *Phlebotomus* are the most important vector, especially in China. *Phlebotomus chinensis* are the major vector of visceral leishmaniasis in China, and *Ph. chinensis longiductus*, *Ph. major wui* and *Ph. alexandri* come next.

Sand fly fever (also called pappataci fever) is a virus disease caused by the pathogen of sand fly fever virus and transmitted by some species of sand flies. The disease distributes in African, Asia and Europe, especially in Mediterranean areas.

Bartonellosis is also called Oroya fever or Carrion's disease, caused by the pathogen of *Bartonella bacilliformis*. It is mainly transmitted through *Ph. nonuchii* and *Ph. verrucarum*, etc.

Control

Sand flies are weak flyers and relatively easy to be controlled. The environment management is usually to improve the sanitation around the dwellings of humans, poultry and livestock. It is necessary to keep the surroundings clean and to remove rubbish to eliminate the breeding habitats of the larvae. Chemical control is often recommended as the major measure and most insecticides (including organochlorides, organophosphates, carbamates and pyrethroid) are usually effective to sand flies. It is often recommended to spray the insecticides such as DDT, malathion or deltamethrin (decamethrin) around the breeding habitats of larvae or the rest areas of adult sand flies. It is also important to avoid the disturbance of sand flies by using mosquito net, door screen, window screen and even repellents, etc.

Section 5 Flea

Fleas are a group of arthropods in order Siphonaptera in zoological taxonomy and they are blood-sucking insects. Over 2,500 species of fleas have been documented in the world and over 600 species and subspecies recorded in China.

Morphology

Fleas are secondarily wingless insects with piercing-sucking mouthparts in their adults. The colour of flea body may be light yellow, yellowish black, brown black or jet-black. The body is highly flattened laterally and is represented by 3 major parts:

head, thorax and abdomen. They have no wings and no compound eyes, the legs are modified for jumping, the antennae are very short and recessed in antennal fossa on the head. Thorax of fleas is provided with three pairs of legs; the hind legs are the longest. The shape of the head, the flat body shape and prehensile claws of legs help it to move easily through host wool. Length of jump some flea species attains 32cm, average body length being from 1 to 5mm (see Figure 14-5-1 and Figure 14-5-2).

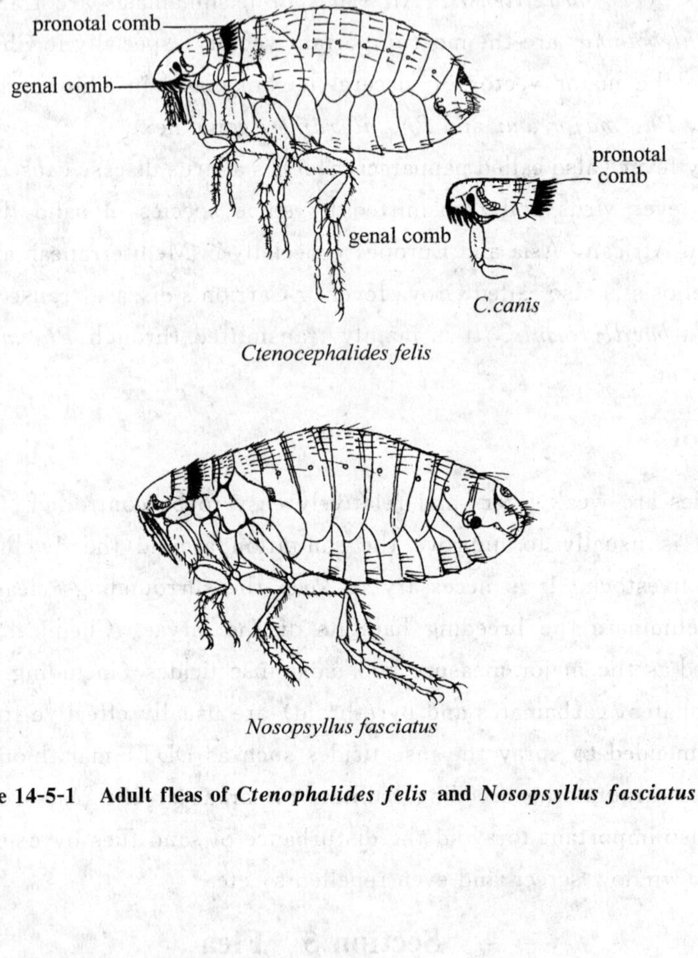

Figure 14-5-1 Adult fleas of *Ctenophalides felis* and *Nosopsyllus fasciatus*

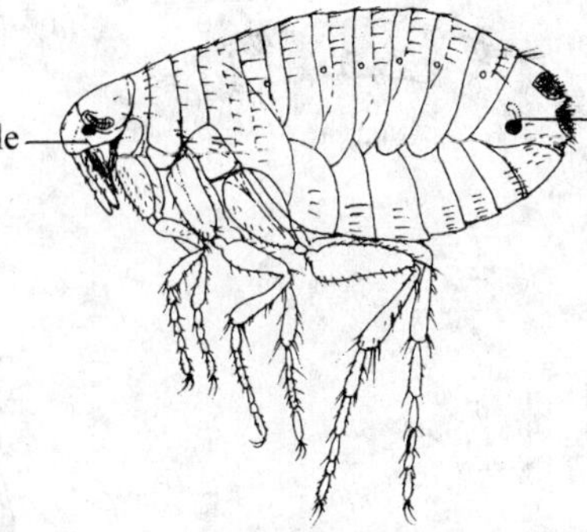

Pulex irritans

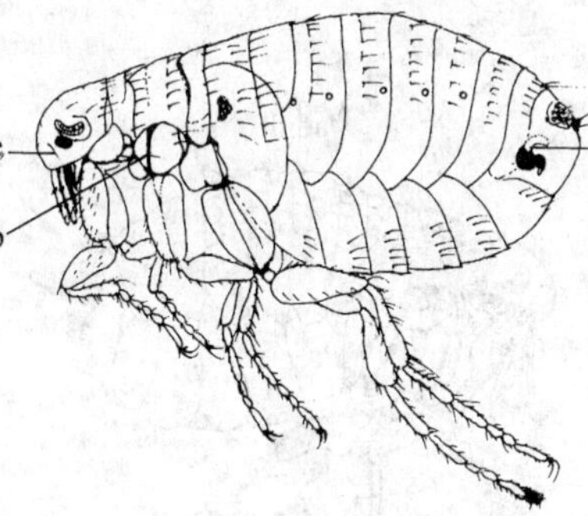

Xenopsylla cheopis

Figure 14-5-2 Adult fleas of *Pulex irritans* and *Xenopsylla cheopis*

Life Cycle

Fleas are obligatory ectoparasites and blood feeders, parasitizing warm-blooded vertebrates. More than 94% of known species are parasites of mammals and only about 5% of them occur on birds. The fleas have 4 phases of development: eggs, free-living larvae, pupae and imagoes or adults. They belong to holometabolic insects with complete metamorphosis. The larva is wormlike, legless and eyeless with biting mouthparts. The larva undergoes 3 instars. Prior to pupation it empties the alimentary canal, and spins a silken cocoon. Wormlike free-living legless flea larva develops in the litter of the host's nest. Although female fleas usually oviposit on the host, the eggs are not sticky and so drop off the host's body. This often happens in the host's nest or lair, where is a supply of detritus and flea feces on which larvae feed. The larvae hatch within 2 to 21 days; the larval instars require 9 to 15 days; and the pupa completes development in as short a time as a week. Fleas can survive long periods as adults without food, particularly under conditions of high humidity (see Figure 14-5-3).

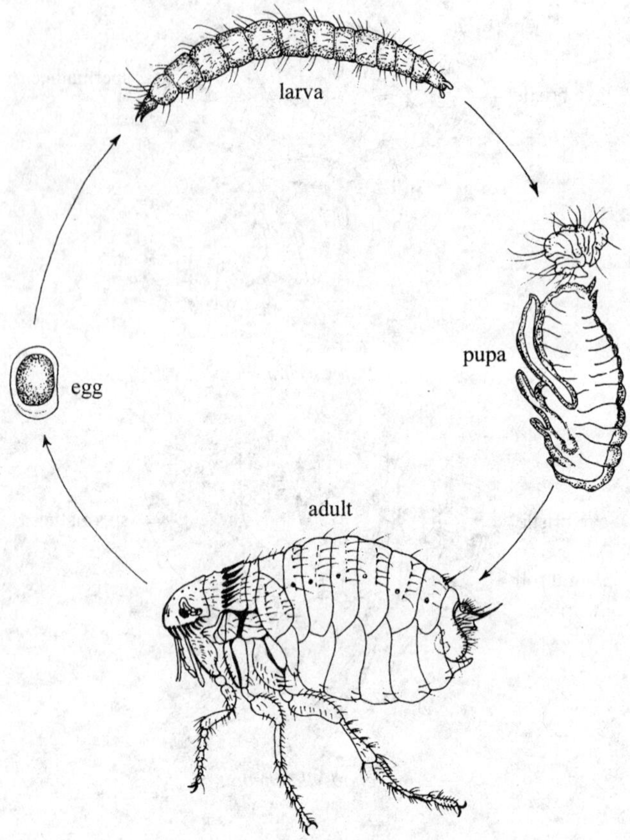

Figure 14-5-3 Life cycle of flea

Ecology

The majority of fleas are closely associated with the host's home (nest, burrow etc.), attacking the host for feeding. Both male and female adults are obligatory hematophages (sucking blood), parasitising warm-blooded animals including mammals and birds. Fleas are very sensitive to the body temperature of hosts. When host animal dies, fleas depart and seek new hosts and this is important in transmitting diseases. Fleas are widely spread on all continents, Antarctica included. They occur on hosts and in their nests in all types of habitats from the equatorial deserts and tropical rainforests to the northernmost regions of Arctic tundra. In general the largest number of species and genera of fleas occur in several regions with temperate subtropical climate and predominance of mountain landscapes.

Relationship with Diseases

Direct injury

Flea's blood sucking activity usually causes harassment (itching and dermatitis, etc.). Females of chigoe, *Tunga penetrans*, can burrow beneath the host skin and cause tungiasis. Tungiasis may happen in some wild animals (rodents for example), but seldom occur in humans.

Indirect injury

Fleas are known as vectors of plague, endemic typhus (murine typhus) and some other diseases.

Plague (or black-death) is caused by a bacterium, *Yersinia pestis*, and it is essentially a disease of rodents. Humans contact this disease through the bite of fleas. During rodent plague outbreaks, many animals die and their hungry fleas seek other sources of blood to survive. Persons and animals that visit places where rodents have recently died from plague risk getting the disease from flea bites. More than 200 species harbor the pathogen of plague (*Yersinia pestis*) in nature. There are chitinous agnails (reverse spine structure) in the proventriculus of flea. Plague bacteria multiply in the proventriculus and then form a bacterium embolus to block flea's digestive canal. The blockage of bacterium embolus gives rise to a reverse flow of blood back to the host's body. The hungry fleas have to frequently change their hosts for new blood meal because of the blockage and this prominently increases the transmission opportunity. Flea species with bacterium embolus are usually powerful vectors. For example, *Xenopsylla cheopis* has been proved to be a powerful effective vector of plague in China, especially in southwest regions.

Endemic typhus (murine typhus) caused by *Rickettsia mooseri* is also transmitted through fleas, mainly by *Xenopsylla cheopis* as well. The pathogen multiplies inside the intestinal epithelium of fleas and then passes out from flea feces. The transmission usually occurs when skin wound is contaminated by flea feces or liquid from crashed flea body.

In addition, some species of fleas can be an intermediate host of some tapeworms, such as *Dipylidium caninum*, *Hymenolepes nana* and *H. diminuta*.

Control

Of many mammals and birds (hosts of fleas), rodents (rats and mice) are the most important hosts. The control of fleas should be considered together with the control of rodents. It is a simple way to eliminate the nests of rodents and birds around the dwelling and to keep the environment (human house and the stable of livestock) clean. To prevent pets from the parasitism of fleas, it is simple and necessary to bathe them. Repellents are also recommended to avoid the disturbance of fleas.

Section 6　Louse

There are over 3, 000 species of louse species in the world and they are all obligate ectoparasites of mammals and birds, excluding monotremes (duck-billed platypus, for example) and bats. All the lice are wingless parasitic insects, belonging to an independent order in zoological taxonomy, order Phthiraptera. There are two groups of lice, that is, the sucking lice (suborder Anoplura) and chewing lice (suborder Mallophaga). Only sucking lice are medical insects (permanent ectoparasites) while chewing lice have little medical significance. Over 500 species of sucking lice have been documented in the world and they are all blood-feeding ectoparasites of mammals. At least two species of Anoplura, human louse (*Pediculus humanus*) and pubic louse (*Phthirus pubis*), are ectoparasites of humans. *Pediculus humanus* is divided into two subspecies, that is, *Pediculus humanus humanus* (body louse) and *Pediculus humanus capitis* (head louse). Apart from causing skin irritations, human lice are the vectors of several blood-borne diseases.

Morphology

Sucking lice (Anoplura) are small, wingless, dorsoventrally flattened, and have piercing-sucking mouthparts with reduced (or no) eyes. The body size of sucking lice ranges from 0.5mm to 8mm, and they have three pairs of legs. Their tarsal claws are often enlarged, which look like pincher claws of a crab, and this is an adaptation for clinging to hair and feathers. Body lice (*Pediculus humanus humanus*) are very similar to head lice (*Pediculus humanus capitis*), but pubic lice (*Phthirus pubis*) are very different. The adult pubic louse resembles a miniature crab (see Figure 14-6-1).

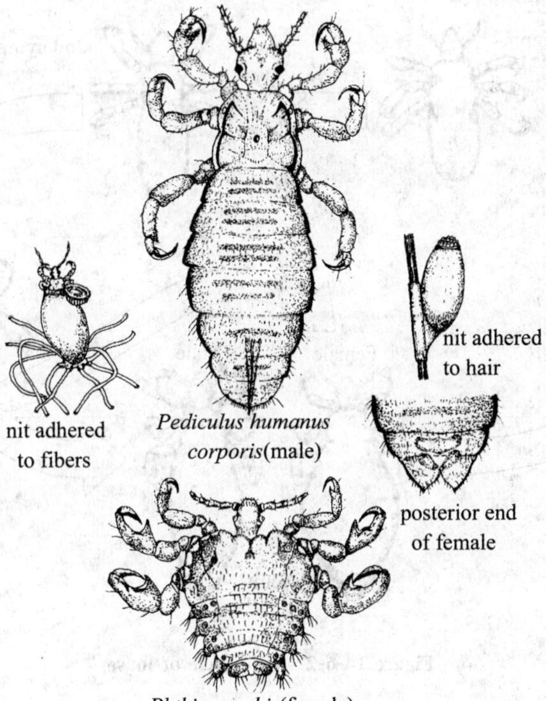

Figure 14-6-1 Human lice

Life Cycle

The life cycle of sucking lice belongs to hemimetabolic type (incomplete metamorphosis) with three stages, that is, egg, nymph and adult. A louse egg (commonly called a nit) is cemented to the hairs of their hosts and there are three nymphal instars. Females, usually larger than males, lay eggs on their hosts. Eggs are oval and usually yellow to white. Eggs take about one week to hatch. The egg hatches into a baby louse called a nymph. The nymph looks like an adult louse, but is smaller. Nymphs mature into adults about 7 days after hatching (see Figure 14-6-2).

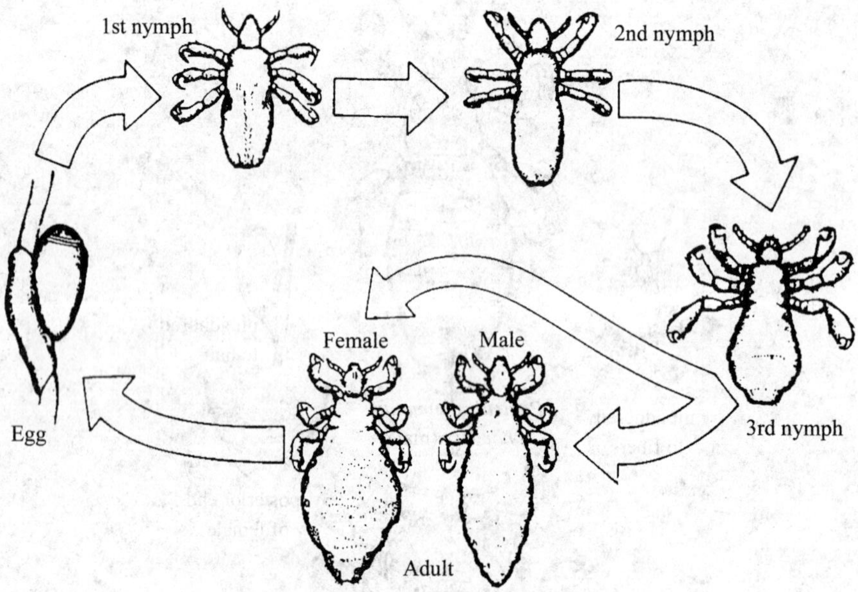

Figure 14-6-2 Life cycle of louse

Ecology

Sucking lice are blood sucking insects. To live, adult lice (both male and female) and three instars of nymphs need to feed on blood. If the louse falls off a person, it dies within 1-2 days. If the host has a high fever or dies, the louse has to leave him and to search for a new host, and this provide an opportunity in the transmission of louse born diseases. The life span of female lice is usually 30-60 days while that of males is shorter. As lice spend their whole life on the host (permanent ectoparasites), they have developed adaptations which enable them to maintain a close contact with the host. These adaptations are reflected in their size (0. 5mm to 8mm), stout legs and claws in order to cling tightly to hairs and cloth fibers, wingless and dorsoventrally flattened. Their colour varies from pale beige to dark grey.

The lice are highly host specific and many species even prefer specific sites on their host's body. Head lice (*Pediculus humanus capitis*) are exquisitely adapted to living mainly on the scalp and neck hairs of their human host. Lice present on other body parts covered by hair are not head lice but are either *Pubic lice* (*Pthirus pubis*) or body lice (*Pediculus humanus humanus*). Pubic lice are specialized to live in the human pubic hair, but may also live in hair on other areas of the body such as hair on the legs, armpit, mustache, beard, eyebrows and eyelashes. Infestations of young children are usually on the eyebrows or eyelashes.

Relationship with Diseases

Direct injury

The louse feeds on human blood and its blood-sucking activity causes itching, which can become secondarily infected when scratching break the skin. The most common symptom is itching. Pubic lice are normally spread by sexual contact and are considered a sexually transmitted disease, but can also be spread by sharing clothes or bedding. Since lice cannot live long away from a warm human body and also lice do not have feet designed to walk or hold onto smooth surfaces such as toilet seats, the infestation isn't likely to be spread by sitting on a toilet seat.

Indirect injury

Apart from direct parasitism on the body and cause direct injury, human louse (*Pediculus humanus*) has long been proved to be the vector of several louse born diseases, epidemic typhus (louse-borne typhus), Trench fever (quintan fever) and epidemic relapsing fever (louse-borne relapsing fever). Nowadays, with the improvement of personal sanitation and health condition, all the louse born diseases are becoming very rare in the developed countries and regions.

Epidemic typhus (louse borne typhus) is caused by the pathogen of *Richettsia prowazekii*. The pathogen multiplies inside the intestinal epithelium of lice and then passes out from louse feces. The transmission usually occurs when skin wound is contaminated by louse feces or liquid from crashed louse body.

Trench fever (quintan fever) is caused by another *rickettsia*, *Bartonella quintana*. The pathogen also multiplies inside the intestinal epithelium of lice and passes out from louse feces. The transmission of trench fever is similar to that of epidemic typhus.

Epidemic relapsing fever (louse borne relapsing fever) is caused by a spirochete, *Borrelia recurrents*. Since the pathogen only multiplies inside louse hemocele, it can not be passed out from louse feces. The transmission only occurs when crashed louse liquid contaminates skin wounds.

Control

Personal sanitation is of great importance in the control of lice, including bath, shower, changing clothes and underwears, etc. Body lice and head lice are easily killed by 1% permethrin or pyrethrin shampoo, but the pubic hair can be shaved off to remove the nits (eggs) of pubic louse. Lice can survive in bedding and clothing, so these items must be treated, sterilized, or contact with them must be avoided for two weeks, after which time any louse will have died. Lindane (1%), another insecticide, is not recommended for pregnant or nursing women or for children less than 2 years old.

Section 7 Other Insects

Bedbug

Bedbugs are red-brown and wingless insects with the size of 4-5mm long and about 3mm wide. Only two species (*Cimex lectularis* and *C. hemipterus*) are of medical importance, which suck human blood. Bedbugs belong to family Cimicidae in order Hemiptera and with incomplete metamorphosis in their life cycle: egg, nymph and adult. Both nymph and adult bedbugs are bloodsucking insects, often disturbing humans. They usually hide in bedding, clothes, and dark spaces. Bed bugs, however, don't transmit diseases, so their bites are merely unpleasant and itchy (see Figure 14-7-1, Figure 14-7-2 and Figure 14-7-3).

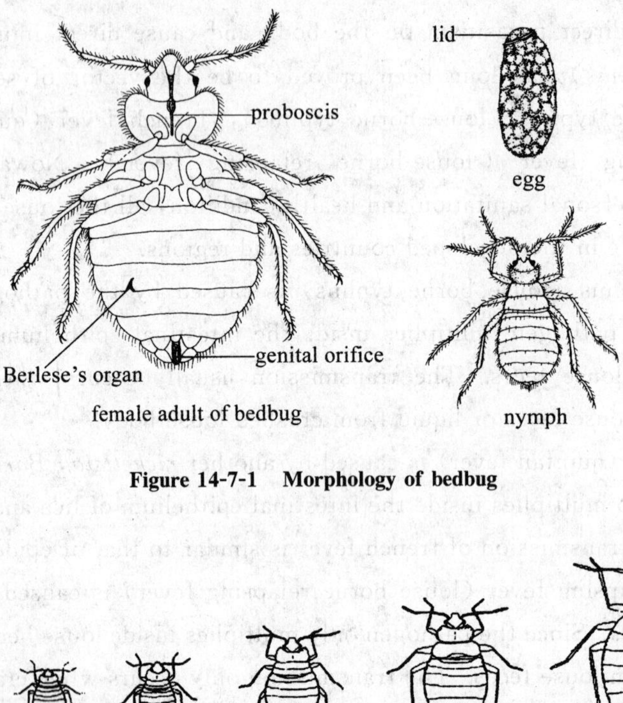

Figure 14-7-1 Morphology of bedbug

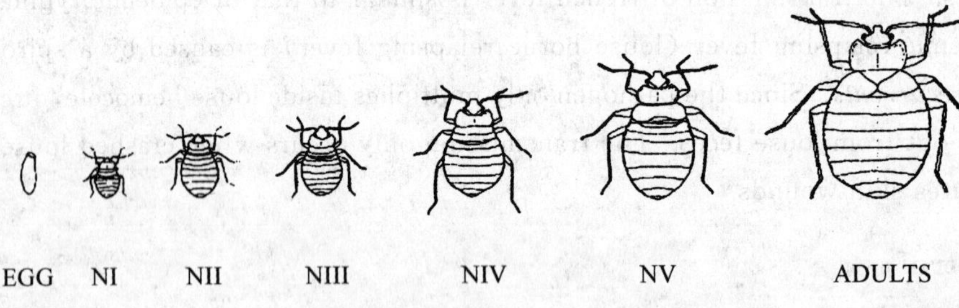

Figure 14-7-2 Life cycle of bedbug

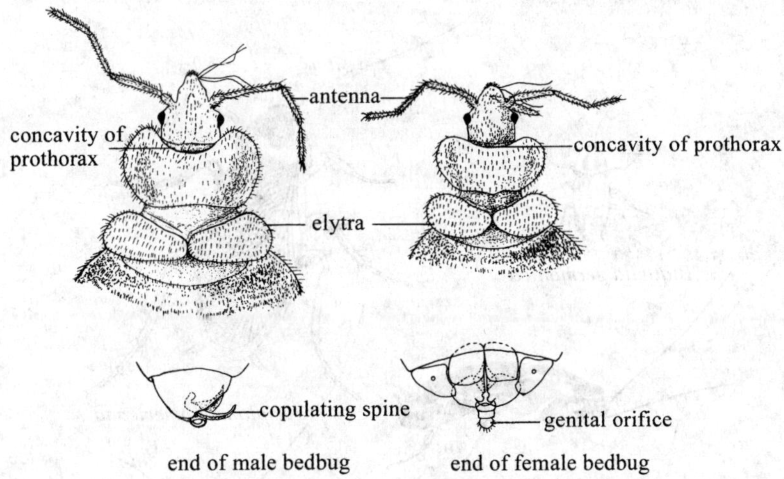

Figure 14-7-3 Important structures of bedbug

Cockroach

Cockroaches belong to order Blattaria in Insecta. There are over 5,000 species in about 350 families in the world, and about 240 species (belonging to 60 genera in 18 families) in China. The adults are dorsal-ventrally flattened with two pairs of wings, and they are quick walker with three pairs of strong legs. Cockroaches are hemimetabolic insects with incomplete metamorphosis and they have three basic stages in their life cycle: egg, nymph and adult. Eggs are usually inside an ootheca. A nymph resembles an adult morphologically (see Figure 14-7-4 and Figure 14-7-5).

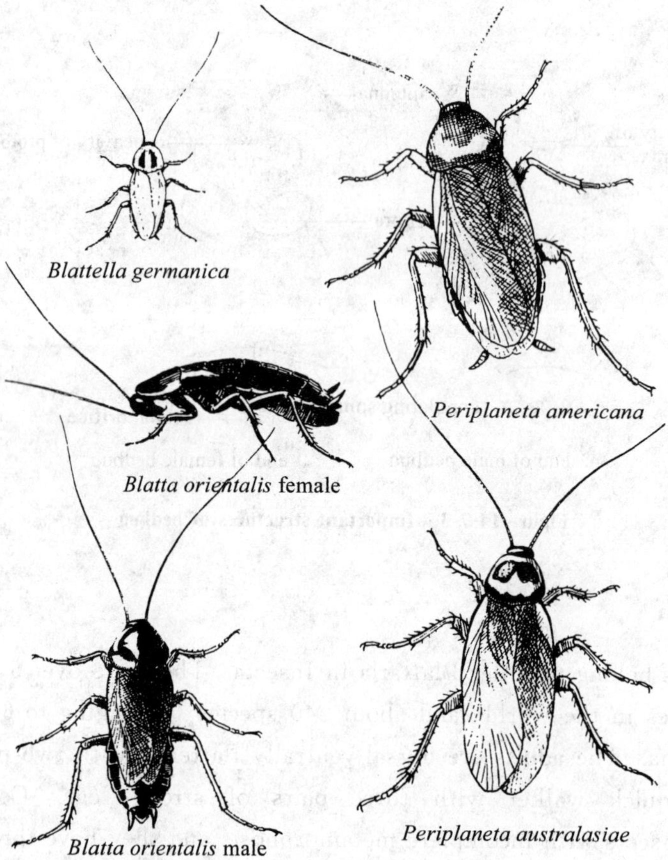

Figure 14-7-4　Common cockroaches

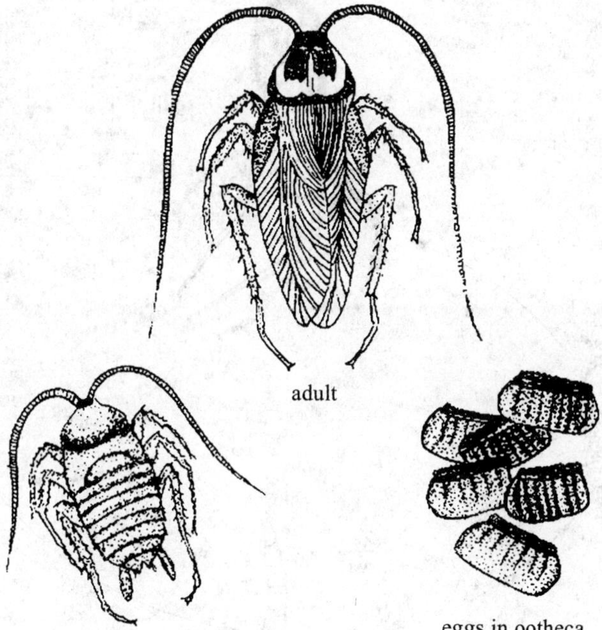

Figure 14-7-5 Life cycle of cockroach

Cockroaches are widely distributed insects and often found in houses, especially kitchen. They are omnivorous insects, feeding on a variety of food such as excretory (or secretory) substance of humans and animals, dead body of animals and humans' food, etc. The medical importance of cockroaches is similar to house flies and focuses on their mechanical transmission of some diseases, including poliomyelitis, salmonellosis, amebic dysentery and even toxoplasmosis, etc. In some instance, cockroaches may be as intermediate hosts of *Gongylonema pulchrum*, *Trichostrongylus orientalis*, *Hymenolepis diminuta* and *Moniliformis moniliformis*, etc. In addition, the antigen of cockroaches can give rise to allergic reaction.

Biting Midge

Biting midges are small insects and their adults range from 1 to 2.5mm with two wings. They belong to an independent family, Ceratoponidae, in order Diptera. Over 4,000 species of biting midges, belonging to 70 genera, have been recorded in the world, and over 300 species in China. The life cycle of biting midges is holometabolic (complete metamorphosis) with four stages, that is, egg, larva with four instars, pupa and adult (see Figure 14-7-6).

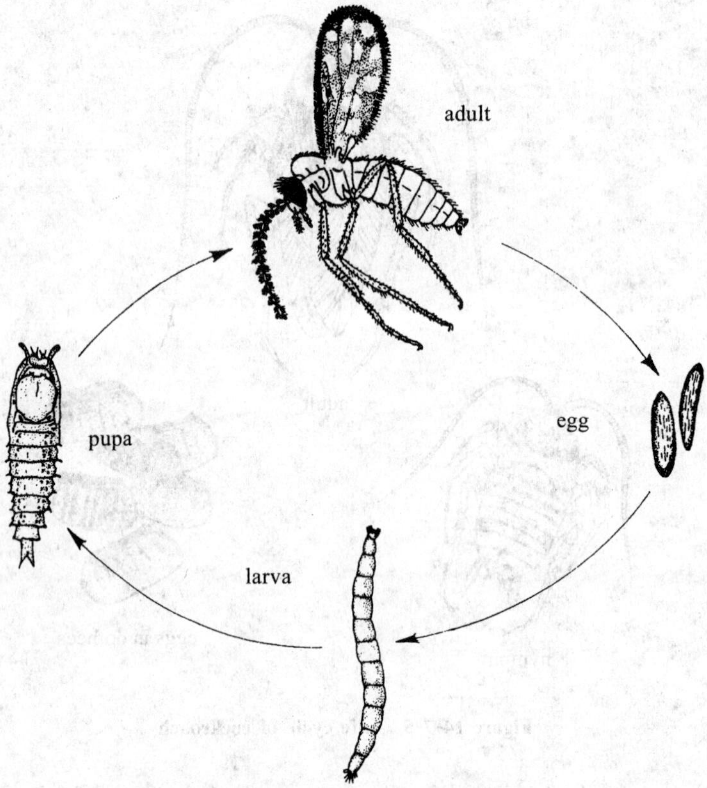

Figure 14-7-6 Life cycle of biting midge

Similar to mosquitoes, only female biting midges are bloodsucking insects while males suck plant liquid instead. Biting midges often cause terrible itching on skin sites where they bite for blood. Some species of biting midges in genus *Culicoides* can biologically transmit some pathogens of filariasis in Africa and South America, including *Dipetalonema perstans*, *D. streptocerca* and *Mansonella ozzardii*. Some species of biting midges in genus *Culicoides* are also the vector of bluetongue (a virus disease) in sheep and horses.

Black Fly

Black flies form a separate family, Simuliidae, belonging to order Diptera in Insecta. More than 1, 200 species are known in the world and about 90 species in China. The size of adults ranges from 3 to 5mm with two wings. Black flies are holometabolic (complete metamorphosis) with four stages in their life cycle: egg, larva, pupa and adult (see Figure 14-7-7 and Figure 14-7-8).

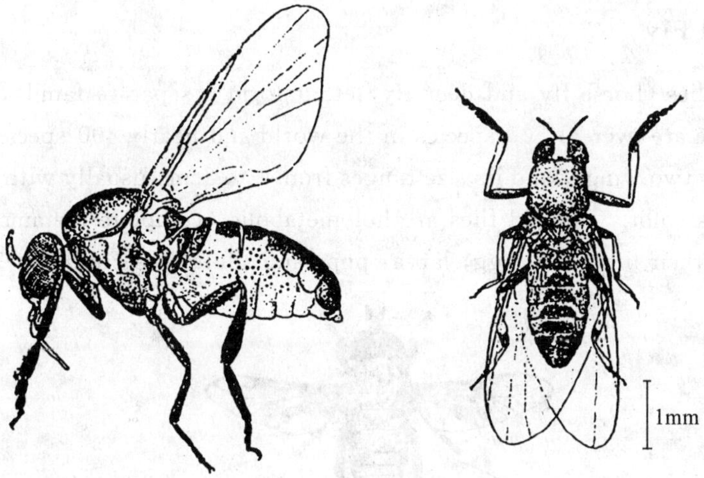

Figure 14-7-7 Female adult of black fly

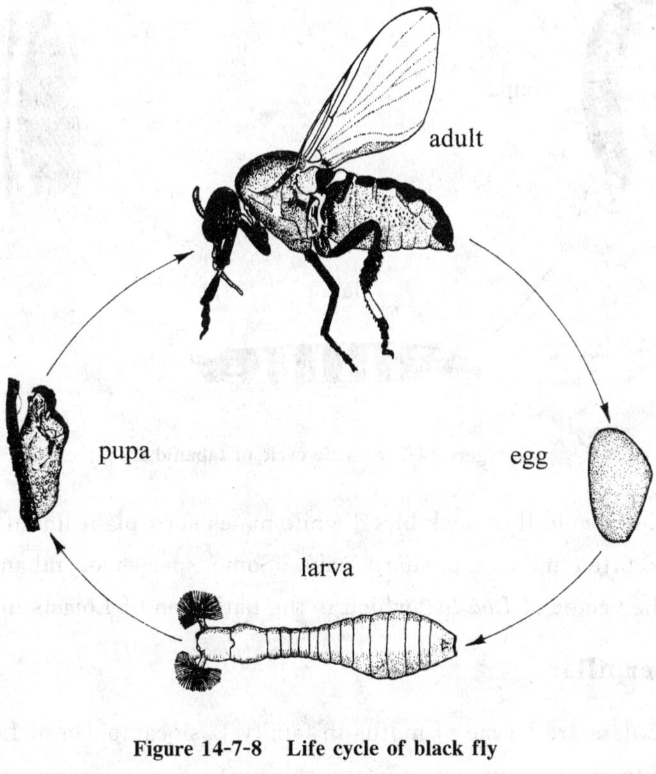

Figure 14-7-8 Life cycle of black fly

Only female black flies are bloodsucking insects, and some species in *Simulium* are the vector of *Onchocerca volvulus* which is the pathogen of Onchocerciasis (river blindness) in Africa and tropical South America.

Tabanid Fly

Tabanid flies (horse fly and deer fly, etc.) form a separate family, Tabanidae in Diptera. There are over 3, 500 species in the world and nearly 400 species in China. A tabanid fly has two wings, and its size ranges from 1 to 3cm, usually with yellow, grey, brown or black color. Tabanid flies are holometabolic (complete metamorphosis) with four stages in their life cycle: egg, larva, pupa and adult (see Figure 14-7-9).

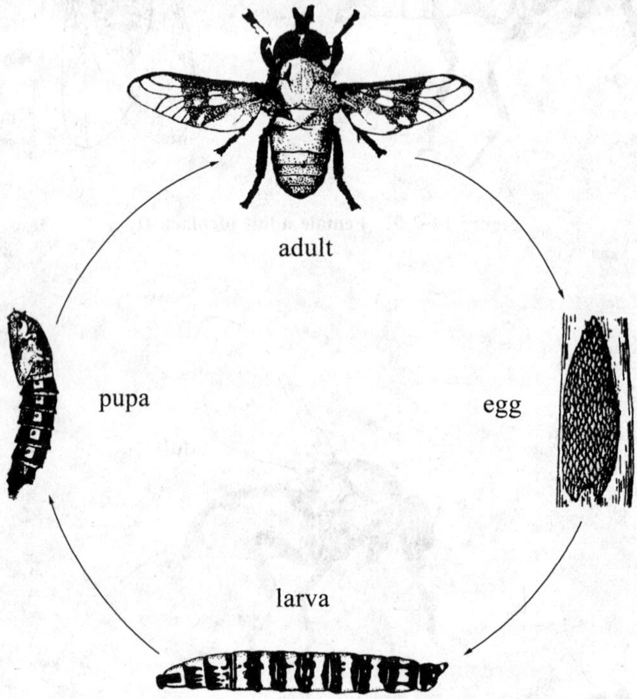

Figure 14-7-9 Life cycle of tabanid fly

Only female tabanid flies suck blood while males suck plant liquid instead. The bite of tabanid flies often induces a sharp pain. Some species of tabanid flies in genus *Chrysops* are the vector of *Loa loa* which is the pathogen of Loiasis in Africa.

Pine Caterpillar

Pine caterpillars are larvae of moths in family Lasiocampidae of Lepidoptera with a holometabolic life cycle (complete metamorphosis): eggs, larvae, pupae and adults. They have many poisonous hairs on their body, which may cause allergic dermatitis when contacting with skin (see Figure 14-7-10).

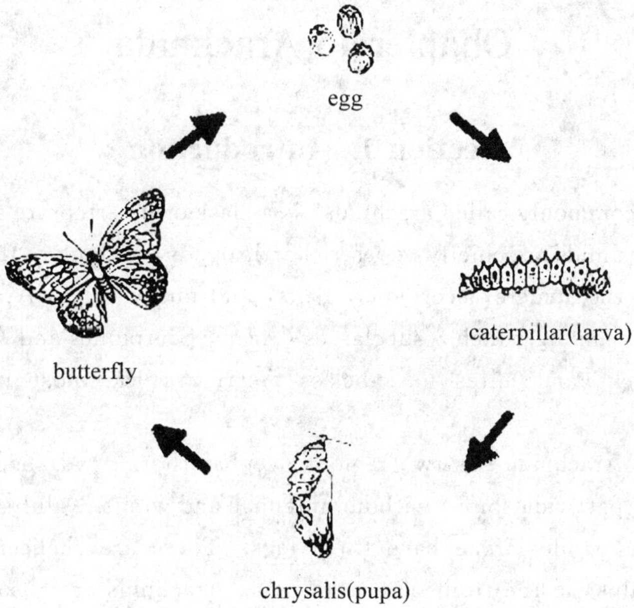

Figure 14-7-10 Life cycle of pine caterpillar

Rove Beetle

Rove beetles belong to Staphylinidae in Coleoptera. They are holometabolic insects with four stages in their life cycle: egg, larva, pupa and adult. Adults of some species (*Paederus fuscipes*, for example) in genus *Paederus* contain toxin which causes a special dermatitis called paederus dermatitis (see Figure 14-7-11).

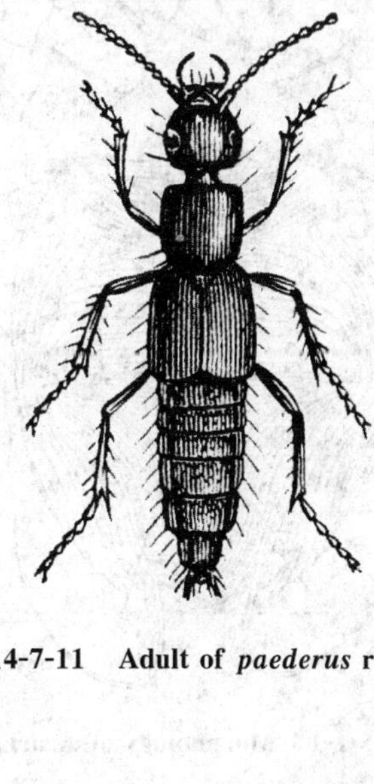

Figure 14-7-11 Adult of *paederus* rove beetle

(Guo Xianguo)

Chapter 15 Arachnida

Section 1 Introduction

Arachnida (commonly called arachnids) is a class of invertebrate animals in phylum Arhtropoda. Arachnids are chiefly terrestrial arthropods, with more than 70,000 known species including the spiders, scorpions, ticks, and mites. Class Arachnida is divided into 9 subclasses, amung which 3 subclasses (Acari, Scorpiones and Araneae) are close to medicine. Ticks and mites in subclass Acari are the most important medical arachnids.

The body of Arachnida has two regions (cephalothorax and abdomen) or is fused together into one part (idiosoma) without antennae and wings. Adults and nymphs have four pairs of legs while larvae have three legs. There are chelicerae and pedipalps (simply called palps) in the front of gnathosoma. Arachnids are absolutely not insects because they are easily distinguished from insects by the fact that they have eight legs instead of six. The pedipalpi (leg-like mouthparts) of some species has instead been adapted for sensory, prey capture or reproductive functions. Larval arachnids only have six legs; they grow their fourth pair when they molt into nymphs (see Figure 15-1-1).

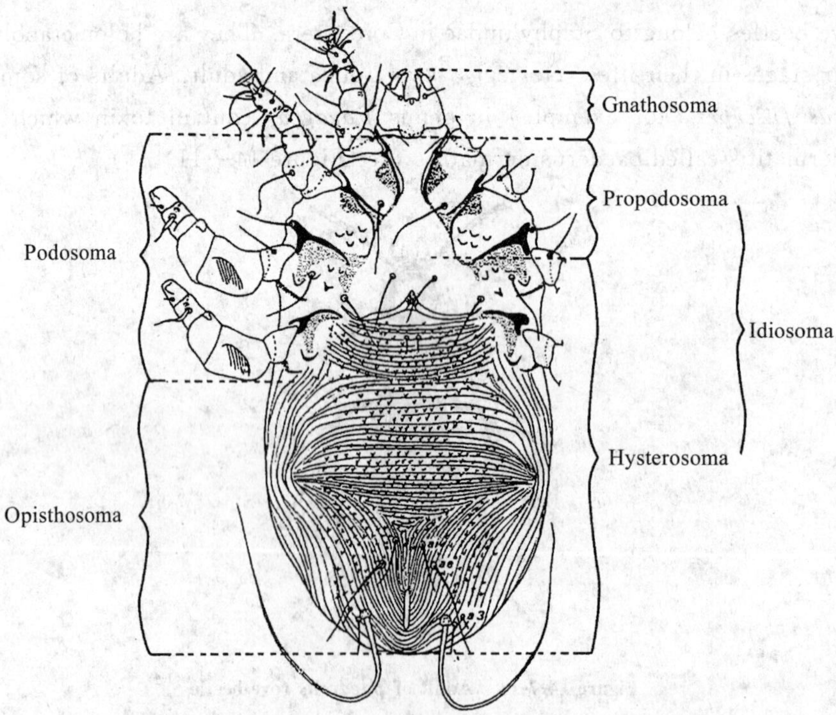

Figure 15-1-1 Morphology of Acari (mite)

Subclass Acari usually includes two groups of arachnids, ticks and mites with about 50, 000 known species in the world. Ticks are obligatory ectoparasites and there are three families of ticks, that is, Ixodidae, Argasidae and Nuttalliellidae. There are about 800 known species (and subspecies) in the world, including more than 700 species in Ixodidae (hard ticks), 150 species in Argasidae (soft ticks) and only one species in Nuttalliellidae, while about 100 hard tick species (Ixodidae) and 10 soft tick species (Argasidae) in China. Of three families of ticks, only hard ticks (family Ixodidae) and soft ticks (family Argasidae) have medical significance. Mites are a big group of arachnids with a variety of species, which belong to many families in Acari, and most species in Acari are actually mites instead of ticks. Most mite species have no medical importance and medical mites are only a small portion in the world of mites. Generally mites can be distinguished from ticks by some visible characteristics (see Table 15-1-1). Major groups of medical ticks and mites (subclass Acari) include hard ticks, soft ticks, chigger mites, gamasid mites, itch mites, follicle mites and dust mites, etc. (see Table 15-1-2).

Table 15-1-1　Major differences between tick and mite

	Tick	Mite
Body size	Usually large, 2-10mm	Usually small, 0.1-1mm
Body hairs	With fewer body hairs or absent	Usually with numerous body hairs
Hypostome	Toothed, exposed	Untoothed, hidden
Position of stigma	Behind coxal IV	In front of coxal IV or absent

Table 15-1-2 Some categories of medical Acari in zoological taxonomy

Category	Order	Suborder	Superfamily	Family	Species number
Tick (Hard tick & Soft tick)	Parasitiformes	Metastigmata	Ixodidea	Ixodidae, Argasidae & Nuttalliellidae	About 800 species (and subspecies) in the world (more than 700 hard tick species, 150 species soft tick species); about 100 hard tick species and 10 soft tick species in China
Chigger mite (Sand mite)	Acariforrmes	Prostigmata	Trombidioidea	Trombiculidae	Over 3,000 species (and subspecies) in the world and more than 400 species in China. About 50 species invading humans.
Gamasid mite	Parasitiformes	Mesostigmata	Several superfamilies	Many families	Over 500 species in China
Itch mite	Acariforrmes	Astigmata	Sarcoptoidea	Sarcoptidae	28 species (and subspecies)
Follicle mite	Acariforrmes	Prostigmata	Cheyletoidea	Demodicidae	140 species (and subspecies)
Dust mite	Acariforrmes	Astigmata	Acaroidea	Pyroglyphidae	34 species

Since arachnids are a large group of arthropods, their ecological behaviors are quite different. Some arachnids are carnivorous, feeding on the pre-digested body of insects and other small animals. Some are venomous—they secrete poison from specialized glands to kill prey or enemies. Others (ticks and medical mites) are parasites, some of which are carriers of disease. The typical life cycle of arachnids (especially ticks and mites) includes basic four stages, that is, egg, larva, nymph and adult, while a nymph may have several stages (see Figure 15-1-2). Ticks and mites (Acari) usually lay eggs, which hatch into immature adults, but some female mites directly produce larvae or nymphs. The female adults in some species can produce eggs, larvae or even nymphs without copulating with males, and this is called parthenogenesis.

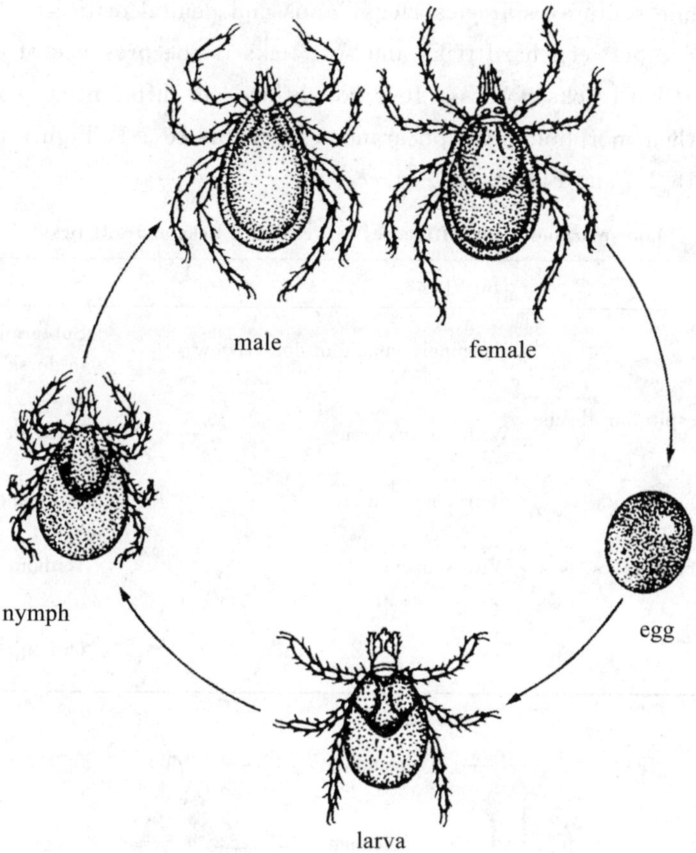

Figure 15-1-2 Life cycle of Acari

The medical significance of ticks and mites focuses on their transmitting diseases, especially zoonoses. The disease transmission by ticks and mites usually shows following characteristics: (1) Nearly all tick-borne and mite-borne diseases are zoonoses; (2) Transovarial transmission (transmission through eggs) is very common; (3) Ticks and mites can be the vector and reservoir at the same time in zoonosis transmission; (4) Most tick-borne and mite-borne diseases are of sporadic prevalence.

Section 2 Hard Tick and Soft Tick

Morphology

Hard ticks in family Ixodidae and soft ticks in family Argasidae are of great medical significance. They have some common morphological features and ecological behaviors. The body of ticks has fused together into a whole part called idiosoma, and the gnathosoma (capitulum) is on the anterior idiosoma. There are capitulum-base with (or without) porous area (in female), chelicerae, hypostome and pedipalps on the ganathosoma while scutum, spiracles, legs, anus and genital orifice on the idiosoma. The key difference between hard ticks and soft ticks is the presence of dorsal scutum (hard plate) that hard ticks possess. It is not difficult to differentiate hard ticks from soft ticks from their morphological appearance (see Table 15-2-1, Figure 15-2-1, Figure 15-2-2, Figure 15-2-3 and Figure 15-2-4).

Table 15-2-1 Major morphological differences between hard ticks and soft ticks

	Hard ticks	Soft ticks
Gnathosoma	Terminal; visible in dorsal view	Subterminal; invisible in dorsal view
Dorsal side of capitulum basis in female	With porous area	Without porous area
Pedipalps (palps)	Short, not nimble	Long and nimble
Dorsal side of idiosoma	With scutum	Without scutum
Distinction between female and male	Easy	Difficult

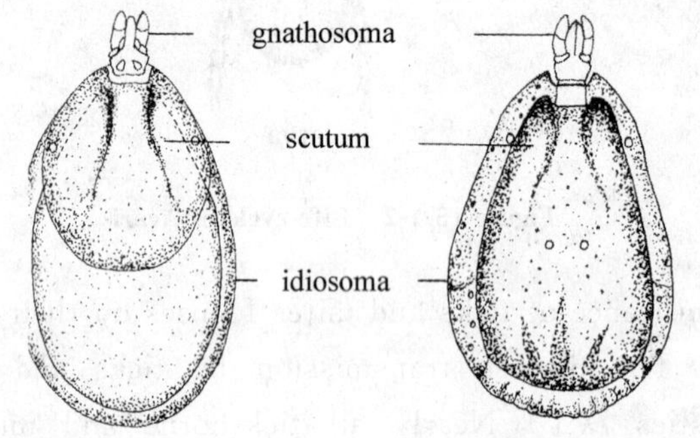

female tick of Ixodes (dorsal view)   male tick of Hyalomma (dorsal view)

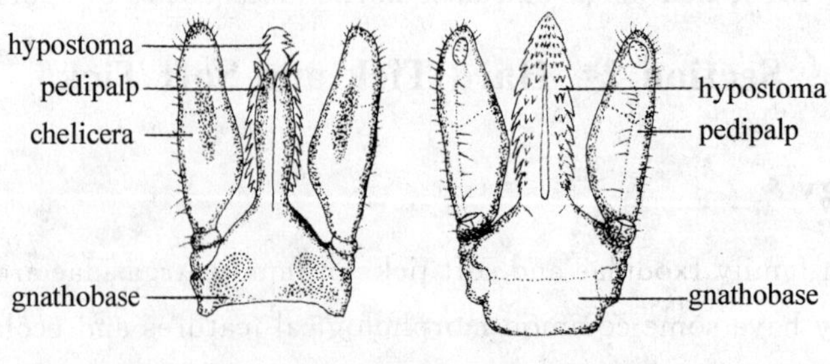

Gnathosoma of *Ixodes persulcatus*

Figure 15-2-1 Morphology of hard tick

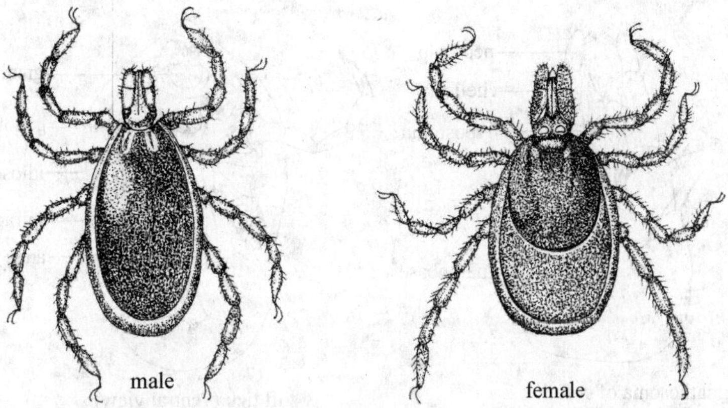

Ixodes persulcatus

Figure 15-2-2 Male and female of hard tick

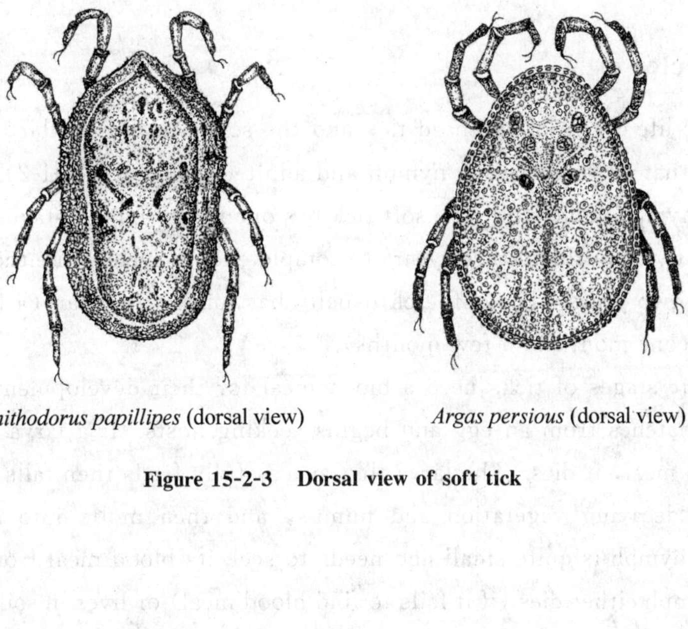

Ornithodorus papillipes (dorsal view) *Argas persious* (dorsal view)

Figure 15-2-3 Dorsal view of soft tick

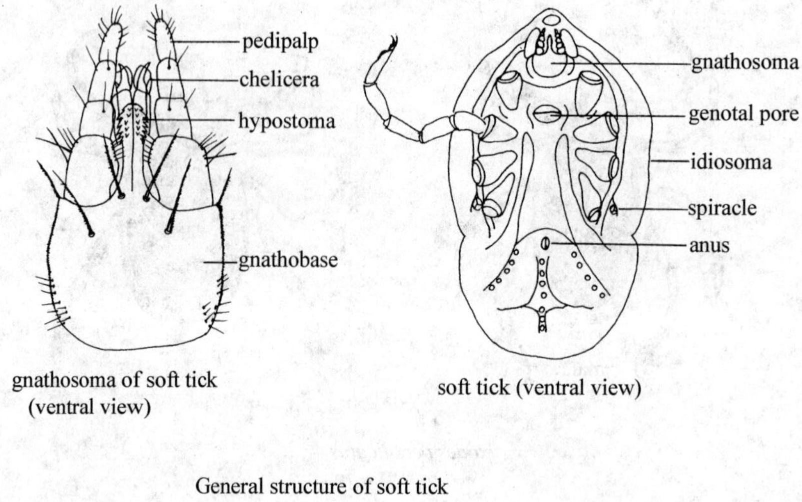

Figure 15-2-4 Ventral view of soft tick

Life Cycle

The basic life cycles of the hard tick and the soft tick are similar and include four basic stages, that is, egg, larva, nymph and adult (see Figure 15-1-2). The hard tick has only one nymph stage while the soft tick has one to six nymph stages. The hard tick usually needs two months to three years to complete a life cycle while the soft tick needs six months to two years. The soft tick usually has longer life span (a few years) than the hard tick (one month to a few months).

All the life stages of ticks need a blood meal for their development. A larva with only six legs hatches from an egg and begins seeking hosts. If a larva does not find a host for blood meal, it dies. The larva that successfully feeds then falls off its host and lives in soil, decaying vegetation and humus, and then molts into an eight-legged nymph. This nymph is quite small and needs to seek its blood meal from a vertebrate. Then, the nymph either dies (if it fails to find blood meal) or lives in soil to molt into an adult. The eight-legged adult tick is somewhat larger and seeks a larger host for its required blood meal. The adult female lays eggs and then dies.

Ecology

Both hard ticks and soft ticks need to ingest a blood meal to transform to their next stage of development. They take their requisite blood meal from all classes of vertebrates (e. g. mammals, reptiles, birds), with the exception of fish. Adults, nymphs and larvae have to suck blood for their development. Ticks feed by perching in low vegetation and waiting (questing) for a susceptible host on which they can attach and feed. Once on a host, the tick attaches its hypostome, a central piercing element with hooks, into the host's skin. Some ticks secrete a cementing material to fasten themselves to the host. In addition, ticks in genus *Ixodes* secrete anticoagulant, immunosuppressive, and anti-inflammatory substances into the area of the tick bite. These substances presumably help the tick to obtain a blood meal without the host's noticing.

Hard ticks often distribute in forests, bushes, pasture and desert, etc. Soft ticks, however, are commonly seen in animals' sheds, birds' nests and humans' houses, etc. Ticks have a variety of hosts (mammals, birds, reptiles and amphibians) for a blood meal. Some ticks only feed on a single host and these ticks are often called "single-host tick" and *Boophilus microplus* (a species of hard tick) is an example. Some ticks have to change hosts for blood meal. For instance, larva and nymph of *Hyalomma detritum* (a species of hard tick) feed on a species of host and adult has to change its host. After the larva and nymph finish a blood and drop off the first host to develop to an adult, the newly emerged adult has to seek another host for a blood meal, and this tick is called "two-host tick". Over 90% of hard ticks are "three-host ticks", and three stages (larva, nymph and adult) feed on three different hosts respectively for blood meal. Soft ticks with several nymphal stages are usually "multiple-host ticks" because they feed on more than three different hosts.

Relationship with Diseases

Direct injury

Besides direct impairment from stinging and secondary infection or allergic reaction to proteins in tick saliva, some hard ticks contain toxin in their saliva which can cause tick paralysis. Tick paralysis is commonly seen in children, and death may happen in a severe situation.

Indirect injury

Ticks are excellent vectors for disease transmission and they can carry and transmit a remarkable array of pathogens, such as bacteria, spirochetes, rickettsiae, protozoa, viruses and nematodes, etc. They are second only to mosquitoes as vectors of human diseases (especially zoonoses). A single tick bite can transmit multiple pathogens, a phenomenon that has led to atypical presentations of some classic tick-borne diseases. In some countries (e. g. the US), ticks are the most common vectors of vector-borne diseases.

(1)Forest encephalitis

Forest encephalitis is also called Russian spring-summer encephalitis, caused by the pathogen of forest encephalitis virus. It widely distributes in Russian, Europe and China (mainly in forest regions in Northeast China). The natural infectious sources are mainly from the infection of wild rodents and birds. The disease is transmitted through the bite of hard ticks and transovarial transmission is also possible. The clinical manifestations of forest encephalitis are similar to epidemic type B encephalitis transmitted by mosquitoes, but with higher mortality (more death). The common clinical manifestations include high fever, nausea, vomiting, severe headache, coma and paralysis, etc. Humans get the diseases by the bite of infected hard ticks. The main vector in China is *Ixodes persulcatus*.

(2)Xinjiang haemorrhagic fever (XHF)

Xinjiang haemorrhagic fever (XHF) is also called Crimean-Congo haemorrhagic fever, caused by the pathogen of XHF virus or CCHF virus. XHF widely distributes in Africa, Asia and Europe, and in China it mainly distributes in Xinjiang. The natural infectious sources are mainly from the infection of livestock and wild animals (wild vertebrates). The disease is transmitted through the bite of hard ticks and transovarial transmission is also possible. The clinical manifestations of Xinjiang haemorrhagic fever are similar to epidemic hemaerrhagic fever, including fever, headache, bleeding tendency (e. g., purpuric spot or petechia on skin), hypotension, hematuria (blood-urine), albuminuria (protein-urine), etc. Humans get the diseases by the bite of infected hard ticks. The main vector in China is *Hyalomma asiaticum kozlovi*.

(3)Lyme disease

Lyme disease is caused by a species of spirochete pathogen, *Borrelia burgdorferi*, and it mainly distributes in the United States and Europe. There are also case reports from China. The natural infectious sources are mainly from wild rodents and other mammals. The disease is transmitted through the bite of hard ticks. The clinical manifestations include chill, fever, headache, movable muscle pain or joint pain, swelling joint and enlargement of lymph nodes, etc. Humans get the diseases by the bite of infected hard ticks. The main vector in China is *Ixodes persulcatus*, but the vectors in foreign countries include *Ixodes dammini*, *I. pacificus*, *I. ricinus* and *I. persulcatus*, etc.

(4)Tick-borne relapsing fever

Tick-borne relapsing fever is also called endemic relapsing fever, caused by an array of pathogens, *Borrelia persica*, *B. latyschevi* and *B. hermsii*, etc. Tick-borne relapsing fever widely distributes in Africa, Asia, Europe, North America and South America, and in China it mainly distributes in Xinjiang and some western provinces. The natural infectious sources are mainly from the infection of wild rodents and infected humans (patients). The disease is transmitted through the bite of soft ticks, and it is also possible for humans to be infected when they contact with the secreted substances from coxal glands of infected soft ticks. The clinical manifestations of the disease are similar to epidemic relapsing fever transmitted by human lice, with intermittent chill and fever. The main vectors in China are *Ornithodorus* ticks, for example, *O. papillipes.*

(5)Other diseases

North Asia tick-borne typhus (also called Siberian typhus), a rickettsial disease, is transmitted through the bite of hard ticks (e. g. *Dermacentor nuttalli*). Q fever (another rickettsial disease) can be transmitted by some hard ticks and soft ticks sometimes. In addition, ticks may be possible to transmit tularemia or rabbit fever (bacterial disease), babesiosis and even plague in some circumstances.

Control

The control of ticks should follow the general principles of medical arthropods and integrated management is recommended. The integrated management of ticks can be achieved by the following ways: (1) environment management through cleaning stalls of livestock, eradicating weeds around houses and stalls, and walling up mouse-holes, etc; (2) chemical control by spraying pesticides to killing ticks; (3) personnel protection by swearing protective clothes, gloves and hoses to keep from the invasion of ticks.

Section 3 Trombiculid Mite (Chigger)

Trombiculid mites are also called chigger mites (chiggers) or sand mites sometimes, which belong to Trombiculidae in Acari. Over 3, 000 species (including 400 species in China) in the world have been recorded.

Morphology

Trombiculid mites are a unique group and only larva stage is ectoparasitic in life cycle and other stages are of free living. Simply because of this reason, the identification of trombiculid mites is mainly based on larva's morphology instead of adult. The larva of trombiculid mite (usually 0. 2mm to 0. 4mm of size) is tiny, rounded, red (or colorless) and it is a hairy creature with a dorsal plate (or called scutum) and three pairs of legs (see Figure 15-3-1).

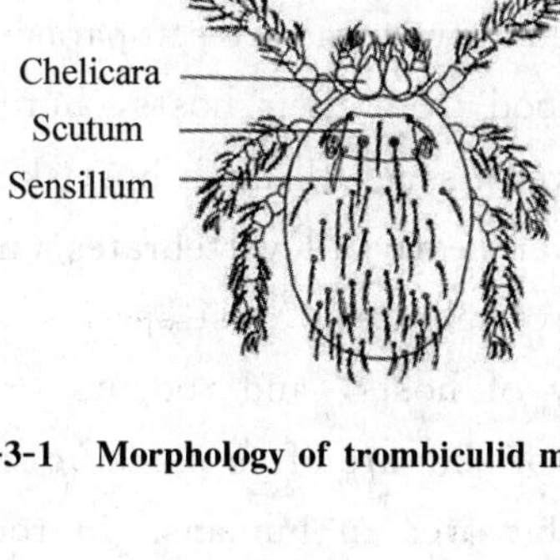

Figure 15-3-1 Morphology of trombiculid mite (larva)

Life Cycle

The life cycle of trombiculid mite is unique with six stages, namely egg, larva, nymphochrysalis, nymph, imagochrysalis and imago (adult). Both adult and nymph are free-living creatures while only larva is ectoparasite (see Figure 15-3-2).

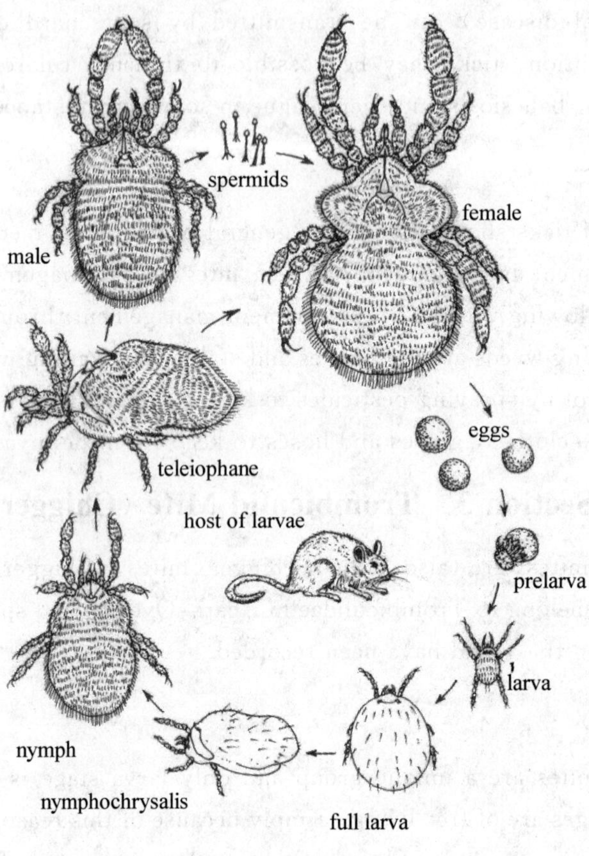

Figure 15-3-2 Life cycle of trombiculid mite

Ecology

Adults and nymphs of trombiculid mites are free-living creatures, feeding on small arthropods and insect eggs, and only larvae are ectoparasites. The larvae of trombiculid mites do not actually suck blood from their hosts, but instead they usually need to ingest body liquid (and dissolved tissue) through host skin for their development. The hosts of trombiculid mites cover nearly all vertebrates (mammals, birds, reptiles and amphibians) and even some invertebrates. Most species of trombiculid mites have low host specificity with a variety of hosts, and rodents (rats and mice) are the most important hosts. Tender sites of skin are often parasitic sites of chiggers, for example, waist, armpit, groin and pubic area in humans. In rodents, however, auricle and external ear canal are mostly common parasitic sites. When chiggers feed, they fix their mouthpart on host skin first and then inject their saliva to dissolve skin tissue to form a specific canal, stylostome. Chiggers suck the dissolved tissue, together with body liquid, as their food through the stylostome. Chiggers are weak walkers and they often move within a definitive narrow realm (usually 10cm to 20cm) without a strong dispersing ability.

Relationship with Diseases

Direct injury

The bite of chiggers often gives rise to local lesion of skin, which is called trombidosis (chigger dermatitis). The infection begins as a red indurated lesion that eventually enlarges to 8-12mm in diameter, vesiculates and ruptures, and becomes dark and necrotic in the center, called eschar. The formation of eschar can be as a specific sign in clinical diagnosis.

Indirect injury

Chiggers are the vector of scrub typhus (or tsutsugamushi disease). Scrub typhus is an acute infectious disease caused by *Rickettsia tsutsugamushi* (*R. orientalis*). It is transmitted through the bite of chiggers and transovarial transmission is common. Wild rodents, particularly rats in genus *Rattus*, are the reservoirs of the disease. Scrub typhus is limited to China, Southeast Asia, India, northern Australia, and the adjacent islands. Clinical characteristics include the formation of eschar (a primary cutaneous lesion at the site of mite's bite), fever lasting about two weeks, and a maculopapular rash. The patients may also experience headaches, shaking chills, enlarged lymph nodes or spleen, anorexia, and general discomfort. Some species of chiggers in genus *Leptotrombidium* are powerful vectors of scrub typhus, such as *Teptotrobidium deliense*, *L. scutellare*, *L. akamushi* and *L. kaohuense*, etc. *L. deliense* is the most important vector in China.

In recent years, some species of chiggers have been proved to be the potential vector of epidemic hemorrhagic fever (EHF).

Control

The integrated control of trombiculid mites focuses on three aspects: (1) environment management, such as environment sanitation, eradication of wild weed, and control of rats and mice; (2) application of pesticides (miticides) thoroughly in breeding areas surrounding humans' dwelling; (3) application of repellent (expellent) to keep skin from the attack of chiggers.

Section 4 Itch Mite (Scabies Mite)

Itch mite is also called scabies mite or mange mite, which belongs to Sarcoptidae in zoological taxonomy. Scabies mites are permanent parasites of humans and other animals with relatively high host specificity. The itch mite for humans is *Sarcoptes scabiei* and it lives within the subcutaneous tissues of skin on humans, causing the condition known as scabies.

Morphology

Itch mites are very small, oval and straw colored mites, measuring 0. 2-0. 5mm in length. Their bodies are covered with fine lines and several long hairs without eyes. They have short and thick legs, with the first two pairs of legs stalked with ambulacra. The posterior two pairs of legs are morphologically different between male and female. The female has a long bristle on the terminal of two posterior legs while the male has ambulacra on the 4th pair of legs instead. The immature stages of scabies mite are comprised of a six legged larval stage, followed by 2 nymphal stages that have eight legs, and each stage resembles the adult mite (see Figure 15-4-1).

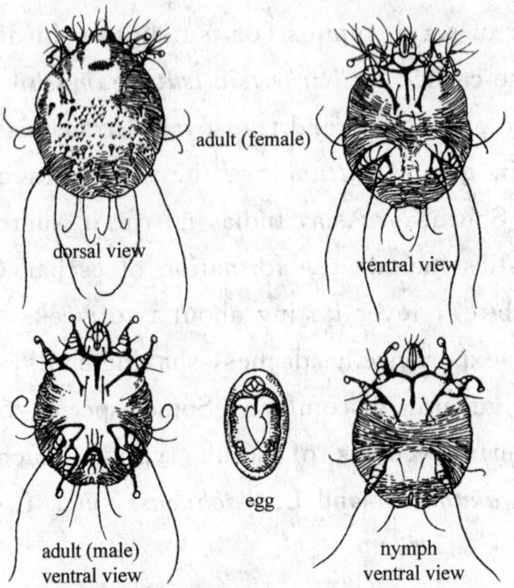

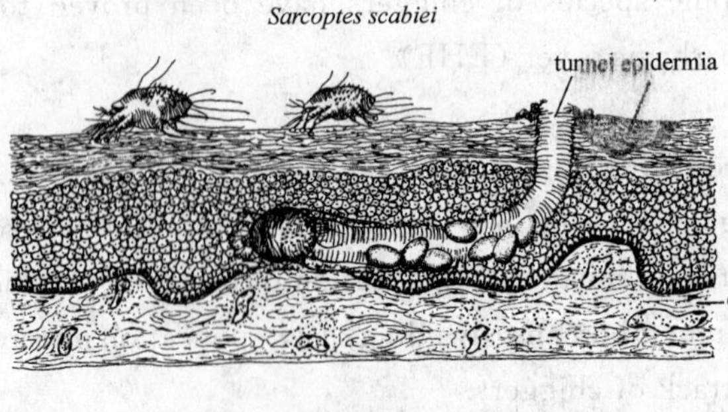

site of inhabitation of *Sarcoptes scabiei*

Figure 15-4-1 Different stages of itch mites

Life Cycle

The life cycle of itch mite includes five stages: egg, larva, protonymph, deutonymph and adult. It takes over 10-17 days to finish the entire life cycle. The mite mates on the skin of its host, male inseminating female. Males die soon after mating. Newly mated females burrow into the outer layer of human skin and excavate a tunnel where they lay their eggs. The mite eats skin and tissue fluid that oozes from its excavation. After fertilization, female mites wander on the skin to seek a suitable site for a permanent burrow. The transfer of a female to another host at this stage will initiate a new infection. Female mites rarely leave their burrows, and if removed by scratching and remain undamaged, they will attempt to burrow again.

Pathogenesis

Human itch mite, *Sarcoptes scabiei*, is the pathogen of scabies, and it is not the vector of diseases. Scabies is an infestation of skin. Scabies infestations can present different clinical manifestations and may be difficult to be diagnosed. The initial infestation may remain undetected for a month or more, before sensitization develops and an immunological response in the host is triggered. The allergic reaction is from components of the mite's feces, skin moults, saliva or moulting fluids diffusing into the tissues of the host from the burrows. The patient can experience severe itching all over the body, and especially at night. Large areas of the body can be covered by a rash that can last for weeks but which will not (or only rarely) coincide with the areas of mite infestation. Eruption of the skin into small itchy lesions may occur in conjunction with the rash. Scabies mites tend to burrow into the skin where there is a natural crease and the host's reaction will be minimal. The hands, and webbing between the fingers, the wrists, and elbows are common areas. From the surface of the skin, the tunnels appear as greyish pencil marks and in darker skin the tunnels appear paler. The severe itching and scratching can lead to secondary infections and, in cases of heavy infestations anemia can develop (see Figure 15-4-2).

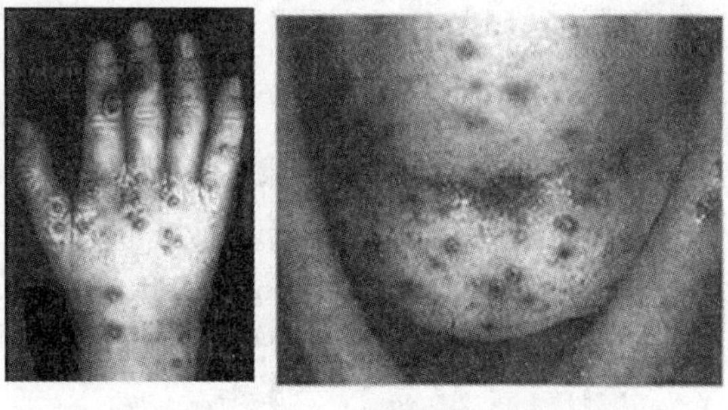

Figure 15-4-2 Skin lesion of scabies

Diagnosis

Diagnosis is most commonly made by looking at the burrows or rash. A skin scraping may be taken to look for mites, eggs, or mite fecal matter to confirm the diagnosis. The skin scrapings are examined under a light microscope for the presence of mites or eggs after a glass slide mount is prepared from the scrapings with sterilized oil or lactic acid. The lactic acid aids in clearing any thick layers of skin cells in the sample to reveal any evidence of scabies mite, but clearing may take some time (hours to days).

Epidemiology

The infestation of *Sarcoptes scabiei* is common, worldwide distributed, and affects people of all races and social classes. Scabies spreads rapidly under crowded conditions where there is frequent skin-to-skin contact between people, such as in hospitals, institutions, child-care facilities, and nursing homes.

Prevention and Control

Scabies is highly contagious in overcrowded situations and close contact with infected individuals should be avoided. Direct body touching, shaking hands, or sharing beds and contaminated objects of an infected person are common modes of transmission. The patient should be isolated and treated after diagnosed with scabies. All individuals that have had significant contact with primary patients should be treated as well.

Most scabies infections are easy to be controlled, providing the directions of the scabicide treatments are followed. The following drugs are recommended as external use: (1) scabies lotions consisting of scabicides such as lindane, permethrin, sulfur and sulfur ointment, etc.; (2) soothing lotion for itching during treatment and recovery; (3) hydrocortisone cream. When administrating the treatment, the lotion should be applied to a clean body from the neck down to the toes and left overnight (eight hours). After eight hours, take a bath or shower to wash off the lotion. A common problem of treatment failure is insufficient coverage of the body with the scabicide, and resistance is rare.

Section 5 Gamasid Mite

Gamasid mites are a large group of arachnids, belonging to suborder Mesostigmata in Acari, with many families such as Dermanyssidae, Laelapidae and Macronyssidae, etc. Though there has been no reports about all known species over the world, over 500 species in China have been reported from China.

Morphology

The adults of gamasid mites are oval-shaped, 8-legged with a brown, yellow, grayish or white color. They usually measure from 0. 2mm to 0. 5mm, but the largest can reach 3mm. The stigma is between coxal III and coxal IV, and therefore gamasid mites are often called mesostigmatid mites, meaning middle-stigma mites (see Figure 15-5-1).

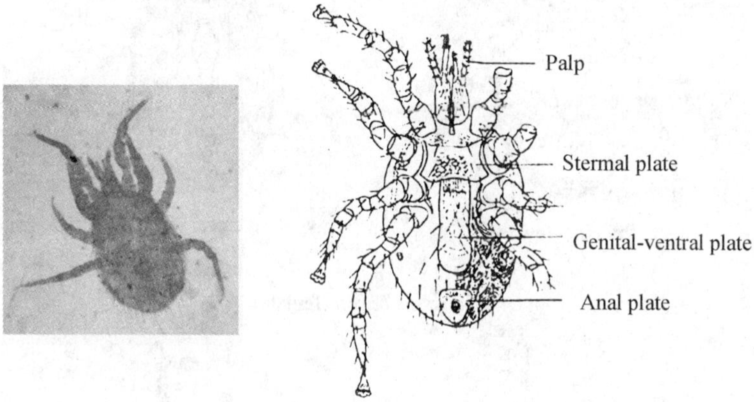

Figure 15-5-1 Female adult of gamasid mite

Life Cycle

The life cycle of gamasid mites includes five stages: egg, larva, protonymph, deutonymph and adult. The minute egg is pearly white while the 6-legged larva is translucent and whitish. The 8-legged nymph is similar to the adult with various colors. The females may lay eggs (oviparity) or directly produce larvae or nymphs (ovoviviparity) and parthenogenesis are common.

Ecology

Most gamasid mites are free-living creatures (some are predators) without medical significance. Some ectoparasitic or endoparasitic gamasid mites are of medical significance, and their hosts cover mammals, birds, reptiles, amphibians and some other invertebrates. Small mammals (rodents, insectivores and bats, etc.) often harbour lots of gamasid mites on their body surface.

Relationship with Diseases

Direct injury

Some ectoparasitic gamasid mites may lead to dermatitis (gamasidosis) through their bite, as seen in *Ornithonyssus bacoti* and *Dermanyssus gallinae* (see Figure 15-5-2). In poultry, the loss of blood (anemia) and irritation caused by gamasid mite infestations lead to decreased vigor and egg production of the host. Young birds and setting hens may actually be killed by mite-induced anemia.

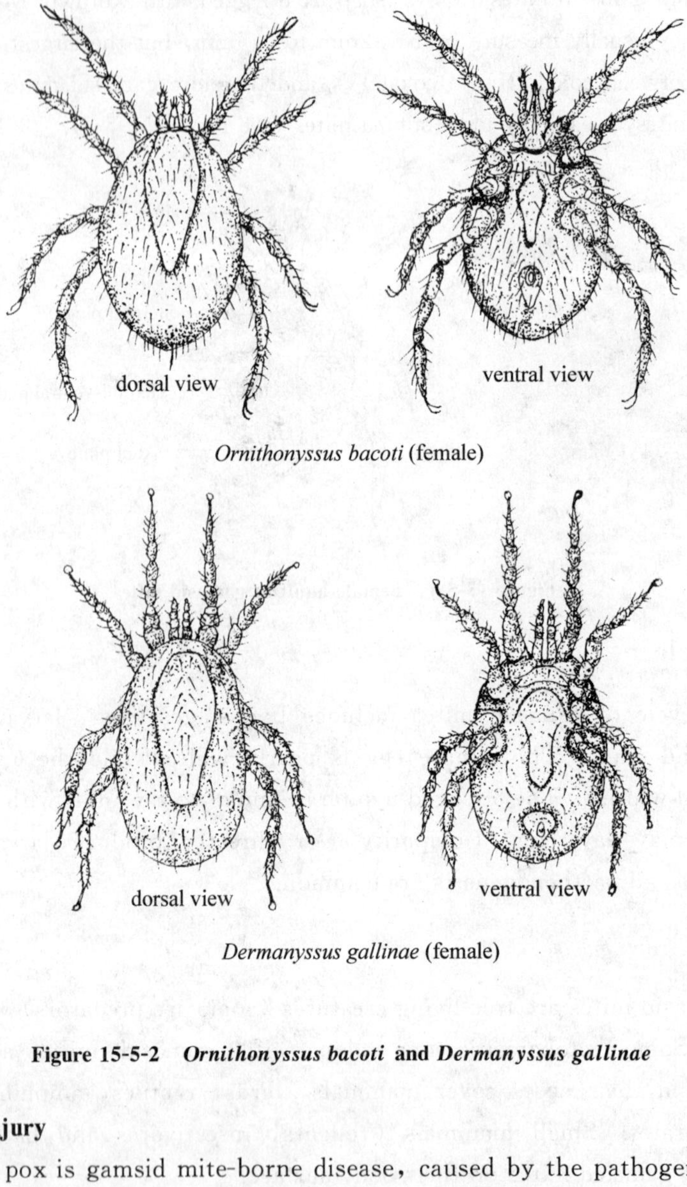

Figure 15-5-2 *Ornithonyssus bacoti* and *Dermanyssus gallinae*

Indirect injury

Rickettsia pox is gamsid mite-borne disease, caused by the pathogen of *Rickettsia akari* and transmitted through the bite of gamasid mites. The disease mainly distributes in the United States. The infectious source is from infected rodents while the main vector is *Allodermanyssus sanguineus*.

Gamasid mites may be the vector of hemorrhagic fever with renal syndrome (HFRS), which is also called epidemic hemorrhagic fever (EHF) in China. HFRS is a world-wide distributed virus disease, caused by the pathogen of hantaan virus. HFRS can be spread by direct contact with infectious sources (mainly rodents) or through the respiratory and alimentary tracts, and it can be transmitted by the bite of mites as well. Some species of gamasid mites (e. g. *O. bacoti* and *Haemolaelaps glasgowi*) are proved to be potential vectors of HFRS.

In addition, it is also reported that gamasid mites can harbor more than 20 kinds of some other pathogens.

Control

The integrated control measures for gamasid mites are similar to those for trombiculid mites. Repeat applications of miticides are necessary sometimes. Pesticides can help suppress mite populations, but must be used in combination with bird or rodent control. Sprays and aerosols containing the active ingredient miticides are recommended since the treatment will remain effective for at most a few days.

(Guo Xianguo)

Section 6 Demodicid Mite

Demodicid mites belong to Family Demodicidae. They are all permanent parasites of human being and mammals. More than 140 species have been known. They cause a disease usually called demodectic mange or demodicidosis. Members of genus have a high degree of both host and site specificity. Two species parasitize human body, that is, *Demodex folliculorum* which lives in hair follicles and *Demodex brevis*, which is found in sebaceous glands.

Morphology

Human demodex mites are generally called the follicle mites and minute carrot or worm shaped. They range in length from 100μm to 400μm. They are translucent and creamy white in color. The females are larger than males. *D. folliculorum* is longer than *D. brevis*. A gnathosoma which is short trapezoid is located at the anterior part of the podosoma. There is a longitudinally oral slit on the central position of ventral side of the hypostome. An oral needle that can stretch out and draw back hides in the oral slit. There is a segmented palpus in each lateral side of the gnathosoma. The end of the palpus is ventrally armed with several sharp claws. The podosoma ventrally has 4 pairs of stubby and five-segmented legs. There are single and forked claws on the end of each leg. *D. folliculorum* has a large backward spur on the femur of each legs. The vulva is between the fourth pair of legs. The male's genital pore is dorsally located between the second pair of legs, in which there is a writing brush-like penis that can stretch out and draw back. The opisthosoma has whorls. Nowadays an anus has not been found (see Figure 15-6-1).

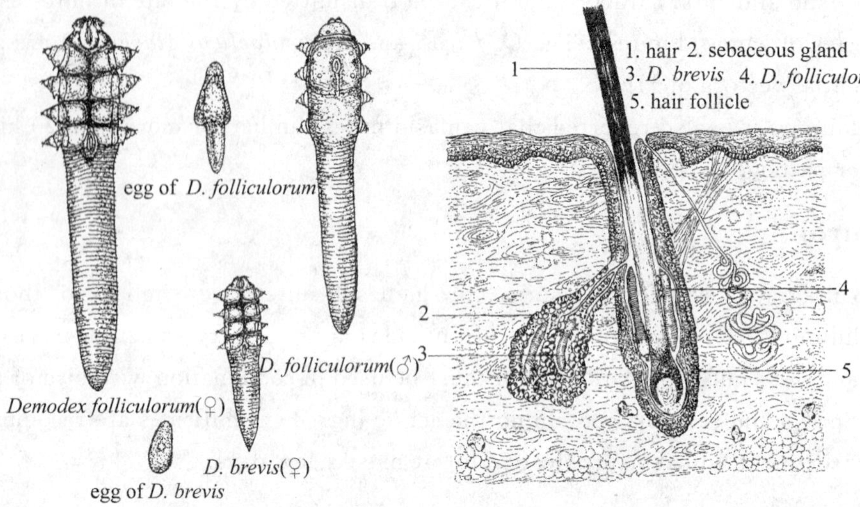

Figure 15-6-1 Morphology of human demodex mites

Table 15-6-1 Morphological difference between *Demodex folliculorum* and *Demodex brevis*

	Demodex folliculorum	*Demodex brevis*
Appearance	fingered, with a plump terminal end	with a tapering end
Length	♀294μm, ♂279.7μm	♀203μm, ♂148.1μm
Gnathosoma(dorsal view)	ahead protruding coxal endite, overstep the level of palpus	shorter than palpus
Palpal claw	seven, thorn-like	five, curved thorn-like
Podosoma seta	♀ no, ♂ two pairs	no, has not been seen
Genital pore	♀ ventrally, between the 4th pair of legs ♂ dorsally, between the 2nd pair of legs	behind the 4th pair of legs has not been seen
Opisthosoma and its whorl	plump terminal end with whorls like concentric circles	tapering end with whorl-like flattened concentric circles
Egg	a narrow mushroom-like	oval in shape

Life Cycle

Human demodex mites are obligate parasites for all stages of their life cycles. *Demodex folliculorum* lives in the hair follicle while *Demodex brevis* in the sebaceous gland. Several mites commonly inhabit a single hair follicle. Both exist in mainly on the forehead and face, particularly around the nose and rim of eyelid. The pattern of the life cycle is as follows: egg—larva—protonymph—nymph—adult.

The life cycle probably requires about 2 weeks in summer, while it takes long in winter. The female life span is more than 4 months, and the male will die after mating. Adults mate and deposit eggs in the hair follicle or gland in which larvae with 3 pairs of leg hatch. The larva and nymph develop through molts. They have special piercing and sucking mouthparts and may feed on tissue fluid and contents of the hair follicle or gland. All life stages may be found in a single hair follicle. Mites can freely migrate among hair follicles. The transmission is accomplished by direct or indirect contact.

Pathogenesis and Clinical Manifestation

Mites may stab or scratch local cells with their piercing mouthparts and sharp claws and feed on tissue fluid and scraps, which injure the protective screen of the skin. Mites and their excreta, secretion and remains also block the drain passage of sebum. It is suspected that follicle mites may be involved in introducing bacteria into the skin follicles. Above agents may cause local nonspecific inflammation, allergic reaction and secondary infection, which result in granulomatous skin eruptions and manifest acne, acne rosacea (brandy nose), loss of eyelashes, seborrhea capitis and dermatitis in susceptible individuals. Most of the infections are asymptomatic, so human demodex mites are considered as opportunistic parasites.

Other demodicids of importance are the goat follicle mite (*D. caprea*), cattle follicle mite (*D. bovis*), the horse follicle mite (*D. equi*) and hog follicle mite (*D. phylloides*). All four cause a pustular dermatitis with nodules and loss of hair. Holes in the skin caused by these mites reduce the value of leathers. Besides, the dog follicle mite (*D. canis*) causes red mange. The skin develops reddish pimples, pustules, hair loss and is covered with a foul-smelling yellow exudate.

Diagnosis

Exact diagnosis depends on demonstrating a mite in skin scrapings. An easy means of inspecting the mite is to examine microscopically some oil expressed from the forehead and nose using nails. Often used diagnostic methods include: (1) get the sample from the forehead or nose with a scraper or special nippers; (2) stick a cellophane tape on the face for a night and then examine microscopically the cellophane tape.

Epidemiology

Human demodex mites are prevalent all over the word. The incidence of these mites is very high, about 90% in persons over 14 years of age using a special scraper inspection. Reported incidences from various districts are from 27% to 95% because various inspecting methods are used. The incidence of the mites in humans is from 20% in persons 20 years of age or younger to nearly 100% in the aged. The incidence and infective density of the mites in males are higher than those in females. The prevalence rate is about 10% in young persons.

Treatment

Sulfur ointment, metronidazole cream, benzyl benzoate and dibutyl phthalate are effective and for external use.

(Yuan Fangshu, Guo Shuling and He Shenyi)

Section 7 Dust Mite

As an important source of allergen, dust mites are cosmopolitan arachnids in human habitation, existing in various dusts. Sometimes dust mites are also called house dust mites, abbreviated by allergists to HDM. Main species of HDM are *Dermatophagoides pteronyssinus*, *Dermatophagoides farinae* and *Euroglyphus maynei* and they are considered to be one of the most common causes of asthma worldwide.

Morphology

As a member of subclass Acari, adult dust mites have eight legs. Both male and female adult dust mites are globular in shape, creamy white and have a striated cuticle. The adult measures approximately 0. 2-0. 4mm in length and 0. 2-0. 3mm in width (see Figure 15-7-1).

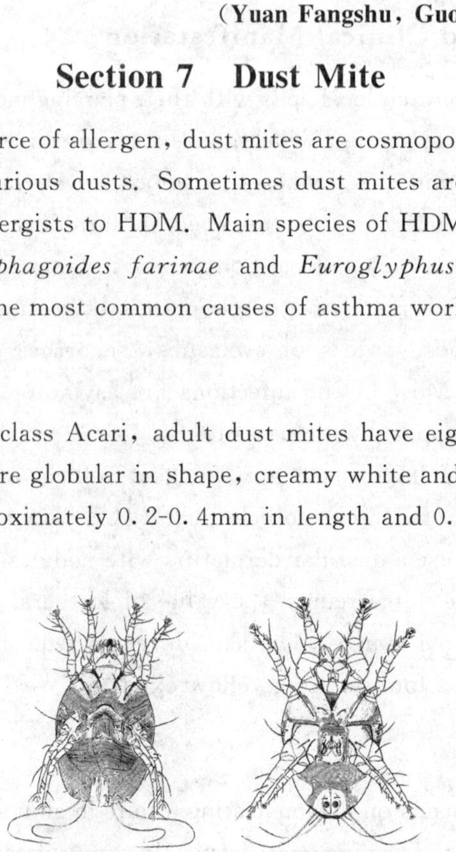

Figure 15-7-1 Adult of house dust mite

Life Cycle

Similar to itch mites, gamasid mites and follicle mites, the life cycle of dust mites also include five stages: egg, larva, protonymph, deutonymph and adult. The whole life cycle from egg to adult takes approximately one month to complete and mature female mites lay 1-2 eggs per day. Adult mites can live up to two months but this is dependent on humidity and temperature of their surrounding environment.

Ecology

Dust mites often live in the fine layer of minute dust particles that continually settles on household items, particularly common in carpets, bedding, pillows and furniture, etc. They usually thrive in the modern environment of fully-carpeted, and are comfortable at 25℃ and 75% relative humidity. They are found almost world wide but their numbers are considerably reduced at high altitudes and dry climates. They feed on human skin scales and secretions, house dust, fungal spores, pollen grains, plant fibres, and insect scales. An average person sheds about 1. 5 grams of skin a day (approximately 3-4. 5kg per year), which is enough to feed roughly a million dust mites.

Pathogenesis

Dust mites do not transmit any disease-causing pathogens (not the vector of diseases), but they are an important source of allergens, leading to direct impairment. They do not bite or sting, but harbour strong allergens in their bodies as well as in their secretions, excreta and shed skins. Constant contact with these allergens can trigger respiratory and dermatological complaints in some humans. As one of the most significant allergens, dust mites are implicated in allergic asthma, rhinitis, conjunctivitis, dermatitis, childhood eczema and other allergic conditions. Allergic asthma and rhinitis are the most common allergic reactions induced by dust mites. The allergic asthma and rhinitis induced by dust mites have no specific presentations in clinics. The patients with allergic asthma may experience dyspnea, chest stuffy (fuggy chest), cyanopathy, etc. The presentations of allergic rhinitis include sneeze, running nose and snuffle, etc.

Diagnosis

The allergic asthma and rhinitis induced by dust mites can be diagnosed from contact history, clinical manifestation, immunological detection and identification of suspicious dust mites. The identification of dust mites is performed with the use of light microscopy and taxonomic keys, after the specimen has been extracted from the dust substrate and especially prepared on a glass slide. A variety of immunological tests can be used to test for allergic responses to dust mites, such as skin prick tests, intradermal tests, ELISA and other immunological tests.

Prevention and Control

It is virtually impossible to eliminate all dust mites from a household, but areas where mites tend to congregate can be targeted. If possible, floor carpet could be replaced with smooth hard surface that is easy to clean. Mattresses and pillows can be encased in especially manufactured "plastic" products that aid in the exclusion of mites. Bedding and curtains should be selected on their ability to withstand frequent laundering. Thorough vacuuming on a regular basis, including all mattresses, especially the seams and framework of the bed, will also help. A reduction in humidity levels by increased air circulation and ventilation throughout the house will assist in maintaining mites at a lower level. Some chemical agents (e. g. 7% of Nipagin, 1% of lindane and other acaricides, etc.) can also be used for killing the mites in the environment. Allergies from house dust mite can be managed by immunotherapy using mite extracts called desensitization therapy, in conjunction with reducing the mite population in the home of the patient. Some anti-allergic medicines can be used for controlling the symptoms of asthma and allergic rhinitis.

Section 8 Other Mites

Acarid Mite

Acarid mites are also called flour mites, which belong to family Acaridae. They are usually free-living creatures, mainly breeding in the storehouses of food (especially flour and other food powder) under the warm and humid environment (see Figure 15-8-1).

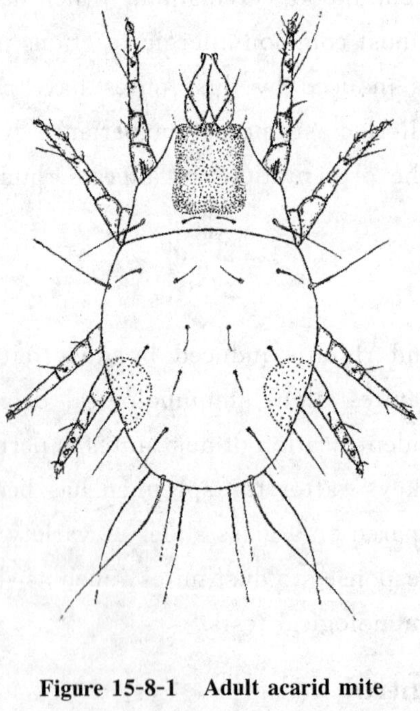

Figure 15-8-1 Adult acarid mite

The direct contact with acarid mites may lead to acarodermatitis. Occasionally acarid mites may be as the pathogen and cause pulmonary acariasis, intestinal acariasis and urinary acariasis if they invade into respiratory, alimentary and urinary systems. The patient with acariasis may experience a variety of symptoms without specific clinical presentations. The confirmation of diagnosis depends upon finding the pathogen, acarid mites.

Pyemotid Mite

The pyemotid mites in family Pyemotidae are mainly found in the cultivated areas and they are actually some predators, feeding on some agricultural pests. Some pyemotid mites can be utilized for the biological control of agricultural pests as the natural enemy of pests (see Figure 15-8-2).

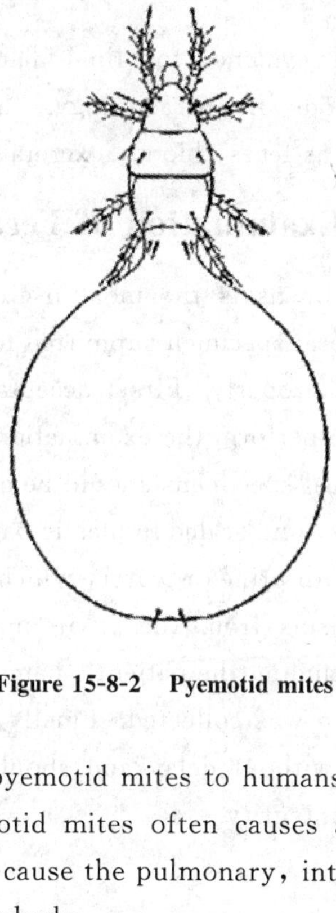

Figure 15-8-2 Pyemotid mites

The direct impairment of pyemotid mites to humans is of its medical significance. The direct contact with pyemotid mites often causes acarodermatitis. On very rare occasions, pyemotid mites may cause the pulmonary, intestinal or urinary acariasis as a pathogen if they invade into the body.

(Guo Xianguo)

Part V Experimental Diagnostic Techniques

Chapter 16 Etiologic Tests

As etiologic tests provide evidence for final diagnosis of parasitosis, they are important experimental methods in parasitology. Etiologic tests mainly include examination of such specimens as feces, blood, excreta and secreta.

Section 1 Examination of Fecal Specimens

Examination of fecal specimens is the most useful and important technique for diagnosis of parasitosis. The fecal specimen submitted to the laboratory for examination for parasites must be collected properly. First, acceptable specimens should contain a sufficient amount of material to perform the examination procedures, approximately 5-7 grams of feces. Second, the fecal specimens should be collected in clean, wide-mouthed containers with tight fitting lids, and sealed in plastic bags for transport. Care should be taken to avoid contamination with urine or water, which might harm existing organisms or introduce free-living organisms from the environment. Third, specimens should always be properly labeled, including the patient's name, identification number and the date and time that the specimen was collected. Finally, the fecal specimens should be transported to the laboratory without delay and should be processed immediately or preserved to maintain parasite integrity.

Direct Smear Method

Direct smear method is used for detection of helminth eggs and trophozoites and cysts of protozoa. It is easy, non time-consuming and three continuous smears may improve the detection rate.

Direct wet film

Direct wet film is suitable for detection of helminth eggs and trophozoites of protozoa. Wet films allow the observer to study the motility of protozoan trophozoites which are often characteristic.

In preparation of a wet film, a small portion of feces is mixed with a drop of sodium chloride on a clean slide. It is best in making the wet film to take small amount of materials from several parts of the stool sample. The film should not be too thick. As a rule, the film should be thin enough so that ordinary newsprint can easily be read through it. Usually the wet film is checked under low power of the microscope. Questionable objects may be subject to further investigation using the high dry objective (400X total magnification) for which a coverglass is placed on the preparation.

Iodine stain

Iodine stain is useful for detection of protozoan cysts. The procedure for preparation of the wet film is same with direct wet film except for substituting a drop of iodine stain for sodium chloride. Iodine stain kills the parasites and enhances the appearance of the nucleus and cytoplasmic structures such as glycogen vacuoles.

Iodine stain:

kalium iodidum 4g,

iodine 2g,

distilled water 100ml.

Store the iodine stain in a brown glass bottle.

Auramine-phenol and modified acid-fast method

The auramine-phenol and modified acid-fast method is most useful for detection of oocysts of *cryptosporidium* at present. In this method, the fresh fecal specimen or preservative fecal specimen (fixed with 10% formaldehyde and stored at 4°C within one month) is stained first by auramine-phenol and then modified acid-fast solution. Under light microscope, the oocyst is stained rose pink and the nonspecific particles dark blue. It is easy for the observer to differentiate the oocyst from other particles.

Auramine-phenol stain:

Solution I: 1g/L auramine-phenol solution

(auramine 0.1g, phenol 5.0g, distilled water 100ml)

Solution II: 3% hydrochloric acid-ethanol

(hydrochloric acid 3ml, 95% ethanol 97ml)

Solution III: 5g/L kalium hypermanganicum

(kalium hypermanganicum 0.5g, distilled water 100ml)

The procedure is: drop Solution I to the dried fecal film, 10-15min later rinse the film with water; drop Solution II and rinse with water 1min later; drop Solution III and rinse with water 1min later; then dry the film and observe under fluorescence microscope.

Modified acid-fast stain:

Solution I: phenol-basic fuchsin solution

(basic fuchsin 4g, 95% ethanol 20ml, phenol 8ml, distilled water 100ml)

Solution II：10% sulphuric acid

(sulphuric acid 10ml，distilled water 90ml)

Solution III：0.2% malachite green

(20g/l malachite green stock solution 1ml，distilled water 10ml)

The procedure is：drop Solution I to the dried fecal film，1.5-10min later rinse the film with water；drop Solution II and rinse with water 1-10min later；drop Solution III and rinse with water 1 min later；then dry the film and observe under light microscope.

Kato's Thick Smear

This method is suitable for detection of helminth eggs. The procedure is：place about 50-60mg fecal sample on a slide，then cover the feces with a 30mm×25mm×40μm transparent cellophane (advanced infiltrated with glycerol-malachite green solution)，incubate the slide at 30℃-36℃ for 30min or at 25℃ for 1h，then dry the fecal film and observe under light microscope. It is important to handle the thickness of the fecal film and the temperature and period of clearing. If the fecal film is too thick or the period of clearing is too short，the helminth eggs are often covered by sediments in feces and cannot be found. Otherwise，the helminth eggs are distorted and hard to be identified.

glycerol-malachite green solution：

glycerol 100ml，

distilled water 100ml，

3% malachite green solution 1ml.

Modified Kato's Thick Smear

This is an improved method and two procedures are added to the Kato's thick smear：first，a 5cm×5cm nylon sieve is used to discard the sediments in feces. Second，the filtered feces are placed in the template pore of a dosing plate. As the size of the dosing plate and the template pore is fixed，we can calculate the number of helminth eggs even the adult parasites in one gram feces in order to evaluate the state of parasite infection (see Figure 16-1-1).

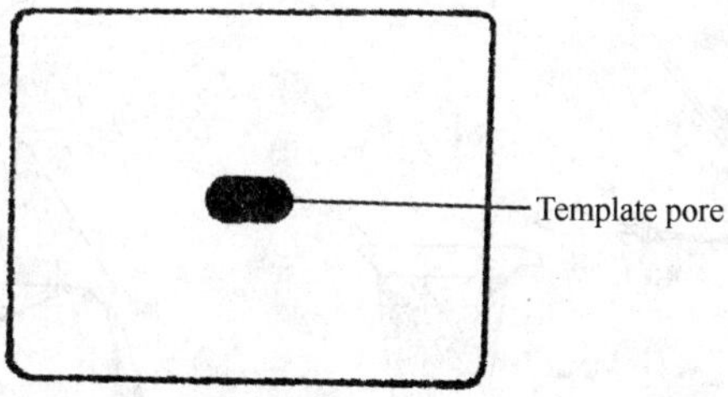

Figure 16-1-1 Modified Kato's thick smear dosing plate

Concentration Method

Concentration methods aid in the removal of debris and allow for the detection of even small numbers of parasites in a specimen. The described methods fall into two general classes: sedimentation and flotation techniques.

Sedimentation method

The density of most of the protozoan cysts and helminth eggs are higher than water and they can be separated from the lighter debris through sedimentation procedure to improve the detection rate.

(1)Nature sedimentation

This method is also called gravity sedimentation. It is especially useful for those helminth eggs whose density is higher than water. The advantage of this method is that the visual field is clear and it is easy for the observer to find the parasite eggs but it also has disadvantages as time-consuming and tedious handling.

The procedure is: suspend about 20-30g fecal specimen with water, filter the sample with wet gauze (2-3 layers) or metallic sieve (40-60 meshes), rinse the fecal residue with water, let the filtered fecal suspension stand for 20-30min, decant the supernatant carefully and slowly. Add water to the fecal residue again and this time let it stand for 15-20min. Then repeat the above procedure 2 or 3 times until the supernatant is clear. Decant the supernatant and place the deposition on a slide for observation (see Figure 16-1-2).

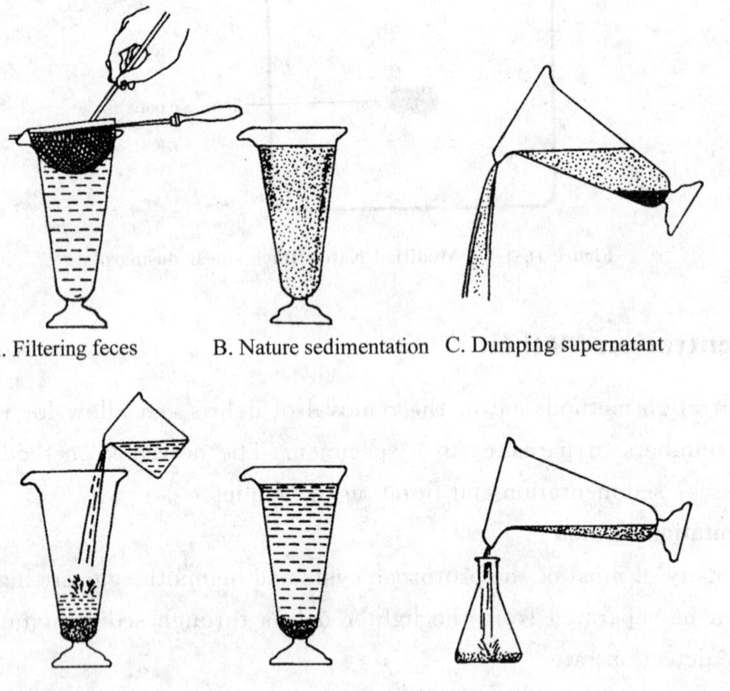

A. Filtering feces B. Nature sedimentation C. Dumping supernatant

D. Adding water again E. Nature sedimentation F. Collecting depositor

Figure 16-1-2 Nature sedimentation of feces

For detection of schistosoma (blood fluke) eggs, we'd better shorten the period of sedimentation as the miracidium in the egg is easy to hatch especially when the room temperature is higher than 15℃. For detection of protozoan cysts, the period for changing water should be extended to 6h.

(2)Centrifugal sedimentation

Using this method, we transfer the filtered fecal suspension mentioned in "nature sedimentation" into a 10ml centrifuge tube, centrifuge at 1,500-2,000rpm for 1-2min, decant the supernatant and add water again. Repeat the centrifuge procedure for 3-4 times until the supernatant is clear. Then decant the supernatant again and place the deposition on a slide for observation.

This method is easy and convenient and is often used in clinic detection.

(3) Formalin-ether sedimentation

The formaldehyde used in this method allows for the recovery of all protozoan cysts, helminth eggs and larvae. The ether may extract the debris and fecal fat which decreases the impurity and improves the concentration effect.

The procedure is: place about 1-2g fecal specimen into a small container, mix the sample with about 10-20ml water, filter the fecal suspension with gauze (2-3 layers) or metallic sieve (100 meshes) into a centrifuge tube, centrifuge at 2,000rpm for 2min. Decant the supernatant, add 7ml 10% formaldehyde, then add 3ml ether 5min later, stopper the tube and shake it vigorously, remove the stopper and centrifuge for 2min. After centrifugation such four layers should result as the ether layer, the debris plug, the formaldehyde layer and the sediment. The eggs or cysts are in the sediment. With an applicator stick, free the debris plug from the sides of the tube. Carefully decant the top three layers. The sediment at the bottom is prepared for observation. For detection of protozoan cysts, we can stain the slide, cover it with a coverglass and then observe the slide under microscope (see Figure 16-1-3).

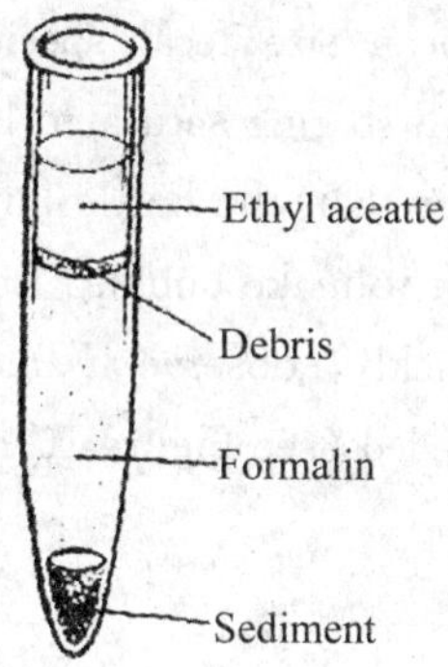

Figure 16-1-3 Sedimentation tube after centrifugation in Formalin-Ethyl Acetate Concentration

(4) Merthiolate-iodine-formaldehyde centrifugal sedimentation

This method can be used for concentration, fixation and stain for helminth eggs and trophozoites and cysts of protozoa. If 1g of fecal specimen is weighed accurately, then the detection of helminth eggs can be quantified.

The procedure is: mix 1g fecal specimen with about 10ml merthiolate-iodine-formaldehyde solution thoroughly, filter the fecal suspension with 2-3 layers gauze into a centrifuge tube, add 4ml ether and mix it for 2min, then centrifuge at 2,000rpm for 1-2min. After centrifuge, also four layers are resulted: the ether layer, the debris plug, the merthiolate-iodine-formaldehyde layer and the sediment. The eggs or cysts are in the sediment. Carefully decant the top three layers. The sediment at the bottom is prepared for observation.

Merthiolate-iodine-formaldehyde solution:

I: Merthiolate-formaldehyde solution:

1/1,000 thimerosal tincture 200ml, 40% formaldehyde 25ml, glycerol 50ml, distilled water 200ml.

II: Lugol's solution

Iodine 5g, Kalium iodidum 10g, distilled water 100ml. (This solution can be kept for no longer than one week.)

Mix 2.35ml merthiolate-formaldehyde solution and 0.15ml 5% Lugol's solution. This solution can be preserved for 8h.

Floatation method

In contrast to the sedimentation technique in which the parasites are denser than the suspending fluid, flotation methods concentrate lighter potential parasites at the surface of a suspending fluid.

(1) Saturated brine floatation

This method is most useful for those eggs with low density such as hookworm eggs and tapeworm eggs.

The procedure is: place soybean size fecal specimen into a floating bottle with an applicator stick, mix the sample with sparing saturated brine, then add saturated brine slowly until the surface of the fluid is upper than the bottle but no fluid overflows. Then cover the bottle with a slide and be careful not to make bubble. Let the bottle stand for 15-20min, then raise the slide and turn it over quickly, observe it under microscope. When the high dry objective is used, a coverglass is needed (see Figure 16-1-4).

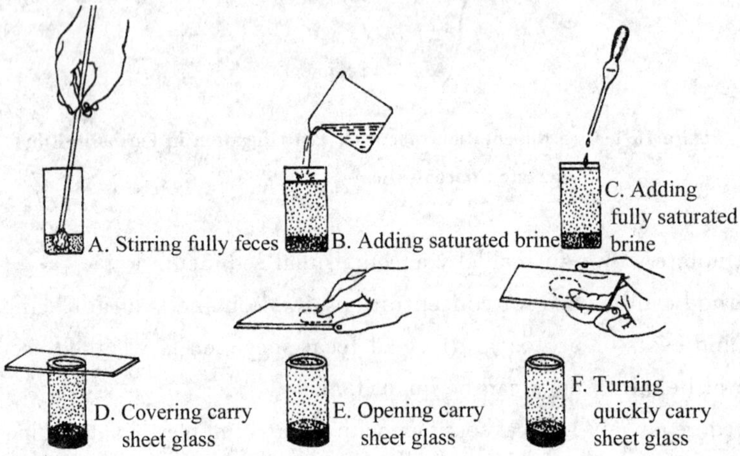

Figure 16-1-4 Saturated brine floatation

(2) Zinc-sulfate centrifugal floatation

This technique works well for the recovery of protozoan cysts, *coccidian* oocysts and some helminth eggs.

The procedure is: transfer about 1g fresh stool into a centrifuge tube, add 10ml water and mix thoroughly, strain and centrifuge the specimen as mentioned above in the method "centrifuge sedimentation". When the supernatant is clear, decant the supernatant, add 33% zinc sulfate into the tube and mix it. Then fill the centrifuge tube with zinc sulfate to within 1cm of the rim and centrifuge the tube for 1min at 2,000rpm. Withdraw 1 or 2 drops of the surface film with a wire loop, transfer it to a slide and observe under microscope.

(3) Floatation method with sucrose solution

This method is particularly effective for the recovery of protozoan cysts, oocysts and sporocysts.

The procedure is: transfer about 5g fresh stool into a container, add 15-20ml water, mix it and strain the specimen as mentioned above in the method "centrifuge sedimentation". Then centrifuge the strained fecal suspension at 1,500rpm for 5-10min. Decant the supernatant, add sucrose solution and centrifuge again. Withdraw 1 or 2 drops of the surface film with a wire loop, transfer it to a slide, add a coverglass and observe using the high dry objective or the oil immersion lens. Oocysts will appear as transparent, rounded structures containing a dark dot and yellow sporozoites.

Sucrose solution:

sucrose 500g,

distilled water 320ml,

phenol 6.5ml.

Concentration with nylon pouch

This method is mainly used for concentration of the blood fluke eggs. When using this technique, two nylon pouches are needed, 120 meshes and 260 meshes respectively. The diameter of blood fluke eggs is just between the pore sizes of these two nylon pouches.

The procedure is: put one nylon pouch (120 meshes) into another nylon pouch (260 meshes) and clamp them respectively. Be careful not to stick the bottom of the two pouches. Transfer about 30g fecal specimen into a glass and mix it with water. After strain with metallic sieve (60 meshes), transfer the fecal residue into the interior nylon pouch. Put these two pouches into water and draw them up and down slowly to rinse the fecal residue until effluent from the pouch is clear. Draw the interior pouch out and discard the debris. Discard the clamp on the outer pouch, transfer the sediment into a measuring glass, let it stand for 15min. Decant the supernatant and detect the sediment with microscope.

This method is non time-consuming, loses few eggs and can avoid discarding the miracidium hatched during handling.

Larva Hatching Method

Culture method for hookworm larva

Under proper temperature and humidity, the hookworm eggs may hatch soon and grow into larva in a few days. The detection rate of hatching method is obvious higher than the direct smear method and the larva hatched benefits us for identification of different species.

The procedure is: add about 2ml distilled water into a clean tube (1cm×10cm), make the filter paper into a "T" size which is as wide as the tube but a little longer. Mark the name and number of the subject with pencil at the trabecules of the filter paper. Pick about 0. 2-0. 4g fecal specimen and smear it evenly in the middle of the filter paper, insert the paper into the tube until the bottom of the paper is soaked in water but the fecal specimen does not contact the water. Incubate the tube at 25℃-30℃ and add water every day in order to keep the fluid surface at the same height. After 3-5 days, hookworm larva moving snake-like may be observed at the bottom of the tube. If no larva observed, the incubation period should be extended to 5 days. If the room temperature is low, we can place the tube into warm water (30℃) before detection (see Figure 16-1-5).

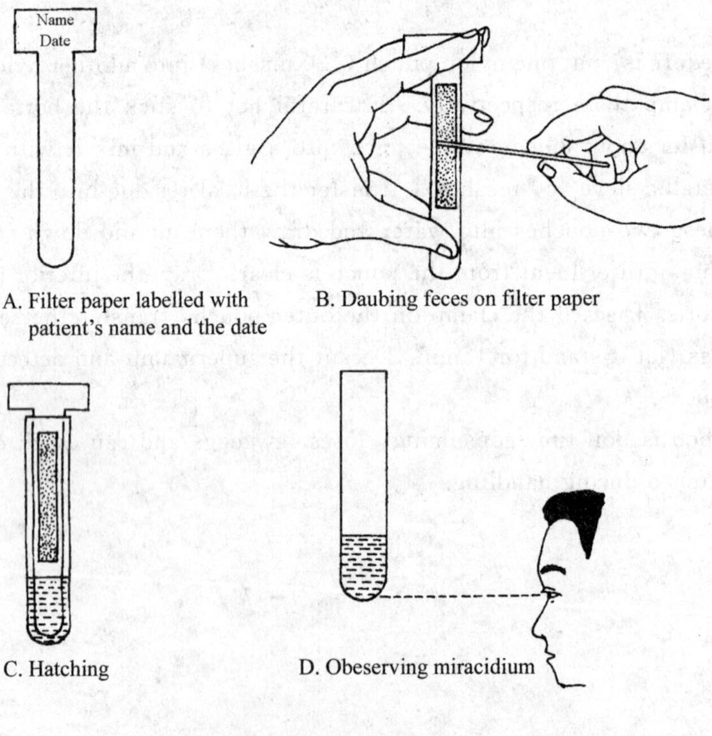

A. Filter paper labelled with patient's name and the date

B. Daubing feces on filter paper

C. Hatching

D. Obeserving miracidium

Figure 16-1-5 Culture method of larva

This method is also useful for identification of trophozoites of *Amoeba* and *Trichomonas hominis*. For this kind of detection, about 1g fecal specimen is needed and the incubation period is 2-4 days, usually 48h.

Miracidium hatching method

If feces containing viable blood fluke eggs are diluted with approximately 10 volumes of water, the eggs hatch within a few hours releasing miracidia. The miracidia are positively phototrophic. This method just takes advantage of this characteristic.

The procedure is: concentrate about 30g fecal specimen by nature sedimentation, transfer the sediment into a conical flask, full the flask with water, hatch the specimen at 20℃-30℃ for 4-6h, then observe directly or with a magnifying glass (see Figure 16-1-6).

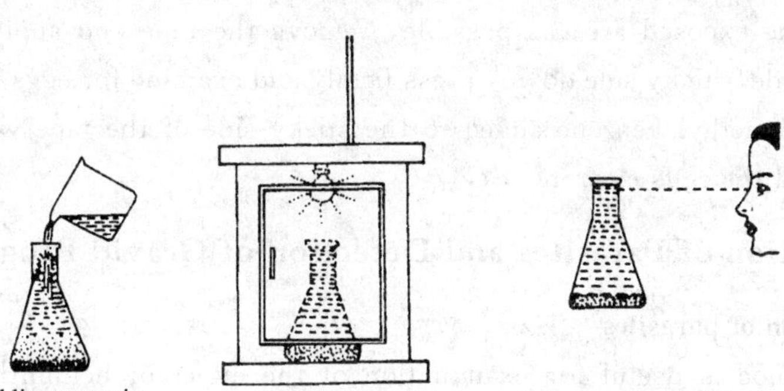

A. Adding water in depositor of feces　　B. Hatching　　C. Observing miracidium

Figure 16-1-6 Culture method of miracidium

The white dots swim straight back and forth at 1 or 2cm under the fluid surface are miracidia. Also we can suck the miracidia out for further detection if necessary. If no miracidia were observed, we can view it every 4-6h within 24h. When the temperature is above 25℃, the eggs hatch soon. So it is better rinse the fecal specimen with 1% brine or cold water and for the last time, rinse with water at room temperature.

Anal Swab

This technique is especially useful for detection of *Enterobius vermicularis* (pinworm) and *Taenia saginata* (beef tapeworm) eggs. During the night, the adult female pinworm migrates out of the anus and deposits her eggs around the perianal region, so the tape should be used in the morning before the patient washes or defecates. When the gravid proglottid of beef tapeworm comes to the anal active or passive, it is often squeezed and the eggs in it are freed and sticked to the perianal region. So anal swab is also used in detection of beef tapeworm.

Cotton swab

The procedure is: soak the applicator stick in saline, discard the saline before use, wipe around the perianal region, put the stick into a tube filled with saturated brine, stir the stick vigorously, discard the stick and add saturated brine until the tube is full, cover the tube with a slide, then 5min later take the slide for detection. Otherwise, discard the stick and let the tube stand for 10min or centrifuge to get sediment for detection.

Cellophane tape

A variety of commercially prepared collection kits are available. Patients are generally children, so parents or caretakers should be given clear instructions regarding the proper collection technique.

The procedure is: cut a piece of clear cellophane tape approximately 2cm×6cm in size, stretch the tape evenly, sticky side out, apply the tape to the anal region covering as much of the exposed area as possible, remove the tape and apply to a clean, dry microscope slide, sticky side down, press firmly and examine for eggs under low power. One drop of dimethyl benzene added to the sticky side of the tape will make the tape more even and the eggs clearer.

Elutriation of Parasites and Detection of Gravid Proglottid

Elutriation of parasites

This method is useful for examination of the effect of helminthicide. The adult elutriated from the fecal specimen benefits for the recovery of species and number of the parasite.

The procedure is: take all the fecal specimen 24-72h after taking helminthicide, mix the sample with water, decant the debris with gauze (2-3 layers) or metallic sieve (40 meshes), rinse with water repeatedly, then transfer the specimen into a glass container with water, put a piece of black paper under the container for examination of the parasite.

Detection of gravid proglottid

The procedure is: rinse the gravid proglottid with water, put it between two slides, press the slides slightly to make the proglottid flat, and then observe the structure facing the light and differentiate the species of the tapeworm according to the uterus branches. Or inject ink or carmine red carefully and slowly into the uterus at the center of the posterior part of the proglottid, count the branches of the uterus trunk after coloration.

Carmine red solution:

aluminum potassium sulfate saturated solution 100ml,

carmine red 3g,

glacial acetic acid 10ml.

Let the mix liquid stand in incubator at 37℃ overnight, and then filter it just before use.

Section 2 Examination of Blood

Microscopic examination of fresh blood is useful for detection of two types of parasites: *Plasmodium* spp. and *filaria*. When fresh blood is examined, it is important to make sufficient preparation. The preparation of good blood film depends to a large extent on the cleanliness of microscope slides and coverglasses employed. It is essential that both slides and coverglasses be washed in cleaning solution, tap water, distilled water and 95% alcohol to make them free of dust and oil. Then dry the slides and coverglasses with a clean towel before use. For specific identification of these organisms, permanent stain is essential.

Detection of *Plasmodium* spp.

Collection of blood specimen

Blood samples may be obtained from the fingertip or earlobe. When collect the blood specimen, first knead the finger or earlobe to make it hyperemia, cleanse the skin with 75% alcohol. Then after the skin dried, knead the part for collection of blood with left thumb and forefinger, sting the skin with blood lancet in right hand to get blood sample. The time of collection is important for the recovery and identification of the *plasmodium*. For *P. vivax* it is better to collect the blood sample 6-8h after stroke, for *P. falciparum* ring form initial stage of stroke and for *P. falciparum* gametocytes 7-10 days after stroke.

Film preparation

When examine the *Plasmodium* spp., we often use the thin and thick blood smear. Thin blood smears are suggested for the observation of morphologic details and species identification. And thick blood smears are typically used for screening purpose particularly when the parasitemia may be low. These two smears can be made on one slide for convenient comparison.

(1) Thin blood smear

The procedure is: place a small drop of blood near one end of a microscope slide, use a second slide as a "push slide" or spreader, back the spreader into the blood at a 30℃-45℃ angle, and draw the blood across the slide in one continuous movement. A properly made smear will have an end taper to a strap-shaped edge. Most of the area of the slide will be a thin layer one cell thick (see Figure 16-2-1A).

(2) Thick blood smear

The procedure is: place 2-3 drops of whole blood close together at one end of a slide, mix the drops together with another slide in a circular motion over an area of 2cm in diameter (the mixing should continue for at least 30 seconds to prevent formation of fibrin strands), allow the slide air dry thoroughly at room temperature, lake the dry slide to remove hemoglobin (see Figure 16-2-1B).

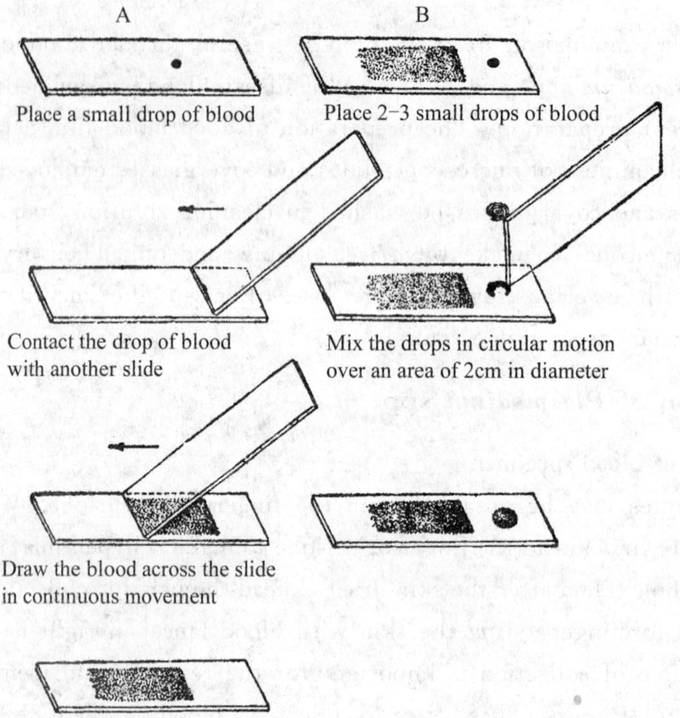

Figure 16-2-1 Preparation of the thin (A) and thick (B) blood smear

Fixation and stain

There are two kinds of permanent stains that are commonly used in the clinical laboratory for the blood smear—Giemsa and Wright's staining. It is better to dilute the stain solution with proper buffer and rinse the slide with buffer after staining.

Buffer: dibasic sodium phosphate solution

(dibasic sodium phosphate 9.464g, metered volume to 1,000ml with distilled water)

potassium dihydrogen phosphate solution

(potassium dihydrogen phosphate 9.073g, metered volume to 1,000ml with distilled water)

Make the buffer just before use and for different pH value prepare the buffer with the ratio listed in Table 16-2-1.

Table 16-2-1 Dispensing of different pH buffer

pH value	KH_2PO_4 (ml)	Na_2HPO_4 (ml)	Distilled water (ml)
6.8	4.9	6.3	90
7.0	6.3	3.7	90
7.2	7.3	27	90
7.4	8.1	1.9	90

(1) Giemsa staining

The procedure is: dilute the Giemsa stain with buffer at the ratio of 1 : 15-20, draw the stain field with wax pencil, fix the thin and thick blood film with methanol (for thick blood film, haematolysis is needed), drop the diluted Giemsa stain on the blood films, stain for 25-30min at room temperature, rinse with buffer or water, observe the slide when the films are dried.

Giemsa staining provides significant morphologic details for the species identification of blood parasites and the slide Giemsa stained can be preserved for a long time, but it is also time-consuming.

Giemsa stain: Giemsa stain powder 1g, methanol 50ml, glycerol 50ml. Triturate the Giemsa stain powder adding glycerol continuously, transfer the suspension into a brown bottle, rinse the triturator with methanol for several times, transfer the methanol into the same bottle, stuff the lid fast, mix thoroughly, incubate the bottle at 65℃ for 24h or at room temperature for 1 week, filter the suspension for use.

(2) Wright's staining

The procedure is: for the thin blood film we can begin with the staining procedure, but for the thick blood film haematolysis, fixation is also needed before staining. Cover the thin and thick blood films with Wright's stain, stain for 1min, add the same amount buffer to the films, shake the slide slightly to mix the stain and the buffer, then a floating film light copper colored appears, 3-5min later rinse the slide from one side with water or buffer, dry the slide and observe under microscope.

As Wright's stain combines the fixative and stain in one solution, it is convenient especially for clinical test. But the stain is easy to adhere to the film, easy to color fading and cannot be preserved for long period.

Wright's stain: Wright's stain powder 0.2-0.5g, methanol 97ml, glycerol 3ml. Mix the Wright's stain powder with glycerol and triturate thoroughly, rinse the triturator with methanol several times and transfer all the suspension into a bottle, mix and filter the suspension 1 or 2 weeks later for use.

Detection of Microfilaria

Collection of blood samples

Wuchereria bancrofti and *Brugia malayi* exhibit nocturnal periodicity, therefore blood samples should be collected between 10 p. m. at night and 2 a. m. on the next morning when the microfilariae are most likely to be present in the peripheral blood.

Examination

(1)Examination of fresh blood samples

Drop one drop of fresh blood on a slide, add a coverglass and observe using lower power. The larvae swimming snake-like are the microfilariae. To differentiate the species, staining is needed.

(2)Thick blood film

The staining method is the same with that of *Plasmodium*. But the 2-3 drops of blood are smeared into a 2cm×3cm rectangle.

(3) Centrifugal concentration

In some patients, the number of microfilariae in peripheral blood is too small. For this instance, we can collect 1-3ml blood from the vein with heparin for anticoagulation, add 9 aliquots of distilled water for haematolysis, centrifuge and take the sediment for microscope examination.

(4)Concentration of living microfilariae

Add 1/2 volume distilled water to a centrifuge tube, add 10-12 drops of blood, then add sodium chloride to the tube, mix them and centrifuge at 3,000rpm for 3min, take the sediment for microscope examination. Or transfer 1ml venous blood into a tube with 0.1ml 3.8% natrium citricum, mix them and add 9ml distilled water, centrifuge for 2min after haematolysis, decant the supernatant and centrifuge again, then take the sediment for microscope examination.

Section 3 Examination of Excreta and Secreta

Detection of Sputum and Aspirates from Lung

Sputum and aspirates from lung are often helpful for diagnosing infections with *Paragonimus westermani* (lung fluke) eggs, trophozoites of *Entamoeba histolytica*, protoscoleces of hydatid, larva of *Strongyloides stercoralis*, *Ascaris lumbricoides* and hookworm, dust mites.

Direct wet mount

This method is used in recovery of lung fluke eggs and trophozoites of *Entamoeba histolytica*. Sputum specimens should be collected in the early morning and a proper specimen should be from the lower respiratory passages, not saliva. Draw 1 or 2 drops of sodium chloride to a clean slide, pick some sputum especially those questionable, make it into a sputum smear, add a coverglass and examine under microscope. Only charcot-leyden crystal and no lung fluke eggs may also indicate there may be an infection of lung fluke. For this instance, several more smears should be made and all negative results may suggest that digestion and concentration method is needed.

Digestion and concentration

Collect all the sputum for 24h in a glass, add the same amount of 10% NaOH, mix by a glass rod, incubate at 37℃ for about 2-3h until the sputum becomes thinner, enclose it into several centrifuge tube separately and centrifuge the tubes at 1,500rpm for 10min, decant the supernatant, take 1 drop of sediment for examination. This is useful for detection of some helminth eggs and mites.

Detection of Duodenal Aspirates and Bile

Duodenal aspirates and bile are most often evaluated for trophozoites of *Giardia lamblia*, eggs of *Clonorchis sinensis* (liver fluke), *Fasciolopsis buski* (intestinal fluke) and *Fasciola hepatica*.

Detection of duodenal aspirates

Transfer the duodenal aspirates to a slide, add a coverglass and examine under microscope. For higher detection rate, we may dilute the duodenal aspirates with sodium chloride, enclose it in several centrifuge tube separately, centrifuge the tubes at 2,000rpm for 5-10min and take the sediment for examination. If the duodenal aspirates are too thick, we'd better digest them with 10% NaOH before centrifuge. But the digestion is not suitable for detection of protozoan trophozoites. The eggs of *Fasciolopsis buski* and *Fasciola hepatica* are hard to differentiate from morphological features, but the former may be found only in duodenal aspirates but not in bile.

Enteric-test capsule method

This method consists of a weighted length of nylon yarn coiled within a gelatin capsule. For adults, the yarn is 140cm in length and for children 90cm. An extended piece of the yarn is taped to the patient's cheek and the capsule is swallowed. The capsule material dissolves in the patient's stomach and the yarn is carried into the duodenum. After 4-6h of incubation, the line is retrieved and the material adhering to the yarn is examined microscopically (see Figure 16-3-1).

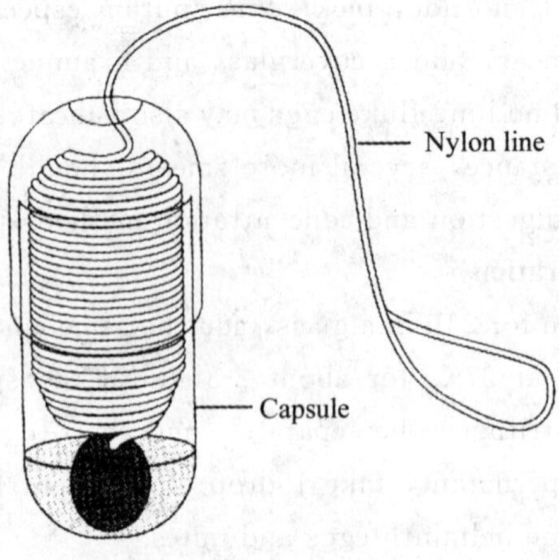

Figure 16-3-1 Entero test

Detection of Urine and Hydrocele

Urine is the specimen of choice for the recovery of *Schistosoma haematobium* eggs and can also be indicated for the detection of microfilariae. Urine is collected into a wide-mouth, sterile container with a tight fitting lid. The specimen is centrifuged and the sediment is examined microscopically. Chyluria should be mixed with the same amount of ether thoroughly in order to dissolve the fat by ether. Then decant the fat layer, centrifuge and take the sediment for examination.

Hydrocele is mainly used for diagnosis of microfilariae of *W. bancrofti*. Cleanse the scrotum skin with iodine-alcohol, aspirate the hydrocele using syringe, then make a direct smear for examination or dilute the aspirates with proper amount of sodium chloride, centrifuge and take the sediment for detection microscopically.

Detection of Vaginal Secretions and Prostatic Fluid

Detection of vaginal secretions

Detection of vaginal secretions is used for examination of *Trichomonas vaginalis* and for eggs and adults of pinworm and trophozoites of *E. histolytica*.

(1) Direct wet mount

Take secretions from posterior fornix, neck of uterus and vaginal wall of the patient, transfer the secretion to a slide dropped with sodium chloride, and then detect the slide microscopically for the parasites.

(2) Suspension method

Smear a coverglass with a thin layer of vaseline at the edge, draw a drop of sodium chloride on the coverglass, transfer the vaginal secretions into the sodium chloride, turnover the coverglass and put it on a slide, press slightly to make these two glass sheets stick together. Now the drop is suspended under the coverglass and ready for examination.

Detection of prostatic fluid

This method is used for detection of *Trichomonas vaginalis* in male genitourinary tract. Take some prostatic fluid by massaging the prostate, transfer it to a slide, draw one drop of sodium chloride, add a coverglass and examine microscopically for *Trichomonas vaginalis*.

Detection of Cerebrospinal Fluid

This technique is mainly useful for detection of *Toxoplasma*, trophozoites of *E. histolytica*, lung fluke, ectopic *S. japonicum*, protoscoleces or hooklets of hydatid, larva of *S. stercoralis*, *Gnathostoma spinigerum* and *Angiostrongylus cantonensis*.

Take about 2ml cerebrospinal fluid, centrifuge at 2,000rpm for 5min and examine the sediment microscopically. For detection of trophozoites of *amoeba*, centrifuge is not suitable as it affects the activity of the pseudopodium. For *Toxoplasma* and *amoeba*, the slide needs to fix with methanol, stain with Giemsa or Wright's method and observe using the oil lens.

As the parasites mentioned above appear in the cerebrospinal fluid on rare occasions, the negative result of this method cannot deplete the infection completely.

Section 4 Biopsy

Biopsy of Skin and Subcutaneous Tissue

Examination of helminth

The larva or adults of some parasites may develop into a node or lump in subcutaneous tissue which includes cysticercus cellulosae, sparganum mansoni, adult of lung fluke and larva of *Pagumogonimus skrjabini*, *Gnathostoma spinigerum* and *Gnathostoma hispidium*. Specimens should be surgically removed and submitted to the laboratory in sterile saline to prevent dehydration. Biopsy materials can be used to prepare touch prep slides for further staining or for histologic processing.

Examination of protozoa

This method is also used for patients suspected with dermal leishmaniasis. Cleanse the skin with a lump or papule, stab the skin and suck tissue fluid with a syringe, make a smear with the tissue fluid, stain it with Giemsa or Wright's stain for examination microscopically. Or we can make smear with skin snips or make histological sections with the node or lump extirpated.

Examination of arthropod

(1)Examination of scab mites

Stab the end of the tunnel with a sterile needle and take out the scab mites for examination. Or draw liquid paraffin to the papule with an sterile operating knife blade, scrape the stratum corneum on the top of the papule, transfer the materials scraped to a slide drawn with liquid paraffin beforehand, add a coverglass for examination microscopically.

(2)Examination of demodicid mites

Scrape the skin with an acne compressor or a bended forceps, transfer the scraped secretion from sebaceous glands to a slide, add some glycerol and examine under microscope. Or apply a piece of cellophane tape approximately 5cm in length to forehead, nose and nasal furrow at night, press the tape evenly with hand, remove the tape next morning, apply it to a slide for examination. This method is easy, convenient and painless which is especially helpful for census.

Biopsy of Muscle

This method is useful for examination of Sparganum mansoni, cysticercus cellulosae, adult of lung fluke and larva of *P. skrjabini* and *T. spiralis*. The lumps removed surgically from the muscle can be observed directly under anatomical lens or a microscope. For morphologic identification, sheeting, fixation, staining and dehydration are also needed. For *T. spiralis*, remove a piece of rice-size muscle from the patient, transfer the piece of muscle to a slide, draw one drop of 50% glycerol-alcohol, add another slide and press these two slides firmly, observe using the lower power. The muscle must be detected right after removed or the larva will be destroyed and hard to be identified.

Biopsy of Lymph Node

This technique is used for detection of adults of filaria, *Leishmania*, *Toxoplasma* and *Trypanosoma*.

Examination of filaria

Usually we suck the adults from the suspected lymph nodes with a syringe or remove the affected lymph nodes and detect directly or make histological sections for examination.

Examination of *Leishmania*

The *Leishmania* in the lymph node tends to be eliminated much lower than the other part, so biopsy of lymph nodes for *Leishmania* is significantly meaningful for radical cure. Usually we choose the inguinal lymph nodes. Cleanse the skin, pinch the lymph node with left thumb and forefinger, stab into the node with a sterile and dry syringe in the right hand and now the tissue fluid from the node can flow into the syringe. Transfer the small amount of tissue fluid to a slide, make a smear, stain it and examine. Smears made from the surface of the lymph node removed are also used.

Biopsy of Bone Marrow

This method is often used for detection of amastigote of *L. donovani* with higher detection rate than biopsy of lymph nodes.

Ilium is usually chosen for stab. Let the patient lie on one side, stab into the skin using a transfixion pin, when the transfixion pin touches the bone surface, pierce the transfixion pin into the bone about 0. 5-1. 0cm, take out the inner part of the transfixion pin and connect the transfixion pin to a syringe (2ml) for sucking of bone marrow. Transfer the bone marrow to a slide, make a smear, fix with methanol, stain just as the thin and thick blood films and then observe with oil immersion lens.

Biopsy of Lung Tissue

This method is used for diagnosis of *Pneumocystis*. Make a smear with the stab or a small piece of lung tissue removed, dry it at room temperature and stain with modified silver staining.

The procedure of modified silver staining is: put the slide into 5% chromic acid at 20℃ for 5min for oxidation, rinse with lotic water for several seconds; soak the slide in 1% sodium bisulfite for 1min, rinse with lotic water and distilled water; transfer the slide to silver methenamine (a solution of 2 parts silver methenamine to 1 part dimethyl sulfoxide), incubate at 60℃ for 90min until the smear turns into yellow brown, rinse with lotic water and distilled water for 5min respectively; stain in 0. 1% auric chloride for 2-5min, rinse with distilled water for 4-5 times; immerse the slide in 2% sodium thiosulfate for 5min, rinse with lotic water for at least 10min; stain with 0. 3% brilliant green for 45s; dehydrate in 95%, 99% and 100% alcohol for 2min step by step; clear with dimethyl benzene for 3 times and mount with neutral gummi.

As a result, the cysts of *Pneumocystis* appear as round, orbicular-ovate or irregular shape, the cyst wall is stained brown. The red cells on the slide are stained light yellow and the background light green.

Biopsy of Liver Tissue

The infected liver can be used for identification of *E. histolytica* trophozoites, *S. japonicum* eggs, *P. skrjabini* larva, hydatid of *Echinococcus granulosus* and *E. multilocularis*. It is a taboo to stab in the last two instances so it is very important to eliminate these two diseases before stab.

Biopsy of Rectum Mucosa

Examination of *S. japonicum*

Remove a piece of rice-size mucosa from the rectum with protoscope, rinse with water, lay it between two slides, press slight to make it evenly, then observe under microscope.

Examination of trophozoites of *E. histolytica*

Scrape mucosa materials with romanoscope from the edge and bottom of the ulcer, transfer the mucosa materials to a slide, drop some sodium chloride, add a coverglass, press slightly and examine immediately. Or take a small piece of mucosa, make histological sections and stain for examination.

(Yang Qing)

Chapter 17 Immunodiagnostic and Molecular Biological Analysis

In the majority of cases, the diagnosis of parasitic disease is made in the clinical laboratory by identification of the parasite itself in body fluids, tissues, or excreta. Clinical signs and symptoms, together with the patient's travel history, may dictate what laboratory tests to employ and may suggest ancillary testing by means such as radiography, ultrasonography, and magnetic resonance imaging. In some case, parasites may not be found despite careful search, and radiologic findings may be equivocal. In such case, we may have to rely on immunodiagnostic or biological diagnosis methods to search for a diagnosis on the basis of clues left either by the parasite itself (antigens) or by the body's response to parasitic invasion (antibodies).

Most special techniques are at present beyond the scope of even the best clinical laboratories, although for a number of the more common infections, tests are available in kit form. The problem is, of course, that the need for test for the less common parasitic diseases is so sporadic that it is both economically impractical for them to be made available at a local level and impossible for the laboratory to become proficient in their use.

Test vary considerably in sensitivity (the percentage of positive results in a group known to have an infection; true positives), in specificity (the percentage of negative reactions in a group known to be uninfected; true negatives), and in reactivity. Reactivity is the amount of antigen or antibody needed to produce a demonstrable serologic reaction. Fortunately, most of the tests in current use have a high degree of reactivity.

The following types of tests are those most frequently used at the present time for diagnosis of parasitic disease.

Section 1 Immunodiagnostic Techniques

Dye Test (DT)

The most reliable of these is the Sabin-Feldman dye test. Live virulent tachyzoites of *T. gondii* are used as antigen and are exposed to dilutions of the test serum and to a complement accessory factor resembling complement that is obtained from *Toxoplasma*-antibody free-human serum. This test is sensitive and so far is the most specific test for toxoplasmosis. Its main disadvantages are its high cost and the human hazard of using live organisms.

Circumoval Precipitin

The circumoval precipitin test is a serological test used for diagnosis of schistosomiasis japonica. Soluble egg antigens of *Schistosoma japonicum* block the formation of the circumoval precipitin by serum from infected humans. Consequently, circumoval precipitin inhibition was used to monitor purification of the soluble egg antigens of *S. japonicum*. Crude egg antigens were separated into protein and glycoprotein fractions by lectin chromatography on concanavalin A sepharose.

Bentonite Flocculation (BF)

This test, of relatively low reactivity, is performed by coating particles of bentonite with the test antigen and observing flocculation on addition of the serum. Titration is achieved by serial dilution of the serum. This test is used primarily for the diagnosis of trichinosis, for which other tests are also available.

Direct Immunofluorescence (DFA)

Fluorescence of parasite antigen is induced by the introduction of monoclonal antibodies (produced *in vitro* against the parasite in question and fluorescently tagged) into a fluid or applied to a slide containing the parasite. The organism fluoresces when viewed by fluorescence microscopy. This test is used for detection of cryptosporidiosis, giardiasis, and trichomoniasis (see Figure 17-1-1).

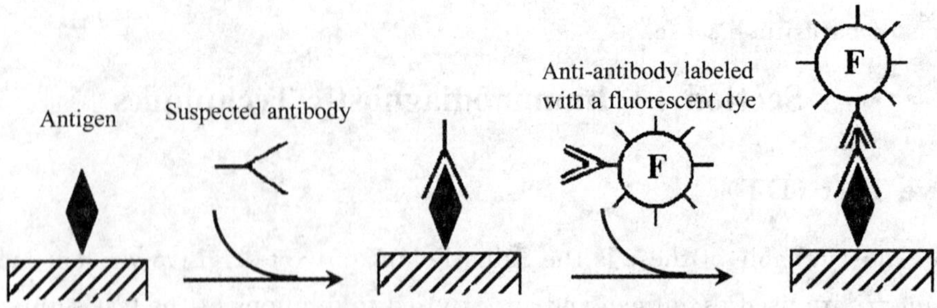

Figure 17-1-1 Abridged general view of direct immunofluorescence

Indirect Fluorescent Antibody (IFA)

A known parasite antigen (for example, blood smears containing *Plasmodium falciparum* obtained from infected *Aotus* monkeys) is exposed to patient serum suspected of containing antibodies to that parasite. Antibodies in the serum bind to antigen of the parasites, the slide is then washed to remove the serum, and the slide is then covered with a solution containing a fluorescent dye. Remaining of the fluorescent dye indicates the presence of the antibody in the serum specimen. By use of appropriate antihuman globulin, one may test for IgG or IgM. This test is used for diagnosis of babesiosis, Chagas' disease, cryptosporidiosis, giardiasis, leishmaniasis, malaria, and toxoplasmosis (see Figure 17-1-2).

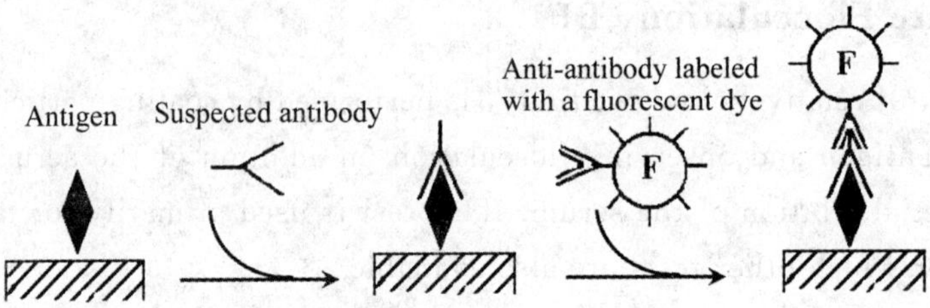

Figure 17-1-2 Abridged general view of indirect fluorescent antibody

Radioimmunoassay (RIA)

Radioimmunoassay is commonly used to measure the levels of hormones in blood and tissue fluids. In RIA for an antigen, pure antibody against that antigen is radioactively labeled, usually with ^{125}I. This test is used for detection of helminthiasis.

Enzyme Immunoassay (EIA)

A general term for several different procedures that determine the presence or absence of a parasite by the reaction between the parasite antigen or antibodies, an enzyme-coupled corresponding antibody or antigen, and the enzyme substrate, with production of a color that may be assayed either qualitatively or quantitatively. Enzyme immunoassay is the most widely used of all the types of tests for detection of parasitic infections.

Enzyme-linked Immunosorbent Assay (ELISA)

A specific variation of enzyme immunoassay, the ELISA has become increasingly popular because of sensitivity and ease of interpretation. The appropriate antigen or antibody is bound to a solid support (microtiter well, beads, test tube walls). The specimen to be tested (serum, cerebrospinal fluid, feces) is added and reacts with the already present antigen or antibody. Washing then removes unbound material, after which enzyme-linked antibody or antigen is added, which reacts with the antigen or antibody of the test material. An additional washing removes all unbound material, and finally a solution that reacts with the remaining enzyme to produce a color change is added. This change may be measured either visually or colorimetrically. ELISA (often listed simply as EIA) is used to diagnose a wide variety of parasitic diseases (see Figure 17-1-3).

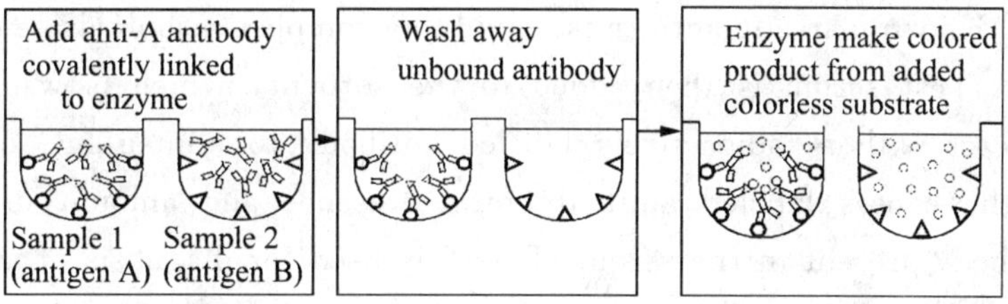

Figure 17-1-3 Principle of enzyme-linked immunosorbent assay

Indirect Hemagglutination (IHA)

One of the older test modalities, indirect hemagglutination depends on the agglutination (clumping) of antigen-coated sheep erythrocytes by antibodies in the test serum. It may be roughly quantitated by dilution of the test serum, and is used for diagnosis of amebiasis (*E. histolytica/dispar* complex), Chagas' disease, cysticercosis, echinococcosis, filariasis, and toxoplasmosis (see Figure 17-1-4).

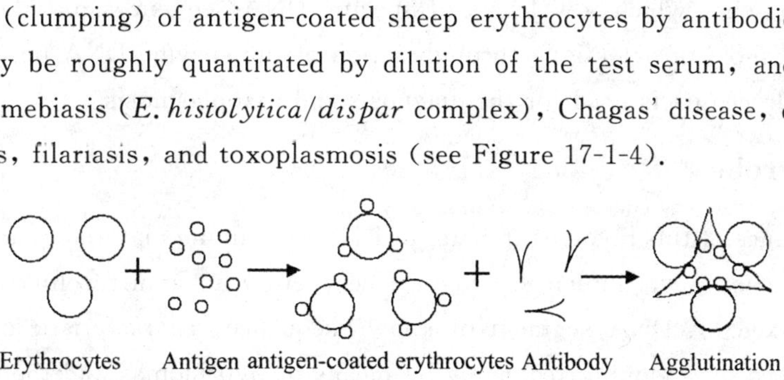

Figure 17-1-4 Abridged general view of indirect hemagglutination

Latex Agglutination (LA)

See Bentonite Flocculation. This procedure is the same, with substitution of latex particles for bentonite. Latex agglutination is an older test, but it is still used for diagnosis of *Trichomonas vaginalis* infection.

Immunoblot (IB)

A more sensitive version of the IHA, in which a sample of protein-containing material from serum, cerebrospinal fluid, or other tissue or excreta is electrophoresed onto a polyacrylamide gel. The electrophoretically separated proteins on the gel are then transferred (by blotting) onto a sheet where they are recognized by radioactively labeled specific antibodies, whose presence can be assayed after the sheet is washed. This technique is used primarily for the detection of cysticercosis, echinococcosis, paragonimiasis, and schistosomiasis.

Radioallergosorbent Test (RAST)

Developed as a test for antibodies to certain allergens, RAST test specifically for IgG and IgE. Known parasite antigen is bound to a complex carbohydrate matrix known as a sorbent. Test serum is then added to the sorbent, which is washed and then allowed to react with a radioactively labeled antibody to human IgG or IgE. After removal of the excess labeled antibody, the presence and amount of radioactivity measure antibody present in the serum. RAST is used for diagnosis of anisakiasis and ascariasis.

Section 2 Molecular Biological Analysis

Polymerase Chain Reaction (PCR)

A method that which low levels of specific DNA sequences may be amplified to reach the threshold of detection, through action of the enzyme DNA polymerase. This complicated procedure is used for the diagnosis and toxoplasmosis.

DNA Probe

Performance of this involves transfer of DNA-containing material of any sort (insect salivary glands or gut, human serum or feces, etc.) to a nitrocellulose membrane, where it is fixed. A DNA segment of known sequence, characteristic of the parasite DNA (produced by a cloning technique by means of hybridomas and then radioactively labeled), is hybridized to the DNA on the membrane. Radioactivity remaining after the membrane is washed signals the presence of the parasite. This procedure is used primarily for the detection of *Trichomonas vaginalis*.

Western Blotting (WB)

This type of immunoblot test is used in diagnosis of cysticercosis, echinococcosis, and schistosomiasis (see Figure 17-2-1).

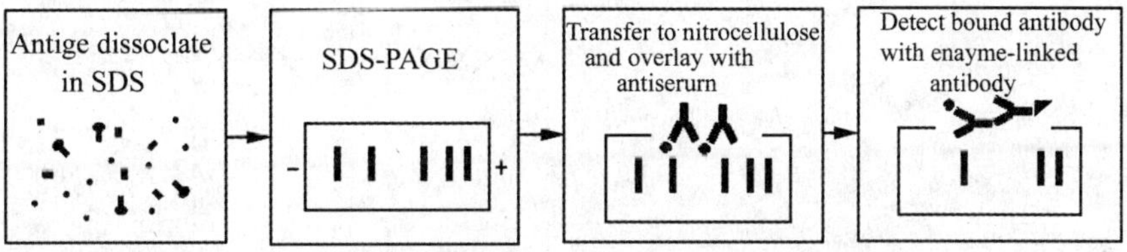

Figure 17-2-1 Principle of Western blotting

Table 17-2-1 Antibody and antigen detection test for parasitic diseases

Disease	antibody test(s)	antigen test(s)
African trypanosomiasis		
Amebiasis	EIA	EIA
Angiostrongyliasis		
Anisakiasis		
Babesiosis	IFA	
Baylis ascariasis		
Chagas' disease	EIA, IFA	
Cryptosporidiosis		EIA, DFA, IFA
Cysticercosis	EIA, IB	
Echinococcosis	EIA, IB	
Fascioliasis	EIA	
Filariasis	EIA	
Giardiasis		EIA, DFA, IFA
Leishmaniasis	EIA, IFA	
Malaria	IFA	
Paragonimiasis	EIA, IB	
Schistosomiasis		EIA, ELISA, IB
Strongyloidiasis	EIA,	
Toxocariasis	EIA,	
Toxoplasmosis	EIA, IFA	
Trichiniasis	BF, EIA,	
Trichomoniasis		DFA, LA, DNA probe

(Liu Hongli)

LABORATORY MANUAL

Regulations for Parasitological Experiments

Purpose

1. Reinforce and enhance the lectures taught in the classroom.

2. Master the preliminary fundamental techniques and the basic skill of parasitology.

3. Teach the practical and realistic attitude of scientific work and overcoming difficulties on one's own, so as to get a solid foundation for further studies and research work in parasitology.

Requirements

1. Study the content of what you will do in the laboratory before the experiment. Coming late or leaving early is not allowed.

2. Wear a white gown in the laboratory. Keep the laboratory clean and silent. Smoking and spitting are strictly prohibited.

3. Handle the microscope and slide specimens with extreme care. Clean the oil-immersion objective and slide with lens paper and xylol after use. Put the slides back into the original slide box. If there is any damage or there are missing specimens or accessories, report to the teacher immediately.

4. In the demonstration room, never move the specimens and mechanical stages of the microscope, otherwise you will make trouble for other's observation.

5. Complete the lab work within the time allowed. Drawings must be clear and accurate. Answers must be concise. Use proper report paper only. Use 2H, HB, or color pencils for drawings. The tip of the pencil must be sharp enough.

6. When the experiment is over, put the microscope and slide box in their proper place. Clean the glassware, etc. The students on duty will do the following work: clean the floor and tables, shut off water supply and electricity, close the windows and the door. Safety first!

The Use of Microscope

Adjustment of illumination

For the best result, the specimen must be correctly illuminated. At first, use low power objective for the adjustment of light. Use plane mirror for natural light and concave mirror for artificial or dim light. Adjust by elevating or lowering the condenser and adjust the diaphragm aperture in order to get a correct intensity of illumination. Too strong or too weak illumination will give you a blurred vision or a dark and hardly visible image.

Specimen observation

Put the slide on the stage. Adjust the focus with the coarse focusing knob, so that the image is visible under low power objective. Then adjust to clearest position with the fine focus.

If observation under high power is desired, move the object to the center of the field. Then turn to the high power objective.

For the use of oil-immersion: add a little drop of cedar wood oil on the slide. Turn down the oil-immersion objective so that the objective is immersed in the oil and nearly touching the slide. Watch carefully with your eyes during this manipulation. Otherwise you may damage the slide or even the objective! Adjust the focus with fine focus until the specimen is clearly visible.

Calculation of magnification

The magnification is engraved on the ocular and objective. Magnification=mag. of ocular×mag. of objective.

Precautions

1. The fine focus is the finest and most delicate mechanical part of the microscope. One full turn of the fine focus may elevate or lower the 0.1mm. Its range of movement is quite limited. Turn the fine focusing knob only in to and fro directions for adjusting. Never turn the fine focus in the same direction too far.

2. During adjustment, pay attention to the objective not touching the fecal specimen and pressing against the slide. Otherwise the slide and objective may be crushed.

3. With the aid of the mechanical stage, examine the blood film or fecal smear thoroughly, so that you will not miss any positive findings.

4. After use of oil-immersion objective, clean it with xylol and lens paper. Wipe off the excessive xylol with dry lens paper.

5. After lab, check the accessories of the microscope. Turn the objectives away from the light path of the microscope. Lower the tube and the condenser. Put the microscope into the box.

Medical Helminthology

The word "helminth" means worm. Helminths include both free-living and parasitic multi-cellular animals. They are bilaterally symmetrical. They have no skeletal system, neither endoskeleton nor exoskeleton. Their motile activity is accomplished by wormy movement. There are at least three important classes concerned in medical helminths, namely nematoda, trematoda and cestoidea.

Nematoda

The nematodes are non-segmented, cylindrical in shape, and covered by a tough cuticle. They have a complete digestive tract. The sexes are separate and generally males are much smaller than female worms. The tail of a male is usually curved or may be expanded into a thin translucent copulatory bursa. Reproductive organs are tubular and lie coiled within the body cavity. In the male there is a single tubule which at its smaller end consists of testicular cells, and terminates in an ejaculatory duct opened into the cloaca. The female worm has two cylindrical ovaries which expand into uteri. The uteri may each open to the exterior through a single vulva or there may be a common vagina between the vulva and uteri. The vulva is frequently located near the middle of the body. The majority of nematodes are free living. Many nematodes are parasites of plants, others are agents of animal diseases, and approximately one dozen are commonly encountered in man.

The parasitic nematodes are generally light creamy-white in color.

Diagnosis of intestinal nematode infection is generally made by demonstration of the characteristic ova in the feces.

Lab. 1 *Ascaris lumbricoides*

The parasite inhabits the small intestine. The *ova* pass out in feces and develop in the external environment to the infective stage. After ingestion, the larvae hatch in the small intestine and migrate to the lung where they stay and develop for about 10 days. Then through respiratory passages, esophagus, and stomach, they go back to the small intestine and grow to adulthood. The adult worms are cylindrical with both ends pointed, creamy-white in color or sometimes with a pinkish cast. The cuticle has fine circular striations. The females are larger than males. The vulva of the female is situated near the junction of the anterior and middle thirds of the body. The terminal end of a male is curved.

Requirements

1. Study the morphological characters of ova and adult worms of *Ascaris*.
2. Learn the inhabiting site, infective stage, and method of transmission.
3. Master the direct smear method in fecal examination.

Procedure

1. Individual observation

In a slide specimen of *Ascaris* eggs, search for eggs under low power. Then study the structure in detail under high power.

a. Fertilized eggs: broadly oval, brown, average size $60 \times 45\mu m$. The thick smooth shell is covered by a coarsely mammillated albuminous coat stained brown by bile. The eggs are unsegmented and contain a mass of coarse lecithin granules when oviposited and discharged in feces. Between the unsegmented embryonic cell and both ends of the shell, there is a new-moon shaped clear space at each end (crescent shaped clear space) (Plate I. 1).

b. Unfertilized eggs (Plate I. 2): unfertilized eggs, measuring 90 by $44\mu m$, are frequently seen in the feces. The shell and albuminous coat are thinner than those of fertilized eggs. Internally their structure consists of a mass of disorganized, highly refractile granules of various sizes. Both fertile and infertile eggs at times lack the outer albuminous coat, and are then called decorticated eggs. Decorticated *Ascaris* eggs are colorless (Plate I. 4).

2. Demonstration

a. Adult worms: notice their size, shape, color, and sexual difference.

b. Life cycle of *Ascaris*: notice the site of infection, infective stage, and method of transmission.

c. Embryonated eggs: There is a coiled larva within the egg shell. This is the infective stage (Plate I. 3).

d. The tip of the head, apical, and side views, under low power; on the tip of the head there are 3 lips, a larger lip on the dorsal side and a pair of smaller ones lying ventro-laterally. This is one of the characteristic features for identifying the order ASCARDIDA.

e. A case of eye ascariasis: 2 adolescent *Ascaris* extracted from the orifice of the right lacrymal duct of a girl 1-year of age. The worms measure 4-5cm in length and 1-2mm in breadth.

f. A jar of *Ascaris* (304 worms): removed by operation from a 6-year-old boy suffering from acute intestinal obstruction by *Ascaris*.

3. Technique

Preparation of a direct fecal film, refer to Page 426. What are the precautions in performing the direct film?

Works

1. Drawings

Draw a fertile and infertile *Ascaris* eggs and mark down their magnifications.

2. Problems

a. Can all *Ascaris* infections be diagnosed by fecal examination? Why?

b. State the physiological features of *Ascaris* eggs and their significance.

Lab. 2 Hookworms

Ancylostoma duodenale and *Necator americanus*

At least two species of hookworms infect men in China. *A. doudenale* and *N. americanus.* They are parasites of the small intestine. The eggs are discharged in feces. Under suitable conditions the eggs develop in the moist sandy soil and hatch into rhabditiform larvae within 1-2 days. The rhabditiform larvae feed on bacteria and organic material, molt, and develop into filariform larvae in about 7 days. The filariform larvae are infective and capable of penetrating through the skin when they are in contact with the human body. Through the blood stream, the larvae go to the lung and through respiratory passages and epiglottis to the intestine. There, they grow up to adults. The adults of the two species are morphologically distinct while the eggs are essentially alike.

How do you discover the hookworm patients? How do you identify the two species of hookworms (adult)? What are the principles of the flotation method for the recovery of hookworm eggs?

Requirements

1. Study the morphology of hookworm eggs and the difference between hookworm eggs and decorticated fertilized *Ascaris* eggs.

2. Identify the shape and body curvature of two species of adult hookworms.

3. Study the site of inhabitation, infective stage, and method of transmission of hookworm disease.

4. Master the brine flotation technique.

Procedure

1. Individual observation

Slide specimen of hookworm eggs: the shells are thin, hyaline, oval in shape. The size of the egg is about the same as that of the fertilized *Ascaris* egg (60μm×40μm). When discharged in normal stool, the hookworm eggs are usually in the early cleavage stages (2-8 cell stage). In constipated stools, the eggs may be in morula or tadpole stage; less commonly the eggs may contain motile first-stage larva. Search for eggs under low power and then identify their structure under high power(Plate I. 6, 7).

2. Demonstration

a. Decorticated fertilized *Ascaris* eggs: notice that the shell is thick and the embryonic cell is unsegmented. The decorticated *Ascaris* egg is also colorless (Plate I. 4).

Lab. Table 2-1 The difference between decorticated *Ascaris* and hookworm eggs

	decorticated *Ascaris* egg	hookworm egg
shell	thick	thin
egg cell	unsegmented	2 to 8 cells
space between shell and cell	new-moon shaped space between cell and ends of shell	empty space surrounding the cells

b. The morphological difference between two species of hookworms

Lab. Table 2-2 The morphological difference between two species of hookworms

	A. *duodenale*	N. *americanus*
size	larger, female 1cm or more, male around 1cm	smaller
shape	single curve, looks like "C"	double curves, looks like "S"
mouth	2 pairs of ventral teeth	1 pair of ventral cutting plates
copulatory spicule	1 pair with separate endings	1 pair which unite to form a terminal hooklet
caudal spine of female	present	no
position of vulva in female	post-equatorial	pre-equatorial

c. A section of small intestine showing hookworms attached to the intestinal mucosa by means of their stout mouthparts.

d. Filariform or infective larvae: the mouth becomes closed, esophagus elongates and the larva now is transformed into the non-feeding filariform type (third stage larva). The old cuticle may be shed or may remain for some time as a protective coat.

e. Life cycle of hookworm: notice the site of inhabitation, infective stage, and method of infection.

f. Geophagia: patients suffering from heavy hookworm infection may show an abnormal appetite. They may like to eat uncooked rice, clay, hair, bricks, paper, charcoal, ashes, etc.

g. Fecal culture for diagnosis of hookworm larvae: spread a thin (1-2mm) film of feces on the middle third (one side only) of a 13mm by 120mm strip of filter paper. Place the paper in a 15ml conical-tip centrifuge tube containing about 3ml of distilled water, the paper being forced to 1cm from the bottom and with the clean side pressed towards the side of the tube. The culture is held at room temperature (20℃-30℃) in the dark for 3-5 days and water is added daily as needed to hold the water level well above the bottom end of the paper but the fecal film is not in direct contact with water. The capillary flow of water upwards through the paper and fecal film keeps the feces moist. Three days later, the larvae migrate to the water pool where they can be seen with a hand lens. If the larvae can not be found, the observation should be continued for 5 days.

3. Technical procedure

Brine flotation method: in a flotation cup (about 3. 5cm in depth, 2cm in diameter) comminute 2-3g of feces with saturated brine. Add more brine and take off the macroscopic debris floating on the fluid. Additional brine is poured into the cup until the cup is almost full. Then add more brine drop by drop with a dropper until the fluid level reaches the rim. On the top of the cup a microscopic slide is superimposed, so that the liquid surface is just in contact with the slide without air bubbles between them. Wait for 15-20 minutes. Turn up the slide, add a coverslip, and examine under a microscope.

Eggs of intestinal nematodes will thus be concentrated and not damaged.

Precaution

1. Stool for diagnosis of hookworm infection must be fresh. In optimal circumstances, hookworm larvae will hatch in 1-2 days.

2. The amount of specimen must not be too small because the eggs may not be concentrated successfully with a little mount of feces.

3. The amount of brine added must be accurate, neither too much so that the liquid will overflow, nor insufficient so that air bubbles occur under the slide.

4. Take care so that during the turning of the slide no fluid will drop from the slide.

Works

1. Drawing

Draw a hookworm egg.

2. Problems

a. What are the morphological differences between the two species of hookworms in the adult stage?

b. From your knowledge of hookworm life cycle, how do you make an early diagnosis, treatment, and determine the efficacy of treatment?

c. Compare the advantages and disadvantages between brine flotation and larval cultivation for the diagnosis of hookworm disease.

d. What are the clinical and epidemiological significance in the hookworm egg counting technique?

Lab. 3 *Enterobius vermicularis*

Enterobius vermicularis is commonly known as pinworm. The adult worms inhabit the cecum and adjacent portions of the large and small intestine. Right after maturity, the worms mate and the male dies soon after mating. Therefore the male worms are rarely seen. The female worms migrate down the intestinal tract and pass out of the anus at midnight. The worms may migrate several inches out of the anus, depositing eggs on the peri-anal skin as they crawl. The eggs become fully embryonated and infective within a few hours of the time they are deposited. Humans become infected by mouth and by auto-infection or retro-infection.

Requirements

1. Study the morphology of pinworm adults and eggs.

2. Learn the site of inhabitation, the site of oviposition, and Graham Scotch tape swab method for recovery of *Enterobius* eggs.

Procedure

1. Individual observation

a. Slide specimen of *Enterobius* eggs: the colorless eggs are embryonated. They are 50-60 micrometers in length and 20-30μm in breadth and have a translucent shell of moderate thickness. They are usually conspicuously flattened on one side (somewhat like the seed of persimmon), and this flattening and shorter breadth, plus the thicker shell, serves to differentiate the eggs from hookworm ova(Plate I. 5).

b. Slide specimen of adult worms: notice their size, shape, and color with naked eyes.

2. Demonstration

a. Anterior end of *Enterobius* adult, slide specimen: notice the cephalic inflation at anterior end and esophageal bulb.

b. Life cycle of *Enterobius*: notice the site of infection, infective stage, and method of transmission.

c. *Enterobius* eggs (collected by Graham Scotch tape swab): notice a larva within the egg.

3. Graham Scotch tape swab (cellophane tape) for *Enterobius* and *Taenia* eggs

a. Fold together sticky surfaces of a piece of Scotch tape, 2 by 8cm in length, for about 1cm at each end.

b. Stretch tape, sticky side out, over butt end of a test tube, holding non-sticky ends firmly with thumb and forefinger.

c. Apply tape to anal area, rocking back and forth to cover as much of the mucosa and mucocutaneous area as possible.

d. Remove tape and apply to microscope slide, sticky side down. Press firmly into position. (Wash hands thoroughly right after the collection of specimen.)

e. Examine for ova under low power of microscope. Pinworm ova, which are generally deposited at night, will be found scattered around the peri-anal region. The examination should be made in the morming, before the patient has washed or defecated.

Works

1. Drawing

Draw an *Enterobius* eggs.

2. Problem

Why is stool examination usually unsuccessful for the recovery of *Enterobius* eggs?

Lab. 4 *Trichuris trichiura*

The adults inhabit human cecum. The eggs are discharged with feces. The eggs develop to the infective stage in the soil. Humans become infected by swallowing the infective eggs. The eggs hatch in the small intestine and become adults in the cecum.

What are the morphological characteristics of adults and eggs of Trichuris?

Requirements

Study the morphology of both adults and eggs of *T. trichiura.* Study the life cycle of *T. trichiura.*

Procedure

1. Individual observation

Trichuris eggs: the eggs are brownish and unsegmented. They measure 50-54 microns in length, with translucent refractile prominences (usually referred to as polar plugs) at either end (Plate I. 8).

2. Demonstration

a. Adults: the adult worms are from 3 to 5cm in length. The females are larger than males. The thin almost colorless anterior three-fifths of the body consist of the much-reduced esophagus. The expanded posterior part of the worm is pinkish-gray in color and contains the intestine and reproductive organs.

b. Life cycle: notice the site of inhabitation, infective stage, and method of transmission. The adult worms attach with their attenuated anterior ends embedded in the mucosa of cecum, adjacent ileum colon.

Works

1. Drawing

Draw a *Trichuris* egg.

2. Problem

Compare the life cycles of *Ascaris* and *Trichuris*.

Lab. 5 *Wuchereria Bancrofti* and *Brugia malayi*

The filariae are long, thread-like nematodes. There are two species found in China, that is, *Wuchereria bancrofti* and *Brugia malayi*. They inhabit the lymphatic system of man. The worms are viviparous, producing microfilariae instead of eggs. The microfilariae are nocturnal in peripheral blood. The mosquito is the agent of transmission of the parasite. An essential developmental cycle takes place within the body of the insect.

How do you diagnose filaria patients?

State the morphological differences between bancroftian and malayan microfilariae.

Requirements

1. Study the morphology of bancroftian and malayan microfilariae.
2. Study the life cycles of *W. bancrofti* and *B. malayi*.
3. Study the site of inhabitation, infective stage, and method of transmission of *W. bancrofti* and *B. malayi*.
4. Master the technique of blood film preparation for examining microfilariae.

Procedure

1. Individual observation

Observe thick blood films searching for bancroftian and malayan microfilariae under low power respectively. Then identify their structures in detail under high power. The microfilariae are thread-like with blunt anterior end and pointed posterior end. The body is sheathed. There are numerous nuclei within the body. The nuclei of bancroftian microfilariae are equal-sized, clearly defined and countable(Plate IV. 6).

Lab. Table 5-1 Differences between *M. bancrofti* and *B. malayi*

	M. bancrofti	*M. malayi*
size	larger 244-290μm×5. 3μm	smaller
body curvatures	graceful, sweeping curves	irregular, kinky curves
cephalic space	shorter, length : width=1 : 1	longer, length : width=2 : 1
nuclei	equal-sized, clearly defined, countable	unequal-sized, coalescing, uncountable
terminal nuclei	no	2

2. Demonstration

a. Malayan microfilariae (Plate IV. 5).

b. Filariform (infective) larvae: filariform larvae (about 1mm in length) emerging from the proboscis of a mosquito.

c. The life cycle of filaria: notice the site of inhabitation, vectors (*Culex pipiens pallens* for *W. bancrofti* and *Anopheles sinensis* for *B. malayi*) and method of transmission.

d. Specimen of scrotal elephantiasis, removed from a late case of bancroftian filariasis.

e. Photographs of late cases of elephantiasis.

3. Preparation of thick blood film (refer to Page 434)

For the recovery of microfilariae, approximately 60 cubic mm of blood (about 3 drops) may be required and the blood must be collected between 9: 00 p. m. and 2:00 a. m.

Works

1. Drawing

Draw a bancroftian microfilariae.

2. Problems

a. What are the precautions in the preparation of the thick blood film?

b. What are the morphological features of bancroftian and malayan microfilariae?

Lab. 6 *Trichinella spiralis* (Trichina Worm)

Trichinella spiralis is a rather unusual species which completes its life cycle in one host. It is common in carnivorous mammals, including rodents and humans. It is the smallest nematode parasite of humans. The males measure 1. 4 to 1. 6mm long and are more slender at the anterior than at the posterior end. The anus is nearly terminal and has a large papilla on each side. The copulatory spicule is absent. Females are about twice the size of males. The vulva is located near the middle of the esophagus, which is about a third the length of the body. The single uterus is filled with developing eggs in its posterior portion, whereas the anterior portion contains fully developed, hatched juveniles. Most juveniles are carried away by the hepatoportal system through the liver, then to the heart, lungs, and arterial system, which distributes them throughout the body. The juveniles form the larval cysts in muscular tissues.

Requirements

1. Recognize the larva in host muscle.
2. Understand the features of parasitization and pathogenesis of the larva.
3. Learn the technique for the detection of the larva.

Procedure

1. Individual observation

Larvae in host muscle section: under low power, search for the larvae in the muscle. Note the lemon-shaped capsule in which the larvae are located.

2. Demonstration

a. Adults, stained: study grossly under low power. Notice their size and differences between both sexes. You can see many larvae inside the body of the female.

b. Biopsy: a small piece of infected mouse muscle is pressed between two slides and examined under low power. Note the larval cysts in muscle tissues, with their long axis parallel to the direction of muscle fibers.

Work

Draw a larva within muscles.

Lab. Table 6-1 Key characteristics of intestinal nematodes

Nematode	Characteristic features
Enterobius vermicularis	Smooth, thick-shelled, persimmon seed shaped egg. Scotch tape test recommended for diagnosis. Adult worm is white with pointy tail and may be seen in feces. Transmission is usually by ingestion of infective eggs.

Ascaris lumbricoides	Mammillated, thick-shelled eggs, fertilized (1-cell stage), or unfertilized (exaggerated bumpy mammillated shell) eggs may be found in feces. Decorticated eggs may be present. Transmission is usually by ingestion of infective eggs.
Trichuris trichiura	Barrel-shaped thick-shelled egg with 2 polar plugs. Adult worm with whiplike shape rarely seen in feces. Transmission is usually by ingestion of infective eggs.
Ancylostoma duodenale/ Necator americanus	Oval, thin-shelled eggs in 4 to 8-cell stage, a clear space exists between the shell and the developing embryo. Larvae may develop from eggs left at room temperature. Adult worms rarely seen in feces. Transmission is usually by skin penetration.
Strongyloides stercoralis	First stage rhabditiform larva, having a short buccal capsule, and a large genital primordium. Thin-shelled eggs are not usually found in feces. Transmission is usually by skin penetration.

Trematoda

Adult trematodes or flukes are parasites of vertebrates. They are generally hermaphroditic. Most adult trematodes are dorsoventrally flattened and leaf-shaped. The body is covered with a resistant cuticle which may be smooth or spiny. There are two suckers, that is, an anterior oral sucker and a more posterior ventral sucker or acetabulum. The digestive tract is composed of a mouth, esophagus, and ceca, which run parallel to each other ending blindly near the posterior end of the worm. There are usually two testes leading by means of long, thin ducts to the genital pore, which usually lies in the region of the ventral sucker. There is a single ovary, from which arises a tubule near its origin to form a seminal receptacle. A series of glandular structures called vitellaria, usually in two masses lying lateral to the intestinal ceca, produces the egg material. Vitelline ducts lead inward from the vitellaria to the region of the ovary; the ducts from the ovary, the seminal receptacle, the vitellaria, and sometimes a Laurer's canal come together at the ootype or Mehlis gland, and here the shell is formed around the ovum. The uterus arises from the Mehlis' gland and winds forward to the genital pore. In most trematodes, the uterus is the largest organ in the body, filled with many thousands of ova.

Trematode ova have a smooth hard shell, which is transparent and generally of a yellow-brown or brown color. Most ova have an operculum or cap at one end. The miracidium is covered with cilia, and in some species may be fully developed when the eggs are passed in the feces. The shell may be smoothly continuous in outline, or there may be a slight flare (eminence; shoulder), making the line of cleavage between shell and operculum. The flared portion of the shell, into which the operculum fits, is known as the opercular shoulder. Spines may be present on the shell.

Lab. 7 *Clonorchis sinensis*

The definitive hosts of *C. sinensis* or the Chinese liver fluke are man, cat, dog, and other carnivorous mammals. The worms inhabit small bile ducts and may inhabit the gall bladder and common bile duct when the infection is heavy. The eggs with miracidium inside are discharged in the feces. The eggs hatch in the first intermediate host, snails of the genus *Parafossarulus*, *Alocinma*, and *Bithynia* when they are ingested by these snails. The miracidia develop and multiply in the snail host to form sporocyst, rediae, and cercariae. The cercariae emerge from the snail host and penetrate into fresh-water fish. They encyst in the muscles, gills, scales, etc. Human infection results from the consumption of fresh-water fish containing the metacercariae. Fish may be eaten raw, smoked, pickled, or dried.

Requirements

1. Study the morphology of the adult and eggs of *C. sinensis*.
2. Study the site of inhabitation, pathogenecity, and diagnosis of clonorchiasis.

Procedure

1. Individual observation

a. Eggs of *C. sinensis*, slide specimen: the brownish operculated eggs of *C. sinensis* are one of the smallest among all eggs of human helminths, being 29μm×17μm in size. The opercular shoulders are evident. A small and inconspicuous spine may be seen at the non-operculated end. A fully developed miracidium is found in the egg when the egg is discharged with feces. Eggs of *C. sinensis*, *Heterophyes heterophyes*, *Metagonimus vokogawai*, and *Opisthorchis felineus* are morphologically alike(Plate I. 10).

b. Adult of *C. sinensis*, slide specimen: the worm is thin and translucent, 10-25mm×3-5mm in size, narrower in the anterior half and broader in the posterior half. The worm is hermaphoditic.

2. Demonstration

a. Adult fluke, unstained specimens: notice their size, shape, and color. Stained specimen: notice the male and female genital organs and digestive tract.

b. Intermediate hosts: the first intermediate host-snails: *Parafossarulus*, *Alocinma*, and *Bithynia*.

The second intermediate host: fresh-water fish: *Ctenopharyngodon*, *Cyprinus*, *Pseudorasbora*.

c. Metacercaria: it is ovoid, about 138μm × 115μm, double cyst wall, excretory bladder visible.

d. Cat's liver infected by *Clonorchis*: notice the site of inhabitation and pathological changes of the liver.

e. Different stages of *C. sinensis* in the life cycle.

Works

1. Drawing

Draw a *Clonorchis* egg.

2. Problems

a. State the life cycle of *C. sinensis*.

b. State the morphology of the eggs and adult *C. sinensis*.

Lab. 8 *Fasciolopsis buski*

The giant intestinal fluke, *Fasciolopsis buski*, is found in China, Viet Nam, Thailand, Indonesia, and the Indian Subcontinent. Adult worms live attached to the bowel wall, primarily in the duodenum and jejunum.

Infection is acquired by ingestion of the metacercariae, encysted on fresh-water vegetation such as water caltrop or water chestnuts, which may be consumed raw or peeled with the teeth. Reservoir hosts include pigs, dogs, and rabbits.

Adult worms are flesh-colored, 2-7.5cm in length by 0.8-2cm in width. The eggs are discharged in feces.

Requirements

1. Study the morphology of the eggs and adult worms.

2. Study the life cycle of the worm, site of inhabitation, intermediate host, larval developmental stages, infective stage (metacercaria), and method of transmission.

Procedure

1. Individual observation

The eggs of *F. buski*, slide specimen: the ellipsoid ova are yellowish-brown in color. The shell is transparent, with a small operculum at the more pointed end. Eggs are unembryonated when passed with feces, containing an ootid and 20-40 yolk cells. They measure 130-140μm in length by 80-85μm in breadth, being the largest among all human helminth eggs(Plate I. 12).

2. Demonstration

a. Adults, unstained specimen: notice the size, shape, color, and position of the oral and ventral suckers of the worm.

b. Adult, stained specimen: study the male and female genital organs and the digestive tract.

c. The intermediate hosts: the first intermediate hosts (snails of the genus *Segmentina*, *Planorbis*). The metacercaria carriers: water vegetation such as water caltrop, water chestnut, water bamboo shoots, and other aquatic vegetation.

d. The metacercaria: the infective stage.

Works

1. Drawing

Draw an *F. buski* egg.

2. Problems

a. Describe the morphological differences between the eggs of *C. sinensis* and *F. buski*.

b. What is the method of transmission of fasciolopsiasis?

c. How do you kill the metacercariae encysted on the aquatic vegetation?

d. From your knowledge of the life cycles of *C. sinensis* and *F. buski*, how do you make a plan for the control of these two worms?

Lab. 9 *Paragonimus westermani*

Human infection with the lung fluke, *Paragonimus westermani*, occurs throughout the Far East, many islands of the Southwest Pacific, Indonesia, Zaire, Cameroon, and Nigeria. Animal infection is extensive. Reservoir hosts include a wide variety of carnivorous mammals.

The eggs are discharged into the bronchi or bronchioles. They may be expectorated, or if swallowed will appear in the feces.

Infection results from the ingestion of raw or improperly cooked and pickled or rice-wine soaked crayfish or fresh-water crabs with metacercariae. The metacercariae excyst in the small intestine, penetrate through its wall into the peritoneal cavity, and make their way through the diaphragm and pleura into the lungs. A cyst-like capsule produced by the host tissue surrounds the developing parasite, which grows to maturity in about six weeks. The circuitous route of migration allows the worms to lodge and mature in ectopic locations such as the mesentery, groin, pleura, subcutaneous tissue or brain. Rupture of the cyst capsule into a bronchiole leads to discharge of eggs, but not the parasite.

Requirements

1. Study the morphology of the eggs and adult worms of *P. westermani*.

2. Study the life cycle, site of inhabitation, intermediate hosts, larval developmental stages, infective stage (metacercaria), and method of transmission.

Procedure

1. Individual observation

Eggs of *P. westermani*, slide specimen: the golden-brown eggs are found in sputum or feces. The ovoid eggs have a flattened operculum, distinctly set off from the rest of the shell by raised opercular shoulders. They measure 80-120μm in length by 48-60μm in breadth, and are immature when found in the sputum or feces (Plate I. 11).

2. Demonstration

a. Adult worms of *P. westermani*: the fresh adult worms are reddish brown in color and very thick bodied. The cuticle is spiny. They are from 0. 8-1. 6cm in length, 0. 4-0. 8cm in width, and from 0. 3-0. 5cm in thickness. The ovary and uterus lie side by side just behind the ventral sucker. Two lobed testes lie side by side in the posterior part of the body. The worms are typically found encapsulated in cystic structures adjacent to the bronchi. There are usually two worms in one capsule.

b. The life cycle: developmental stages—egg, miracidium, sporocyst, mother rediae, daughter rediae, cercariae, and metacercaria.

The first intermediate host—snails of the genus *Melania*. The second intermediate host—fresh-water crabs of the genus *Eriocheir*, *Potamon*, *Seasarma*, and crayfish of the genus *Cambaroides* and *Procambarus*.

c. Cat's lungs infected by *P. westermani*.

d. Charcot-Leyden's crystals in sputum.

3. Technique for recovery of *Paragonimus* eggs in sputum

a. Direct smear method: same as for fecal direct smear method. Refer to Page 427. It is better to select the bloody or rusty portion of sputum for examination. Trophozoite of *E. histolytica*, fragments of germinal layer of hydatid cyst wall and scolices of Echinococcus granulosus, eggs of *P. westermani* and Charcot-Leyden's crystals may be recovered by this method. Occasionally eggs of blood flukes or *Strongyloides* larvae may be coughed up.

b. Sodium hydroxide digestion technique: put 1-3ml of sputum into a centrifuge tube. Add equal amount of 10% NaOH solution. Shake the mixture and let stand for 2 hours until the mucus is dissolved. Centrifuge for 1-2 minutes. Examine for sediment under a microscope.

Works

1. Drawing

Draw a *Paragonimus* egg.

2. Problem

How do you diagnose a case of paragonimiasis clinically?

Lab. 10 *Schistosoma japonicum*

Three species of schistosomes parasitize man, namely *Schistosoma japonicum*, *S. mansoni*, and *S. haamatobium*. There is only one species, *S. japonicum*, found in China. Although the adult schistosome worms live in the mesenteric veins, their eggs are generally found in the feces. The adults of *S. japonicum* live in the small branches of superior mesenteric veins adjacent to the small intestine. The inferior mesenterics and caval system may also be invaded.

The schistosomes differ in a number of ways from other trematodes. They are diecious, and the two sexes are rather dissimilar in appearance. Female worms are long and slender, 1.2-2.6cm in length, with a body almost circular in cross section, and 0.3mm or less in diameter. Male worms are from 1.0-2.2cm long, and while the body is flattened behind the ventral sucker, it looks cylindrical as it is characteristically curved inward ventrally to form a gynecophoral canal in which the female reposes.

The females leave the male worms to deposit their ova in small venules, close to the lumen of the intestine. An enzyme is elaborated by the miracidium, and this diffuses through the egg shell and helps to digest the overlying tissue. The action of this enzyme, plus necrosis of the tissue caused by pressure of the egg, works together to liberate the egg from the tissues into the lumen of the intestine. Schistosome eggs are not operculated, and hatch by rupture if liberated into fresh water. The miracidium swims in search of an appropriate snail host—*Oncomelania*. It penetrates the snail where it undergoes a cycle of development (mother sporocyst, daughter sporocysts), giving rise to a large number of cercariae infective to man.

Human infection takes place by direct penetration of the cercariae through the skin to invade the circulatory system. The young flukes are carried by the blood stream to the liver sinusoids, where they begin their growth. Two weeks or longer after infection the maturing worms commence a migration against the flow of blood in the portal system to their final location in mesenteric veins.

Cercariae of the schistosome parasites, both of man and of lower animals, have a forked tail, and glands at the anterior end which assist penetration of the skin.

Requirements

1. Study the morphology of eggs and adult *S. japonicum*.
2. Study the intermediate host (*Oncomelania*) and the infective stage—cercaria.
3. Learn the diagnostic methods.

Procedure

1. Individual observation

a. *S. japonicum* eggs, slide specimen: the eggs are oval in shape and light yellow in color. Size 74-106μm× 55-80μm, being larger than *Ascaris* eggs. The eggs may have a minute lateral spine, but this structure is difficult to see. The host's blood and tissue may adhere on the shell. When discharged in feces, a mature miracidium is found in the shell(Plate I. 13).

b. Cercaria, slide specimen: this is the infective stage. The tail is forked.

2. Demonstration

a. Adult worms: the male worms are creamy white. Behind the ventral sucker, there is a gynecophoral canal in which the female reposes. The female worms are more slender and darker (brown) in color.

b. The life cycle: the developmental stages—miracidium, mother sporocyst, daughter sporocyst, cercaria, and adolescent worm.

c. Gross specimens of rabbit's lungs and liver to show numerous organized pseudo-tubercles.

d. A rabbit's mesentery to show the adult schistosome in the mesenteric veins.

3. Techniques

Concentration of eggs by sedimentation

a. A stool specimen (about 30g) is homogenized by shaking in normal saline (about 500ml) and is then strained through two layers of gauze.

b. The material is allowed to sediment for 30 minutes, the supernatant decanted, and the sediment resuspended in saline. The process is repeated at least twice.

c. Examine the sediment under a microscope.

Schistosomal hatching test:

The first two steps are the same as a. and b. stated above.

d. The saline is decanted and replaced with tap or distilled water, and the suspension is placed in an Erlenmeyer flask. Additional water is added if necessary. The fluid level should reach to 3cm below the rim of the flask.

e. The water in the neck of the flask is then illuminated strongly from the side.

f. The illuminated area is then examined with a magnifying glass to detect the presence of free-swimming miracidia.

Works

1. Drawing

Draw an S. *japonicum* egg.

2. Problems

a. State the life cycle and epidemiology of S. *japonicum*.

b. The pathological changes of schistosomiasis are chiefly due to the effect of the eggs. Why?

Lab. Table 10-1 Key Characteristics of Trematodes

Trematode	Characteristic features
Fasciolopsis buski (Giant intestinal fluke)	Largest fluke inhabiting humans. Large, operculated eggs found in feces. Transmission is by ingestion of metacercariae encysted on freshwater vegetation.
Heterophyes, Metagonimus	Small, virtually indistinguishable intesinal flukes. Small, operculated eggs found in feces. Transmission is by ingestion of metacercariae encysted in freshwater fish.
Fasciola hepatica (Sheep liver fluke)	Large, operculated eggs (indistinguishable from those of F. buski) found feces. Transmission is by ingestion of metacercariae encysted on freshwater vegetation.
Clonorchis sinensis (Chinese liver fluke)	Small, delicate, operculated eggs with prominent shoulders found in feces. Transmission is by ingestion of metacercariae encysted in freshwater fish.
Paragonmus westermani (Oriental lung fluke)	Large, operculated eggs. Found in sputum or feces. Transmission is by ingestion of metacercariae encysted in freshwater crab and crayfish.
Schistosoma mansoni (Blood fluke)	Oval egg with a large lateral spine found in feces. Transmission by skin penetration of cercariae from freshwater snail.
Schstosoma japonicum (Blood fluke)	Round egg with a small lateral spine found in feces. Transmission by skin penetration of cercariae from freshwater snail.
Schistosoma haematobium (Blood fluke)	Oval egg with a large terminal spine found in urine. Transmission by skin penetration of cercariae from freshwater snail.

Cestoidea (Cestoda)

The Cestoidea or tapeworms comprise a class of the phylum platyhelminths. All tapeworms are parasitic, bilaterally symmetrical dorsoventrally flat and ribbon-like. Living worms are white or light yellowish in color. The cestode body consists of an anterior attachment organ or scolex, followed by a chain of segments or proglottids (strobila). The strobila grows throughout the life of the tapeworm by continuous proliferation of new segments or proglottids in the region immediately posterior to the scolex. The new segments are referred to as immature proglottids. The mature ones are found near the middle of the chain. Each mature proglottid may contain one or two sets of both male and female reproductive organs. The terminal portion of strobila contains the gravid segments usually filled with eggs. The cestodes do not have a digestive system.

All adult cestodes inhabit the small intestine of vertebrates. The cestodes generally require a second or intermediate host. The embryo in the cestode's egg is called an oncosphere and bears six elongated hooks.

Lab. 11 *Taenia solium* and *Taenia saginata*

The pork and beef tapeworms inhabit the human small intestine. After passing out of the host, the gravid proglottids rupture and set eggs free. The eggs are ingested by the intermediate host (pig or cattle) and hatch in the digestive tract. The oncospheres penetrate the small intestinal wall and grow to cysticercus in the muscles or connective tissue. Humans become infected by eating raw or not well cooked, infected pork or beef.

Infection with the larval stage of cysticercus of pork tapeworm occurs upon ingestion of eggs, either from exogenous sources or from his own stools. It is thought that reverse peristalsis may carry intestinal contents with eggs to the upper portion of the duodenum, where after hatching, the oncospheres penetrate the intestinal wall. For these reasons, infection with adults of *T. solium* is dangerous both to the patient and to those with whom he comes in contact. Cysticercosis of man due to *T. saginata* apparently occurs quite rarely.

Requirements

1. Study the morphology of *Taenia* eggs.
2. Study the morphology of adult, gravid segment, and cysticerci of *T. solium* and *T. saginata*.
3. Learn the diagnostic methods and pathogenesis of taeniasis.

Procedure

1. Individual observation

a. *Taenia* eggs, slide specimen: the eggs of the two tapeworms are alike. The eggs may be found free in the feces. They may also be recovered by means of a Scotch tape swab (refer to enterobiasis). They are spherical, 31-43μm in diameter. The oncosphere is enclosed in a thick, radially striated coat called embryophore, usually dark brown in color. The six-hooked larva can be easily seen in living eggs, but frequently becomes shriveled and opaque in preserved material. The radially striated coat is, however, sufficiently characteristic so that *Taenia* eggs cannot be confused with any other eggs of human helminthes(Plate I. 17).

b. The gravid proglottid of *T. solium*, slide specimen: gravid segments are usually longer than wide, and contain a branched uterus filled with eggs. A central uterine stem extends throughout the length of the gravid segment. From this stem arise side branches which project laterally and extend toward the lateral margin of the proglottid. These main side branches may have a variable number of smaller secondary branches. In *T. solium*, the main branches on one side of the central stem vary from 7 to 13. Specific diagnosis of *T. solium* is made by counting the number of uterine side branches.

c. *Cysticercus cellulosae*: it is the larval stage of *T. solium*. It is semi-transparent, an opalescent white in color, elongate-oval in shape, and may reach a length of 0.6-1.8cm. The bladder is fluid filled, and on one side is seen a denser area containing the scolex with four suckers and hooklets.

2. Demonstration

a. Adult tapeworms of the two species:

Lab. Table 11-1 Differences between *T. solium* and *T. seginata*

		T. solium	*T. seginata*
Adult	length	2-4m	4-8m
	scolex	1mm in diameter with hooks and 4 suckers	2mm with 4 suckers only
	no. of proglottids	800-1,000	1,000-2,000
	uterine lateral branches	7-13 on one side	15-30
No. of segments detached		1 or several at one time, passively passed	usually single, may actively migrate out
cysticercus		scolex with hooks found in hog & man	without hooks found in cattle

b. The life cycles of the two species.

c. *Cysticercus cellulosae* and *C. bovis* encysted in the pork and beef, respectively, gross specimen.

d. Scolices of *T. solium* and *T. saginata*: notice the four suckers and presence or absence of hooks.

3. Technique

a. Examination of the cysticercus: tear the fibrous tissue away from the cysticercus with dissecting needles or forceps. Place the specimen between two microscope slides which are separated at the edges by thin pieces of cardboard. Fasten the slides by means of rubber bands at each of the slide. Examine under the dissecting microscope and search for the suckers and hooklets.

b. Examination of gravid proglottids: if gravid proglottids are found in a stool specimen, they should be rinsed in tap water and placed between two microscope slides which are separated at the edges by thin pieces of cardboard. The preparation may then be fastened by means of rubber bands at the end of the slides so that the segments become somewhat flattened. The uterine branches should be clearly visible under the low power of a dissecting microscope.

Works

1. Drawing

Draw a *Taenia* egg.

2. Problems

a. What are the differences between the two *Taeniae* in their morphology and life cycle?

b. Which one is more dangerous to man? Why?

Lab. 12 *Hymenolepis nana*

Hymenolepis nana, the dwarf tapeworm of man, is a common parasite of the house mouse and is found in man all over the world. Infection with *H. nana* is seen frequently in children but occurs in adults as well. The adults inhabit the ileum.

H. nana is unique in that the adult worm develops following the ingestion of the eggs by man. Thus the intermediate host may not be necessary in its life cycle. In this manner, a second generation of adult worms may be produced from the initial infection within the same person. This phenomenon is called hyper-infection.

H. nana may also develop into infective cysticercoids in various intermediate hosts such as grain beetles and fleas. When ingested with contaminated grain products, the larvae will grow into adult worms in mice and man.

Requirements

Study the morphology of *H. nana* eggs and adults.

Procedure

1. Individual observation

Eggs of *H. nana*, slide specimen: the eggs are broadly ovoid, have a thin and smooth outer, and measure 30-47μm. They contain the six-hooked oncosphere within a rigid membrane. This membrane has two polar thickenings from which project four to eight long and thin filaments called polar filaments. The presence of these polar filaments is diagnostic and serves to differentiate *H. nana* (Plate I. 19) from *H. diminuta* (Plate I. 20).

2. Demonstration

The adult of *H. nana*: 10-25mm in length, 1mm in breadth, 100-200 segments in total. Scolex globular or rhomboid with four suckers and a retractile rostellum equipped with hooklets.

Works

1. Drawing

Draw an *H. nana* egg.

2. Problem

Describe the life cycle, pathogenesis, and control of *H. nana*.

Lab. 13 *Echinococcus granulosus* (The hydatid tapeworm)

The minute tapeworm, *E. granulosus*, lives as an adult in the intestine of dogs and other canines (definitive hosts). The larval stage of *E. granulosus*, the hydatid cyst, may be found in many animals, chiefly herbivores, i. e., sheep, cattle, camels, etc. (intermediate hosts). Man is an accidental intermediate host of the larval stage. Human infections result from the ingestion of eggs of *E. granulosus*. In man the hexacanth embryo hatches in the small intestine and penetrates the intestinal mucosa, losing the six hooklets in the process. The embryo reaches the blood or lymph vessels, most frequently the portal vessels, and is carried to the liver or other tissues. In the tissues, the hexacanth larva develops rather slowly into a hydatid cyst. The head is invaginated and the four suckers and the crown of hooklets are visible inside the scolex.

Requirements

1. Recognize the basic structures of adult and larva.
2. Understand the pathogenesis and the site of inhabitation.

Procedure

1. Individual observation

a. Adult of *E. granulosus*, stained specimen on a slide: study grossly under low power. Notice it is characterized by having only three proglottids—one immature, one mature, and one gravid. The head has a pyriform scolex with four suckers and a crown of hooklets.

b. Hydatid sand: notice scolex size, suckers, and hooklets.

2. Demonstration

a. Adult, stained: it has four major segments, a scolex and three proglottids. The terminal proglottid is gravid and contains mature eggs which are released from it. Notice the hooklets and suckers on the scolex.

b. Adult, preserved specimen: attached to the intestinal wall of a dog. A great many adults are attached by their scoleces to the mucosa. They have the appearance of a layer of villi.

c. Hydatid sand: find a scolex and identify the invaginated rostellum and hooklets by focusing up and down on this scolex.

d. A camel's liver infected with hydatid cyst: the hydatid cyst is round. The fluid within the cyst has been lost due to the incision. Notice the layers of wall and a lot of white granulation on the inner edge, called a brood capsule.

Lab. Table 13-1 Key characteristics of cestodes

Cestode	Characteristic features
Diphyllobothrium latum (Broad fish tapeworm)	Scolex has lateral sucking grooves (bothria). Operculated eggs, embryo is a ciliated coraciedium. Gravid proglottid wider than long; rosette-shaped uterus. Procercoid and plerocercoid larvae. Transmission by ingestion of poorly cooked fish. Ingestion of first intermediate host may result in sparganosis
Taenia saginata (Beef tapeworm)	Scolex has 4 suckers, but no hooks. Spherical to oval, striated eggs, typical of Taenia species. Embryo is a 6-hooked oncosphere. Greater than 1, 000 proglottids. Lateral uterine branches number 15-25. Cysticercus larvae. Transmission by ingestion of poorly cooked beef.
Taenia solium (Pork tapeworm)	Scolex has 4 suckers with 2 rows of hooks. Spherical to oval, striated eggs, typical of Taenia species. Embryo is a 6-hooked oncosphere. Fewer than 1,000 proglottids. Lateral uterine branches number 7-14, Cysticercus larvae. Transmission by ingestion of poorly cooked pork. Ingestion of eggs may result in cysticercosis

Hymenolepis nana (Dwarf tapeworm)	Scolex bears a short rostellum with 4 suckers and 1 row of hooks. Thin-shelled round to oval egg contains concosphere and polar filaments. Embryo is a 6-hooked concosphere. Proglottid contains sac-like gravid uterus full of eggs. Cysticercoid larvae. Transmission by ingestion of infective eggs
Hymenolepis diminuta (Rat tapeworm)	Scolex bears rostellum, but lacks hooks seen in *H. nana*. Eggs resemble those of *H. nana* without polar filaments. Embryo is a 6-hooked oncosphere. Proglottids indistinguishable from those of *H. nana*. Cysticercoid larvae. Transmission by ingestion of infected arthropods
Dipylidium caninum (Dog and cat tapeworm)	Scolex has 4 suckers, and rows of tiny, hooklike spines. Eggs enclosed in membrane-bound packets. Embryo is a 6-hooked oncosphere. Progottid contains uterus with packets of eggs. Cysticercoid larvae. Transmission by ingestion of cysticercoid larvae
Echinococcus granulosus (Hydatid tapeworm)	Scolex has 4 suckers and numerous hooks. Eggs identical to Taenia species. Hydatid cyst larvae. Transmission by accidental ingestion of eggs. Hydatid cysts develop in tissues
Multiceps species	Parasitizes dogs, foxes, and wolves. Coenurus larvae, intermediate between cysticercus and hydatid cyst. Transmission by accidental ingestion of eggs

Medical Protozoology

General Considerations

There are four important classes in medical protozoology.

1. Class ZOOMASTIGOPHOREA. Flagellum (a) for locomotion, multiplication by asexual binary fission.

2. Class RHIZOPODEA. Pseudopodium (a) for locomotion, multiplication asexual. Example: *Entamoeba histolytica*, *E. coli*.

3. Class TELOSPOREA. No obvious organelle for locomotion; multiplication by alternation of generations (sporogony and schizogony), exclusively parasitic. Example: *Plasmodium* spp.

4. Class CILIATEA. Cilia for locomotion, containing two kinds of nuclei, a macro- and a micro-nucleus, reproduction by binary fission and conjugation. Example: *Balantidium coli*.

Lab. 14 *Entamoeba histolytica*

E. histolytica is a pathogenic amoeba. There are trophozoite and cyst stages in its life cycle. Only the mature cyst (with 4 nuclei) is infective. Men get infection by mouth. The amoebae inhabit the human colon. They multiply by binary fission. The cysts pass out with feces. The life cycle of *E. histolytica* is cyst—trophozoite—cyst. The trophozoites may invade the intestinal wall or even liver and lung tissues by blood dissemination and induce pathological changes.

What are the morphological characters of trophozoites living in tissue (trophozoites)? Are there any morphological differences between cysts and trophozoites? Are there any technical differences for the examination of cysts and trophozoites? Why?

Requirements

1. Master the morphological characters of *E. histolytica* cysts and trophozoites. Differentiate *E. histolytica* from the non-pathogenic amoebae.

2. Learn the technique of fecal examination for *E. histolytica* trophozoites and cysts.

Procedure

1. Individual observation

a. Cyst of *E. histolytica* in iron-haematoxylin stain.

Search for the cyst under low power. It is easier to search for the organisms in the portion of the specimen where it is neither too thick nor too thin. Then move the cyst to the center of the field. Turn to high power or oil-immersion to identify the structures in detail. The cyst is spherical. Its surrounding is usually clear and transparent. There are 1-4 nuclei in a cyst. The spherical nucleus is covered by a delicate, dark nuclear membrane. There are numerous fine chromatin granules evenly distributed on the inner side of the nuclear membrane. There is a fine and dense nucleolus (karyosome) located in the center of the nucleus. There are usually no dark rod-shaped chromatoid bodies and glycogen vacuoles in mature cysts(Plate II. 3, 4).

b. Living trophozoites

Keep the stage of the microscope in a horizontal position. Put one drop of dilute fluid and one drop of normal saline on a slide. Mix well. Look for the living trophozoites under low power. Never use oil-immersion in this procedure. The amoeba is transparent and mobile. Note the type of movement resulting from pseudopodium formation. The motility will slow down in low temperature or prolonged examination. Watch for the mobility with patience. There is no RBC in artificially cultivated trophozozites.

c. Cyst of *E. coli* in iron-haematoxylin stain.

E. coli is non-pathogenic. They usually exist simultaneously with *E. histolytica*. Search for the cyst as for *E. histolytica* stated in a. The size of *E. coli* is larger than that of *E. histolytica*. There are 1-8 nuclei in a cyst. The cyst with 8 nuclei is a mature cyst. Morphological characters of nuclei: a thicker nuclear membrane, unequal sized chromatin granules irregularly distributed on inner side of nuclear membrane; eccentrically located larger karyosome; chromatoid bodies resemble splinter-like sticks or fragments(Plate II. 6).

2. Demonstration

a. Trophozoite of *E. histolytica* in iron-haematoxylin stain, under oil-immersion.

They are pathogenic and found in the intestinal wall, and liver or lung tissues. They are larger in size, about 20-40μm in diameter. The cytoplasm is bluish grey, ectoplasm hyaline, pseudopodium finger or tongue-like, endoplasm granular, RBC bluish black and varying in size (due to digestion). The features of nucleus are the same as that of the cyst.

b. Trophozoite of *E. hartmanni*, iron-haematoxylin stain, under oil-immersion.

They are non-pathogenic, small in size (3-12μm). Ectoplasm and endoplasm are evident. Only bacteria but no RBC is found in food vacuoles. Fine nucleolus, centrally or eccentrically located, peripheral nuclear chromatins are fine and evenly distributed.

c. Trophozoite of *E. coli*, iron-haematoxylin stain, under oil-immersion.

Non-pathogenic. About 20-50μm in size (larger than *E. histolytica*). Ectoplasm and endoplasm cannot be easily differentiated. Many food vacuoles with bacteria but no RBC is present in the endoplasm. The nuclear structure is the same as the nucleus of the cyst.

d. Living trophozoite of *E. histolytica* under high power.

Notice that there are RBCs in the trophozoite obtained from dysenteric stools, but no RBC in the trophozoite from artificial culture.

Lab. Table 14-1 Morphological differentiations of *E. histolytica* cyst and other non-pathogenic cysts

		E. histolytica	*E hartmanni*	*E. coli*	*I. butschlii*	*E. nana*
Iodine stain	size(μm)	5-20	4-10	10-30	8-10	4-10
	spheroid or elliptic	shapc	spherical	spherical	spherical	spheroid, ovoid or irregular
	number of nucleus	1-4	1-4	1-8	1	1-4
	Glycogen vacuoles	found in immature cyst	found in immature cyst	found in immature cyst	1-2, large	occasionally found in immature cyst
Iron haematoxylin stain	nucleus	samc as trophozoite	same as trophozoite	same as trophozoite	Nucleolus big, eccentric	same as trophozoite Chromatoid bodies
	one or a few, rod shaped	many, short rod shaped or fragments	rare, splinter-like sticks or fragments	none	none	

e. Charcot-leyden crystals, iron-haematoxylin stain. The crystals are colorless, transparent, rhomboids when unstained. They are deep blue in iron haematoxylin stain. They usually appear in acute amoebic dysenteric stools. Their appearance is of diagnostic value. If present, you must search for *E. histolytica* carefully.

f. A section of intestinal wall showing amoebic ulcers, gross inspection. Note the morphological features of nucleus.

Lab. Table 14-2 **Key characteristics of intestinal amebae**

Species	Trophoszoite	Cyst
Entamoeba histolytica	10-60μm, finely granular cytoplasm, evenly distributed peripheral nuclear chromatin; small, central karyosome; Inclusions: ingestion of RBC is diagnostic, progressive motility	10-20μm, mature cyst contains 4 nuclei, elongated chromatoidal bars with blunt, smooth ends. Small, central karyosome
Entamoeba hartmanni	5-12μm, finely granular cytoplasm, evenly distributed peripheral nuclear chromatin; small, central karyosome. Inclusions: bacteria, no RBC, non-progressive motility	5-10μm, mature cyst contains 4 nuclei, elongated chromatoidal bars with blunt, smooth ends. Central karyosome
Entamoeba coli	15-50μm, coarsely granular cytoplasm; unevenly distributed peripheral nuclear chromatin; large, discrete, eccentric karyosome; inclusions: bacteria, yeast, debris; sluggish, non-progressive motility	10-35μm, mature cyst contains 4 nuclei; elongated chromatoidal bars with blunt, smooth ends; central karyosome
Endolimax nana	6-12μm, granular cytoplasm; no peripheral nuclear chromatin; karyosomes are large and blotlike; inclusions: bacteria; sluggish, non-progressive motility	5-10μm, mature cyst contains 4 nuclei; no peripheral nuclear chromatin; large karyosomes, but smaller than trophozoite; no visible chromatoidal bars
Iodamoeba butschlii	8-20μm, granular, vacuolated cytoplasm; no peripheral nuclear chromatin; large karyosomes; inclusions: bacteria, yeast; sluggish, non-progressive motility	5-20μm, mature cyst contains 1 nucleus; no peripheral nuclear chromatin; large karyosome, with granules on one side; no visible chromatoidal bars; prominent glycogen vacuole

Technique of Stool Examination

Direct film

At first, examine the entire stool specimen grossly to determine its consistency and component elements (viz., feces, mucus, blood, tissue elements, and undigested food) and look for macroscopic parasite objects such as roundworms, tapeworm proglottids, etc. Comminute 1-2mg of feces (preferably with blood and mucus) in a drop or two of physiologic saline on a slide. Cover the specimen with a cover glass. This film should be free of air bubbles and macroscopic debris. The film thus prepared ought to be adequate for examination yet not so thick that ordinary newsprint cannot be read through it. This unstained film is particularly valuable for the study of living parasites such as motile protozoan trophozoites, helminth eggs, and nematode larvae.

Iodine-stained film

Prepare the film as stated above, but use iodine solution instead of physiological saline. The iodine film is employed primarily to study the diagnostic features of protozoan cysts.

In iodine stain, the protozoan cyst is light yellowish, nucleus visible though not stained, glycogen bodies brownish, chromatin granules and chromatoid bodies unstained.

After examination, use forceps to put the cover glass into Lysol dish and the slide into the Lysol jar. Wash your hands.

Zinc sulfate centrifugation-flotation method

1. Prepare a fecal suspension by comminuting about 10 parts of tap water with 1 part of the stool specimen (about 1-2g).

2. Approximately 10ml of the suspension is strained through 1 layer of wet cheese cloth (in a small funnel) into a Wassermann tube.

3. The preparation in the tube is then centrifuged for 45-60 seconds at a speed of 2,000 rpm. The supernatant fluid is poured off, 2ml or 3ml of water added to fill the tube.

4. Repeat 3 (usually 2 or 3 times) until the supernatant fluid is clear.

5. The last supernatant fluid is poured off, 3-4ml of zinc sulfate (c. p.) solution of specific gravity 1. 180 added, the packed sediment broken up and enough zinc sulfate solution added to fill the tube to within about one-half inch of the rim.

6. The tube is centrifuged for 45-60 seconds at 2,000 rpm and is brought to a stop for 1 or 2 minutes.

7. Several loopfuls of diagnostic material floating in the surface film are removed by means of a bacteriologic loop onto a clean slide, a drop of iodine stain is added, and the preparation agitated manually to insure uniform staining. The preparation is mounted with a cover glass and is now ready for examination.

Formalin-ether concentration method

1. Emulsify approximately 1gm of feces in 10-12ml of normal saline.

2. Filter through 2 layers of moist gauze into a centrifuge tube.

3. Centrifuge 1 minute at 1,500 rpm; pour off supernatant, and resuspend in fresh saline.

4. Centrifuge 1 minute at 1,500 rpm; if supernatant is still cloudy, repeat.

5. Add 10ml of 10% formalin to sediment, and allow standing for 5 minutes.

6. Add 3ml of ether, shake vigorously.

7. Centrifuge, loosen "plug" between formalin and ether layer, decant supernatant, and examine sediment.

Works

1. Drawing

Draw the cyst of *E. histolytica* and *E. coli* in proportion (iron-haematoxylin stain), showing their microscopic features. Draw a trophozoite of *E. histolytica*.

2. Problems

a. How do you differentiate the pathogenic amoeba and non-pathogenic amoebae from their morphological features?

b. How do you examine trophozoites and cysts of amoebae? What are the important points you must pay attention to during these examinations?

Lab. 15 *Leishmania donovani*

L. donovani is the causative organism of visceral leishmaniasis, commonly known as kala-azar. They are parasites of the reticulo-endothelial system of man. There are leishmanial forms (L. D. bodies) known as amastigote in human and other mammalian hosts and leptomonas forms (promastigote) in sandflies and cultures. The sand flies (*Phlebotomus* spp.) are transmitting vectors.

Procedure

1. Individual observation

a. Amastigotes (L. D. bodies) prepared from bone marrow. Lymph node, liver or spleen punctures of patient or infected hamster, Giemsa stain. Search for the parasite under oil-immersion. L. D. bodies are round or ovoid in shape, 2μm-3μm in diameter. The cytoplasm is light bluish. The nucleus is relatively big and reddish violet in color. The small kinetoplast is rod shaped and also reddish violet in color (Plate II. 15, 16).

Amastigotes are usually present within the macrophages. But they may be set free owing to the rupture of the parasitized cells. They must be differentiated from blood platelets. The blood platelets are usually irregular in form and clumped in a mass and stained light reddish violet. There are no internal structures in the platelets.

b. Promastigotes (leptomonas) Giemsa stain. The promastigotes are infective. They multiply in the digestive tract of sandflies and culture medium. They are spindle shaped, 10-20μm × 1.5-4μm in size. The nucleus is relatively big and round, and is located in the middle of the cell. The parabasal body is located in the anterior end of the cell. Both nucleus and parabasal body are reddish violet after staining. A fine flagellum arises from the anterior end. Its length is just as long as the body length (Plate II. 17).

2. Demonstration

a. Living promastigotes from culture medium, under low or high power. The promastigotes may grow in clumps with their flagella mingled in the center, just like a chrysanthemum flower.

b. *Phlebotomus chinensis*, under dissecting microscope. Sandflies are hairy, humped small flies. Their size is only one-third of a mosquito.

c. Specimens of infected and normal hamsters showing abdominal organs (hepatosplenomegaly). Compare the differences of the color and size of the liver and spleen between infected and normal hamsters.

Works

1. Drawing

Draw several leptomonad and leishmanial forms with color pencils.

2. Problems

a. How do you identify the leishmanial forms free in the blood film?

b. From which organs or tissues can you collect the specimen for the laboratory diagnosis of kala-azar? Why?

Lab. 16 *Trichomonas vaginalis* *T. hominis* *T. buccalis* (including other trichomonads)

T. vavinalis invades the urogenital tract of the human body. It is one of the causative agents of vaginitis and urethritis. There is only a trophozoite stage in *T. vavinalis*. The trophozoite is the infective stage. How do you make a definitive diagnosis for trichomoniasis vaginalis?

Requirements

1. Become familiar with the morphology and motility features of *T. vaginalis*.
2. Learn the diagnostic technique for trichomoniasis.

Demonstration

1. Stained *T. vaginalis*, under oil-immersion.

Pear shaped, 10-30μm $\times$ 5-10μm, 4 anterior flagella, short undulating membrane (one half the length of the body), axostyle protruding posteriorly outside of the body, no cytostome (Plate II. 21, 22).

2. Living *T. vavinalis*, hanging drop or direct film prepared from discharges of Trichomonas vaginitis.

Search under low or high power for living trichomonads. Notice their jerky movement. You will see the activities of flagella and undulating membrane under high power. The trichomonad is actively motile so that it is difficult to see its structures in detail. The motility will slow down by adding one drop of blood serum (1 : 10 dilution) to the specimen. You may find large polygonal vaginal epithelial cells, small round WBC, and clusters of pus cells in the vaginal discharge.

Problem

What is the characteristic feature of locomotion of *T. vaginalis*?

T. hominis

T. hominis inhabits the human colon. There is only a trophozoite form. The parasite is usually found in diarrheic stools. Its pathogenicity is not yet clear.

Demonstration, stained *T. hominis*

Pear shaped, 8-15μm × 3-5μm, 3-5 anterior flagella, 1 posterior flagellum, a long undulating membrane.

It is very active in fresh specimen.

T. buccalis

It also has only a trophozoite stage. *T. buccalis* and *T. hominis* are morphologically alike, with a fine axostyle. The parasite inhabits the calculi and cavities of teeth caries. It is usually found in the suppurative fistula of alveolar process.

Demonstration, *T. buccalis*(Plate II. 24)

Lab. 17 *Giardia lamblia*

The parasite inhabits the small intestine (mainly in duodenum) and gall bladder. It may induce diarrhea. There are trophozoite and cyst forms. The trophozoites are usually found in diarrheic stools. The cysts are usually found in formed stools. The cyst is the infective stage.

Requirements

Learn the morphological features of the trophozoites and cysts.

Demonstration

1. Trophozoite, hematoxylin stain.

The trophozoite is bilaterally symmetrical. About 10-18μm in length, pear shaped, dorsoventrally flattened, broader in the anterior half and narrower in the posterior half with a pointed terminal. On the ventral surface of the anterior half, there is a round hollow sucker. There is 1 pair of nuclei situated bilaterally along the center of the sucker. There are 4 pairs of flagella, 1 pair of axostyles, and 1 pair of parabasal bodies (Plate II. 13).

2. Cyst, hematoxylin stain.

About 10-14μm×7-10μm, elliptical in shape, thick cyst wall, 2-4 nuclei situated in one end of the cyst, and the axostyles and parabasal bodics in the other half(Plate II. 14).

In iodine stain, the cyst is brownish, and the nuclei and axostyles are visible.

Lab. Table 17-1　　Key characteristics of intestinal and atrial flagellates and ciliates

Flagellates/Ciliates	Trophozoite	Cyst
Giardia lamblia	9-20μm by 5-15μm, pear-shaped or teardrop shaped with 2 nuclei, linear axonemes, curved median bodies, and 8 flagella; sucking disc. Falling leaf motility	8-18μm by 7-10μm, round to oval with 4 nuclei, axonemes and median bodies
Chilomastix mesnili	5-24μm by 5-8μm, teardrop shaped, prominent cytostome, 1 nucleus, 4 flagella. Stiff, rotary motility	5-10μm by 4-6μm, lemon shaped with 1 nucleus, and anterior knob or "nipple" cytostome
Enteromonas hominis	4-10μm by 3-6μm, oval shape, 1 nucleus, 4 flagella. Jerky motility	4-10μm by 4-6μm, oval shape, 1-4 nuclei
Retortamonas intestinalis	4-8μm by 5-6μm, oval or pear shaped, 1 nucleus, 2 flagella. Jerky motility	4-8μm by 4-5μm, pear shaped, 1 nucleus
Trichomonas hominis	7-18μm by 5-8μm, pear-shaped, 4-6 flagella, 1 nucleus, undulating membrane extends the full length of the organism, axostyle present. Rapid, jerky motility	No cyst form

续表

Dientamoeba fragilis	5-16μm, ameba-like shape, 1 or 2 nuclei, no visible flagella, debris in cytoplasm; pale staining. Active motility and pseudopod present	No cyst form
Trichomonas vaginalis	8-23μm by 5-12μm, pear-shaped, 1nucleus, 4-6 flagella, prominent axostyle. Undulating membrane extends halfway down the length of the organism. Rapid, jerky motility	No cyst form
Trichomonas tenax	5-12μm by 7-9μm, pear-shaped, 1nucleus, 5 flagella, undulating membrane extends the full length of the organism, axostyle protrudes beyond posterior end. Rapid, jerky motility	No cyst form
Balantidium coli	30-100μm by 30-80μm, very large ovoid shape, large bean-shaped macronucleus, numerous cilia, cytostome/cytopyge	45-65μm, oval or spherical shape, large macronucleus

Lab. 18 *Plasmodium*

There are four species of human malaria. They are *Plasmodium vivax*, *P. falciparum*, *P. malariae*, and *P. ovale*. *P. vivax* and *P. falciparum* are common agents of malaria. *P. malariae* is less common, while *P. ovale* is a rare species. The malaria parasites require two different hosts, man and anopheline mosquito, in order to complete their life cycle. There are schizogony (including exoerythrocytic and erythrocytic) and gametocytogony in man and sporogony in anopheline mosquito.

What are the morphological characteristics of the three malaria species in the erythrocytic stage?

In ordinary conditions, you can only find the ring forms and gametocytes of *P. falciparum* in the peripheral blood. Where are the erythrocytes infected by immature and mature schizonts of *P. falciparum*? Are there any clinical and diagnostic significances for this condition?

Requirements

1. Individual observation

a. *P. vivax*, thin blood film, stained (Plate III).

Under low power, search a portion of the film where the red blood cells are evenly distributed, neither too thick nor too scanty. Then adjust the illumination and search that portion for malaria parasites under oil-immersion, row by row. In stained film the malaria parasites show reddish nuclei, bluish cytoplasm, and yellowish brown pigment.

(1) Ring form. In this stage the parasitized red cells show no changes. The dot-like, reddish nucleus is situated on one side of the ring. The size of the ring is about one-fourth to one-third of the diameter of a red cell.

(2) Ameboid trophozoite. This is the advanced stage of ring form. The parasitized red cells have become enlarged and pale, and may be seen to contain a number of fine red granules known as schüffner's dots. Both cytoplasm and nucleus of the parasite increase in mass. There may be pseudopodia extending out from the cytoplasm. Brownish malaria pigment begins to appear in this stage.

(3) Schizont. This is an advanced stage of trophozoite. The parasite very nearly fills the infected cell. This mature trophozoite ceases its ameboid activity and becomes compact. The single nucleus divides repeatedly to give rise to a total of 12-24 nuclear masses. The cytoplasm finally segments to form separate small masses around each nucleus. The malaria pigment has condensed. The individual parasites thus produced are known as merozoites, and upon rupture of the infected cell, they are released to infect new red cells. As the cycle is never entirely synchronous, parasites at more than one stage of development will usually be seen in a single blood film.

(4) Gametocyte. In addition to asexual forms, gametocytes may usually be seen during the first few paroxysms. The rounded gametocytes contain more pigment. The infected cells enlarge, and schüffner's dots may be seen. Fully mature gametocytes fill the red cell more completely and contain more pigment than schizonts. The nucleus of macrogametocytes is dense and eccentrically located, while that of microgametocytes forms a pale, loose network and is centrally located.

b. *P. falciparum*, thin blood film, stained(Plate III).

The young trophozoites are minute rings. The ring may have 2 small chromatin dots. Double or even triple infection of red cells is not uncommon. Occasionally the earliest stages do not assume a ring form but lie spread out along the periphery of red cells. Such parasites are referred to as applique (marginal) or accole (gliding bird) forms. The infected red cells may develop a few dark-red markings known as Maurer's dots.

The gametocytes of *P. falciparum* are elongate crescent or sausage shaped. The ends of the gametocyte may be pointed, or bluntly rounded, and the remains of the red cell may be seen in the concavity formed by the arched body of the parasite.

2. Demonstration

a. *P. vivax*, different erythrocytic stages, oil-immersion. Notice their morphological features and enlarged infected red cells.

b. *P. falciparum*, ring forms and gametocytes.

c. *P. malariae*, different stages of schizogony and gametocytes. The parasitized red cells do not enlarge. Notice the morphological differences between *P. malariae* and *P. vivax*.

d. Sporozoites, salivary gland smear of an infected mosquito. They are spindle shaped with a nucleus in the middle of the body.

e. Occysts, on the stomach of an infected mosquito. Notice that the rounded oocysts rest on the outer surface of the stomach wall.

f. Exoerythrocytic stage of chicken malaria, stained smear of chicken's brain, oil-immersion. You can see numerous merozoites in a mature exoerythrocytic schizont.

g. *P. vivax*: thick film, stained, under oil-immersion. All red cells are hemolyzed. Most of the malaria parasites may be broken, collapsed or distorted, except for gametocytes.

3. Manipulation

a. Preparation of blood film and staining technique. The blood film is prepared for demonstration of parasites in the blood. The slide should be smooth and free of all blemishes, oil, lint (linen fibers) and fingerprints. In making a thin film, a small drop of blood from a cleaned finger, toe (of children) or ear lobe is brought in contact with one end of the slide and is immediately drawn out into a smooth film 1-cell thick with the smooth, straight edge of another slide. In making the thick film, a somewhat larger drop of blood is deposited near the other end of the slide and is spread out evenly to the size of about 20mm diameter. Both films must be allowed to dry thoroughly, if necessary in a drying oven at about 37℃-40℃ overnight, without contamination from dust or excreta of flies or roaches. Unless the slide is extremely clean, the thick film is likely to flake off. Freshly prepared film always stains best.

b. Giemsa's stain

The procedure for use of Giemsa's stain with thin film is as follows:

(1) Fix blood films in absolute methyl alcohol for 1 minute.

(2) Allow slides to dry.

(3) Immerse slides in a solution of 1 part of Giemsa stock to 30-50 parts of buffered water (pH 6.8-7.2). Stain 30 minutes to 1 hour.

(4) Dip slides briefly in buffered water, drain quickly and thoroughly, and air-dry.

The procedure to be used with thick films is the same, except that steps 1 and 2 are omitted. If the slide has a thick film at one and a thin film at the other, fix only the thin portion, then stain both parts of the film simultaneously.

c. Wright's stain.

The procedure for staining is as follows:

(1) Cover blood film with a measured number of drops of Wright's stain; allow to remain for 1 minute.

(2) Add an equal number of drops of buffered water (pH 6.8-7.2); blow on slide to mix water with stain.

(3) Stain for 3 to 5 minutes; for malaria parasites up to 15 minutes may give better results.

(4) Flood off the stain with buffered water, drain quickly and thoroughly, and air-dry.

Wright's stain is not suitable for thick films.

Works

1. Prepare a thick and thin blood film and stain with Giemsa's stain as stated above.

2. Draw a few erythrocytic stages of *P. vivax* with color pencils.

3. Problems

a. How do you prepare a good thick and thin blood film on one slide? What are the advantages and disadvantages of searching for malaria parasites in thick and thin blood film? What are the precautions for the Wright's and Giemsa's staining techniques?

b. What are the morphological features of erythrocytic stages of malaria parasites?

Lab. 19 *Toxoplasma*

Toxoplasma has a worldwide distribution and is able to develop in a wide variety of vertebrate hosts, but its definitive hosts are the domestic house cat and certain other felidae. With the mucosal cells of the small intestine of the cat, the organisms develop first to produce schizonts and gametocytes and finally oocysts which are passed in the feces. The oocysts become infective when they are swallowed with food or water which are contaminated by sporulated oocysts. These oocysts, 9μm to 11μm in width by 11μm to 14μm in length, are similar in appearance to those of *Isospora belli* but smaller, containing 2 sporocysts, each of which encloses 4 sporozoites.

Toxoplasma trophozoites may be found in the mesenteric lymph nodes and in other organs of the cat, while in other vertebrates these non-intestinal forms are the only stages seen. They are crescentic in shape and may be seen in the peritoneal exudate of experimentally infected mice. Some organisms can be seen in the cytoplasm of macrophages while others have been freed from ruptured cells. They vary in length from

4μm to 6μm and in breadth from 2μm to 3μm.

Requirements

1. Master the morphological characteristics of *Toxoplasma* trophozoites and oocysts.

2. Understand the life cycle of *Toxoplasma*.

Procedure

Individual observation

Toxoplasma trophozoites film, Giemsa stain, from the peritoneal exudate of experimentally infected mice under oil-immersion. They are crescentic in shape, 4-6μm × 2-3μm in size. The organism has a reddish stained nucleus in the middle of the body and the cytoplasm is stained bluish(Plate II. 27, 28).

Demonstration

1. The trophozoite of *Toxoplasma*.

2. The oocyst 9-11μm×11-14μm in size, round shape, contains 2 sporocysts, each of which encloses 4 sporozoites.

Lab. 20 *Balantidium coli*

There are cyst and trophozoite stages in the life cycle of *B. coli*. The trophozoites inhabit human colon, and terminal ileum. They are chiefly lumen dwellers, subsisting on bacteria, but may penetrate the intestinal mucosa to cause ulceration. They multiply by binary fission. The cyst is the infective stage.

Demonstration

1. Trophozoites, hematoxylin stain, oil-immersion

Average size 50-100μm×40-70μm. The body shape is ovoid, somewhat flattened on one side. A cytostome opens on the flattened side near the anterior end. The body is covered with cilia. There are two deeply stained nuclei in the body. The macronucleus, situated near the middle of the body, may be spherical, ellipsoid, elongate, curved, or kidney shaped. The micronucleus is spherical and small, and lies quite close to the macronucleus. Food vacuoles and contractile vacuoles may be seen in the cytoplasm.

2. Cysts

The spherical or ellipsoid cysts are about 50μm to 75μm in length. There is a thick refractile cyst wall, within which a motile organism may be seen in fresh specimens. In stained specimens the macronucleus can usually be seen within the cyst wall, but other structures are usually not observed.

Medical Arthropodology

General Considerations

Members of the phylum ARTHROPODA constitute the largest assemblage of species in the Animal Kingdom. They are elongated, multicellular invertebrates with bilateral symmetry, true segmentation (metamerism), jointed true appendages and a chitinous exoskeleton, which in many species is impregnated with calcium carbonate. Sexes are separate.

The life cycles of arthropods may be grouped into two main forms, complete metamorphosis (holometabola) and partial or incomplete metamorphosis (hemimetabola). In complete metamorphosis there are egg, larvae (one to several stages), pupa, and adult. In partial metamorphosis there are egg, larvae (one to several stages), nymph (more or less resembling adults), and adult.

There are four classes of medical importance in the phylum ARTHROPODA.

Class EUCRUSTACEA. Usually lacking abdominal appendages. Species of *Diaptomus* and *Cyclops* are intermediate hosts of important human worm parasites. Several species of crabs and crayfishes are the second intermediate hosts of *Paragonimus westermani*.

Class CHILOPODA (Centipedes). Usually with one pair of legs for each segment behind the head; first pair of head appendages modified as poison claws.

Class ARACHNIDA. Body divided into head-thorax (cephalothorax) and abdomen; with chelicerae and lacking antennae; adults with four pairs of thoracic legs. Scorpions, spiders, and acari are representatives of the class.

In the order ACARI (ticks and mites) the head, thorax, and abdomen unite without superficial evidence of segmentations; mouth provided with a median sub-oral piercing organ, the hypostome; adults with four pairs of legs, larvae with three pairs of legs.

Class INSECTA. With distinct head, thorax and abdomen, and three pairs of thoracic legs. Many species are of medical importance.

Lab. 21 Mosquitoes

The mosquito is one of "the pests". They transmit malaria, filariasis, epidemic encephalitis B, etc. The life cycle of the mosquito is complete metamorphosis. The egg, larva, and pupa reside in water. Only female mosquitoes are blood sucking and transmit pathogens. Three mosquito genera are of medical importance. They are *Anopheles*, *Culex*, and *Aedes*. They differ in morphology, ecology, and transmission of diseases.

Requirements

1. Master the different features of adult *Culex pipiens pallens*, *Anopheles hyrcanus sinensis*, and *Aedes albopictus*.

2. Study the general morphology of mosquitoes in different developmental stages and the piercing mouthparts of the adults.

3. Study the generic features of mosquitoes and the use of "key to the adult female mosquitoes".

Procedure

1. Individual observation

Adult mosquitoes, mounted on an insect needle. Observe with a hand lens.

(1) *Culex pipiens pallens*

Head: subglobose. A pair of prominent compound eyes bilaterally located, deep in color. A pair of antennae, whip-like, extending bilaterally, with 15 segments each ornamented with whorled hairs, which are long and numerous in males and scanty in females. One proboscis protrudes from the front lower part of the head. The proboscis consists of a labium, labrum, hypopharynx, and one pair of both mandibles and maxillae. The tip of the labium is called the labella. A pair of maxillary palpi is located bilaterally to the proboscis. They are short (about one-fifth that of the proboscis) in females and long in males. There are numerous fine hairs on the male palpi. Thorax: including three segments, pro-, meso-, and meta-thorax. The mesothorax is the most developed. The mesoscutum is important for classification. There are three pairs of legs (one pair on each segment). The leg consists of five parts: coxa, trochanter, femur, and tibia with one joint each, and the distal tarsus consisting of five segments with a pair of terminal articulated claws and pulvilli.

The wings arise from the posterolateral angle of the mesonotum. The scales of the wing provide distinctive color patterns of diagnostic importance. The third thoracic segment has a pair of halters. Abdomen: the abdomen is elongated, cylindrical and consists of ten segments, although only eight are clearly visible, due to sexual modification of the terminal two. In the female the ninth is greatly reduced and, at its junction with the eighth, bears the genital opening, while the tenth, which is also reduced and narrowed, bears the anus and the terminal cerci. The eighth, ninth, and tenth segments of the male are twisted and are modified into the external genital organs, i. e., the terminalia (grasping organ or hypopygium), which have a relatively complicated structure. The abdominal segments are covered by tergal and sternal plates, separated by an expandable pleural membrane on each side.

(2) *Anopheles hyrcanus sinensis*

Grayish brown in color. The length of maxillary palpi is equal to the proboscis both in male and female; the terminal part is enlarged in the male. Usually there are white bands of palpi and black and white scales on the wing. Black and white spots may be present on the fringe.

(3) *Aedes albopictus*

Black in color with silvery white spots, a median longitudinal white stripe on the mesonotum. With white bands on legs.

Lab. Table 21-1 Generic identification of mosquitoes in egg, larval, pupal, and adult stages

	Anopheles	*Culex*	*Aedes*
Eggs	naviculate with air sacs (floats), laid singly on water	laid in rafts floating on water	laid singly in or near water
Larvae	lie parallel to surface film, possess palmate hairs, no siphon	lie obliquely to water surface, siphon long and slender, several pairs of siphon hairs	lie obliquely to water surface, siphon short and broad, 1 pair of siphon hairs
Pupae	breathing trumpets short and broad	long and tubular	short and truncated
Adults	rest with proboscis in a straight line with body, at an resting surface	rest with proboscis not in line with body, body is parallel to resting surface	same as *Culex*
	wing usually spotted or dappled	wing not usually spotted or dappled	same as *Culex*
	palpi usually as long as proboscis	palpi of female less than half length of proboscis	same as *Culex*
	body brownish or grayish in color, without spots	body brownish or grayish in color, no spots	body blackish with white bands or spots
		legs without bands; thorax without distinct markings	legs with white bands; thorax with stripes or patches of silvery or golden scales

2. Demonstration

a. Larvae, slide specimen: the larva consists of head, thorax, and abdomen.

(1) *Culex* larva: there are tufts of hairs on the body.

Head: there are antennae, eyes, and mouthparts.

Thorax: 3 segments fused together. It is broader than head and abdomen.

Abdomen: 9 segments. There is a long and slender siphon originating from the dorsum of the 8th segment.

(2) *Anopheles* larva: no siphon, a pair of spiracles arising from the dorsum of the 8th segment. From lst to 7th abdominal segment there is a pair of palmate hairs on each segment.

(3) *Aedes* larva: the siphon is relatively short and broad.

b. Eggs:

(1) *Culex* eggs.

(2) *Anopheles* eggs.

(3) *Aedes* eggs.

c. Pupae, slide specimen:

(1) *Culex* pupa: composed of cephalothorax and abdomen.

There is a pair or slender breathing trumpets on the cephalothorax.

(2) *Anopheles* pupa: trumpets short and broad, a cleft in front.

(3) Aedes pupa: trumpets short and broad, opening triangular.

Works

1. Drawing

Draw a mosquito wing, showing its venation.

2. Problems

a. Tabulate the differences of 3 mosquito genera in egg, larval, pupal, and adult stages.

b. Describe the general features of all insects and the specific features of a mosquito.

c. Enumerate the human diseases transmitted by 3 mosquito genera.

d. State the mosquito-pathogen relationships.

e. State the distributions of mosquitoes in the city and in the countryside. Why are they different in distribution?

Key to the adult female mosquitoes most frequently found in China

1. Palpi and proboscis equal in length, with no scales on abdomen, with dark and pale scales on the wing ·· 2

Palpi shorter than proboscis, with scales on abdomen wings dark ················ 3

2. Costa with only 2 pale spots, palpus with 4 white bands ························
·· Anopheles hyrcarius sinensis

Costa with at least 4 pale spots, palpus with 3 white bands, relatively small in size
·· *A. minimus*

3. Mesonotum black, with silvery white scale spots, tarsus with obvious white bands ·· 4

Mesonotum brownish, tarsus with no obvious or without white bands ············ 5

4. Mesonotum with an obvious white longitudinal stripe in the middle ············

Aedes albopictus Mesonotum with 2 large white spots bilaterally ………………………………………………………………………………………………… *Ae. chemulpoensis*

5. Proboscis with a white band and in the middle, tarsus with no obvious white bands ……………………………………………………………… Culex tritaeniorhynchus

Proboscis and tarsus both without white band ……………… Culex pipiens pallens

Lab. 22 Flies

The filth flies are one of "the four pests". They transmit many kinds of infectious diseases, including infections of digestive, respiratory, nervous systems, and sense organs. They transmit pathogens by mechanical means. The life cycle of flies is complete metamorphosis. The fly larvae of some species are agents of myiasis in man and other vertebrates. The breeding places are widespread and varied in different species. The pupae are found in the ground near the breeding place. The adult flies are omnivorous. The majority of flies have lapping type mouthparts. The flies regurgitate and defecate all the time when they take food. The transmission of infectious disease will be greatly aggravated by this characteristic.

Requirements

1. Study the general characteristics of common house flies and different stages in the life cycle.

2. Study the relationships between the morphology of flies and transmission of disease.

Procedure

1. Individual observation

a. Adult mounted on insect needle: observe with a hand lens.

Many bristles cover the entire body. The body is divided into head, thorax, and abdomen.

Head: with one pair of compound eyes. With the exception of Bellieria, the compound eyes of female flies are separated from each other, while in males the compound eyes are contiguous.

Thorax: with three pairs of legs; mesothorax well developed, with a pair of wings; three to four longitudinal blackish strips on the mesonotum.

Abdomen: 10 segments, first to fifth segments visible; the remainder are modified to form external genitalia and are hidden in the abdomen.

b. Adult, slide specimen.

Head of *Musca vicina*: two compound eyes composed of many hexagonal shaped ocelli; three ocelli (simple eyes) on the apex, located at the angles of an inverted triangle; a pair of antennae below the compound eyes, composed of three segments; feather-shaped arista arising from the middle of the third segment; mouthparts are of lapping type, composed of rostrum, haustellum, and labella; a pair of maxillary palpi arising from antero-lateral aspects of rostrum. The haustellum, which is contiguous with and distal to the rostrum, consists of a labrum-epipharynx (upper lip), hypopharynx, and labium. At its distal extremity the labium ends in a pair of oval lobes, the labella, each provided with numerous pseudotracheae, are actually chitinous food troughs. When at rest, the labella approximate each other; when feeding, they are separated and can be molded to the feeding surface.

Legs: Covered with numerous bristles. At the distal end, the terminal tarsus ends in a pair of claws and pulvilli with numerous fine hairs.

Wings: six longitudinal veins, unbranched. The form of curvature of the fourth vein and the distance between terminal ends of the third and fourth veins are important in classification.

c. Larva, posterior spiracles, slide specimen: at the posterior end, there is a pair of D-shaped posterior spiracles with long sinuous slits and a central button (in *Musca*).

2. Demonstration

a. House flies frequently found in China:

(1) *Musca vicina*: medium-sized (males 5.8-6.5mm, females 6.5-7.5mm in length), gray, mesonotum with four equally broad, dark, longitudinal stripes. The fourth longitudinal vein of the wing bends abruptly upwards, nearly meeting the third longitudinal vein. The arista is feather-like.

(2) *Lucilia sericata*: medium-sized, metallic green, cheeks with silvery white fine hairs. The fourth vein of the wing bends abruptly upwards as in *Musca*.

(3) *Chrysomyia megalocephala*: large, brilliant metallic golden green or blue-green, compound eyes bright red in color, cheeks with yellowish fine hairs, fourth vein of the wing same as in *Musca*.

(4) *Aldrichina grahami*: large, stout, thorax grayish black, with long and thick bristles, metallic deep blue abdomen.

(5) *Muscina stabulans*: relatively big medium-sized, dark gray non-metallic, mesonotum with four longitudinal black stripes (two medial strips long and evident, two lateral ones interrupted), fourth vein of the wing curves gently upwards.

(6) *Stomoxys calcitrans*: medium-sized, dark gray, more or less like *Musca vicina*, mouthparts of piercing type, arista feather-like on one side only, mesonotum and fourth vein the same as in Muscina stabulans.

(7) *Bellieria melanura*: large (10-14mm), arista feather-like on basic part only, mesonotum with three longitudinal black stripes, fourth vein of the wing same as in *M. vicina*, and a checkered light and dark upper abdominal surface.

(8) *Fannia canicularis*: small-sized (5-6mm), dark gray, arista without hairs, fourth vein of the wing is almost parallel to the third vein.

b. Different stages in the life cycle: egg, larva, pupa, and adult.

Work

1. Drawings

a. Draw a tarsal terminalia of *Musca vicina*.

b. Draw a wing of *Musca vicina* showing its venation.

2. Problem

Design a plan for the control of flies in a village.

Lab. 23 Lice

Lice are dorsoventrally flattened, relatively small, wingless insects, which have three pairs of stout legs, each ending in a tarsal claw. The mouthparts have adapted to sucking host's blood and cutaneous juices. They are exclusively ectoparasites of mammals. Lice have partial metamorphosis—egg, nymph and adult. They spend their entire life on their hosts.

Human lice consist of three types: (1) head louse, *Pediculus humanus* var. *capitis*. (2) body louse, *p. h.* var. *corporis*; *P. humanus* var. *capitis* is at present a hybrid breed. (3) pubic or "crab" louse, *Phthirus pubis*.

Lice play a twofold role in the production of disease in man: (1) body lice, and to a lesser extent head lice and pubic lice, transmit louse-borne typhus fever, trench fever, relapsing fever, and other diseases from man to man; (2) lice produce an irritating dermatitis (pediculosis).

Requirements

Study the general morphology of lice.

Procedure

1. Individual observation

Adults (body lice and pubic lice):

a. Body louse, slide specimen: observe under low power. Grayish white in color, dorsoventrally flattened, wingless; Female larger than the male.

Head: rectangular-ovoidal from dorsal aspect, a pair of eye spots, a pair of five-jointed antennae (anterior to the eye spots), mouthparts of piercing type, hidden in the head when not in use.

Thorax: three pairs of strong legs provided with claws adapted for clinging to hairs or fibers.

Abdomen: the abdomen of the male is narrower than that of the female and is rounded posteriorly. In the female the terminal segment is inverted V-shaped.

b. Head louse, slide specimen: dark grayish, smaller than the body louse.

c. Pubic louse, slide specimen: crab-like, distinctive in appearance(Plate IV. 7).

2. Demonstration

a. Eggs: elongated ovoid, operculated, light yellow in color, cemented to hair or clothing(Plate IV. 8).

b. Nymph: closely resembling the adult but smaller in size and sexually immature.

Work

What diseases are transmitted or induced by lice?

Lab. 24 Fleas

Fleas are partially host-specific ectoparasites, which are temporarily attached to the skin of mammals and birds for sucking blood and are particularly abundant on nest-building rodents.

Adults are small, wingless, brown, glistening insects, which are compressed laterally, have piercing mouthparts, and conspicuous legs, of which the hind pair is especially developed and is adapted for jumping.

The head is usually longer than high, and is divided into two portions, which are obliquely separated by antennal grooves. In front, the dorsal portion is called the frons; the ventral portion is termed the gena (cheek). The region behind the antennal groove is the occiput.

The life cycle of fleas is complete metamorphosis—egg, larva, pupa, and adult.

Fleas are harmful to man in two capacities: (1) they are hosts and transmitters of important diseases (plague, murine typhus fever and tapeworms); (2) their bites produce an irritating dermatitis.

Requirements

1. Study the general feature of fleas in different developmental stages.
2. Study the morphology of some common fleas.

Procedure

1. Individual observation

Adult flea, slide specimen: body laterally compressed, wingless, divided into head, thorax, and abdomen.

Head: 1 pair of antennae, with 3 segments, situated in the antennal groove; a pair of eyes in front of antennae. The presence or absence of genal comb and pronotal comb and position of ocular bristal are important in identification.

Thorax: composed of 3 segments—pro-, meso-, and meta-thorax, each of which consists of tergal, sternal, and pleural plates; 3 pairs of strong legs, each of which is attached to the pleural plate; the mesopleuron may have chitinous suture.

Abdomen: composed of 10 segments; from 1st to 8th segment with a pair of spiracles on each segment; a saddle-shaped pygidium on the 9th segment (possibly a sensory organ); in the 7th segment there is a chitinous spermatheca (seminal receptacle) in females; in males there are 2 pairs of small claspers on the 9th segment; extending inward from the region between 9th segment; extending inward from the region between the 9th and 10th segment is the long, coiled, chitinous aedeagus or cirrus organ.

Remark: presence or absence of eyes, genal, and pronotal combs, position of ocular bristle, shape of spermatheca and male external genitalia are important in the identification.

2. Demonstration

Developmental stages, slide specimen:

Egg: ovoid, non-operculated, 0.5mm×0.34mm.

Larva: creamy white, slender, without legs and eyes, chewing type mouthparts.

Pupa: the mature third stage larvae spin a cocoon around itself and pupate.

3. Some fleas commonly found in China:

Pulex irritans: without genal and pronotal comb; ocular bristle under the eye, mesopleuron narrow and without suture(Plate IV. 3).

Xenopsylla cheopis: with no genal and pronotal comb; ocular bristle in front of eyes; mesopleuron broad, with vertical suture.

Citellophilus tesquorum sungaris: with pronotal comb only; spermatheca ovoid in anterior part, banana-shaped at the tail.

Ctenophalides felis: with both genal and pronotal combs; head narrow and elongated; C-shaped spermatheca(Plate IV. 4).

C. canis: with both genal and pronotal combs; head short; frons rounded; tail of spermatheca elongated.

Works

1. State the relationships between the epidemic plague and ecology of fleas.
2. Why can we control plague since liberation?

Lab. 25 *Phlebotomus* (Sand Flies)

The sand flies are blood-sucking insects belonging to the genus *Phlebotomus*. The adults are small, hump-backed, tawny in color, with conspicuous black eyes and hairy body, wings, and legs. The oval-lanceolate wings are carried erect and the male terminalia are long and prominent. They are poor fliers but take characteristic hops. Only females feed on blood.

The life cycle is complete metamorphosis.

Phlebotomus may transmit sand fly fever, bartonellosis and kala-azar. *P. chinensis* is the transmitter of kala-azar in China.

Requirements

1. Study the general features of sand flies in different developmental stages.
2. Study the morphology of adult *P. chinensis*.

Procedure

1. Individual observation

P. chinensis—adult, pharyngeal armature and spermatheca, slide specimen: from 2nd-6th segments of abdomen the hair is erect; pharyngeal armature is not well developed, with numerous fine spines on the surface and with ridges on the terminal part; spermatheca with 9-13 segments and maize-shaped; 5 bristles (setae) on the terminal segment of the superior clasper (in males).

2. Demonstration

a. Sand fly in different developmental stages:

(1) Adult, slide specimen: about 3mm in length.

Head: a pair of compound eyes, a pair of antennae, a pair of palpi, piercing mouthparts; palpus with 5 segments, 4th and 5th segments turning downwards and backwards.

Thorax: humped back; mesothorax well developed; with a pair of hairy wings; wing venation lst, 3rd, and 6th longitudinal veins unbranched, 2nd with 3 branches, 4th and 5th veins 2 branches each; 3 pairs of slender legs.

Abdomen: 10 segments, hairy.

(2) Egg, slide specimen: elongate ovoid, 0.4mm in length, brownish or black in color, usually with net-like decorations.

(3) Larva, slide specimen: 4 stages; divided into head, thorax, and abdomen; without eyes; chewing type mouthparts. lst stage larva with 1 pair of bristles at terminal end; 2nd-4th stage larvae with 2 pairs of bristles.

(4) Pupa, slide specimen: the mature 4th stage larva pupates with its shed-skin, so, there are 2 pairs of terminal bristles at one end of the cocoon.

b. *P. sergenti* mongolensis: notice its difference from *P. chinensis*.

Spermatheca: short and small, with 4 segments. Pharyngeal armature: with many patches, without ridges. External genitalia of male: superior clasper stout, with 4 bristles on the terminal segment.

Works

1. Drawing

Draw a spermatheca and a superior clasper of *P. chinensis*.

2. Problems

a. What are morphological and ecological feature of sand flies? Are they related to the control of sand flies?

b. State the relationship between the sand flies and human disease.

Lab. 26 *Cimex* (Bed Bugs)

Only two species, *Cimex lectularius* and *C. hemiptera*, commonly invade human habitations. *C. lectularius* is common in Temperate Zones and *C. hemiptera* in the Tropics. They are mahogany-brown in color, about 5mm long by 3mm broad, and covered with fine hairs.

The easiest differentiation of the two species is the distinct antero-lateral expansions of the pronotum in *C. lectularius*, which is lacking in *C. hemiptera*.

The life cycle of bed bugs is incomplete metamorphosis—egg, nymph, and adult.

There is no convincing evidence that they are natural biological vectors for the transmission of disease-producing agents.

Requirements

Study the general morphology of bed bugs.

Procedure

1. Individual observation

Adult, slide specimen:

Head: 1 pair of compound eyes, without ocelli; 1 pair of antennae with 4 segments; piercing type mouthparts.

Thorax: prothorax comprises the greatest part of the thorax; 3 pairs of legs; 1 pair of vestigial wings.

Abdomen: composed of 10 segments; a lambdoid copulatory orifice (organ of Berlese) on the right side of the 5th sternal plate of the female; the 9th and 10th segments are modified to genital organs in both sexes.

2. Demonstration

Cimex in different developmental stages.

Adult

Eggs: operculated; elongate ovoid; 1mm in length; white colored with dark network ornaments.

Nymph: smaller than adult and sexually immature.

Work

State the control of bed bugs.

Lab. 27 Ticks

All ticks are parasitic. They are large mites with a leathery integument and adapted to suck blood from mammals, birds, and reptiles. As adults they usually measure a centimeter or more in length. They are differentiated from mites by having an armed hypostome and a definite pair of tracheal spiracular openings situated just behind the basal segment of the 3rd or 4th pair of legs.

They are divided into two families, the *ARGASIDAE* (soft-bodied ticks) and the *IXODIDAE* (hard-bodied ticks).

Ticks are important agents and vectors of human disease: (1) several species of ticks are required host and transmitters to man, of important pathogenic organisms (Rocky Mountain spotted fever and related rickettsiosis, tick-borne relapsing fever, Russian spring-summer encephalitis, tularemia, and plague); (2) the salivary secretions of certain ticks produce systemic toxemia (tick paralysis), which may cause death, and (3) tick bites produce appreciable pain and traumatic injury. Besides, ticks are the agents of diseases of great economic significance in domestic animals.

Requirements

1. Study the morphology of ticks in different developmental stages.
2. Identify soft-bodied ticks and hard-bodied ticks.

Procedure

Demonstration—slide specimens:

1. Hard-bodied ticks—*Dermacentor andersoni*: the dorsal plate or shield covers the entire surface of the male, but only the anterior portion of the female; the capitulum extends forward beyond the dorsal shield. Pay attention to its size and shape, position of capitulum, shape and number of legs, and difference between male and female(Plate IV. 10).

a. Capitulum: the capitulum or false head is attached to the anterior of the body of the hard-bodied tick.

The basal portion of the capitulum consists of a broad chitinous ring, the posterior constricted portion of which constitutes the connection with the body (basis capitulum). The basis capitulum carries the mouthparts, consisting of the toothed hypostome, a more or less median, finger-like process, ventral to the mouth in position; a pair of chelicerae, arising directly from the oral opening on the dorso-lateral aspects of the hypostome and situated in a sheath which is the direct continuation of the capitular base; and a pair of pedipalps, or palps, which arise from the ventrolateral margin of the capitular base. The paired palps each consist of 4 segments, of which the terminal one is small and is set into a depression of the 3rd segment.

b. Body: ovoid, dorsoventrally flattened with elastic, leathery skin. The dorsal surface is characterized by having sculpturing, furrows or color patterns. From the lateral aspects of the anterior half or three-fifths of the body, the 4 walking legs arise, their basal (coxal) segments forming shield-like plates. On the ventral surface the genital orifice lies in the mid-line in the anterior half, while the anal pore is situated a short distance in front of the posterior extremity. The spiracular opening on each side is found posterior to the 4th coxal segment. The openings are located on chitinized stigmal plates. There are grooves which divide the venter more or less into fields.

2. Soft-bodied ticks: brownish in color. They are different from hard-bodied ticks in the following: without shield; capitulum is underneath the anterior dorsal surface; spiracular opening on each side is found posterior to the 3rd coxal segments.

Work

State the chief morphological difference between hard-bodied ticks and soft-bodied ticks.

Lab. 28 *Sarcoptes scabiei*

The itch mite, *Sarcoptes scabiei*, is cosmopolitan in distribution. It parasitizes both man and other mammals. It is a permanent ectoparasite.

The development of *S. scabiei* is incomplete metamophosis—egg, larva, nymph (2 stages), and adult.

Requirements

Study the morphology of *S. scabiei*.

Procedure

1. Individual observation

Adult, slide specimen: pay attention to its size. It is a microscopic arthropod of ovoid contour, with minute mouthparts (chelicerae and palps, 1 pair each) superficially resembling a turtle's head, no special respiratory apparatus, and with its anterior 2 pairs of legs well separated from its posterior 2 pairs. The anterior legs terminate in delicate sucking pads (pulvilli); the posterior legs both end in long hair bristles in the female, while in the male the 3rd pair has bristles and the 4th pair pulvilli. The female measures 330-450μm$\times$350μm and the male, 200-240μm$\times$200μm. On the dorsal surface there are numerous parallel ridges, except for a small, smooth median area just behind the head, and in addition, several mid-dorsal tooth-like spines, and in other areas longer, finger-like spines and long and short hair. The anal pore is situated at the terminal end of the body. The female genital pore is in the center of the ventral surface. The male external genitalia is situated between the 2 hind pairs of legs.

2. Demonstration

Larva, slide specimen: smaller than adult, with 3 pairs of legs.

Work

How do you treat and prevent scabies.

Vocabulary of Parasitology

abates 双硫磷
Acanthamoeba 棘阿米巴属
Acanthamoeba castellanii 卡氏棘阿米巴
Ancylostoma caninum 犬钩口线虫
acanthella 棘头体
acanthopodia 棘状伪足
acanthor 棘头蚴
Acari 螨亚纲(蜱螨亚纲)
Acariformes 真螨目
accidental parasite 偶然寄生虫
acetabulum 腹吸盘
acquired immunity 获得性免疫
adult 成虫
Aedes aegypti 埃及伊蚊
Aedes albopictus 白纹伊蚊
African sleeping sickness 非洲昏睡病(非洲睡眠病)
African trypanosomiasis 非洲锥虫病
agglutinin 凝集素
AIDS 艾滋病
albendazole 阿苯达唑(丙硫咪唑)
Aldrichina grahami 巨尾阿丽蝇
allethrin 丙烯菊酯
Alocinma longicornis 长角涵螺
alternation of generations 世代交替
alveolar hydatid cyst 泡球蚴
amastigote 无鞭毛体
ambulacra 吸垫
ameba 阿米巴
American trypanosomiasis 美洲锥虫病
aminoquinoline 氨基喹啉
Amiota variegata 变色纵眼果蝇
amoeba pores 阿米巴穿孔素
amoebic colitis 阿米巴性结肠炎
amoebic dysentery 阿米巴痢疾
amoebic keratitis (AK)阿米巴性角膜炎

amoebic liver abscess 阿米巴肝脓肿
amoeboma 阿米巴肿
ampulla 壶腹
anal swab 肛门拭子法
anchoring disc 固定盘
Ancylostoma braziliense 巴西钩口线虫
Ancylostoma ceylanicum 锡兰钩口线虫
Ancylostoma duodenale 十二指肠钩口线虫
Ancylostoma-secreted antigen-1（ASP-1）钩虫分泌抗原-1
anemia 贫血
Angiostrongylus cantonensis 广州管圆线虫
anisakiasis 异尖线虫病
Anisakis 异尖线虫
Anopheles anthropophagus 嗜人按蚊
Anopheles dirus 大劣按蚊
Anopheles minimus 微小按蚊
Anopheles sinensis 中华按蚊
Anoplura 虱目
antenna 触角
antennal fossa 触角窝
antepygidial bristle 臀前鬃
anticoagulin 抗血凝素
antigen determinant 抗原决定簇
antigen disguise 抗原伪装
antigenic diversity 抗原差异
antigenic variation 抗原变异
anti-idiotypic antibody 抗独特型抗体
apical membrane antigen（AMA）顶端膜抗原
apical prominence 顶突
apoptosis 细胞凋亡
appendicitis caused by Enterobius vermicularis 蛲虫性阑尾炎
Arachnida 蛛形纲
Araneae 蜘蛛亚纲
arbo-disease 虫媒病
Argasidae 软蜱科
Aristichthys nobilis 鳙鱼(大头鱼)
arrested telophase 分裂停滞期
artemether 蒿甲醚

artemisinin (quinghaosu)青蒿素
artesunate 青蒿琥酯
auramine-phenol 金胺一酚(染色法)
ascariasis 蛔虫病
Ascaris lumbricoides 似蚓蛔线虫
ascaroside 蛔甙层
asexual generation 无性生殖
atovaquone 阿托喹酮
balantidial dysentery 结肠小袋纤毛虫痢疾
Balantidiidae 小袋科
Balantidium coli 结肠小袋纤毛虫
Bandicota bengalensis 小板齿鼠
basal body 基体
basal lamella 基质膜
basal plasma membrane 基质膜
basement layer 基层
basoquin 氨酚喹,阿莫地喹
baytex 倍硫磷
beaver 河狸(水獭)
bed bug 臭虫
bentonite flocculation test (BFT) 皂土絮状试验
Bertiella studeri 司氏伯特绦虫
bifunctional antibody 双功能抗体
binominal system 二名制
biological transmission 生物性传播
bispecific antibody (BsAb) 双特异抗体
bithionol 硫双二氯酚
Bithynia fuchsianus 赤豆螺(傅氏豆螺)
biting midge 蠓
black fly 蚋(黑蝇)
bladderworm 囊虫
Blastocystidea 芽囊原虫纲
Blastocystis 芽囊原虫属
Blastocystis hominis 人芽囊原虫
blastocystosis hominis 人芽囊原虫病
Blattaria 蜚蠊目
Blattella germanica 德国小蠊
blephearoplast 毛基体

blood-inhabiting flagellate 血居鞭毛虫
Boettcherisca peregrina 棕尾别麻蝇
Boophilus microplus 微小牛蜱
Borrelia burgdorferi 伯氏包柔氏螺旋体
Borrelia latyshevyi 拉氏包柔氏螺旋体
Borrelia persica 波氏包柔氏螺旋体
Borrelia recurrentis 回归热包柔氏螺旋体
bothridium 突盘
bothrium 沟槽
bradysporozoites (BS) 迟发型子孢子
bradyzoite 缓殖子
brine flotation 饱和盐水浮聚法
Brugia malayi 马来布鲁线虫
Brugia timori 帝纹布鲁丝虫
buccal capsule 口囊
budding 芽生
Calabar swelling 卡拉巴丝虫性肿块
calcareous body 石灰小体
Calliphoridae 丽蝇科
Cambaroides spp. 蝲蛄
Capillaria hepatica 肝毛细线虫
capillary tubule 毛细管
capitulum 假头
Carassius auratus 鲫鱼
carbon dioxide fixation 二氧化碳固定
Caridina nilotica gracilipes 细足米虾
carrier 带虫者
caveola-vesicle complex 凹窝小泡复合体
cecum 肠支
cell coat 细胞被
cell-detaching factor 细胞离散因子
cellophane tape 透明胶纸法
centrifugal sedimentation method 离心沉淀法
Centrocestus formosanus 台湾棘带吸虫
cephalic alae 头翼
Ceratopogonidae 蠓科
cercaria 尾蚴
cercarial dermatitis 尾蚴性皮炎

cercomere 小尾
cerebral malaria 脑型疟
Cerithecea 蟹守螺超科
cestode 绦虫
cestodiasis 绦虫病
Chagas' disease 恰加斯病(美洲锥虫病)
Chagoma 恰加氏肿
chemokine family 趋化因子家族
chigger mite 恙螨
Chilopoda 唇足纲
Chiniofon 喹碘方
chip microarray 芯片微阵技术
chitin 壳质
chloroquine 氯喹
chlorothiazide 氯丙嗪
chromatin granules 核周染色质粒
chromatoid body 拟染色体
Chrysomyia megacephala 大头金蝇
Chrysops vanderwulpi 广斑虻
Chrysops 斑虻
chyluria 乳糜尿
ciliate 纤毛
Ciliophora 纤毛门
Cimex hemipterus 热带臭虫
Cimex lectularius 温带臭虫
Cimicidae 臭虫科
cinchona 金鸡纳
circular muscle 外环肌
circulating antigen (CAg)循环抗原
circumlarval precipitin test (CPT) 环蚴沉淀试验
circumoval precipitin test (COPT)环卵沉淀试验
Cirrhinus molitorella 鲮鱼
cirrus 阴茎
cirrus pouch 阴茎袋
Class Lobosea 叶足纲
Class Metacanthocephala 后棘头虫纲
Class Nematoda 线虫纲
Class Sporozoa 孢子虫纲

Class Trematoda 吸虫纲
Class Zoomastigophorea 动鞭纲
classical Dengue 典型登革热
claw 爪
clonorchiasis 华支睾吸虫病
Clonorchis sinensis 华支睾吸虫
cluster analysis 聚类分析技术
cockroach 蜚蠊
coenurus 多头蚴
collecting tubule 集合管
commensalism 共栖
common vitelline duct 总卵黄管
compact nucleus 实质核
complete metamorphosis 全变态
compound eyes 复眼
concentration method 浓聚法
concomitant immunity 伴随免疫
conjugation 结合生殖
conoid 类锥体
contact-dependent cytopathic effect 接触依赖性细胞病变效应
contractile vacuole 伸缩泡
coracidium 钩球蚴
Coxiella burneti 贝氏立克次体
Crimean-Xinjiang haemorrhagic fever 新疆-克里米亚出血热
Crustacea 甲壳纲
cryptosporidiosis 隐孢子虫病
Cryptosporidium parvum 微小隐孢子虫
Cryptosporidium 隐孢子虫
Ctenopharyngodon idellus 草鱼(白鲩)
Culex pipiens pallens 淡色库蚊
Culex pipiens quinquefasciatus 致倦库蚊
Culex tritaeniorhynchus 三带喙库蚊
Culicidae 蚊科
Culicoides homotomus 同体库蠓
culture method for hookworm larvae 钩蚴培养法
cutaneous larva migrans (CLM) 皮肤幼虫移行症
cutaneous leishmaniasis (CL) 皮肤利什曼病
cuticle 角皮

cycloguanil 环氯胍
Cyclophyllidea 圆叶目
Cyclorrhapha 环裂亚目
Cyprinus carpio 鲤鱼
cyst 包囊
cyst carriers or cyst passengers 包囊携带者
cystacanth 感染性棘头体
cysteine-rich proteins (CRP) 富含半胱胺酸蛋白
cysticercoid 似囊尾蚴
cysticercoid larva 似囊尾蚴
cysticercus 囊尾蚴
cysticercus bovis 牛囊尾蚴
cysticercus cellulosae 猪囊尾蚴
cysticercus racemosus 葡萄状囊尾蚴
cytoadherence reverse antibody 使细胞粘连现象逆转的抗体
cytochrome c oxidase subunit I 细胞色素 C 氧化酶亚单位 I
cytokine 细胞因子
cytolytic type 细胞溶解型
cyton region 细胞体区
cytopharynx 胞咽
cytoplasmic connective 胞浆连接部
cytostome 胞口
cytotoxic type 细胞毒型
damage of urogenital system 泌尿生殖系统损害
dapsone 氨苯砜
Davaineidae 代凡科
definitive host 终宿主
delayed type hypersensitivity (DTH) 迟发型超敏反应
deltamethrin 溴氰菊酯
Demodex brevis 皮脂蠕形螨
Demodex folliculorum 毛囊蠕形螨
Demodicidae 蠕形螨科
Dengue fever 登革热
Dengue haemorrhagic fever 登革出血热
Dengue virus 登革病毒
Dermacentor nuttalli 草原革蜱
Dermanyssus gallinae 鸡皮刺螨
Dermatitis caused by hookworm larvae 钩蚴性皮炎

Dermatophagoides farinae 粉尘螨
Dermatophagoides pteronyssinus 屋尘螨
Diamond's 戴蒙德氏
diarrhea and allotriophagy 腹泻和异嗜症
dichlorvos(DDVP) 敌敌畏
Dientamoeba fragilis 脆弱双核阿米巴
diethyl carbamazine (DEC) 乙胺嗪
digenetic trematode 复殖吸虫
diiodohydroxyquinoline 双碘喹啉
diloxanide 二氯尼特
diltiazem 硫氮卓酮
Dinobdella ferox 凶恶怖蛭
Dioctophyma renale 肾膨结线虫
dioctophymiasis renale 肾膨结膨线虫病
Dipetalonema perstans 常现唇棘线虫
Dipetalonema streptocerca 链尾唇棘线虫
Diphyllbothrium Pacifidum 太平洋裂头绦虫
Diphyllobothrium latum 阔节裂头绦虫
Diplogonoporus grandis 大复殖孔绦虫
Diplopoda 倍足纲
Dipylidium caninum 犬复殖孔绦虫
dipstick assay 快速试纸法
dip-stick 试条法，试纸条法
Diptera 双翅目
direct smear method 直接涂片法
disseminated hyperinfection 播散性超度感染
distal cytoplasm 远端胞浆
Dracunculidae 龙线虫科
Dracunculus 龙线虫属
Dracunculus medinensis 麦地那龙线虫
dust mite 尘螨
ecdysis 蜕皮
Echinochasmus japonicus 日本棘隙吸虫
Echinochasmus liliputanus 藐小棘隙吸虫
Echinostomatidae 棘口科
ectoparasite 体外寄生虫
ectopic lesion 异位损害
ectopic lesion 异位病变

ectopic parasitism 异位寄生
egg count 虫卵计数
egg per gram (EPG)每克粪便虫卵数
Eimeriidae 爱美虫科
ejaculatory duct 射精管
elephantiasis 象皮肿
embryo 胚胎
emergence 羽化
Encephalitozoon 脑炎微孢子虫属
Encephalophilus silvestris 森林脑炎病毒
encystation 成囊
metacercaria 囊蚴
endemic relapsing fever 地方性回归热
endemic typhus 地方性斑疹伤寒
endo-autoinfection 自身体内感染
endodyogeny 内二芽殖法
endogenous budding 内出芽
Endolimax nana 微小内蜒阿米巴
endoparasite 体内寄生虫
endoplasmic reticulum 内质网
Entamoeba coli 结肠内阿米巴
Entamoeba dispar 迪斯帕内阿米巴
Entamoeba gingivalis 齿龈内阿米巴
Entamoeba hartmanni 哈门氏内阿米巴
Entamoeba histolytica 溶组织内阿米巴
Enterobius vermicularis 蠕形住肠线虫(蛲虫)
Enterocytozoon 肠上皮细胞微孢子虫属
entro-test 肠内试验
environmental manipulation 环境处理
environmental modification 环境改造
enzyme-linked immunoblotting (ELIB)酶联免疫印渍技术
eosinophilia 嗜酸性粒细胞增多症
epidemic typhus 流行性斑疹伤寒
epimastigotes 上鞭毛体
epitope 表位
Erhaiini 洱海螺族
Eriocheir spp. 绒螯蟹
erythrocyte binding antigen (EBA)红细胞结合抗原

erythrocytic stage 红细胞内期
esophageal commissure 背索
esophagus 食管
Eucoccidiida 真球虫目
Euroglyphus maynei 埋内欧螨
excretory bladder 排泄囊
excretory factor (EF) 排泌因子
excretory-secretary product (ESP) 排泄—分泌物
exo-autoinfection 自身体外感染
exo-erythrocytic stage 红细胞外期
exogenous budding 外出芽
exoskeleton 外骨骼
external plasma membrane 外质膜
extraintestinal amoebiasis 肠外阿米巴病
extranuclear spindle 核外纺锤体
extrinsic incubation period 外潜伏期
facilitated diffusion 易化扩散
facultative parasite 兼性寄生虫
Family Oligacanthorhynchidae 稀棘棘头虫科
Family Trypanosomatidae 锥虫科
Fasciola hepatica 肝片形吸虫
fascioliasis 片形吸虫病
fasciolopsiasis 姜片虫病
Fasciolopsis buski 布氏姜片虫
female gamete 雌配子
festoon 缘垛
fibril 纤丝
filaria 丝虫
filariasis 丝虫病
flagellated protozoon 鞭毛虫
flagellum 鞭毛，鞭节
flame cell pattern 焰细胞式
flame cell 焰细胞
flea 蚤
float hair 掌状毛
flotation method 浮聚法
fluid mosaic model 液态镶嵌模型
fly 蝇

follicle mite 毛囊虫
follicle 卵泡
food-borne parasitosis 食源性寄生虫病
food vacuole 食物泡
foregut 前肠
Forcipomyia（L）taiwana 台湾铗蠓
forest encephalitis 森林脑炎
formalin-ether sedimentation 醛醚沉淀法
furapyrimidone 呋喃嘧酮
Gal/GalNAC lectin 半乳糖/乙酰氨基半乳糖凝集素
galea 螯盔
gamasid mite 革螨
Gamasoidea 革螨总科
gametocyte 配子体
gametogony 配子生殖
ganglion 神经节
gastrointestinal blooding 消化道出血
Gastropoda 腹足纲
gastropod 腹足类
gel-like 凝胶状
genal comb 颊栉
gene knock out 基因敲除
Gene family 基因家族
genital atrium 生殖窦
genuine infection 真性感染
Genus Leishmania 利什曼属
Genus Macracanthorhynchus 巨吻棘头虫属
genus name 属名
germinal cell 生发细胞
germinal layer 生发层
Giardia duodenalis 十二指肠贾第虫（蓝氏贾第鞭毛虫的别名）
Giardia intestinalis 肠贾第虫（蓝氏贾第鞭毛虫的别名）
Giardia lamblia 蓝氏贾第鞭毛虫，贾第鞭毛虫
giardiasis 贾第虫病
Glossina morsitans 刺舌蝇
Glossina pallidipes 淡足舌蝇
Glossina palpalis 须舌蝇
glycocalyx 糖萼

glycogen vacuole 糖原泡
glycophorin-binding protein (GBP)血型糖蛋白结合蛋白
gnathosoma 颚体
Gnathostoma doloresi 杜氏颚口线虫
Gnathostoma hispidum 刚刺颚口线虫
Gnathostoma spinigerum 棘颚口线虫
gnathostomiasis 颚口线虫病
Golgi complexes 高尔基复合体
Gongylonema neoplasticum 癌筒线虫
Gongylonema orientale 东方筒线虫
Gongylonema pulchrum 美丽筒线虫
Gongylonema 筒线虫
gonotrophic cycle 生殖营养周期
Gordiacea 铁线虫
Gordiidae 铁线虫科
Gordioidea 铁线虫目
Gordius 铁线虫属
Granulomatous amoebic encephalitis (GAE)肉芽肿性阿米巴性脑炎
gravid proglottid 孕节
group dancing 群舞
gut-associated antigens (GAA) 肠相关抗原
gynecophoral canal 抱雌沟
Haemolaelaps glasgowi 格氏血厉螨
haemolysin 溶血素
hair snake 发形蛇
Haller's organ 哈氏器
Halofantrine 卤泛曲林
halter 平衡棒
Haplorchis pumilio 钩棘单睾吸虫
Haplorchis yokogawai 多棘单睾吸虫
hard tick 硬蜱
helminth 蠕虫
Hemiculter kneri 克氏鲦鱼
Hemiptera 半翅目
hemoflagellate protozoa 血鞭毛虫
hepatic capillariasis 肝毛细线虫病
hermaphrodite 雌雄同体
hermit crabs 寄生蟹

Heterophyes heterophyes 异形异形吸虫
Heterophyid trematodes 异形吸虫
Heterophyidae 异形科
hetrazan 海群生
histidine-rich protein (HRP)富含组氨酸蛋白
Hoeppli phenomenon 何博礼现象
holdfast 附着器
holomyarian type 细肌型
homolactic fermentation 同乳酸酵解(纯乳酸酵解)
hookworm 钩虫
hookworm disease 钩虫病
hookworm infection 钩虫感染
host 宿主
human mammomonogamosis 人体兽比翼线虫病
Human Genome Project (HGP)人类基因组研究计划
human immunodeficiency virus (HIV)人类免疫缺陷病毒
human parasitology 人体寄生虫学
Hyalomma detritum 残缘璃眼蜱
Hyalomma asiaticum kozlovi 亚东璃眼蜱
hycanthone 海蒽酮
hydatid cyst 棘球蚴
hydrocele testis 睾丸鞘膜积液
hydrogenosome 氢化酶体
Hymenolepis nana 微小膜壳绦虫
hypersensitivity 超敏反应
hypnozoite 休眠子
Hypoderma bovis 牛皮蝇
Hypoderma lineatum 纹皮蝇
Hypodermatidae 皮下蝇科
hypopharynx 舌
Hypophthalmichthys molitrixs 鲢鱼
idiosoma 躯体
IFN-γ γ-干扰素
IL-2 白介素-2
imagochrysalis 成蛹
imipramine 丙咪嗪
immature proglottid 幼节
immune evasion 免疫逃避

immune response 免疫应答
Immunoenzymatic staining test (IEST) 免疫酶染色试验
immunologic memory 免疫记忆
immunotoxin 免疫毒素
incomplete metamorphosis 不完全变态
incubation period 潜伏期
Indirect fluorescent antibody test (IFT)间接荧光抗体试验
Indirect haemagglutination test (IHA) 间接红细胞凝集试验
Inermicapsifer madagascariensis 马达加斯加绦虫
Infantile hookworm disease 婴儿钩虫病
inflation 膨大部
insect 昆虫
Insecta 昆虫纲
insecticide resistance management (IRM) 杀虫剂抗性管理
insecticide resistance 抗药性
insecticide 杀虫剂
instar 龄
integrated control 综合防制
interferon (IFN)干扰素
interleukin 白细胞介素
intermediate host 中间宿主
internet 互联网
intestinal amoebiasis 肠阿米巴病
intracystic bodies 囊内小体
Iodamoeba butschlii 布氏嗜碘阿米巴
iodoquinol 碘化喹宁
Isolapotamon spp. 石蟹
Isolapotamon nasicum 鼻肢石蟹
Isolapotamon physalicum 僧帽石蟹
Isospora 等孢球虫
Isospora belli 贝氏等孢球虫
Isospora natalensis 纳塔尔等孢球虫
itch mite 疥螨
itraconazole 依曲康唑
ivermectin (IVM) 伊维菌素
Ixodes persulcatus 全沟硬蜱
Ixodidae 硬蜱科
Ixododea 蜱总科

Japanese B encephalitis virus 流行性乙型脑炎病毒
Japanese B encephalitis 日本乙型脑炎
kala-azar 黑热病
Kerandel sign 克兰德耳氏征
Kinetofragminophorea 动基裂纲
kinetoplast 动基体
Kinetoplastida 动基体目
Kingdom Animal 动物界
Kingdom Protista 原生生物界
knob 节结
labella 唇瓣
labial palp 下唇须
labium 下唇
labrum 上唇
Laelaps echidninus 毒厉螨
landrin 混灭威
larva migrans 幼虫移行症
latex agglutination (LA) test 胶乳凝集试验
Laurer's canal 劳氏管
leeches 水蛭
Leishman-Donovan body (LD body) 利杜体
Leishmania braziliensis 巴西利什曼原虫
Leishmania donovani 杜氏利什曼原虫
Leishmania major 硕大利什曼原虫
Leishmania mexicana 墨西哥利什曼原虫
Leishmania tropica 热带利什曼原虫
leishmaniasis 利什曼病
Leptotrombidium deliense 地里纤恙螨
Leptotrombidium scutellare 小盾纤恙螨
levamisole 左旋咪唑
life cycle 生活史
ligand 配体
liver fluke 肝吸虫
liver-schizont specific antigen (LSA) 肝裂殖体特异性抗原
Loa loa 罗阿罗阿丝虫
loiasis 罗阿丝虫病
longitudinal muscle 内纵肌
louse 虱

louse-borne relapsing fever 虱媒回归热
Lucilia sericata 丝光绿蝇
lumefantrine 卤泛群
Lyme disease 莱姆病
lymph glands visceral leishmaniasis (LGVL) 淋巴结型黑热病
lymphocytotoxic antibody 毒杀淋巴细胞抗体
lysosome 溶酶体
macracanthorhynchosis 猪巨吻棘头虫病
Macracanthorhynchus hirudinaceus 猪巨吻棘头虫
Macrobrachium superbum 巨掌沼虾
malarial pigment 疟色素
malaria 疟疾
malathion 马拉硫磷
Malayopotamon fukienense 福建马来溪蟹
male gamete 雄配子
malate dehydrogenase (ME)苹果酸脱氢酶
Mammomonogamus 兽比翼线虫
Mammomonogamus gangguiensis 港归兽比翼线虫
Mammomonogamus laryngeus 喉比翼线虫
mandible 上颚
Mansonella ozzardi 奥氏曼森线虫
mepacrine 阿的平
mass drug administration (MDA) 群体治疗
mature proglottid 成节
Maurer's dots 茂氏小点
maxicircle 大环
maxilla 下颚
maxillary palp 下颚须
mebendazole 甲苯咪唑
mechanical transmission 机械性传播
median body 中体
medical arthropod 医学节肢动物
medical arthropodology 医学节肢动物学
medical entomology 医学昆虫学
medical parasitology 医学寄生虫学
medicated salt 药盐
mefloquine 甲氟喹
megacolon 巨结肠

megaesophagus 巨食管

Mehlis gland 梅氏腺

membrane-associated antigens (MAA) 膜相关抗原

meromyarian type 少肌型

merozoite surface antigen 1 (MSA)裂殖子表面抗原 1

merozoite 裂殖子

merthiolate-iodine-formaldehyde centrifugation sedimentation method (MIFC) 汞醛碘离心沉淀法

Mesocestoides lineatus 线中殖孔绦虫

mesothorax 中胸

metacercaria 后尾蚴

metacestode 中绦期

metacyclic trypomastigotes 循环后期锥鞭毛体

Metagonimus yokogawai 横川后殖吸虫

metamorphosis 变态

metathorax 后胸

methoprene 烯虫酯

metraterm 子宫末段

metronidazole 甲硝咪唑，甲硝唑

microarray 微点阵技术

micronemes 微线体

Microspora 微孢子门

Microsporida 微孢子虫目

Microsporidiosis 微孢子虫病

Microsporidium 微孢子虫，微孢子虫属

microthrix 微毛

microvilli 微绒毛

minicircle 微环

miracidium hatch method 毛蚴孵化法

miracidium 毛蚴

miraxone 毛蚴松

mite island 螨岛

mitochondrion 线粒体

modified acid-fast method 改良抗酸染色法

modified Kato's thick smear 改良加藤法

molecular mimicry 分子模拟

molt 蜕皮

Moniliformis moniliformis 念珠棘头虫

mosquito 蚊
mosquito-borne disease 蚊媒病
mouthparts 口器
mucocutaneous leishmaniasis (MCL) 皮肤粘膜利什曼病
multilocular hydatid cyst 多房棘球蚴
multiple regulatory action 多重调节作用
multivalent 多价
murine typhus 鼠型斑疹伤寒
Musca domestica vicina 舍蝇
Muscidae 蝇科
mutualism 互利共生
myiasis 蝇蛆病
Mylopharyngodon piceus 青鱼(黑鲩)
Naegleria fowleri 福氏耐格里阿米巴
Naegleria spp. 耐格里属阿米巴
Nanhaipotamon angulatum 角肢南海溪蟹
natrium stibogluconicum 葡萄糖酸锑钠
natural immunity 天然免疫
natural resistance 先天抵抗力
Necator americanus 美洲板口线虫
nematomorphiasis 铁线虫病
nerve process 神经突
nerve trunk 神经干
neutralization antibody 中和抗体
neutralizing 中和作用
nick translation 缺口翻译
niclosamide 氯硝柳胺
nipagin 尼帕净
nocturnal periodicity 夜现周期性
non-pathogenic zymodemes 非致病性酶株群
non-specific immunity 非特异性免疫
non-sterilizing immunity 非消除性免疫
Nosema 小孢子虫属
nymph 若虫
nymphochrysalis 若蛹
obligatory parasite 专性寄生虫
ocular larva migrans (OLM) 眼幼虫移行症
Oestridae 狂蝇科

Oestrus ovis 羊狂蝇
Oestrus 狂蝇
Onchocerca volvulus 旋盘尾丝虫
onchosphere 六钩蚴
Oncomelania hupensis 湖北钉螺
ontogenetic migration 移行
oocyst 卵囊
ookinete 动合子
ootype 卵模
opercular plug 盖塞
opportunistic parasite 机会致病寄生虫
opportunistic parasitosis 机会致病性寄生虫病
opportunistic protozoa 机会致病原虫
opsonic antibody 调理素抗体
oral sucker 口吸盘
Order Archiacanthocephala 原棘头虫目
Order Digenea 复殖目
Order Kinetoplastida 动基体目
organ of Berlese 柏氏器
Orientia tsutsugamushi 恙虫病东方体
Orientobilharzia 东毕吸虫
ornidazole 奥硝唑
Ornithodoros papillipes 乳突钝缘蜱
Ornithonyssus bacoti 柏氏禽刺螨
ovary 卵巢
overlapping regulatory action 重叠的调节作用
oviduct 输卵管
oviparity 卵生
ovoviviparity 卵胎生
ovum 卵
oxamniquine 奥沙尼喹
Pachydrobiini 厚鳃螺族
Pagumogonimus skrjabini 斯氏狸殖吸虫
pamaquine 巴马喹
Panstrongylus megistus 大锥蝽
Parabramis pekinensis 鳊鱼
Parafossarulus striatulus 纹沼螺
Paragonimiasis 并殖病(肺吸虫病)，并殖吸虫病

paragonimus pulmonanis 肺生并殖吸虫
paragonimus westermani 卫氏并殖吸虫
Parapotamon spp. 拟溪蟹
parasite 寄生物
parasitic infection 寄生虫感染
Parasitiformes 寄螨目
parasitism 寄生
parasitophorous vacuole antigen (PVA) 纳虫空泡抗原
parasitophorous vacuole 纳虫空泡
parasitosis 寄生虫病
paratenic host (transport host) 转续宿主
parenchymal tissue 实质组织
Paromomycin (Humatin) 巴龙霉素
paroxysm 发作
pathogenic zymodemes 致病性酶株群
Pediculus humanus capitis 人头虱
Pediculus humanus corporis 人体虱
Pediculus humanus 人虱
pellicle 表膜
pelvic inflammation 盆腔炎症
penetration enhancing factor (PEF) 穿透增强因子
Pentamidine 戊脘脒
perikarya 核周体
Periplaneta americana 美洲大蠊
permanent parasite 长期寄生虫
permethrin 二氯苯醚菊酯
peroxiredoxin 过氧化氢酶(过氧还原素)
persisting migrans 迁延移行
Peyer patches 派伊尔小结
phagocytosis 吞噬
pharyngeal bulb 咽管球
pharynx 咽
pheromone 信息素
Phlebotominae 白蛉亚科
Phlebotomus chinensis chinensis 中华白蛉指名亚种
Phlebotomus chinensis longiductus 中华白蛉长管亚种
phosphoenolpyruvate carboxykinase (PEPCK) 磷酸烯醇丙酮酸激酶
phoxin 辛硫磷

Phylum Acanthocephala 棘头动物门
Phylum Apicomplexa 顶复门
Phylum Arthropoda 节肢动物门
Phylum Ciliophora 纤毛门
Phylum Nemathelminthes 线形动物门
Phylum Platyhelminthes 扁形动物门
Phylum Protozoa 原生动物门
Phylum Sarcomastigophora 肉足鞭毛门
physiological age 生理龄期
pinocytosis 胞饮
piperazine 哌嗪
pirimiphos methyl 甲嘧硫磷
plague 鼠疫
plasmalemma 质膜
plasmochin 扑疟喹啉
Plasmodidae 疟原虫科
Plasmodium cynomolgi 食蟹猴疟原虫
Plasmodium falciparum（*P. f*）恶性疟原虫
Plasmodium inui 猪尾猴疟原虫
Plasmodium knowlesi 诺氏疟原虫
Plasmodium malariae（*P. m*）三日疟原虫
Plasmodium ovale（*P. o*）卵形疟原虫
Plasmodium schwetzi 许氏疟原虫
Plasmodium shortti 疟原虫肖氏种
Plasmodium simium 猴疟原虫
Plasmodium vivax（*P. v*）间日疟原虫
Plasmodium 疟原虫
Pleistophora 匹里虫属
Pleomorphism 多形性
Plerocercoid 裂头蚴
Pleuroceridae 黑贝科
Pneumocystis carinii 卡氏肺孢子虫
Pneumocystosis 肺孢子虫病
Pneumocystis carinii pneumonia（PCP）卡氏肺孢子虫肺炎
polar ring 顶端极坏
polyembryonic proliferation 多胚繁殖
polymerase chain reaction（PCR）聚合酶链反应
polymyarian type 多肌型

Pomatiopsidae 圆口螺科
Pomatiopsinae 圆口螺亚科
Pomatiopsini 圆口螺族
population 种群
post-kala-azar dermal leishmaniasis (PKDL) 皮肤型黑热病
Potamon spp. 溪蟹
Praziquantel 吡喹酮
Preadaptation 前适应
precyst 囊前期
prelarva 前幼虫
premunition 带虫免疫
prepharynx 前咽
primaquine 伯氨喹
Primary amoebic meningoencephalitis (PAM)原发性阿米巴性脑膜脑炎
proboscis 喙
procercoid 原尾蚴
proglottid 节片
proguanil 氯胍
proliferative sparganosis 增殖裂头蚴病
proliferative type 增殖型
promastigote 前鞭毛体
pronotal comb 前胸栉
Prosimulium hirtipes 毛足原蚋
prostatic gland 前列腺
prothorax 前胸
protocoele 原体腔
protoscolex 原头节
protonephron 原肾
proximal cytoplasm 近端胞浆区
pseudocyst 假包囊
Pseudophyllidea 假叶目
Pseudopodium 伪足
pseudopod 伪足
Pseudorasbora parva 麦穗鱼
Psychodidae 毛蛉科
Pthirus pubis 耻阴虱
Pulex irritans 致痒蚤
Pulmonema cantonensis 广州肺线虫

pupation 化蛹
pygidium 臀板
pyrantel 噻嘧啶
pyrimethamine 乙胺嘧啶
Pyroglyphidae 蚍螨科
pyronaridine 咯萘啶
Q fever Q 热
quantitative buffy coat (QBC)血沉棕黄层定量分析法
quinine 奎宁
quinone tanned protein 醌单宁蛋白
Raillietina 瑞列属
Raillietina celebensis 西里伯瑞列绦虫
Raillietina demerariensis 德墨拉瑞列绦虫
Rattus norvegicus 褐家鼠
Rattus rattus 黑家鼠
Reactive oxygen system 活性氧系统
Receptor 受体
recrudescence 再燃
redia 雷蚴
relapse 复发
repellent 驱避剂
reservoir host 储存宿主(保虫宿主)
residual body 残留体
resmethrin 苄呋菊酯
rhabditelliasis axei 艾氏小杆线虫病
Rhabditidae 小杆科
Rhabditis (*Rhabditella*) *axei* 艾氏小杆线虫
rhizoplast 根丝体
Rhodnius prolixus 长红锥蝽
rhoptry 棒状体
ribozyme 核酶
rhoptry antigen (RA)裂殖子棒状体抗原
Rickettsia mooseri 莫氏立克次体
Rickettsia prowazekii 普氏立克次体
Rickettsia siberica 西伯利亚立克次体
Rickettsia tsutsugamushi 恙虫病立克次体
ring form 环状体
ring-infected erythrocyte surface antigen (RESA)环状体感染红细胞表膜抗原

river blindness 河盲症
rostellum 顶突
Russian spring summer encephalitis 俄罗斯春夏脑炎
Salmonella-Schistosome syndrome 沙门氏菌－血吸虫综合征
sand fly 白蛉
Sarcocyst 肉孢子虫囊
Sarcocystin 肉孢子毒素
Sarcocystis 肉孢子虫
Sarcocystis hominis 人肉孢子虫
Sarcocystis lindemanni 林氏肉孢子虫
Sarcocystis suihominis 猪人肉孢子虫
Sarcophagidae 麻蝇科
Sarcoptes scabiei 人疥螨
Sarcoptidae 疥螨科
scabies 疥疮
scape 柄节
Schistosoma haematobium 埃及血吸虫
Schistosoma intercalatum 间插血吸虫
Schistosoma japonicum 日本血吸虫
Schistosoma malayensis 马来血吸虫
Schistosoma mansoni 曼氏血吸虫
Schistosoma mekongi 湄公血吸虫
Schistosome 血吸虫,裂体吸虫
schistosomiasis haematobium 埃及血吸虫病
schistosomiasis mansoni 曼氏血吸虫病
schistosomiasis 血吸虫病
schistosomula 血吸虫童虫
schizogony 裂体增殖
schizont-infected cell agglutination antigen (SICA)裂殖体感染红细胞凝集抗体
schizont 裂殖体
Schüffner's dots 薛氏小点
scientific name 学名
scolex 头节
Scorpiones 蝎亚纲
sea anemones 海葵
secnidazole 塞克硝唑
secretory granule 分泌颗粒
sedimentation method 沉淀法

Segmentina 扁卷螺属
self-limitation 自我限制
seminal receptacle 受精囊
seminal vesicle 储精囊
sensillary base 感器基
sensillum 感器
serine rich Entamoeba histolytica protein (SREHP)溶组织内阿米巴多丝氨酸蛋白
sexual generation 有性生殖
sexually transmitted disease (STD)性传染的疾病
shotgun sequencing 猎枪测序法
Siberian tick-borne typhus 西伯利亚蜱媒斑疹伤寒
Simuliidae 蚋科
Simulium 蚋
Simulium subvariegatum 北蚋
Sinopotamon spp. 华溪蟹
Sinopotamon denticulatum 锯齿华溪蟹
Sinopotamon honanese 河南华溪蟹
Sinopotamon yaanensis 雅安溪蟹
Siphonaptera 蚤目
soft tick 软蜱
sol-like 溶胶状
soluble eggs antigen (SEA) 可溶性虫卵抗原
sparganosis mansoni 曼氏裂头蚴病
Sparganum mansoni 曼氏裂头蚴
sparganum proliferum 增殖裂头蚴
species 种
specific immunity 特异性免疫
species name 种名
spermatheca 受精囊
spheromastigote 球鞭毛体
spiramycin 螺旋霉素
Spirometra mansoni 曼氏迭宫绦虫
Spirurata 旋尾目
sporoblast 孢子细胞
sporocyst 孢子囊，胞蚴
sporogony 孢子增殖
sporont 孢子体
sporozoite 子孢子

spurious infection 假性感染
stadium 龄期
sterilizing immunity 消除性免疫
stibiihexonas 斯锑黑克
stichocyte 杆细胞
stichosome 杆状体
stilbamidine 二脒替
Stomoxys calcitrans 厩螯蝇
strobilus 链体
strongyloidiasis 粪类圆线虫病
stylostome 茎口
Subkingdom Protozoa 原生动物亚界
Suborder Trypanosomatina 锥虫亚目
subpellicular microtubule 膜下微管，表膜下微管
subspecies name 亚种名
sucker 吸盘
sulfadoxine 磺胺多辛
sumithion 杀螟松
sunside (propoxur) 残杀威
superfacial muscle 表层肌
suppressive infection 隐性感染
suramin 苏拉明
surface coat 表被，表面外膜
susceptibility 易感性
symbiosis 共生
symptoms in respiratory system 呼吸道症状
syncytium 合胞体
Syngamidae 比翼科
Syngamiasis 比翼线虫病
tabanid fly 虻
Tabanidae 虻科
Tabanus mandarinus 华虻
tachysporozoites (TS)速发型子孢子
tachyzoite 速殖子
Taenia confusa 混杂绦虫
Taenia hydatigena 水泡带绦虫
Taenia saginata 肥胖带绦虫
Taenia solium 猪肉绦虫

Taenia taeniaeformis 巨颈绦虫
Taenia taiwanensis 台湾带绦虫
tan 鞣化
tapeworm 带虫
TDR 热带病特别规划
tegument 皮层，体被
temporary parasite 暂时性寄生虫
termite 白蚁
testis 睾丸
tetramethrin 胺菊酯
the giant kidney worm 巨肾虫
Thelazia callipaeda 结膜吸吮线虫
thelaziasis 结膜吸吮线虫病
Thiaridae 蜷科
Threshold 界限，发热阈值
tick paralysis 蜱瘫痪
tick 蜱
tick-borne disease 蜱媒病
tick-borne encephalitis 蜱媒脑炎
tick-borne relapsing fever 蜱媒回归热
tick-borne rickettsiosis in Northern Asia 北亚蜱媒立克次体病
tinidazole 替硝唑
torus 梗节
Toxocara canis 犬弓首线虫
Toxocara cati 猫弓首线虫
Toxofactor（TF）弓形虫因子
Toxoplasma gondii 刚地弓形虫
Toxoplasma 弓形虫
Toxoplasmin 弓形虫素
Toxoplasmosis 弓形虫病
Toxotoxin 弓形虫毒素
trabeculae 连接小管
transmission-blocking antigen 阻断传播抗体
transverse commissure 横索
trematoda 吸虫
Triatoma infestans 骚扰蝽
Triatoma sordida 泥色锥蝽
Trichinella spiralis 旋毛形线虫

trichinelliasis 旋毛虫病
Trichobilharzia 毛毕吸虫
Trichomonas hominis 人毛滴虫
Trichomonas tenax 口腔毛滴虫
Trichomonas vaginalis 阴道毛滴虫
Trichostrongylus spp. 毛圆线虫属线虫
trichostrongyliasis 毛圆线虫病
Trichostrongylus 毛圆线虫
Trichostrongylus orientalis 东方毛圆线虫
trichuriasis 鞭虫病
Trichuris trichiura 毛首鞭形线虫(鞭虫)
Triculinae 拟钉螺亚科
Triculini 拟钉螺族
trimetrexate 三甲曲星
Trombiculidae 恙螨科
Trophozoite 滋养体
Trypanosoma brucei brucei 布氏布氏锥虫
Trypanosoma brucei complex 布氏锥虫复合体
Trypanosoma brucei gambiense 布氏冈比亚锥虫
Trypanosoma brucei rhodesiense 布氏罗得西亚锥虫
Trypanosoma Cruzi 克氏锥虫
trypanosomal chancre 锥虫下疳
trypanosomiasis 锥虫病
trypomastigote 锥鞭毛体
Tunga penetrans 穿皮潜蚤
tungiasis 潜蚤病
undulating membrane 波动膜
uterus 子宫
vaccine immunity 疫苗免疫
variant 变异体
variant surface protein (VSP) 表面变异蛋白
vas deferens 输精管
vas efferens 输出管
ventro-genital sucker complex 腹殖吸盘复合器
verapamil 异搏定
vesicles 小泡
vesicular nucleus 泡状核
visceral larva migrans (VLM) 内脏幼虫移行症

visceral leishmaniasis（VL）内脏利什曼病
vitellaria reservior 卵黄囊
vitellaria 卵黄腺
vitelline duct 卵黄管
water born disease 水源性疾病
wing 翅
Winterbottom sign 温特博特姆氏征
Wuchereria bancrofti 班氏吴策线虫
wuchereriasis 班氏丝虫病
Xenopsylla cheopis 印度客蚤
Xinjiang haemorrhagic fever 新疆出血热
yellow fever virus 黄热病病毒
yellow fever 黄热病
Yersinia pestis 鼠疫耶尔森菌
zinc sulfate centrifugal flotation method 硫酸锌离心浮聚法
zygote 合子

（Guo Shuling）

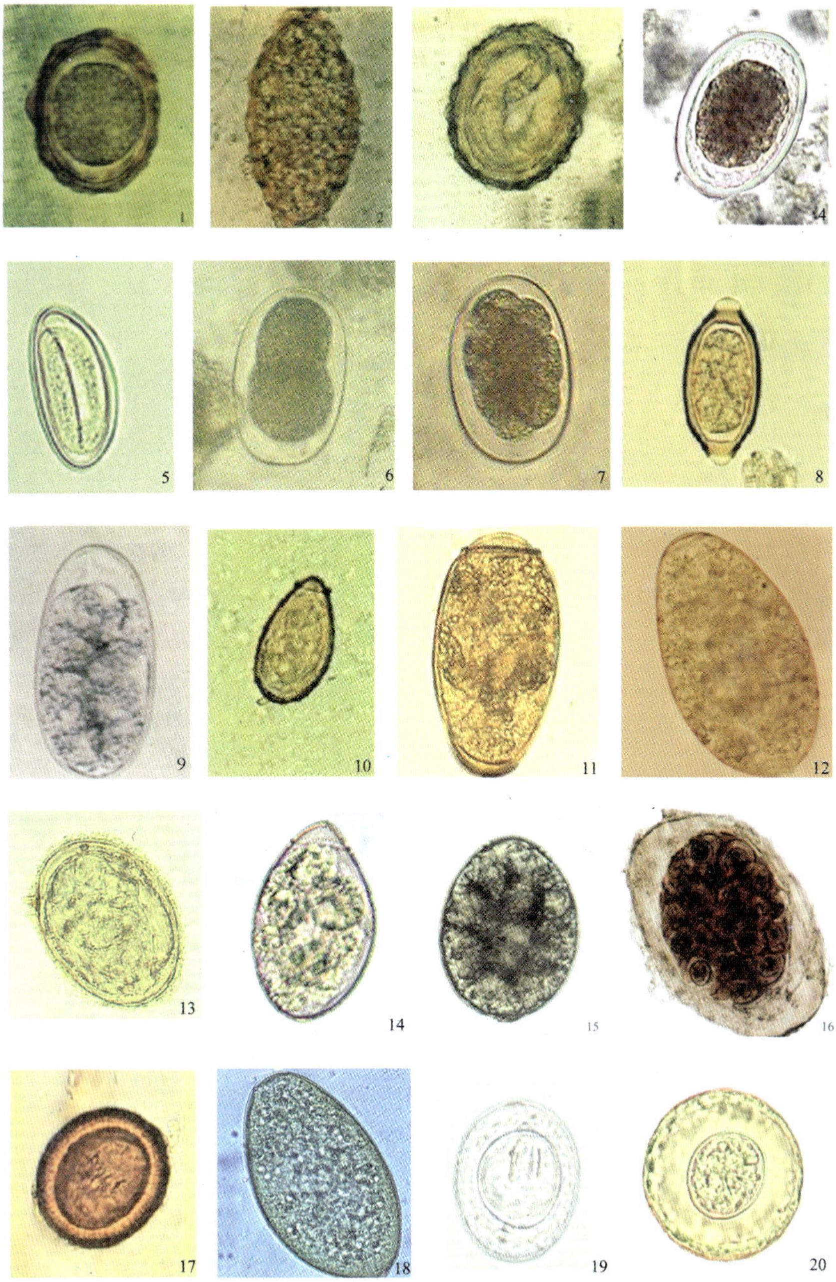

Plate I　Human helminth eggs

1. fertilized ascarid egg　2. unfertilized ascarid egg　3. embryonated ascarid egg　4. decorticated ascarid egg　5. egg of *Enterobius vermicularis*　6, 7. hookworm egg　8. egg of *Trichuris trichiura*　9. egg of *Trichostrongylus orientalis*　10. egg of *Clonorchis sinensis*　11. egg of *Paragonimus westermani*　12. egg of *Fasciolopsis buski*　13. egg of *Schistosoma japonicum*　14. egg of *Spirometra mansoni*　15. egg of *Diphyllobothrium latum*　16. egg of *Dipylidium caninum*　17. tapeworm egg　18. egg of *Fasciola hepatica*　19. egg of *Hymenolepis nana*　20. egg of *Hymenolepis diminuta*

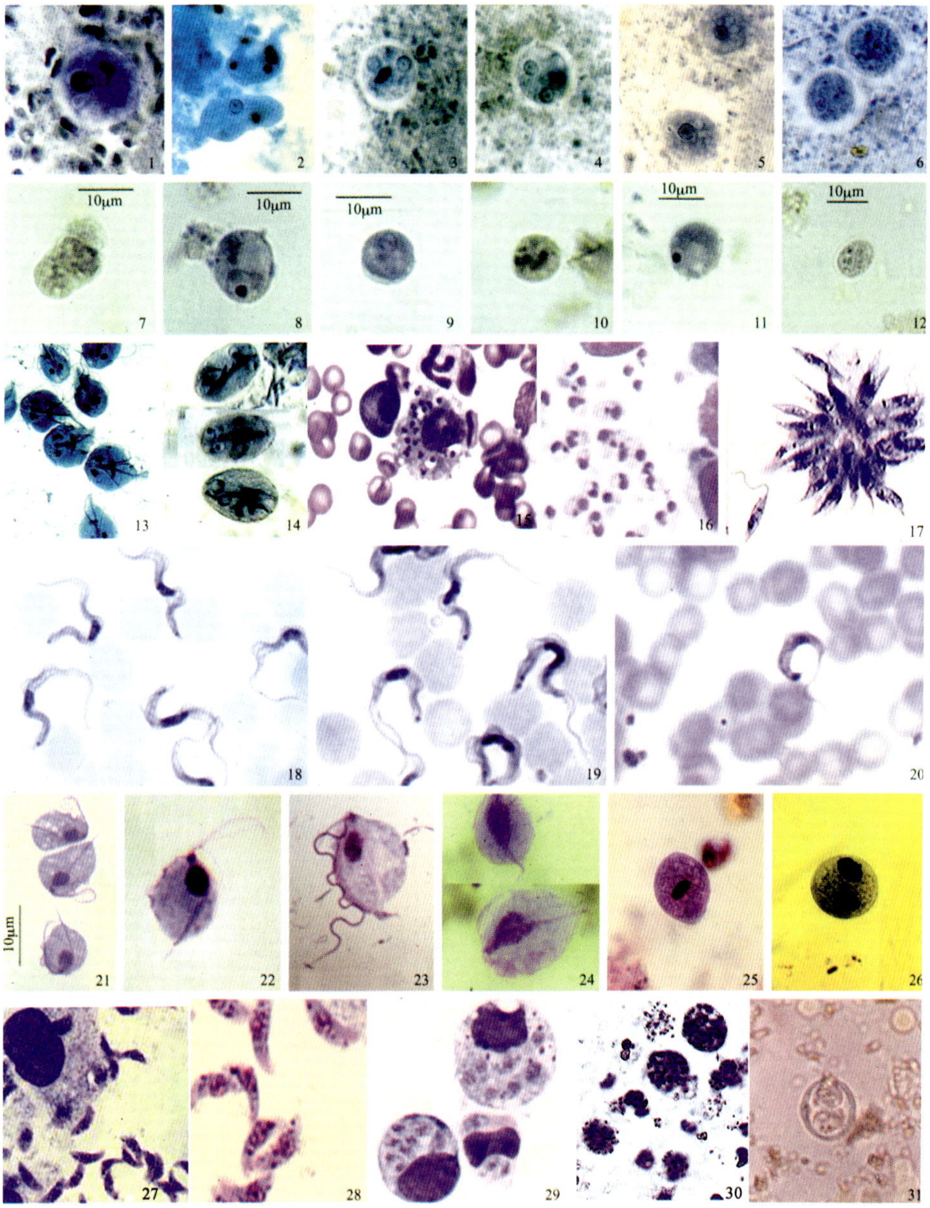

Plate II Medical protozoa

1, 2. trophozoite of *E. histolytica* 3, 4. cyst of *E. histolytica* 5, 6. trophozoite of *E. coli* 7. trophozoite of *Iodamoeba butschlii* 8. cyst of *Iodamoeba butschlii* 9. trophozoite of *E. hartmanni* 10. cyst of *E. hartmanni* 11. trophozoite of *E. nana* 12. cyst of *E. nana* 13. trophozoite of *G. lamblia* 14. cyst of *G. lamblia* 15,16. amastigote of *L. donovani* 17. promastigote of *L. donovani* 18. trypomastigote of *T. brucei rhodesiense* 19. trypomastigote of *T. brucei gamabiense* 20. trypomastigote of *T. cruzi* 21, 22. trophozoite of *T. vaginalis* 23. trophozoite of *P. hominis* 24. trophozoite of *T. tenax* 25. trophozoite of *B. coli* 26. cyst of *B. coli* 27, 28. tachyzoite of *T. gondii* 29. pseudocyst of *T. gondii* 30. cyst of *T. gondii* 31. oocyst of *T. gondii*

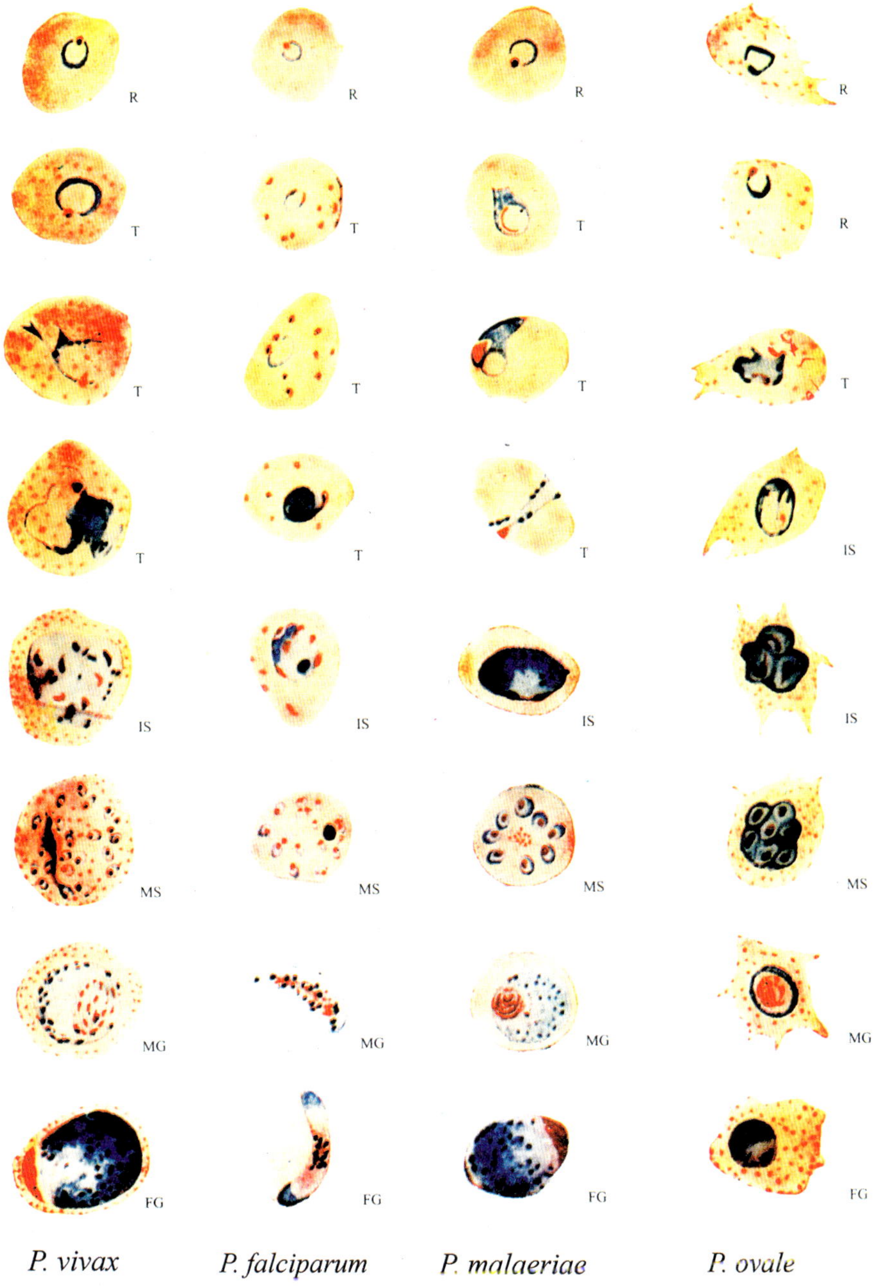

Plate III ***Plasmodium***

R: ring form T: large trophozoite IS: immature schizont MS: mature schizont MG: male gametocyte FG: female gametocyte

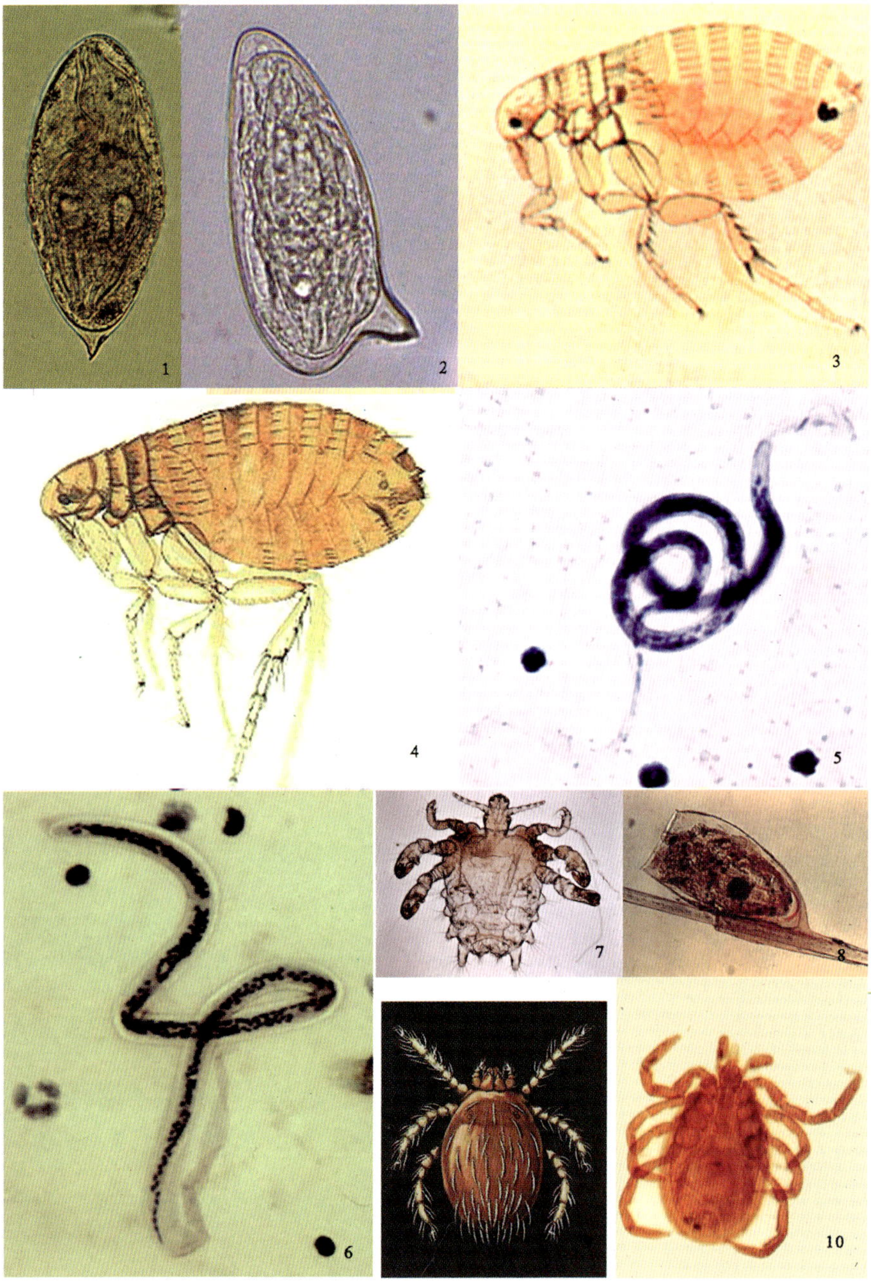

Plate IV

1. *Schistosoma haematobium* 2. *Schistosoma mansoni* 3. *Xenopsylla cheopis* 4. *Pulex irritans* 5. microfilaria of *Brugia malayi* 6. microfilaria of *Wuchereria bancrofti* 7. *Pthirus pubis* 8. nit 9. larva of *Leptotrombidium deliense* 10. ventral view of *Ixodes persulcatus*